# Basic
# Medical Laboratory
# Techniques

*4th Edition*

*To Ron and George*
for their
continuing
support and understanding

# Basic Medical Laboratory Techniques

## 4th Edition

**Barbara H. Estridge, B.S., MT(ASCP)**
COLLEGE OF SCIENCES AND MATHEMATICS
AUBURN UNIVERSITY
AUBURN, ALABAMA 36849

**Anna P. Reynolds, M.S., MT(ASCP)**
COLLEGE OF AGRICULTURE
AUBURN UNIVERSITY
AUBURN, ALABAMA 36849

**Norma J. Walters, R.N., PH.D.**
(RETIRED)
COLLEGE OF EDUCATION
AUBURN UNIVERSITY
AUBURN, ALABAMA 36849

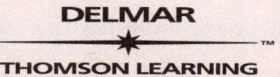

**DELMAR**

**THOMSON LEARNING**

Africa • Australia • Canada • Denmark • Japan • Mexico • New Zealand • Philipines
Puerto Rico • Singapore • Spain • United Kingdom • United States

**Delmar Staff:**

Health Care Publishing Director: William Brottmiller
ACDevelopment Editor: Jill Rembetski
Executive Marketing Manager: Dawn Gerrain
Project Editor: Christopher Leonard

Production Coordinator: John Mickelbank
Art/Design Coordinator: Timothy J. Conners
Cover Design: Cummings Advertising

COPYRIGHT © 2000
Delmar is a division of Thomson Learning. The Thomson Learning logo is a registered trademark used herein under license.

Printed in the United States of America
3 4 5 6 7 8 9 10 XXX 05 04 03 02 01

For more information, contact Delmar, 3 Columbia Circle, PO Box 15015, Albany, NY 12212-0515; or find us on the World Wide Web at http://www.delmar.com

**Asia:**
Thomson Learning
60 Albert Street, #15-01
Albert Complex
Singapore 189969
Tel: 65 336 6411
Fax: 65 336 7411

**Japan:**
Thomson Learning
Palaceside Building 5F
111 Hitotsubashi, Chiyoda-ku
Tokyo 100 0003 Japan
Tel: 813 5218 6544
Fax: 813 5218 6551

**Australia/New Zealand:**
Nelson/Thomson Learning
102 Dodds Street
South Melbourne, Victoria 3205
Australia
Tel: 61 39 685 4111
Fax: 61 39 685 4199

**UK/Europe/Middle East**
Thomson Learning
Berkshire House
168-173 High Holborn
London
WC 1V 7AA United Kingdom
Tel: 44 171 497 1422
Fax: 44 171 497 1426
Thomas Nelson & Sons LTD
Nelson House
Mayfield Road
Walton-on-Thames
KT 12 5PL United Kingdom
Tel: 44 1932 2522111
Fax: 44 1932 246574

**Latin America:**
Thomson Learning
Seneca, 53
Colonia Polanco
11560 Mexico D.F. Mexico
Tel: 525-281-2906
Fax: 525-281-2656

**Canada:**
Nelson/Thomson Learning
1120 Birchmount Road
Scarborough, Ontario
Canada M1K 5G4
Tel: 416-752-9100
Fax: 416-752-8102

**Spain:**
Thomson Learning
Calle Magallanes, 25
28015-MADRID
ESPANA
Tel: 34 91 446 33 50
Fax: 34 91 445 62 18

**International Headquarters:**
Thomson Learning
International Division
290 Harbor Drive, 2nd Floor
Stamford, CT 06902-7477
Tel: 203-969-8700
Fax: 203-969-8751

**Library of Congress Cataloging-in-Publication Data:**
Estridge, Barbara H.
   Basic medical laboratory techniques / Barbara H. Estridge, Anna P. Reynolds, Norma J. Walters.—4th ed.
      p. ; cm.
   Walters' name appears first on previous editions.
   Includes bibliographical references and indexes.
   ISBN 0-7668-1206-5
      1. Diagnosis, Laboratory. 2. Medical laboratory technology. I. Reynolds, Anna P. II. Walters, Norma J. III. Title.
   [DNLM: 1. Laboratory Techniques and Procedures. 2. Technology, Medical. QY 25 E825b 2000]
RB37.W25 2000
616.07'56—dc21
                                                                                              99-054759

# Contents

# List of Color Plates

**ACKNOWLEDGEMENTS FOR COLOR PLATES**

Color Plate 10.  All rights reserved by Abbott Laboratories, Abbott Park, IL. From Diggs, L. W., Sturm, D., & Bell, A. (1985) *The Morphology of Human Blood Cells.*

Color Plates 20, 22, 24-29.  Courtesy of Ames Division of Miles Laboratories, Inc., Elkhart, IN. From *Modern Urine Chemistry.* 1982.

Color Plates 21 and 23.  Courtesy of W. B. Saunders Co., Philadelphia, PA. From Henry, J. *Clinical Diagnosis by Laboratory Methods.* 17th ed. 1984.

Color Plates 28 (right) and 39.  Courtesy of Delmar Publishers, Albany, NY. From Grover-Lakomia, L. I. & Fong, E. *Microbiology for Health Careers.* 6th ed. 1999.

Color Plates 32, 34, 36, 42-45, and 47-48.  Courtesy of Delmar Publishers. Albany, NY. From Shimeld, L. A. *Essentials of Diagnostic Microbiology.* 1999.

Color Plate 46.  Courtesy of W. B. Saunders Co., Philadelphia, PA. From Markell, E. K. & Voge, M. *Medical Parasitology.* 1976.

# List of Figures and Tables

## UNIT 2:   BASIC HEMATOLOGY
### Figures

## TABLES

## UNIT 6: BASIC CLINICAL CHEMISTRY
**FIGURES**

## UNIT 7: BASIC CLINICAL MICROBIOLOGY
### FIGURES

# Preface

*Basic Medical Laboratory Techniques*, 4th edition, is a performance-based text designed for use in allied health programs at the post-secondary and vocational school levels. It is appropriate for medical laboratory technician programs, medical assistant programs, medical laboratory assistant programs, and introductory survey courses in medical technology programs.

## TEXT ORGANIZATION

*Basic Medical Laboratory Techniques* explains the theory and techniques of essential medical laboratory procedures. The content and organization of the eight units (containing sixty lessons) provide for flexibility in teaching and learning. Manual procedures that illustrate fundamental principles are included, along with information about instruments that may be found in smaller laboratories or used in point-of-care testing (POCT). Lessons are short and to the point, covering the basic concepts, and emphasizing safety and quality assurance. The topics covered in the eight units are:

- Introduction to the Medical Laboratory
- Basic Hematology
- Basic Hemostasis
- Basic Immunology and Serology
- Urinalysis
- Basic Clinical Chemistry
- Basic Clinical Microbiology
- Basic Parasitology

After Unit 1, Introduction to the Medical Laboratory, has been completed, Units 2, 4, 5, 6, 7,or 8 may be studied in the instructor's order of preference based on program requirements, time limitations, and laboratory space and equipment. Unit 3, Basic Hemostasis, should be used as a sequel to Unit 2, Basic Hematology.

*Basic Medical Laboratory Techniques*, 4th edition, contains more than 325 illustrations and photographs and 120 tables to enhance the reader's understanding. Forty-eight color plates assist the student in identifying blood cells, components of urine sediment, bacteria, parasites, and bacteriological media. A Glossary, Appendices, and an Index are placed at the end of the text for quick, easy reference. The Glossary includes definitions for the glossary terms from all sixty lessons and pronunciations of some difficult terms. The Appendices contain important reference information, such as addresses of health care regulatory agencies, credentialing agencies, governmental agencies, and professional societies; a guide to Standard and Universal Precautions; metric conversion charts; a list of abbreviations commonly used in the medical laboratory; and a table of laboratory reference values.

## Unit Organization

Each unit contains a list of unit objectives, a brief overview of the unit, a list of References and Resources, and several lessons. The first lesson in each unit is an introduction to the unit subject, with subsequent lessons devoted to a related laboratory procedure, test, or topic. Each lesson contains:

- A list of learning objectives to help students know what is expected of them as they study the lesson.
- A glossary containing new terms and definitions; each term is highlighted the first time it is used in a lesson.
- Introductory material, including principle and rationale of the procedure or test.
- Safety Information pertinent to the procedure.
- Quality assurance and quality control information.
- Basic theoretical and technical information.
- Reminders: Procedural Notes and Safety Precautions.
- Lesson review questions to test students on the material they have just studied.
- Suggested student activities.
- Student Performance Guide, a step-by-step guide to performing the laboratory procedure, including worksheets when appropriate. The Student Performance Guide enables the student to practice the procedure taught in the lesson before being observed and graded by the instructor.

## NEW IN THE FOURTH EDITION

The fourth edition is in a larger format and is in two colors, which aids in visual organization and adds emphasis to the content, and interest to the artwork. The color plates have been revised and expanded to eight pages.

The fourth edition has been revised and updated to include the latest information on instrumentation designed for use in point-of-care testing (POCT). Two lessons on safety have been expanded, with emphasis on Standard Precautions and Bloodborne Pathogen rules. In addition, CDC's Transmission-Based Precautions have been included in the infection control lesson.

Icons representing chemical hazards ✏ and biological hazards ☣ are used in the lessons and Student Performance Guides to emphasize procedures important to student safety. Bulletin boards listing Procedural Notes and Safety Precautions serve as reminders at the end of each lesson, reinforcing safety and technique.

## New Lessons in This Edition

- Morphology of Abnormal Blood Cells in Peripheral Blood
- Disorders of Hemostasis
- Rapid Tests for Hemostasis Disorders
- Specimen Collection and Processing for Clinical Chemistry
- Point-of-Care Testing
- Measuring Electrolytes

## Reorganization of Previous Edition

- Unit 1–The quality assurance lesson has been placed here to emphasize its importance in all areas of the laboratory.
- Unit 2–The platelet count has been moved to this unit. The hemacytometer, red blood cell count, and white blood cell count have been combined into one lesson. Preparing and staining blood smears have been combined into one lesson.
- Unit 4–ABO slide and tube typing have been combined into one lesson that includes forward and reverse typing.
- Unit 5–The pregnancy test lesson has been moved to this unit.
- Unit 7–Transmission-Based Precautions have been added to the lesson on infection control. The fecal occult blood test lesson has been moved to this unit.

## INSTRUCTOR'S RESOURCES/SUPPLEMENTS

An updated Instructor's Manual is available that includes unit objectives, unit overview, and suggested readings and references for each unit. The lesson plans contain objectives, glossary terms, lesson outline, teaching aids and resources, student learning activities, lesson review questions and answers, and instructor's performance check sheets, worksheets, and report forms. A sample test and test key are provided for each lesson.

## ABOUT THE AUTHORS

Barbara H. Estridge, BS, MT(ASCP) and Anna P. Reynolds, MS, BS, MT(ASCP) have several years' experience as instructors in both hospital and university Medical Technology, Medical Laboratory Technician, and Medical Laboratory Assistant programs. They have many combined years of clinical and research experience in hospital and university laboratories in the fields of hematology, chemistry, urinalysis, microbiology, parasitology, and immunology. They are currently involved in biological research, teaching, and analytical chemistry at Auburn University. Norma J. Walters, RN, PhD, now retired, was teacher educator and coordinator of Health Occupations Education at Auburn University for many years.

## ACKNOWLEDGMENTS

We wish to thank the Delmar editorial and production staff for their assistance with this revision. We also wish to thank those individuals who reviewed the manuscript and offered helpful suggestions, especially

Sharlene Aasen, CMA-C
Globe College
Bloominton, MN

Tese Gorszwick, MT(ASCP), CPT(ASPT)
Instructor
Oceanside Unified School District
Carlsbad, CA

Marty Hitchcock, CMA
Program Director, Medical Assisting
Gwinnett Technical Institute
Lawrenceville, GA

Cathy Kelley, CMA, MLT, AS
Program Director, Medical Assisting
National Business College
Bluefield, VA

Mary Ratliff, RN, CMA
Medical Director, Medical Assisting
National Business College
Bristol, VA

We would also like to thank our colleagues and the following companies or individuals for information and/or photographs used in this text.

Abbott Laboratories, Abbott Park, IL

Alpha Scientific Corporation, Southeastern, PA

American Society for Clinical Laboratory Science (ASCLS), Bethesda, MD

AVL Scientific Corp., Roswell, GA

Bayer Corporation, Tarrytown, NY

Beckman Coulter, Fullerton, CA

Becton Dickinson and Company, Franklin Lakes, NJ

bioMerieux, Inc., Hazelwood, MO

Brevis Corp., Salt Lake City, UT

Brinkmann Instruments, Inc., Westbury, NY

Butterfield, M., W. A. Foote Memorial Hospital, Jackson, MI

CDC, U.S. Dept. Health and Human Services, Atlanta, GA

Cholestech Corporation, Hayward, CA

Estridge, John, Los Angeles, CA

Fisher Scientific, Pittsburgh, PA

Folkerts, Dr. Debbie, Auburn, AL

Helena Laboratories, Beaumont, TX

HemoCue, Inc., Mission Viejo, CA

Hoeltke, L. B. *Phlebotomy: The Clinical Laboratory Manual Series*. Delmar Publishers, Inc. 1995.

i-STAT Corp, Princeton, NJ

Integrated Separation Systems, Natick, MA

International Equipment Company, Needham Heights, MA

International Technidyne Corp, Edison, NJ

ISOLAB, Inc., Akron, OH

Leica, Inc., Buffalo, NY

Marshall, J., *Fundamental Skills for the Clinical Laboratory Professional*, Delmar Publishers, Inc. 1993.

Miles Laboratories, Elkhart, IN

Milton Roy Company, Rochester, NY

Nova Biomedical Corp, Waltham MA

NUAIRE, Plymouth, MN

Polymedco, Cortlandt Manor, NY

Reichert Scientific Instruments, Buffalo, NY

Roche Diagnostics Corporation, Branchburg, NJ

Shimeld, L.A. *Essentials of Diagnostic Microbiology*. Delmar Publishers, Inc. 1999.

Sigma Diagnostics, St. Louis, MO

StatSpin, Inc., Norwood, MA

Whitlock, S.A., *Immunohematology: The Clinical Laboratory Manual Series*. Delmar Publishers, Inc. 1997.

Barbara H. Estridge
Anna P. Reynolds

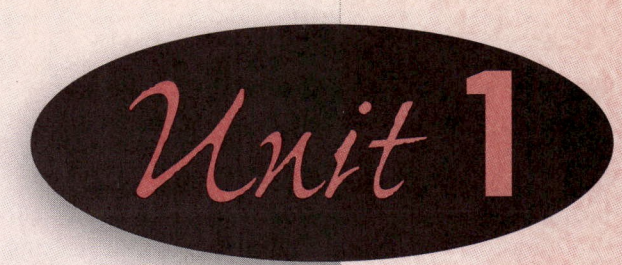

# Unit 1

# Introduction to the Medical Laboratory

## **UNIT** OBJECTIVES

**After studying this unit, you should be able to:**
- *Discuss the organization and function of the medical laboratory.*
- *Discuss the qualifications, job functions, and ethical responsibilities of medical laboratory personnel.*
- *Identify and define selected abbreviations commonly used in the medical laboratory.*
- *Identify and define prefixes, suffixes, and stems in selected medical terms.*
- *Use the metric system to perform measurements.*
- *Discuss laboratory safety rules that must be followed to guard against chemical, physical, and biological hazards.*
- *Discuss the role of quality assurance in the clinical laboratory.*

## **UNIT** OVERVIEW

The medical lab is a place where blood, body fluids, and other biological specimens are tested, analyzed, or evaluated. The observations may be macroscopic or microscopic. The tests may be performed manually or using specialized instruments. Precise measurements are made and the results are calculated and interpreted. Because of this, laboratory workers must have the skills necessary to perform a variety of tasks.

Unit 1 is an introduction to the laboratory environment as a workplace and to the profession of medical technology, which is more commonly called clinical laboratory science. Key concepts and procedures laboratory workers need to know are described. The organization and function of the medical laboratory are addressed in Lesson 1-1. Qualifications and job functions of laboratory personnel are reviewed in Lesson 1-2.

As an introduction to the structure of medical terms, Lesson 1-3 gives basic information about medical terminology and abbreviations of laboratory terms. As other units are studied, additional vocabulary terms will be introduced and defined.

Because laboratory analyses use metric units, a brief introduction to the metric system is given in Lesson 1-4. Knowledge of the metric system is required for some exercises in Units 2 and 6.

Lessons on laboratory safety (Lessons 1-5 and 1-6) are included in this unit because every worker in the medical laboratory must be thoroughly aware of potential hazards in the workplace. Workers must understand and folllow all safety procedures and practices before any laboratory exercises can be conducted.

Methods and procedures for assuring the reliability and accuracy of laboratory analyses are presented in Lesson 1-7, Quality Assurance in the Laboratory. These quality control and quality assurance principles are included in this introductory unit because they must be integrated into all aspects of laboratory operations, from employee training and evaluation, specimen collection and processing, to test analysis, and interpretation and reporting of results.

The use of general laboratory equipment, such as centrifuges, automatic pipets, pH meters, incubators, autoclaves, and laboratory balances, is described in Lesson 1-8. The care, use, and cleaning of frequently used laboratory glassware, such as beakers, test tubes, pipets, and flasks, are explained in Lesson 1-9. The proper care and use of the microscope is included in Unit 1 (Lesson 1-10) because its use is required in the microbiology, hematology, urinalysis, and parasitology units.

Unit 1 is an introduction to the techniques, rules, and skills needed to perform the exercises in Units 2-8. Unit 1 may also be used alone as an introduction to the profession of clinical laboratory science. After Unit 1 has been completed, the remaining units may be studied in order of the instructor's preference depending on available time, laboratory space, and equipment.

## SUGGESTED READINGS AND REFERENCES

Addison, L. A. & Fischer, P. M. (2nd ed.). (1990). *The office laboratory*. East Norwalk, CT: Appleton & Lange.

American Hospital Association, Division of Quality Resources. (February 1992). "OSHA's final bloodborne pathogens standard: A special briefing."

Baker, F. J., Silverton, R. E. & Pallister, C. J., Eds. (7th ed.). (1998). *Baker & Silverton's introduction to medical laboratory technology*. London: Butterworth-Heinemann Medical.

Burtis, C. A., Ashwood, E. R., & Tietz, N.W. (3rd ed.). (1998). *Textbook of clinical chemistry*. Philadelphia: W.B. Saunders Company.

Coastal Health Care, Division of Coastal Video Communications Corp. *Bloodbourne pathogens exposure control manual*. Virginia Beach, VA.

Chabner, D. & Biblis, M. (Eds.). (1996). *The language of medicine: A write-in text explaining medical terms*. Philadelphia: W. B. Saunders Company.

Clerc, J. M., Hammerberg, G., Renk, C., & Dingler, S. (1991). *An introduction to clinical laboratory science*. St. Louis: Mosby-Year Book, Inc.

"Clinical Laboratory Improvement Amendments of 1988," *Federal Register*, Vol. 57, No. 40: 7001–7288. February 28, 1992.

Code of Ethics of the American Society for Clinical Laboratory Science, adopted June 1988, unpublished.

Collins, C. H., Ed. (2nd ed.). (1993). *Safety in clinical and biomedical laboratories*. London: Chapman and Hall.

Dennerll, J. T. (1993). *Medical terminology made easy*. Albany, NY: Delmar Publishers.

Dorland, W. A. N. (Ed.) (28th ed.). (1994). *Dorland's illustrated medical dictionary*. Philadelphia: W. B. Saunders Company.

Ehrlich, A. (3rd Ed.). (1997). *Medical terminology for health professions*. Albany NY: Delmar Publishers.

"Exposure to Hazardous Chemicals in Laboratories," U.S. Department of Labor. Occupational Safety and Health Administration. 1989.

"Hazard Communication," Occupational Safety and Health Administration, Labor, *Federal Register*, Vol. 52, No. 163: 31852–31886, August 24, 1987.

Henry, J. B., Ed. (19th ed.). (1996). *Clinical diagnosis & management by laboratory methods*. Philadelphia: W. B. Saunders Company.

Howanitz, J. H. & Howanitz, P. J. Eds. (1991). *Laboratory medicine: Test selection and interpretation*. New York: Churchill Livingstone, Inc.

Kaplan, A. & Rhona, J. (4th ed.). (1994). *Clinical chemistry: Interpretation and techniques*. Baltimore: Williams & Wilkins.

Karni, K. (1996). *Opportunities in medical technology careers: Clinical laboratory science*. Lincolnwood, IL: VGM Career Horizons.

Kovanda, Beverly M. (1998). *Point of care testing—Capillary puncture*. Albany, NY: Delmar Publishers.

Laposata, M. (1992). *SI unit conversion guide*. Boston: NEJM Books.

Lindh, W. Q., Pooler, M. S., Tamparo, C. D., & Cerrato, J. U. (1998). *Comprehensive medical assisting*. Albany, NY: Delmar Publishers.

Lippert, H. (1978). *SI units in medicine: An introduction to the International System of Units with conversion tables and normal ranges*. Baltimore: Urban & Schwarzenberg.

Marshall, J. (1993). *Fundamental skills for the clinical laboratory professional*. Albany, NY: Delmar Publishers.

Marshall, J. (1995). *Microbiology*. Albany, NY: Delmar Publishers, Inc.

"Occupational Exposure to Bloodborne Pathogens," Final Rule, Occupational Safety and Health Administration (OSHA), Labor, *Federal Register*, Vol. 56, No. 235, Rules and regulations (often referred to as 29 CFR Part 1910.0130).

Passey, R. L. "How to meet the new personnel requirements" in *Medical Laboratory Observer*, September 1992, 47–51.

Pedone, M. J., "Chemical Hygiene Plans: Guidelines for Compliance" in *American Laboratory*, June 1992. 25–28.

Rayburn, S. R. (1990). *The foundations of laboratory safety: A guide for the biomedical laboratory*. New York: Springer-Verlag.

Rice, J. Spellright. (1990). *A medical word book*. Norwalk, CT: Appleton & Lange.

Simmers, L. (4th ed.). (1998). *Diversified health occupations*. Albany, NY: Delmar Publishers.

Simmers, L. (4th ed.). (1998). *Diversified health occupations essentials*. Albany, NY: Delmar Publishers.

Sormunen, C. & Jones, R. F. (4th ed.). (1998). *Terminology for allied health professionals*. Albany, NY: Delmar Publishers.

Thomas, C. L., Ed. (18th ed.). (1997). *Taber's cyclopedic medical dictionary*. Phildelphia: F. A. Davis Company.

Tilton, R. C., et al., Ed. (1992). *Clinical laboratory medicine*. St. Louis: Mosby-Yearbook.

# The Medical Laboratory

## LESSON OBJECTIVES

**After studying this lesson, you should be able to:**

- *Explain the function of a medical or clinical laboratory.*
- *Draw an organizational chart of a typical hospital laboratory.*
- *Describe the functions of the different levels of laboratory personnel.*
- *List the major departments of a typical medical laboratory and name a test that would be performed in each department.*
- *List three examples of nonhospital medical laboratories.*
- *Explain how medical laboratories are regulated.*
- *Explain the purpose of proficiency testing.*
- *Explain the purpose of laboratory accreditation.*
- *Define the glossary terms.*

## GLOSSARY

**AABB** / American Association of Blood Banks

**accessioning** / the process by which specimens are logged in, labeled, and assigned a specimen number

**accreditation** / a voluntary process in which a private, independent agency grants recognition to institutions or programs that meet or exceed established standards of quality

**CAP** / college of American Pathologists

**CDC** / centers for Disease Control and Prevention

**CLIA '88** / clinical Laboratory Improvement Amendments of 1988

**COLA** / Commission on Office Laboratory Accreditation

**DHHS** / Department of Health and Human Services

**epidemiology** / the study of the factors that cause disease and determine disease frequency and distribution

**HCFA** / Health Care Financing Administration

**hematology** / the study of blood and the blood-forming tissues

**immunohematology** / the study of blood group antigens and antibodies; blood banking

**JCAHO** / Joint Commission on Accreditation of Healthcare Organizations, an independent accrediting agency

**microbiology** / a branch of biology dealing with microscopic forms of life

**mycology** / the study of fungi

**NCCLS** / National Committee for Clinical Laboratory Standards; a nonprofit, educational organization that establishes standards of best current practice for clinical laboratories

**pathologist** / a physician specially trained in the nature and cause of disease

**phlebotomist** / one trained to draw blood; venipuncturist

**plasma** / the liquid portion of blood in which the blood cells are suspended; the straw-colored liquid remaining after blood cells are removed from anticoagulated blood

**POCT** / point-of-care test(ing); testing outside the traditional laboratory setting; also called bedside testing, off-site testing, or alternate-site testing

**POL** / physician office laboratory

**reference laboratory** / an independent regional laboratory that offers routine and specialized testing to hospitals and physicians

**serum** / the liquid obtained from blood that has been allowed to clot

**stat test** / a test that must be performed immediately

**virology** / the study of viruses

**whole blood** / blood that contains all components

# INTRODUCTION

Facilities that perform chemical and microscopic tests on blood, other body fluids, and tissues are called medical or clinical laboratories. These laboratories are found in a variety of settings, both government and private. A medical laboratory may be large, offering sophisticated services and employing many skilled workers, or it may be small with only one employee.

This lesson surveys the types of medical laboratories and describes their organization, function, and regulation.

# TYPES OF MEDICAL LABORATORIES

Medical or clinical laboratories can be placed into two groups: hospital laboratories and nonhospital laboratories. Although most people think of hospitals when they think of medical laboratories, laboratories may also be in clinics, group practices, physician offices, veterinary offices, government agencies, and military installations. Some medical laboratories, such as regional reference laboratories, are independent of medical facilities.

## Hospital Laboratories

Medical laboratories are found in private hospitals as well as government-operated hospitals such as veterans' hospitals and hospitals on military bases. The type of medical laboratory found in a hospital depends largely on the hospital's size. A laboratory in a small hospital (less than 100 beds) may perform only very routine test procedures. Complicated or infrequently requested tests may be sent to reference laboratories.

In a medical laboratory in a medium-size hospital (up to 300 beds), routine tests and many more compli-

cated test procedures are performed. Only the most recently developed tests or tests with high levels of complexity would need to be sent to reference laboratories.

Most medical laboratories in large hospitals (more than 300 beds) handle large volumes of work and perform complex tests (Figure 1-1).

## Nonhospital Medical Laboratories

Nonhospital medical laboratories may be publicly operated (government) or privately operated. They provide many services and employment for many skilled workers. In the United States in 1992, more than 50% of all laboratory services were obtained from nonhospital laboratories.

### Physician Office Laboratories

**Physician Office Laboratories** (**POLs**) are medical laboratories in a physician's office or small clinic. The increased availability of rapid-test kits and small, easy-to-operate analyzers has broadened the scope of testing in the POL. Several common laboratory tests, such as hemoglobin, hematocrit, urine reagent strip, pregnancy, blood glucose, and occult blood, can be performed in the POL by multiskilled personnel such as medical assistants. Many POLs perform only CLIA-waived tests (Table 1-1); others may perform tests of moderate complexity. POLs, and all medical laboratories, must obtain permission to operate from HCFA (see Regulation of Medical Laboratories).

### Reference Laboratories

**Reference laboratories** are usually privately owned, regional laboratories that do high-volume testing and offer a wide variety of tests. Large hospitals use reference laboratories primarily to perform complex or infre-

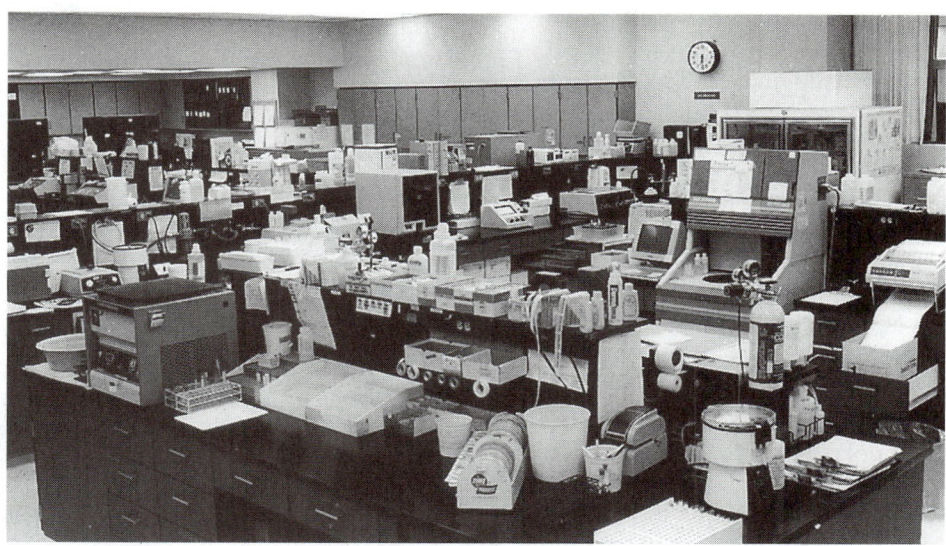

**FIGURE 1-1** A medical laboratory in a large hospital

quently ordered tests. Small hospitals or physicians' offices may use their services for a wide range of tests. Reference laboratories provide courier service to transport specimens from the collection site to the testing laboratory.

### Government Laboratories—Federal

The central laboratory for the national public health system is the Centers for Disease Control and Prevention (**CDC**) in Atlanta, Georgia. This facility provides consulting services to state public health laboratories as well as to individual physicians. **Epidemiology** is an important function of CDC. Data is gathered concerning the cause, distribution, and occurrence of various diseases throughout the United States. The CDC also investigates disease outbreaks throughout the world.

### Government Laboratories—State

Each U.S. state and territory has a medical laboratory operated, usually, by the state's department of public health. These state laboratories provide testing and consulting services to hospitals, physicians, and clinics within the state.

Services available from state laboratories vary from state to state. In general, state laboratories perform tests mandated by state regulations; for example, premarital blood tests and phenylketonuria (PKU) testing of newborns. State laboratories also often offer tests not routinely available in other medical laboratories such as culture of fungi, viruses, and mycobacteria (the agent causing tuberculosis); tests for parasites; tests for reportable infectious diseases such as AIDS; and some environmental testing. Special-case specimens to be sent to CDC for testing are usually sent via state public health laboratories.

## REGULATION OF MEDICAL LABORATORIES

Medical laboratories are regulated by both federal and state agencies. The Clinical Laboratory Improvement Amendments of 1988 (**CLIA '88**), a revision of the

| **Table 1-1.** Examples of tests granted waived status under CLIA (as published by DHHS, June 1999) |
|---|
| Hemoglobin by copper sulfate |
| Hemoglobin by single instrument with direct readout |
| Blood glucose by meters cleared for home use |
| Glycosylated hemoglobin (Hb A1c) |
| Fecal occult blood |
| Spun hematocrit |
| Ovulation tests by color comparison |
| Urine pregnancy tests by visual color comparison |
| Urinalysis reagent strip |
| Microalbumin |
| Rapid Strep test from throat swab |
| Erythrocyte sedimentation rate |
| Immunoassay for *Helicobacter pylori* |
| Prothrombin time |
| Fructosamine |
| Cholesterol |
| Immunoassay for infectious mononucleosis |

Clinical Laboratory Improvement Act of 1967, specifies the standards medical laboratories must meet. CLIA '88 was enacted to improve the quality of medical laboratory testing.

The Health Care Financing Administration (**HCFA**), an agency within the Department of Health and Human Services (**DHHS**), is responsible for implementing CLIA '88. All laboratories performing tests on human specimens, except research laboratories, must obtain a certificate from HCFA to be allowed to perform tests.

Under CLIA '88 rules, laboratories may be classified as those performing (1) waived tests only, (2) tests of moderate and high complexity, and (3) physician-performed microscopy. The classifications are based on the difficulty or complexity of the test procedures and the level of training required to accurately perform the tests. Laboratory personnel standards differ for each of these categories. The more complex the test, the more highly trained the testing personnel must be.

Most hospital laboratories perform moderate- to high-complexity tests. This means that to comply with the law, they must adhere to mandated personnel guidelines and comprehensive recordkeeping and quality assurance programs, participate in proficiency testing programs, and be subject to government inspections.

## ORGANIZATION OF THE HOSPITAL MEDICAL LABORATORY

The organization schemes of most hospital laboratories follow a general outline (Figure 1-2) that may vary slightly depending, usually, on the size of the laboratory. In the last few years, some laboratories have changed department and personnel titles to reflect the terminology used in the CLIA '88 rules. Table 1-2 lists personnel titles as stated in CLIA '88 and gives the commonly used equivalent titles. The personnel qualifications for each category are specified in the Clinical Laboratory Improvement Amendments of 1988, Final Rule, *Federal Register*, Vol. 7, No. 40, February 28, 1992.

### Medical Laboratory Personnel

#### Laboratory Director

The director of the hospital laboratory has customarily been a **pathologist**, a physician specially trained in the nature and cause of disease. Under current regulations, others, such as medical doctors, doctoral scientists (bioanalysts), or doctors of osteopathy, may qualify to be directors. The level of complexity of tests performed in the laboratory determines what qualifications a laboratory director must have. The laboratory director has ultimate responsibility for all laboratory operations.

### Technical Supervisor/Laboratory Manager

Directly under the laboratory director's authority is the technical supervisor or laboratory manager. This is usually someone educated in the medical laboratory sciences who has additional business or management training.

The technical supervisor (laboratory manager) is responsible for the day-to-day operation of the laboratory. The technical supervisor is also responsible for setting personnel standards, establishing training and evaluation procedures, establishing appropriate quality assurance programs, and observing and documenting employee performance and competence. The supervisor is responsible for making available to all personnel an up-to-date procedure manual containing instructions for every procedure performed in the laboratory. The National Committee for Clinical Laboratory Standards (**NCCLS**) develops standards of current best practice for clinical laboratory procedures. Laboratory procedure manuals must follow NCCLS standards.

### General Supervisor/Department Head

Each department has a general supervisor or department head responsible for the quantity and quality of work performed in his or her departments, training employees, and evaluating employee performance. General supervisors report to the technical supervisor.

### Testing Personnel/Bench Technologists

Testing personnel perform the laboratory analyses. These include medical technologists (clinical laboratory scientists) and medical laboratory technicians (clinical

| **Table 1-2.** Job titles of medical laboratory personnel as listed in CLIA '88 Final Rule and commonly used equivalent titles | |
|---|---|
| **CLIA '88 JOB TITLE** | **EQUIVALENT JOB TITLE** |
| Laboratory Director | Laboratory Director (usually a pathologist) |
| Technical Supervisor | Laboratory Manager, Chief Technologist |
| Clinical Consultant | Consultant |
| Technical Consultant or General Supervisor | Department Head, Section Head, Section Supervisor, Technical Specialist |
| Testing Personnel | Bench Technologist, Medical Technologist, Clinical Laboratory Scientist, Medical Laboratory Technician, Clinical Laboratory Technician, Laboratory Assistant |

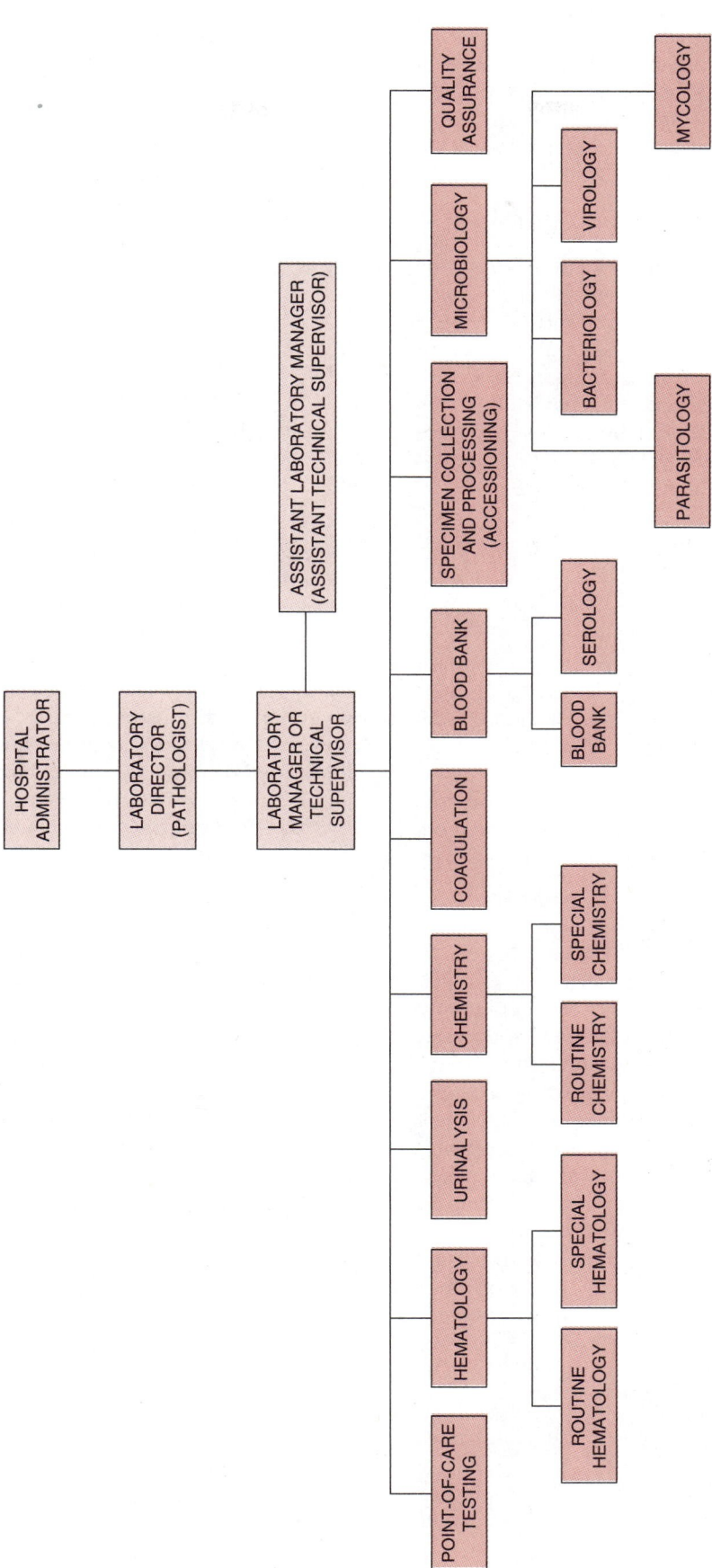

**FIGURE 1-2** Organizational chart of a typical hospital laboratory

laboratory technicians). Non-laboratory personnel such as medical assistants and nurses may perform tests in POLs or other settings outside the laboratory proper. Medical laboratory personnel qualifications are discussed in Lesson 1-2, The Medical Laboratory Professional.

## Departments of the Medical Laboratory

The number of departments in medical laboratories varies. Clinical chemistry, hematology, microbiology, blood bank, and specimen collection and processing usually operate as departments or sections, each with its own department head or general supervisor. The subdivisions within each department may differ from one laboratory to another. Large laboratories may have separate departments for urinalysis, coagulation, serology, parasitology, quality assurance, and off-site testing.

### Quality Assurance

Many laboratories have a section that is responsible for coordinating Total Quality Management (TQM) or quality assurance (QA) for all other sections of the laboratory. Every aspect of a test procedure from specimen collection to reporting of results falls under the umbrella of quality assurance. Responsibilities of the QA section may also include management of off-site testing; personnel training; updating procedure manuals; monitoring compliance with regulatory agencies; record-keeping; documentation of equipment maintenance, calibration and repairs; and participation in proficiency testing.

### Specimen Collection and Processing (Accessioning)

Most hospital laboratories have a separate department responsible for collecting and processing the specimens for testing. This may be called the phlebotomy department. **Phlebotomists** are the personnel who collect the blood specimens. In many laboratories, some or all of the testing or nursing personnel share this responsibility.

In small laboratories, specimens are usually taken directly to the appropriate department for testing. In larger laboratories, specimens may be taken to a central **accessioning** area where they are processed, logged into the computer, and given a specimen number before being distributed to the departments for testing.

### Hematology

Most **hematology** tests involve studying the cellular components of blood. **Whole blood** is used for most procedures.

Hematology procedures can be qualitative or quantitative. The quantitative procedures include counts of the various blood components, such as the number of leukocytes (white blood cells), erythrocytes (red blood cells), or platelets. These counts can be performed manually or using automated systems.

In qualitative procedures, the various blood components are observed for qualities such as cell size, shape, and maturity. Using a microscope, a laboratory worker can view a blood smear, to determine the types of leukocytes present; estimate the size, shape, and hemoglobin content of erythrocytes; or estimate the number of platelets. Any abnormalities are noted during microscopic examination of the blood smear, including immature leukocytes or erythrocytes. Hematocrit, blood indices, and hemoglobin are tests commonly performed to help diagnose anemia. Many companies make sophisticated instruments capable of performing several hematological procedures simultaneously.

*Coagulation.* Coagulation tests may be performed in the hematology department or, in large laboratories, in a separate department. Coagulation tests are performed to diagnose and monitor patients who have defects in their blood-clotting mechanism or are being treated with anti-clotting drugs. Until recently automated coagulation testing systems were used primarily in larger laboratories. However, the development of small, easy-to-use coagulation analyzers allows even small POLs to have the capability of performing coagulation procedures. **Plasma**, the liquid portion of anticoagulated blood, is the specimen used for most coagulation studies.

*Urinalysis.* Like coagulation, urinalysis may be a separate department in a large laboratory, or may be a subdivision of another department, usually hematology or chemistry. In the urinalysis department, physical, chemical, and microscopic examinations of urine specimens are performed. These tests may be performed manually or using automated methods.

### Clinical Chemistry

In the clinical chemistry department, test procedures are usually performed on **serum**, the liquid part of blood remaining after a clot has formed. Tests may also be performed on plasma, urine, and other body fluids, such as spinal fluid and joint fluid.

Procedures performed in the clinical chemistry department include blood glucose, cholesterol, assays of heart and liver enzymes, and electrolytes (chloride, bicarbonate, potassium, and sodium).

The chemistry department is the largest department in most laboratories, and usually has one or more subdivisions. Common subdivisions are special chemistry or toxicology. Here, patients' blood or urine may be analyzed to determine the drug involved in an overdose, blood levels of prescribed drugs, and hormone levels.

The number of instruments available for clinical chemistry analysis has grown rapidly in the last several years (see Lesson 6-4). Many of these instruments provide a wide range of test procedures and are also simple to operate. Thus, it is possible for almost every laboratory to perform a few routine chemistry procedures.

## Microbiology

The **microbiology** department is responsible for culturing and identifying microorganisms, usually bacteria, isolated from a patient's blood, urine, or other body fluid, sputum, or wound. After the organism is cultured from a specimen, susceptibility testing is performed. Susceptibility testing involves exposing the organism to different antibiotics and observing the effect on the organism's growth. This helps to determine which antibiotic would be most effective in treating the infection. **Virology**, the study of viruses, and **mycology**, the study of fungi, are usually a part of the microbiology laboratory.

Traditionally, the microbiology department has been less automated than other departments. However, this has changed. Automated systems are available that can detect growth of an organism, identify an organism, and determine the most effective antibiotic for treatment.

***Parasitology.*** The parasitology laboratory, often a part of the microbiology department, is where patient specimens are examined for parasites. Fecal samples may be examined for evidence of intestinal parasites such as tapeworms or hookworms. Examination of blood for parasites such as the malaria parasite is usually performed in the hematology department.

## Blood Bank

The blood bank department may also be called transfusion services or **immunohematology**. Several procedures are performed in this department. If a transfusion is required, the patient's ABO group and Rh blood type are determined by blood bank technologists. The technologists then test the blood units in storage to determine which would be compatible to transfuse into the patient. The blood bank department may also have the capability of processing donated blood into specialized components such as concentrated red blood cells and plasma.

***Serology/Immunology.*** Serology, or immunology, may be a subdivision of the blood bank or microbiology departments if it is not a separate department. Serum is the specimen usually used for serological tests; sometimes urine is tested. In serology, specimens are tested using antigen-antibody methods. Among tests performed in this section are those for pregnancy, arthritis, infectious mononucleosis, HIV, hepatitis, sexually transmitted diseases, and other infectious diseases.

### Point-of-Care Testing

Changes are occurring rapidly in all aspects of health care delivery systems. One of the major changes occurring in the clinical laboratory is the implementation of Point-of-Care Testing (**POCT**). POCT brings the laboratory test to the patient rather than obtaining a specimen from the patient and sending it to the laboratory for testing. This means laboratory test results are available more rapidly, providing improved patient care.

POCT is used in settings such as clinics, HMOs, nursing homes, physician offices, emergency rooms, intensive care units, and surgery suites. POCT is also referred to as bedside testing, near-patient testing, off-site testing, or alternate-site testing.

The evolution of small, simple-to-use analyzers that require only a tiny amount of specimen has led to widespread POCT implementation. Handheld portable analyzers can measure substances such as hemoglobin, glucose, blood gases, cholesterol, and electrolytes. Most require only a drop of blood, usually obtained by fingerstick. Most POCT tests are CLIA-waived.

The advent of POCT has created the opportunity for more collaboration between the laboratory and other components of the health care team. Although nonlaboratory personnel from the nursing service or surgery or ER teams may perform the tests, the laboratory is usually responsible for selecting instrumentation, training personnel, developing procedure manuals, and monitoring quality assurance procedures and instrument maintenance.

## PROFICIENCY TESTING

CLIA '88 requires that laboratories performing moderate- or high-complexity testing participate in an approved proficiency-testing program in which samples are sent to the laboratory for analysis at regular intervals. After the samples are tested, the laboratory reports results to the proficiency-testing agency, which evaluates them for accuracy and for the laboratory's performance compared to other laboratories. Participation in a proficiency-testing program is an important part of a laboratory's quality assurance program and allows the laboratory to have confidence in testing methods, identify deficient areas, and provides documentation of performance for accrediting and regulatory agencies.

## ACCREDITATION OF MEDICAL LABORATORIES

**Accreditation** is a voluntary process in which an independent agency grants recognition to institutions or programs that meet or exceed established standards of quality. Most health care institutions seek accreditation because it enhances the institution's reputation and gives the public a way to assess the institution's quality of care.

An institution desiring accreditation invites the accrediting agency to inspect its facility to determine if established standards are being met.

Some of the many agencies that accredit health care institutions and laboratories include the Joint Commission on Accreditation of Healthcare Organizations (**JCAHO**), which accredits hospitals; the College of American Pathologists (**CAP**), which offers accreditation to medical laboratories; the American Association of Blood Banks (**AABB**), which accredits blood bank departments; and the Commission on Office Laboratory Accreditation (**COLA**), which accredits physician office laboratories. A list of some accrediting agencies for clinical laboratories is included in Appendix A.

## REQUESTING A LABORATORY TEST

Laboratory personnel perform test procedures only after a proper laboratory request form has been received. Only a physician may initiate the request by writing the order in the patient's chart. Nursing staff will then send a written request or computer-generated request to the laboratory. After the request is received, the laboratory will collect the proper specimen, perform the test, and record, report, and chart the results.

A **stat test** must be performed as rapidly as possible because of an emergency or life-threatening situation. In these cases, all personnel must see that test requests and specimens are transported to the laboratory as quickly as possible. Laboratory personnel must perform the test and report the results as rapidly as possible without sacrificing the accuracy and reliability of results.

Outpatient laboratory testing is carried out when a patient brings a written physician's request to the laboratory. Some outpatients may have "standing orders." For example, patients on certain medications may come

in at regular intervals for tests to monitor the effectiveness or dosage of the drug.

## COMMUNICATIONS

It is important to have good channels of communication within the laboratory and among the laboratory and physicians, other departments in the hospital, and other health care providers. Good communication and cooperation between the laboratory and these groups helps ensure the best possible care for patients.

Much communication in laboratories and health care institutions is facilitated by computers. It is possible to request laboratory tests, analyze findings, and report patient results by computer. The widespread use of computers in health care contributes to efficiency and improved patient care. However, although patient information is available through computers, that information is still confidential.

### SUMMARY

The clinical or medical laboratory is a dynamic workplace. Many changes are occurring as the roles of medical laboratory personnel are redefined and as technology advances. The need for cost containment in providing health care and the promise of major changes in our health care delivery systems mean laboratories must be flexible in adjusting to future trends.

### LESSON REVIEW

1. What is the function of a medical or clinical laboratory?
2. Draw an organizational chart of a typical hospital laboratory.
3. Name five major departments found in a hospital medical laboratory.
4. Name two procedures performed in the hematology department.
5. Name two tests performed in the chemistry department.
6. Why is cooperation between laboratory personnel and other medical or hospital personnel so important?
7. List three locations of medical laboratory facilities other than a hospital.

8. Explain the job functions of the laboratory director, laboratory manager, and department head or general supervisor.
9. How are medical laboratories regulated?
10. How do laboratories become accredited?
11. Define AABB, accessioning, accreditation, CAP, CDC, CLIA '88, COLA, DHHS, epidemiology, HCFA, hematology, immunohematology, JCAHO, microbiology, mycology, NCCLS, pathologist, phlebotomist, plasma, POCT, POL, reference laboratory, serum, stat test, virology, and whole blood.

## STUDENT ACTIVITIES

1. Reread the information on the medical laboratory.
2. Review the glossary terms.
3. Interview an employee of a medical laboratory. Inquire about the laboratory's organization and the types of tests performed. Obtain various laboratory test report forms and note the types of tests performed in each department.
4. Tour a medical laboratory.

# The Medical Laboratory Professional

## LESSON OBJECTIVES

**After studying this lesson, you should be able to:**

- *Give a brief history of medical technology.*
- *List five personal qualities that are desirable in a medical laboratory professional.*
- *Describe the educational requirements for medical technologists (clinical laboratory scientists) and medical laboratory technicians (clinical laboratory technicians).*
- *Discuss the relationship between the medical laboratory professional and the patient.*
- *Explain the functions of accrediting agencies and credentialing agencies.*
- *Explain the purpose of professional societies.*
- *Discuss rules of ethical conduct for laboratory professionals.*
- *Name five areas of employment for medical laboratory professionals other than in hospital laboratories.*
- *Define the glossary terms.*

## GLOSSARY

**AAMA** / American Association of Medical Assistants

**AMT** / American Medical Technologists

**ASCLS** / American Society for Clinical Laboratory Science (formerly American Society for Medical Technology, ASMT)

**ASCP** / American Society of Clinical Pathologists

**ASPT** / American Society of Phlebotomy Technicians

**CAAHEP** / Commission on Accreditation of Allied Health Education Programs (formerly CAHEA)

**clinical laboratory science** / the field of medical laboratory technology

**clinical laboratory scientist (CLS)** / medical technologist

**clinical laboratory technician (CLT)** / medical laboratory technician

**ethics** / a system of conduct or behavior; rules of professional conduct

**ISCLT** / International Society for Clinical Laboratory Technology

**medical laboratory technician (MLT)** /a professional who has completed a minimum of two years of specific training in an accredited medical laboratory technician program and has passed a national certifying examination; clinical laboratory technician

**medical technologist (MT)** / a professional who has a baccalaureate degree from an accredited college or university, has completed clinical training in an accredited medical technology program, and has passed a national certifying examination; clinical laboratory scientist

**medical technology** / the health profession concerned with performing laboratory analyses used in diagnosing and treating disease, as well as in maintaining good health; clinical laboratory science

**NAACLS** / National Accrediting Agency for Clinical Laboratory Sciences

**NCA** / National Credentialing Agency for Laboratory Personnel

## INTRODUCTION

**Medical technology**, or **clinical laboratory science**, is the health profession concerned with performing laboratory analyses. Information gained from the analyses is used in diagnosing and treating disease, as well as in maintaining good health. The analyses are performed by trained, skilled medical laboratory personnel.

What do these medical laboratory personnel do? They work as medical detectives. They use microscopes to observe changes in cells. They test blood to find compatible blood for transfusions. They use special stains to identify microorganisms and analyze cells. They measure substances such as glucose and cholesterol in the blood. They discover and identify organisms causing infections. They operate complex instruments. They use standards and controls to ensure reliable results. They work under pressure. They work with speed, accuracy, and precision. They adhere to high ethical standards.

This lesson examines the medical laboratory profession, the personal and educational qualifications required, job responsibilities, employment opportunities, ethics, and professionalism.

## HISTORY OF MEDICAL TECHNOLOGY

Medical technology can be traced back several centuries. Papyrus writings dating before 1000 B.C. record descriptions of intestinal parasites, an early example of parasitology. Before medieval times, Hindu doctors performed crude urinalyses when they observed that some urine had a sweet taste and attracted ants. With the invention of the microscope in the seventeenth century, the study of biological specimens progressed from simple visual examination to microscopic examination.

### Early Clinical Laboratories

The first clinical laboratories in the United States appeared in the late nineteenth century and were very crude. Some consisted of only a table and a microscope. They were staffed mostly by doctors who had a special interest in "laboratory medicine." The 1900 U.S. census listed only one hundred laboratory technicians, all male.

### Modern Clinical Laboratories

After World War I, laboratories grew in size and number. It soon became clear that there was a need for (1) educating laboratory workers, (2) defining educational requirements, and (3) identifying adequately trained persons. By the 1930s, basic educational requirements had been established and schools of medical technology were training laboratory workers. Certifying examinations were given to measure the knowledge and ability of workers.

Since World War II, the technology for laboratory testing has become increasingly complex. Laboratory tests now play an essential role in medicine. Specially trained workers comprise most of the work force in the medical laboratory. Today's technology provides a level of health care only imagined a few years ago. The field is constantly changing and broadening in response to new technologies, new federal regulations, and changes in health care needs. Terminology is also changing to reflect these changes. The term "clinical laboratory science" is replacing the term "medical technology" because it more accurately reflects the profession and the field today.

## THE MEDICAL LABORATORY PROFESSION TODAY

There are thousands of medical laboratories in the United States, both large and small. Many laboratories are highly sophisticated and offer complex tests. The personnel staffing of these laboratories include highly skilled professionals who perform complicated analyses (Figure 1-3). These professionals may also be laboratory directors, consultants, teachers, supervisors, and administrators. To become a qualified medical laboratory professional requires certain personal characteristics, completion of a specialized course of study, and successful completion of a national examination.

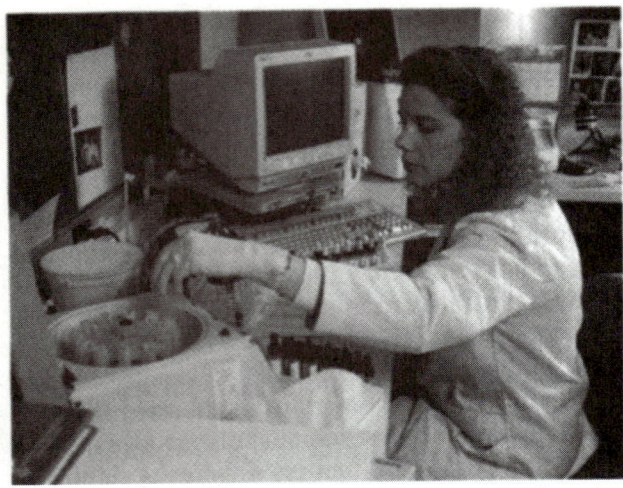

**FIGURE 1-3** A medical laboratory professional at work (Photo by Marcia Butterfield, courtesy of W. A. Foote Memorial Hospital, Jackson, MI)

Several agencies and organizations are involved in establishing and maintaining the principles and standards of the profession. Examples of agencies that accredit educational programs, agencies that certify personnel, and professional organizations and societies that contribute to continued professional development of the medical laboratory professional are listed in Tables 1-3, 1-4, and 1-5. Addresses of these groups are provided in Appendix A.

## Programs for Educating Medical Laboratory Professionals

Several levels of employment, each requiring different skill levels, exist in most medical laboratories. Educational and regulatory requirements for these positions differ. Some positions require only a high school education and documented on-the-job training. However, most laboratories performing moderate- to high-complexity testing desire employees who have completed a prescribed program of study in clinical laboratory science. Several types of programs of study are available through hospitals, colleges and universities, technical schools, and private, independent schools. The programs usually consist of an academic component and a clinical component. Upon completion of a program, the student may become certified by passing a certifying examination.

**Table 1-3.** Examples of accrediting agencies for educational programs for medical laboratory personnel

| | |
|---|---|
| **CAAHEP** | Commission on Accreditation of Allied Health Education Programs (formerly CAHEA) |
| **NAACLS** | National Accrediting Agency for Clinical Laboratory Sciences |

**Table 1-4.** Some credentialing/certifying agencies for medical laboratory and other allied health personnel

| | |
|---|---|
| **AAB** | American Association of Bioanalysts Board of Registry |
| **AAMA** | American Association of Medical Assistants |
| **ABB** | American Board of Bioanalysis |
| **AMT** | American Medical Technologists |
| **ASCP** | American Society of Clinical Pathologists |
| **ASPT** | American Society of Phlebotomy Technicians |
| **DHHS** | U.S. Department of Health and Human Services |
| **ISCLT** | International Society for Clinical Laboratory Technology |
| **NCA** | National Credentialing Agency (for Laboratory Personnel) |
| **NPA** | National Phlebotomy Association |

**Table 1-5.** Professional societies for medical laboratory and other allied health personnel

| | |
|---|---|
| **AAB** | American Association of Bioanalysts |
| **AABB** | American Association of Blood Banks |
| **AACC** | American Association of Clinical Chemistry |
| **AAMA** | American Association of Medical Assistants |
| **AMT** | American Medical Technologists |
| **APIC** | Association of Practitioners in Infection Control |
| **ASCLS** | American Society for Clinical Laboratory Science |
| **ASCP** | American Society of Clinical Pathologists |
| **ASM** | American Society for Microbiology |
| **ASPT** | American Society of Phlebotomy Technicians |
| **CLMA** | Clinical Laboratory Management Association |
| **IAMLT** | International Association of Medical Laboratory Technologists |
| **ISCLT** | International Society for Clinical Laboratory Technology |
| **NPA** | National Phlebotomy Association |

## Accreditation of Educational Programs

Independent agencies provide accreditation for medical laboratory professional programs. Two such agencies are the Commission on Accreditation of Allied Health Education Programs (**CAAHEP**) and the National Accrediting Agency for Clinical Laboratory Sciences (**NAACLS**) (Table 1-3). Programs accredited by these agencies must meet nationally established standards. Addresses of accrediting agencies are given in Appendix A.

## Educational Requirements for Medical Laboratory Professionals

The two most common levels of professionals working in the hospital or reference laboratory are:

- medical technologist (MT) or clinical laboratory scientist (CLS)
- medical laboratory technician (MLT) or clinical laboratory technician (CLT)

### Medical Technologist/Clinical Laboratory Scientist

The **medical technologist (MT)**, or **clinical laboratory scientist (CLS)**, generally has a baccalaureate degree from a college or university and has completed specified clinical training in an accredited medical technology program. To become certified, the individual must also pass a national examination. Certified medical technologists are qualified to perform analyses in all departments of the laboratory. These individuals may also be supervisors or work in other leadership positions in the laboratory.

### Medical Laboratory Technician/Clinical Laboratory Technician

The **medical laboratory technician (MLT)**, or **clinical laboratory technician (CLT)**, generally has an associate's degree from a college or a certificate from an accredited medical laboratory technician program. Upon passing a national certifying examination, the medical laboratory technician is certified.

### Areas of Specialization

Employees may specialize in one area of laboratory work such as microbiology, hematology, or blood banking. To obtain specialist rank, such as specialist in hematology or specialist in blood bank, the employee must complete appropriate academic work, obtain the required number of years of clinical experience, and pass an examination in the specialty area.

## Other Medical Laboratory and Allied Health Personnel

### Phlebotomist (Phlebotomy Technician, Clinical Laboratory Phlebotomist)

Training programs are available for laboratory phlebotomists. These programs require a high school diploma or general equivalency diploma (GED) for entrance. After the training program is complete, certification is available through several organizations following successful completion of a national examination. Examples of certifying organizations and professional designations are:

**AMT**, American Medical Technologists
  RPT, Registered Phlebotomy Technician

**ASCP**, American Society of Clinical Pathologists
  PBT, Phlebotomy Technician

**ASPT**, American Society of Phlebotomy Technicians

**NCA**, National Credentialing Agency (for Laboratory Personnel)
  CLPlb, Clinical Laboratory Phlebotomist

**NPA**, National Phlebotomy Association
  CPT, Certified Phlebotomy Technician

### Medical Assistant (Certified Medical Assistant, Registered Medical Assistant)

The emergence of POCT as an important part of the health care delivery system has resulted in an expansion of the categories of personnel that perform laboratory analyses. Where traditionally only laboratory personnel performed these tests, testing is now being performed by non-laboratory personnel, such as paramedics, medical assistants, licensed practical nurses, and registered nurses, who provide health care in a variety of settings from the patient's home to a physician's office to an emergency room.

Medical assistants are allied health professionals who are frequently employed in ambulatory care settings such as POLs and who have been trained in administrative, clerical, nursing, and laboratory skills. They perform phlebotomy, collect specimens, and perform some waived tests such as hemoglobin, hematocrit, chemical urine testing, pregnancy tests, blood glucose, and fecal occult blood.

Training for medical assistants is available through community colleges, vocational-technical, and private schools. A high school diploma or general equivalency diploma (GED) is required for entrance. There are two levels of education for medical assistants. One is a diploma program requiring one year of post-secondary education; the other is an Associate of Science degree, consisting of two years of post-secondary education.

**Table 1–6.** NCA certification categories and equivalent ASCP certification categories

| NCA DESIGNATION | ASCP DESIGNATION |
|---|---|
| CLS, clinical laboratory scientist | MT, medical technologist |
| CLT, clinical laboratory technician | MLT, medical laboratory technician |
| CLSp, clinical laboratory specialist | S, specialist |
| CLSup, clinical laboratory supervisor | DLM, diplomate in laboratory management |
| CLPlb, clinical laboratory phlebotomist | PBT, phlebotomy technician |

Upon completion of the course of study, certification may be obtained by passing a national examination administered by a certifying organization. Two such organizations and their certification designations are:

**AAMA**, American Association of Medical Assistants

CMA, Certified Medical Assistant

**AMT**, American Medical Technologists

RMA, Registered Medical Assistant

## Credentialing and Certification of Medical Laboratory Personnel

Credentialing or certifying agencies are independent organizations that administer examinations for different levels of medical laboratory professionals. These include the American Society of Clinical Pathologists (**ASCP**), the National Credentialing Agency for Medical Laboratory Personnel (**NCA**), the American Medical Technologists (**AMT**), and the International Society for Clinical Laboratory Technology (**ISCLT**) (Table 1-4).

Agencies differ somewhat in titles used for equivalent training. For instance, the qualifications are the same for CLS (NCA) and MT (ASCP), although the professional designations differ. Table 1-6 gives the designations used by the NCA and the equivalent designations used by the ASCP. Designations are sometimes confusing because there are several certifying agencies. Information about specific eligibility requirements for certification categories can be obtained from the individual certifying agencies. Addresses of these organizations are given in Appendix A.

## Licensing of Medical Laboratory Personnel

Although certification is usually sufficient to meet most employment requirements, some states regulate laboratory personnel by requiring workers to obtain a state license. Licensing laws vary from state to state and are nonexistent in some states. Some states require a fee to obtain a license, or that a test be taken before the license is issued; some states require both.

# ETHICS AND PROFESSIONALISM

## Ethics and the Medical Laboratory Professional

Medical laboratory personnel are health care professionals. They must observe professional **ethics**, a prescribed code of conduct and behavior. Organizations that credential health care professionals have a code of ethics to which their members are expected to subscribe. One example is the code of ethics for laboratory professionals adopted by the **ASCLS**, American Society of Clinical Laboratory Scientists (formerly the ASMT, American Society for Medical Technology). The principles in the code stress that the professional has a duty to his or her patient, colleagues, profession, and society. A portion of this code is given in Table 1-7.

## Privacy/Confidentiality

Laboratory professionals carry out their duty to the patient by providing competent service and maintaining high standards. One important principle that *must* be adhered to is that of patient privacy. Patient information

**Table 1-7.** Portion of Code of Ethics of the American Society for Clinical Laboratory Science (Reprinted with permission of American Society for Clinical Laboratory Science, Bethesda, MD)

As a clinical laboratory professional, I acknowledge my professional responsibility to:

- Maintain and promote standards of excellence in performing and advancing the art and science of my profession;
- Safeguard the dignity and privacy of patients;
- Hold my colleagues and my profession in high esteem and regard;
- Contribute to the general well-being of the community; and
- Actively demonstrate my commitment to these responsibilities throughout my professional life.

is confidential. It must only be discussed with health care employees directly related to the case who have a "need to know." Confidential patient information cannot be released without patient consent unless required by law.

Test results should not be discussed with patients, their relatives, or other inappropriate persons. Test results should be reported only to the physician or other appropriate designated employee. Elevators, cafeterias, and lounges are not appropriate places to discuss patient results or unusual findings.

The increased use of computers in health care has made access to patient information easier for all health care workers. Although these advances facilitate information transfer, workers must realize that it is ethical to access the information only when they have a real need (not a desire) to know. Appropriate security must be in place to protect patient information stored in computer databases from inappropriate access.

## PROFESSIONALISM

### Personal Qualities Desirable in Medical Laboratory Professionals

Dedication, dependability, cooperation, good hygiene, neatness, and a caring attitude are some essential qualities desirable in all health care professionals. In addition, persons working in medical laboratories need special characteristics.

To succeed in the medical laboratory profession, a person needs physical stamina, good eyesight, normal color vision, manual dexterity, a good intellect, and an aptitude for the biological sciences. Communication skills, reliability, honesty, and the ability to relate well to fellow workers are also necessary. Laboratory workers must be observant, motivated, able to perform precise manipulations and calculations, and have good organizational skills.

### Interaction Between Medical Laboratory Personnel and Patients

As in all other areas of health care, the field of medical technology exists for the patient. For a patient to receive the best possible care, a physician must make the proper diagnosis. To make this diagnosis, physicians rely on laboratory analyses, along with information gained from the medical history, physical examination, and clinical symptoms. Therefore, it is imperative that laboratory analyses be performed carefully and accurately, using the best techniques available.

Often, the only contact patients have with the laboratory is through the laboratory assistant, technologist,

or phlebotomist who collects a blood sample from them. At best, it is not pleasant to have blood taken from a vein or finger. At all times, the health care professional needs to be aware of the stress the patient is feeling when hospitalized or ill. The employee must be professional, courteous, and considerate of patients.

### Professional Organizations

There are several professional societies for medical laboratory professionals. These societies provide opportunities for professional growth and continuing education by offering workshops and seminars, and by publishing journals (Table 1-5). Examples of journals for laboratory professionals are *Laboratory Medicine* and *ADVANCE for Medical Laboratory Professionals*.

Membership in a national society usually also includes membership in that society's state affiliate. A listing of several professional societies can be found in Appendix A. Membership and participation in the activities of a professional society contribute to the continuing competence of the medical laboratory professional.

Medical laboratory professionals carry out their duty to colleagues and their profession through professional improvement activities, cooperation, and respect for their colleagues. Through competent practice of their profession, they contribute to the well-being of the community.

## EMPLOYMENT OPPORTUNITIES

Many employment opportunities exist for medical laboratory professionals. Many of the nation's medical laboratory workers are employed in hospitals. Other areas of employment include physician offices, clinics, public health agencies, reference laboratories, the military, research, education, veterinary medicine, and pharmaceuticals. Laboratory professionals are also employed in sales, product development, and technical service departments of medical suppliers and manufacturers.

## RESPONSIBILITIES OF MEDICAL LABORATORY PROFESSIONALS

Set rules and regulations govern health care in all states. Health care agencies have very specific standards, rules, and regulations governing the responsibilities of various health care employees. All health care workers must assume the responsibility of learning exactly what activities are expected and permitted in their jobs. They should understand their job responsibilities fully for their protection, the protection of their employer, and the safety of their patients.

## LESSON REVIEW

1. What is medical laboratory technology? What is the other term used for this field?

2. Describe the beginnings of medical laboratory technology.

3. What are five personal qualities desirable in medical laboratory personnel?

4. What are the educational requirements for medical technologists? For medical laboratory technicians?

5. List five places of nonhospital employment for laboratory personnel.

6. Explain the importance of ethical standards in the practice of medical technology.

7. Explain the laboratory professional's obligation to the patient.

8. How do laboratory professionals become certified?

9. What is the importance of professional societies to the medical laboratory professional?

10. Define AAMA, AMT, ASCLS, ASCP, ASPT, CAAHEP, clinical laboratory science, clinical laboratory scientist, clinical laboratory technician, ethics, ISCLT, medical laboratory technician, medical technologist, medical technology, NAACLS, and NCA.

## STUDENT ACTIVITIES

1. Reread the information on the medical laboratory professional.

2. Review the glossary terms.

3. Complete a Career Information Fact Sheet on the medical laboratory technician and the medical technologist. This should include educational training, cost of program, nature of job, advantages and disadvantages, employment opportunities, and salary range.

4. Use the Interview Fact Sheet and interview a medical laboratory professional. Be sure to consider the following areas: job functions, relationships with coworkers and patients, advantages and disadvantages of job, satisfactions, dissatisfactions, salary, and opportunities for advancement. Describe the benefits of talking to the laboratory worker in person rather than reading the information in a book.

## *Career Information Fact Sheet*

## **LESSON 1-2** The Medical Laboratory Professional

Name _____    Date _____

Job Title:

Legal Requirement:

Name of Program:

Educational Institution:

Cost of Program:

Length of Program:

Admission Requirements:

Nature of the Job:

Earnings:

Advancement:

Related Occupation(s):

Advantages:

Disadvantages:

## *Interview Fact Sheet*

## **LESSON 1-2** The Medical Laboratory Professional

Name _____ Date _____

Job Title:

Educational Preparation:

Approximate Cost of Education Program:

Job Functions:

Approximate Salary:

Job Satisfaction:

Job Dissatisfaction:

Opportunities for Advancement:

Options Available to Broaden Employment Opportunities:

# Introduction to Medical Terminology

## LESSON OBJECTIVES

**After studying this lesson, you should be able to:**

- *Discuss the importance of health care workers understanding and correctly using medical terms.*
- *Define stem words from a selected list.*
- *Define prefixes from a selected list.*
- *Define suffixes from a selected list.*
- *Identify common abbreviations of medical laboratory terms from a selected list.*
- *Pronounce commonly used medical terms from a selected list.*
- *Define the glossary terms.*

## GLOSSARY

**prefix** / modifying word or syllable(s) placed at the beginning of a word

**stem** / main part of a word; root word; the part of a word remaining after removing the prefix or suffix

**suffix** / modifying word or syllable(s) placed at the end of a word

**terminology** / terms used in any specialized field

## INTRODUCTION

Most specialized fields have a unique vocabulary or **terminology**. Medical terminology is the study of terms or words used in medicine. Health care workers must know, understand, and be able to correctly use medical terms to carry out instructions and communicate effectively.

This lesson is only an introduction to the structure of medical terms and to abbreviations frequently used in the medical laboratory. Learning medical vocabulary is a long process. Knowledge of medical terms evolves and expands as the terms are used while working in health care delivery systems. Proper use of medical terminology is as much a part of the job of laboratory and health care workers as other job functions. Each individual can gain confidence in using medical terminology by using the terms in daily activities.

## STRUCTURE OF MEDICAL TERMS

Most medical terms are a combination of word parts—prefixes, suffixes, and stems—that are clues to the meaning of the word. A **prefix** is a word or syllable(s) that modifies the stem and is placed at the beginning of the word. A **suffix** is a word or syllable(s) placed at the end of the word and usually describes what happens to the stem. The **stem** or root is the main part of the word. These word parts are usually connected by a vowel (such as *a, i,* or *o*).

Most of the stems, prefixes, and suffixes used in medical terms are derived from Latin or Greek words and have a specific meaning. By combining various prefixes, stems, and suffixes, many medical terms with precise meanings may be formed.

Not all terms have all three word parts. Some words may have only a prefix and a stem or a stem and suffix. All terms, though, will have a stem, or root, word.

If the meanings of commonly used word parts are known, then a new term can often be analyzed to determine the general idea of its meaning. For example, hyperproteinuria can be divided into three word parts: hyper, protein, uria. "Hyper" means an increased amount. "Uria" refers to "in the urine." Therefore, the term means a condition with an increased amount of protein in the urine. By combining these parts to make a word, a medical shortcut has been created. One word can describe what would normally take a sentence or sometimes a paragraph.

Medical terms, although shorter than sentences, have precise meanings. Sometimes a slight modification, such as alteration of one or two letters, can change the meaning of a word. For example, a macrocyte is a cell larger than normal, while a microcyte is a cell smaller than normal. It is very important to spell, pronounce, and use medical terms correctly so the intended meaning is conveyed.

## Prefixes

Prefixes placed before stem words give more information about the stem, such as location, time, size, or number. For example, *intra*vascular means inside the vessel and *pre*natal refers to something that happens before birth. Table 1-8 contains a list of commonly used prefixes and the definition of each. A sample term using the prefix is also given.

## Stems

The stem or root word gives the major subject of the term. For example, in the term *appendi*citis, the stem is "appendi." Therefore, appendicitis means an inflammation of the appendix. In the term endo*card*itis, the root or stem is "card," referring to heart; the term literally means an inflammation (itis) within (endo) the heart. Commonly used stem words, their definitions, and examples of usage are listed in Table 1-9.

## Suffixes

Suffixes are modifiers attached to the end of a stem word. Suffixes usually tell what is happening to the subject of the stem. They often indicate a condition, operation, or symptom. For example, in the term append*ectomy*, "ectomy" is a suffix that means to cut out or remove by excision. Therefore, an appendectomy is the surgical removal of the appendix. Commonly used suffixes, their definitions, and examples of usage are listed in Table 1-10.

## PRONUNCIATION OF MEDICAL TERMS

It is not enough to just understand written medical terms. You must also be able to pronounce them correctly to communicate effectively with others. Correct pronunciation may be easy for some frequently used or short terms, but is often more difficult for longer terms.

Although most medical terms are derived from Greek and Latin, Latin and Greek pronunciation is not always used. Your medical dictionary can guide you but different authors sometimes disagree on pronunciations. By listening to others who work with you, you can learn how words are commonly pronounced in your area. Pronunciation will be improved and confidence gained by practice.

## ABBREVIATIONS COMMONLY USED IN THE MEDICAL LABORATORY

Abbreviations are used commonly in medicine to avoid having to repeatedly write or say several syllables. Workers should be familiar with frequently used abbreviations so physician's orders or instructions can be carried out correctly.

Some common abbreviations used in the medical laboratory are listed in Table 1-11. Many of these abbreviations will be used in other lessons in this text. (This table does not include abbreviations used in prescriptions, nursing, or other areas of health care.)

**Table 1-8.** Selected prefixes commonly used in medical terminology

| PREFIX | DEFINITION | EXAMPLE OF USAGE | PREFIX | DEFINITION | EXAMPLE OF USAGE |
|---|---|---|---|---|---|
| a, an | absent, deficient | anemia | medi | middle | medicephalic |
| ab | away from | absent | mega | huge, great | megaloblast |
| ad | toward | adrenal | melan | black | melanoma |
| ambi | both | ambidextrous | meta | after, next | metamorphosis |
| aniso | unequal | anisocytosis | micro | small, one-millionth | microscope, microgram |
| ante | before | antenatal | milli | one-thousandth | millimeter |
| ant(i) | against | antibiotic | mon(o) | one, single | monocyte |
| auto | self | autograft | morph | shape | morphogenesis |
| baso | blue | basophil | necro | dead | necrophobia |
| bi | two | binuclear | neo | new | neoplasm |
| bio | life | biochemistry | neutro | neutral, neither | neutrophil |
| brady | slow | bradycardia | olig | few | oliguria |
| circum | around | circumnuclear | orth | straight, normal | orthopedic |
| co, com, con | with, together | concentrate | pan | all | pandemic |
| contra | against | contraception | para | beside, accessory to | paramedic |
| de | down, from | decay | per | through | percutaneous |
| di | two | dimorphic | peri | around | pericardium |
| dia | through | dialysis | phago | to eat | phagocyte |
| dipl | double | diplococcus | poly | many | polyuria |
| dis | apart, away from | disease | post | after | postoperative |
| dys | bad, difficult, improper | dysphagia | pre, pro | before | prenatal |
| e, ecto, ex | out from | ectoparasite | pseudo | false | pseudo-appendicitis |
| end(o) | inside, within | endoparasite | | | |
| enter(o) | intestine | enterotoxin | psycho(o) | mind | psychoanalyst |
| epi | upon, after | epidermis | py(o) | pus | pyuria |
| equi | equal | equilibrium | quad(r) | four | quadrangle |
| glyco | sweet | glycosuria | retro | backward | retroactive |
| hemi | half | hemisphere | semi | half | semiconscious |
| hyper | above, excessive | hyperglycemia | steno | narrow | stenothorax |
| hypo | under, deficient | hypoventilation | sub | under | subcutaneous |
| infra | beneath | infracostal | super, supra | above | superinfection |
| inter | among, between | intercostal | syn | together | synergistic |
| intra | within | intracranial | tachy | swift | tachycardia |
| iso | equal | isotonic | therm | heat | thermometer |
| kilo | one thousand | kilogram | trans | through | transport |
| macr | large | macrocyte | tri | three | trimester |
| mal | bad, abnormal | malformation | uni | one | unicellular |

**Table 1-9.** Selected stems commonly used in medical terminology

| STEM | DEFINITION | EXAMPLE OF USAGE | STEM | DEFINITION | EXAMPLE OF USAGE |
|---|---|---|---|---|---|
| adeno | gland | lymphadenitis | lip | fat | lipoma |
| alg | pain | analgesic | lith | stone | cholelithiasis |
| arter | artery | arteriogram | mening | membrane covering brain | meningitis |
| arthr | joint | arthritis | | | |
| audio | hearing | auditory | morph | shape, form | morphology |
| brachi | arm | brachial | myel | marrow | myelogram |
| bronch(i) | air tube in lungs | bronchitis | myo | muscle | myositis |
| card | heart | myocardium | nephro | kidney | nephrectomy |
| calc | stone | calcify | neur | nerve | neurectomy |
| carcin | cancer | carcinogen | onc | tumor | oncology |
| caud | tail | caudate | ophthal | eye | ophthalmologist |
| ceph(al) | head | encephalitis | os | mouth | ostium |
| chol | bile, gall bladder | cholesterol | os, osteo | bone | osteitis |
| chondr | cartilage | chondroplasia | oto | ear | otitis |
| chrom | color | chromogen | path | disease | pathogen |
| cran | skull | craniotomy | phleb | vein | phlebitis |
| cut | skin | subcutaneous | phob | fear | phobia |
| cyan | blue | cyanosis | phot | light | photometer |
| cyst | bladder, bag | cystocele | pneum | air | pneumonitis |
| cyt(o) | cell | monocyte | pod | foot | pseudopod |
| dactyl | finger | arachnodactyly | pulm | lung | pulmonary |
| dent, dont | tooth | orthodontist | ren | kidney | adrenal |
| derm | skin | dermatitis | rhin | nose | rhinoplasty |
| edema | swelling | edematous | scler | hard | sclerosis |
| erythro | red | erythrocyte | sep | poison | septic |
| febr | fever | afebrile | soma(t) | body | somatic |
| gastro(o) | stomach | gastritis | sperm | seed | spermatogenesis |
| genito | reproductive | genital | stoma | mouth, opening | stomatitis |
| gloss | tongue | glossitis | thorac | chest | thoracotomy |
| hem(a), haem | blood | hematology | tome | knife | microtome |
| hepat(o) | liver | hepatitis | tox(ic) | poison | toxicology |
| histo | tissue | histology | ur(o), uria | urine | hematuria |
| hystero | uterus | hysterectomy | vas | vessel | intravascular |
| iatro | physician | podiatrist | ven | vein | intravenous |

**Table 1-10.** Selected suffixes commonly used in medical terminology

| SUFFIX | DEFINITION | EXAMPLE OF USAGE | SUFFIX | DEFINITION | EXAMPLE OF USAGE |
|---|---|---|---|---|---|
| algia | pain | neuralgia | osis | state, condition, | |
| blast | primitive, germ | erythroblast | | increase | leukocytosis |
| centesis | puncture, aspiration | amniocentesis | ostomy | create an opening | ileostomy |
| cide | death, killer | bacteriocide | otomy | cut into | phlebotomy |
| ectomy | excision, cut out | gastrectomy | opathy, | | |
| emesis | vomiting | hematemesis | pathia | disease | adenopathy |
| emia | in the, or of the, blood | bilirubinemia | penia | lack of | leukopenia |
| genic | origin, producing | pyogenic | phil | affinity for, liking | eosinophil |
| ia | state, condition | anuria | phyte | plant | dermatophyte |
| iasis | process, condition | amebiasis | plastic, plasia | to form or mold | hyperplasia |
| iole | small | bronchiole | poiesis | to make | hemopoiesis |
| itis | inflammation | pharyngitis | rrhage | excessive flow | hemorrhage |
| lysis | free, breaking down | hemolysis | rrhea | flow | diarrhea |
| oid | resembling, similar to | blastoid | scope, scopy | view | arthroscope |
| (o)logy | study of | pathology | stasis | same, standing still | hemostasis |
| oma | tumor | hepatoma | troph(y) | nourishment | hypertrophy |

**Table 1-11.** Abbreviations commonly used in medical laboratories

| | | | |
|---|---|---|---|
| A | absorbance | GC | gonococcus, gonorrhea |
| Ab | antibody | GGT | gamma glutamyl transferase |
| ACT | activated clotting time | GI | gastrointestinal |
| AFB | acid-fast bacillus | GTT | glucose tolerance test |
| Ag | antigen | GU | genitourinary |
| AIDS | acquired immunodeficiency syndrome | HAV | Hepatitis A virus |
| ALL | acute lymphocytic leukemia | Hb, Hgb | hemoglobin |
| ALP, AP | alkaline phosphatase | HBV | Hepatitis B virus |
| ALT | alanine aminotransferase (formerly SGPT) | hCG | human chorionic gonadotropin |
| AML | acute myelogenous leukemia | HCl | hydrochloric acid |
| APTT | activated partial thromboplastin time | $HCO_3^-$ | bicarbonate |
| ARC | AIDS-related complex | Hct | hematocrit |
| AST | aspartate aminotransferase (formerly SGOT) | HCV | hepatitis C virus |
| bacti | bacteriology | HDL Chol | high-density lipoprotein cholesterol |
| BBP | blood-borne pathogen | HDN | hemolytic disease of newborn |
| BP | blood pressure | H & H | hemoglobin and hematocrit |
| BT | bleeding time | HIV | human immunodeficiency virus |
| BUN | blood urea nitrogen | $H_2O$ | water |
| C | centigrade, Celsius | HPF | high-power field |
| CBC | complete blood count | HSV | herpes simplex virus |
| cc, ccm | cubic centimeter | ICU | intensive care unit |
| CCU | coronary care unit | IgG | immunoglobulin G |
| CGL | chronic granulocytic leukemia | IgM | immunoglobulin M |
| CK | creatine kinase | IM | infectious mononucleosis |
| Cl | chloride | i.m. | intramuscular |
| CLL | chronic lymphocytic leukemia | ITP | idiopathic thrombocytopenic purpura |
| cm | centimeter | IU | international unit |
| CNS | central nervous system | IV, i.v. | intravenous |
| C & S | culture and sensitivity | K | potassium |
| CO | carbon monoxide | kg | kilogram |
| $CO_2$ | carbon dioxide | L | liter |
| CPK | creatine phosphokinase | LD, LDH | lactate dehydrogenase |
| crit | hematocrit | LDL Chol | low-density lipoprotein cholesterol |
| CSF | cerebrospinal fluid | LPF | low-power field |
| cu mm | cubic millimeter, $mm^3$ | M | molar |
| diff | leukocyte differential | MCH | mean corpuscular hemoglobin |
| EBV | Epstein-Barr virus | MCHC | mean corpuscular hemoglobin concentration |
| EIA | enzyme immunoassay | MCV | mean corpuscular volume |
| ESR | erythrocyte sedimentation rate | μg | microgram |
| E.U. | Ehrlich units | μL, μl | microliter |
| F | Fahrenheit | mEq | milliequivalent |
| FBS | fasting blood sugar | mg | milligram |
| FDP | fibrinogen-degradation products | MI | myocardial infarction |
| FUO | fever of unknown origin | mL, ml | milliliter |
| g, gm | gram | MLT | medical laboratory technician |

## Table 1-11 (Continued). Abbreviations commonly used in medical laboratories

| | | | | |
|---|---|---|---|---|
| mm | millimeter | | RNA | ribonucleic acid |
| mmol | millimole | | RPR | rapid plasma reagin |
| MRI | magnetic resonance imaging | | sed rate | erythrocyte sedimentation rate |
| MT | medical technologist | | SGOT | serum glutamic oxaloacetic transaminase |
| N | normal, normality | | SGPT | serum glutamic-pyruvic transaminase |
| Na | sodium | | S.I. | international units (Le Système International d'Unités) |
| NaCl | sodium chloride | | | |
| nm | nanometer | | SICU | surgical intensive care unit |
| O.D. | optical density | | sp. gr. | specific gravity |
| O & P | ova and parasites | | Staph | *Staphylococcus* |
| OPIM | other potentially infectious material | | stat | immediately |
| PCV | packed-cell volume | | STD | sexually transmitted disease |
| pH | hydrogen ion concentration | | STI | sexually transmitted infection |
| PMN | polymorphonuclear neutrophil | | Strep | *Streptococcus* |
| POCT | point-of-care test | | STS | serological tests for syphilis |
| POL | physician office laboratory | | TIBC | total iron-binding capacity |
| PP | postprandial | | TIA | transient ischemic attack |
| PPE | personal protective equipment | | UA | urinalysis, uric acid |
| PRC | packed red cells | | URI | upper respiratory infection |
| PSA | prostate specific antigen | | UTI | urinary tract infection |
| PT | prothrombin time, pro-time | | μmol | micromole |
| qns | quantity not sufficient | | UV | ultraviolet |
| qs | quantity sufficient | | VD | venereal disease |
| RA | rheumatoid arthritis | | VDRL | Venereal Disease Research Laboratory |
| RBC | red blood cell | | VLDL | very low-density lipoproteins |
| RF | rheumatoid factors | | WBC | white blood cell |
| RIA | radioimmunoassay | | XDP | fibrin degradation products |

## LESSON REVIEW

1. Why is it important for health care workers to understand medical terminology?
2. What languages are the basis for most medical terms?
3. How can one learn to correctly pronounce medical terms?
4. Name the stems for cell, heart, head, skin, chest, kidney, muscle, liver, and stomach.
5. Name ten common suffixes and give a meaning for each.
6. Name ten common prefixes and give a meaning for each.
7. List ten abbreviations frequently used in the medical laboratory and give the meaning of each.
8. Define prefix, stem, suffix, and terminology.

## STUDENT ACTIVITIES

1. Reread the lesson on medical terminology.
2. Review the glossary terms.
3. Practice pronouncing the word parts and medical terms in Tables 1-8 through 1-10. Look up pronunciations of ten terms from each table and practice saying them out loud.
4. Study the definitions for prefixes, suffixes, and stems listed in the tables.
5. Use each of the prefixes, suffixes or stems in a word not on the list.
6. Study the abbreviations listed in Table 1-11.
7. Look up the definitions of the examples of medical terms listed in Tables 1-8 and 1-9.

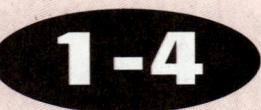
# The Metric System

## LESSON OBJECTIVES

**After studying this lesson, you should be able to:**

- *Discuss the importance of properly using metric units.*
- *Name common prefixes used to denote small and large metric units.*
- *Convert English units to metric units.*
- *Convert metric units to English units.*
- *Convert units within the metric system.*
- *Perform measurements of distance, volume, and weight using the metric system.*
- *Define the glossary terms.*

## GLOSSARY

**centi** / prefix used to indicate one-hundredth of a unit; $10^{-2}$

**gram (g)** / basic metric unit of weight or mass

**kilo** / prefix used to indicate one thousand units; $10^{3}$

**liter (L)** / basic metric unit of volume

**meter (m)** / basic metric unit of length or distance

**micro** / prefix used to indicate one-millionth of a unit; $10^{-6}$

**milli** / prefix used to indicate one-thousandth of a unit; $10^{-3}$

**nano** / prefix used to indicate one-billionth of a unit; $10^{-9}$

**SI units** / standardized units of measure; international units

## INTRODUCTION

Units of measurement are used frequently in medicine. They are used to measure vital statistics such as height, weight, and temperature; the amount of fluid intake and output; and dosages of medication. In the laboratory, measurements are used to indicate numbers of cells or quantities of substances in a patient's blood, serum, or other body fluids. These measurements are then compared to reference (normal) values and the patient's condition is assessed. The results may be used to help establish a diagnosis and prescribe therapy. Therefore, it is important to make all measurements correctly and accurately.

## THE METRIC SYSTEM

The metric system of measurement is used internationally for scientific work. In most countries, the metric system is also used in everyday life. Gasoline is purchased by the liter, body weight is measured in kilograms, and distance is expressed in meters or kilometers.

In the United States, although use of the metric system is increasing, the English system of measurement is still used for most measurements and observations made in everyday life. Weight is reported in pounds, and height in feet and inches. Cooks use measures such as teaspoon, cup, and pint. Speed is measured in miles per hour.

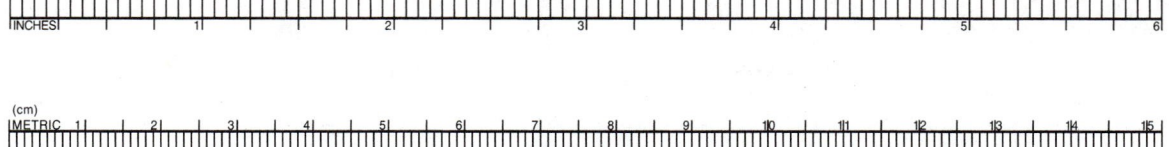

**FIGURE 1-4** Comparison of nonmetric (top) and metric (bottom) rulers

The English system of measurement is not accurate enough for most scientific measurements. The metric system, however, because it is a decimal system, can be used to measure very small quantities accurately and easily (Figure 1-4).

The International System of Units (SI) is the modern, expanded version of the metric system, based on seven fundamental units (Table 1-12). These units have internationally agreed-upon values and were selected because they allow precise, reproducible measurements. The health sciences have been slow to adopt the use of **SI units** in place of some of the more common metric units, but that is beginning to change. In the United States, the National Bureau of Standards sets units of measurement by law. Science students must know and be able to use the metric system and SI units in laboratory observations and measurements.

## TYPES OF MEASUREMENTS

Measurements that are commonly made in the laboratory include the:

- concentration of a substance
- weight of a substance or object
- volume of a solution or object
- size or length of an object
- temperature
- time

The concentrations of substances and weights, volumes, and sizes of objects can be most accurately measured using the metric system. Temperature is measured using the Fahrenheit or the Celsius scale. Laboratory time can be recorded in military time (24-hour clock) or using a 12-hour clock (AM/PM).

## UNITS OF THE METRIC SYSTEM

The metric system is based on a fundamental unit of distance, the **meter (m)**. In the metric system, the **gram (g)** is the basic unit used to measure mass or weight, and the **liter (L)** is the basic unit used to measure volume.

The metric system uses decimal notations and the units are divided into increments of ten. This means that units larger or smaller than the basic units (meter, liter, and gram) can be obtained by multiplying or dividing by increments of ten (or by a power of ten).

## Terminology

Prefixes are added to the terms used for basic metric units to indicate larger or smaller units (Table 1-13). For example, **kilo** means 1000. Therefore, a *kilometer* (km) is 1000 meters or $10^3$ meter, a *kilogram* (kg) is 1000 grams, and a *kiloliter* (kL) is 1000 liters. Although "kilo" is the prefix most commonly used for large units, "deca" may be used to indicate the unit times ten, as in decaliter. Or, "hecto" may indicate the unit times one hundred. The prefixes and their definitions are the same for the three basic units.

In laboratory analyses, it is more common to measure units smaller than the basic units. Table 1-13 lists the prefixes and the multiples of the basic unit that each represents. Two common prefixes are **milli**, which means one-thousandth (.001 or $10^{-3}$), and **centi**, which means one-hundredth (.01 or $10^{-2}$). A *milliliter* is .001 liter, or $10^{-3}$ liter. In chemistry, solutions may be made by adding *milligrams* (mg) of substances to milliliters (mL) of solvent. Substances such as glucose may

**Table 1-12.** The seven basic SI units of measurement

| PROPERTY | UNIT NAME | ABBREVIATION |
|---|---|---|
| Length | meter | m |
| Mass | kilogram | kg |
| Time | second | s |
| Electric current | ampere | A |
| Temperature | Kelvin | K |
| Luminous intensity | candela | cd |
| Quantity of substance | mole | mol |

**Table 1-13.** Commonly used prefixes in the metric system

| ABBREVIATION | PREFIX | MEANING | MULTIPLE OF BASIC UNIT | WEIGHT GRAM (G) | LENGTH METER (M) | VOLUME LITER (L) |
|---|---|---|---|---|---|---|
| k | kilo | 1000 | $10^3$ | kg | km | kL |
| h | hecto | 100 | $10^2$ | hg* | hm* | hL* |
| da | deca | 10 | $10^1$ | dag* | dam* | daL* |
| d | deci | .1 | $10^{-1}$ | dg* | dm* | dL |
| c | centi | .01 | $10^{-2}$ | cg* | cm | cL* |
| m | milli | .001 | $10^{-3}$ | mg | mm | mL |
| μ | micro | .000001 | $10^{-6}$ | μg | μm | μL |
| n | nano | | $10^{-9}$ | ng | nm | nL* |
| p | pico | | $10^{-12}$ | pg | pm* | pL* |

*Units not commonly used in the laboratory

be measured in mg per 100 mL (mg % or mg per deciliter) of serum. In hematology, blood cells are counted per microliter or liter of blood.

Other prefixes commonly used to denote size are **micro**, which denotes one-millionth or $10^{-6}$, and **nano**, which is $10^{-9}$. (See Table 1-13 for abbreviations and prefixes.) Small samples are measured in microliters (μL), which is $10^{-6}$ liter. Wavelengths of light are measured in nanometers (nm), or $10^{-9}$ meter.

## Converting English Units to Metric Units

It may be necessary to convert units within the metric system or to convert English units to metric or metric units to English. For this reason, it is helpful to have a general idea of the metric equivalents of commonly used English measures. Some of these equivalents are listed in Tables 1-14 and 1-15. To convert units from one system to another, simply multiply by the factor listed. For example, since one inch is equal to 2.54 centimeters (cm), twelve inches would equal 12 x 2.54, or 30.48 cm (Table 1-14). To convert metric units to English units, use Table 1-15 in the same manner. Since one kg equals 2.2 pounds, the weight in pounds of a patient weighing 70 kg may be determined by multiplying 70 x 2.2 to equal 154 pounds.

## Converting Units Within the Metric System

In laboratory work, it is more common to need to convert units within the metric system. To make these conversions, the worker needs to know equivalents, such

**Table 1-14.** Conversion of English units to metric units

| | ENGLISH UNIT | ENGLISH ABBREVIATION | | MULTIPLY BY | TO GET METRIC UNIT | METRIC ABBREVIATION |
|---|---|---|---|---|---|---|
| **Distance** | 1 mile | mi | = | 1.6 | kilometers | km |
| | 1 yard | yd | = | 0.9 | meters | m |
| | 1 inch | in | = | 2.54 | centimeters | cm |
| **Mass** | 1 pound | lb | = | 0.454 | kilograms | kg |
| | 1 pound | lb | = | 454 | grams | g |
| | 1 ounce | oz | = | 28 | grams | g |
| **Volume** | 1 quart | qt | = | 0.95 | liters | L |
| | 1 fluid ounce | fl oz | = | 30 | milliliters | mL |
| | 1 teaspoon | tsp | = | 5 | milliliters | mL |

**Table 1-15.** Conversion of metric units to English units

| | METRIC UNIT | METRIC ABBREVIATION | | MULTIPLY BY | TO FIND ENGLISH UNIT | ENGLISH ABBREVIATION |
|---|---|---|---|---|---|---|
| **Distance** | 1 kilometer | km | = | 0.6 | miles | mi |
| | 1 meter | m | = | 3.3 | feet | ft |
| | 1 meter | m | = | 39.37 | inches | in |
| | 1 centimeter | cm | = | 0.4 | inches | in |
| | 1 millimeter | mm | = | .04 | inches | in |
| **Mass** | 1 gram | g | = | .0022 | pounds | lb |
| | 1 kilogram | kg | = | 2.2 | pounds | lb |
| **Volume** | 1 liter | L | = | 1.06 | quarts | qt |
| | 1 milliliter | mL | = | .03 | fluid ounces | fl oz |

as how many milliliters or microliters are in a liter, or how many milligrams are in a gram. These conversions can be made by using the information in Table 1-16.

### Converting to Larger Units

To convert metric units to larger units, such as grams to kilograms or milliliters to liters, the decimal in the original unit is moved to the left for the appropriate number of spaces. Examples: To convert 50 g to kg, multiply by .001, or move the decimal to the left three places: 50 g = .050 kg. To convert centimeters to meters, multiply by .01, or move the decimal two places to the left: 160 cm = 1.6 meters.

### Converting to Smaller Units

To convert metric units to smaller units, such as g to mg or liters to microliters, the decimal in the number is moved to the right the appropriate number of spaces.

**Table 1-16.** Common metric equivalents

| **Mass** | $10^{-3}$ kg | = 1 gram | = $10^3$ mg | = $10^6$ µg |
|---|---|---|---|---|
| | $10^{-3}$ g | = 1 mg | = $10^3$ µg | = $10^6$ ng |
| | $10^{-9}$ g | = 1 ng | = $10^3$ pg | |
| **Volume** | $10^{-3}$ kL | = 1 liter | = $10^3$ mL | = $10^6$ µL |
| | $10^{-3}$ L | = 1 mL | = $10^3$ µL | = $10^6$ nL |
| | $10^{-1}$ L | = 1 dL | = $10^2$ mL | |
| **Length** | $10^{-3}$ km | = 1 meter | = $10^3$ mm | = $10^6$ µm |
| | $10^{-3}$ m | = 1 mm | = $10^3$ µm | = $10^6$ nm |
| | $10^{-2}$ m | = 1 cm | = 10 mm | = $10^4$ µm |
| | $10^{-3}$ mm | = 1 nm | = 10 Å | |

Example: To convert 5 g to mg, multiply by 1000, or move the decimal to the right three places: 5 g = 5000 mg. Scientific notation is often used to make the numbers less bulky and easier to compute. For example, five grams equals 5,000,000 µg or $5.0 \times 10^6$ µg.

## INTERNATIONAL SYSTEM OF UNITS: SI UNITS

Even though the metric system is used internationally for laboratory measurements, the method of reporting results differs from country to country or even within countries. This can be confusing when trying to compare laboratory data. For example, the concentration of protein may be expressed as g/L in some laboratories or g/dL in others.

An effort is being made to standardize the reporting of laboratory values by using **SI units** or the international system of units, Tables 1-17 and 1-18. For example, blood cell counts have traditionally been expressed as the number of cells per cubic millimeter (cu mm) of blood. In the SI system, however, cell counts are expressed as number of cells per liter of blood. Chemical substances such as bilirubin or glucose, which were expressed as mg per deciliter (dL) or per 100 mL, are now expressed as mg or g per liter, or as micromoles (µmol) or millimoles (mmol) per liter.

Units of measurement must be included when reporting all laboratory results. For example, a glucose test result reported as 5.6 would cause great concern to a physician accustomed to blood glucose measurements in mg/dL. Normal blood glucose should be 70-100 mg/dL and 5.6 would be dangerously low (a critical value). However, in laboratories where blood glucose is measured in mmol/liter, 5.6 would be a normal finding.

**Table 1-17.** SI equivalents recommended for use in reporting laboratory results

| COMMON USAGE | SI EQUIVALENT |
|---|---|
| micron (μ) | micrometer (μm; $10^{-6}$ meter) |
| cubic micron (μ³) | femtoliter (fl; $10^{-15}$ liter) |
| micromicrogram (μμg) | picogram (pg; $10^{-12}$ gram) |
| microgram (mcg) | microgram (μg; $10^{-6}$ gram) |
| angstrom (Å) | nm x $10^{-1}$ |
| millimicron (mμ) | nanometer (nm; $10^{-9}$ meter) |
| lambda (λ) | microliter (μL; $10^{-6}$ liter) |

**Table 1-18.** Examples of using SI units in reporting laboratory test results

| TEST | OLD UNIT | SI UNIT |
|---|---|---|
| Cell counts | cells/mm³ or cells/cu mm | cells/μL or cells/liter |
| Hematocrit | % (ex: 41%) | percentage expressed as decimal (ex: 0.41) |
| Hemoglobin | g/dL | g/liter |
| MCV | μ³ | fl |
| MCH | μμg | pg |
| MCHC | % | g/dL (or g/L) |

The National Committee for Clinical Laboratory Standards (NCCLS) has published guidelines defining terminology for uniform reporting of clinical laboratory results. (The address for NCCLS is given in Appendix A.)

## Common Equivalents

To standardize reporting, some metric units previously in common laboratory use are being phased out. Since these units are still used by some laboratories and appear in older books or manuals, it is important to understand the equivalents of these units (Table 1-17). A milliliter (mL) may also be called a cc (cubic centimeter), especially when referring to dosages. A cubic centimeter may be written as cc, cu cm, or cm³. A microliter (μL), which is one-thousandth of a mL, was formerly called a cubic millimeter (cu mm or mm³). Micron is the old term referring to micrometer. Lambda (λ) is the term previously used both for microliter and for wavelength of light; nanometer is now used for wavelength.

## TEMPERATURE MEASUREMENTS

In the United States, the Celsius scale is used for most scientific temperature measurements, while the Fahrenheit scale is used for cooking and for measuring body temperature and weather conditions. Most other countries use the Celsius scale for measuring temperatures in everyday life, as well as for scientific laboratory measurements such as temperatures of reactions, incubation, and boiling points. The formulas for converting from one temperature scale to another are discussed in Lesson 6-3, Laboratory Math and Reagent Preparation.

## LESSON REVIEW

1. What is the basic metric unit of distance or length?
2. What is the basic metric unit of volume?
3. What is the basic metric unit of weight?
4. What are the meanings of centi, deca, hecto, and deci?
5. Why is the metric system preferred over the English system for scientific measurements?
6. Convert the following English measurements to metric units:

   3 inches = _____ cm or _____ mm
   5 qt = _____ liters or _____ mL
   64 oz = _____ g or _____ kg or _____ mg
7. Convert the following units:

   12 mg = _____ μg or _____ g
   50 mL = _____ μL or _____ cc or _____ dL
8. Define centi, gram, kilo, liter, meter, micro, milli, nano, and SI units.

## STUDENT ACTIVITIES

1. Reread the information on the metric system.
2. Review the glossary terms.
3. Practice measuring metric volumes, lengths, and weights and converting metric units using the worksheets.

## *Worksheet—Distance*

### **LESSON 1-4** The Metric System

Name _____   Date _____

Obtain a meter stick or metric ruler and an English ruler from the instructor.  Use the information in Tables 1-13 through 1-17 to answer the questions below.

1. Look at the meter stick. Locate the cm and mm divisions. How many centimeters are in a meter? _____
   How many mm in a cm? _____  How many mm in a meter? _____

2. Draw the indicated length of line beside each number, beginning at the dot.

   35 mm     .

   6 cm     .

   83 mm     .

   1.2 dm     .

3. Measure the lines above using a ruler marked in English units (inches):

   35 mm     =     _____ inches

   6 cm     =     _____ inches

   83 mm     =     _____ inches

   1.2 dm     =     _____ inches

   Which of the measurements (English or metric) do you feel is the most accurate? _____

4. How many mm in one inch? _____  one mm = _____ inch

   How many cm in one inch? _____  one cm = _____ inch

   Convert the following units:

   4 inches     =     _____ cm

   0.5 inches     =     _____ cm

   38 cm     =     _____ inches

   7 cm     =     _____ inches

   3.5 inches     =     _____ mm

   35 mm     =     _____ inches

5. How many inches are in a meter? _____  What English unit of measurement is closest in size to the meter? _____

6. Measure your height or the height of another student using the meter stick.  What is the height in cm? _____
   in meters? _____ Convert the height in cm to inches: _____ Now measure the height in inches and compare the results.

## *Worksheet—Weight*

### **LESSON 1-4** The Metric System

Name _____   Date _____

Use Tables 1-13 through 1-17 to answer the questions below.

1. What is the basic metric unit of weight? _____

2. How many mg in a g? _____ How many μg in a g? _____ How many g in a kg? _____

3. Convert the following units:

    300 mg    =    _____ g   =   _____ kg

    50 mg     =    _____ g   =   _____ kg

    4000 mg   =    _____ g   =   _____ kg

    200 μg    =    _____ g

    750 μg    =    _____ mg

    80 g      =    _____ kg

    What decimal rule did you follow to make the conversions? _____

    _____

4. Convert the following units:

    0.4 kg    =    _____ mg   =   _____ μg

    9.2 kg    =    _____ mg   =   _____ μg

    0.6 g     =    _____ μg

    10 mg     =    _____ μg   =   _____ pg

    280 mg    =    _____ μg   =   _____ pg

    What decimal rule did you follow to make the conversions? _____

    _____

5. Weigh yourself or another student.  What is the weight in g?    _____ in kg? _____

6. A man who weighs 165 pounds would weigh _____ kg.

7. A child who weighs 32 pounds would weigh _____ kg or _____ g.

8. Is a man who is 178 cm tall and weighs 135 kg overweight, underweight, or of normal weight? _____

9. If scales are available, weigh a container, add 10 mL of water, and weigh again.  How much does the water weigh? _____ Does one milliliter of water weigh approximately 1 gram? Yes _____   No _____

## *Worksheet—Volume*

## **LESSON 1-4** The Metric System

Name _____    Date _____

Obtain a medicine cup, a 50 mL graduated cylinder, and a 50 mL beaker from the instructor.  Use Tables 1-13 through 1-17 to answer the questions below.

1. What is the basic unit of volume in the metric system? _____

2. How many mL in a liter? _____ dL in a liter? _____ μL in a liter? _____

3. Convert the following units:

   45 cc      =      _____ liter  =  _____ mL

   550 mL     =      _____ liter

   4 dL       =      _____ liter

   60 μL      =      _____ liter  =  _____ mL

   0.1 dL     =      _____ liter

   6,700 mL   =      _____ liter

   What decimal rule did you follow to make the conversions? _____
   _____

4. Convert the following units:

   0.3 liter  =      _____ dL   =  _____ mL

   5 liters   =      _____ mL

   7 mL       =      _____ μL

   3 dL       =      _____ mL   =  _____ μL

   0.1 dL     =      _____ mL

   What decimal rule did you follow to make the conversions? _____
   _____

5. What English unit is closest in volume to the liter? _____

6. Convert the following English units:

   3.5 pints  =      _____ mL = _____ L

   3 quarts   =      _____ mL = _____ L

   5 fl. oz.  =      _____ mL = _____ L

7. If gasoline is $1.20 per gallon at station A and 30 cents a liter at station B, which has the cheapest gasoline?
   _____

8. Fill the medicine cup to the one fl oz mark with water.  Transfer the water to a 50 mL graduated cylinder.  How many milliliters of water are in one fl oz? _____

   Fill the medicine cup again with water and transfer the one fl oz to a 50 mL beaker.  Which gives the most accurate measurement, the beaker or the graduated cylinder? _____

# Laboratory Safety: Physical and Chemical Hazards

## LESSON OBJECTIVES

After studying this lesson, you should be able to:

- Describe the evolution of the Occupational Safety and Health Administration (OSHA) safety laws.
- Explain the "right to know" provisions of OSHA.
- Explain why safety rules must be observed.
- List three classifications of laboratory hazards.
- Give two examples of physical hazards and ways to prevent or correct each one.
- Give two examples of chemical hazards and ways to prevent or correct each one.
- Explain what should be done if an accident occurs in the laboratory.
- Describe proper laboratory apparel.
- State sixteen basic rules for laboratory safety.
- Define the glossary terms.

## GLOSSARY

**acquired immunodeficiency syndrome (AIDS)** / a form of immune deficiency induced by infection with human immunodeficiency virus (HIV)

**autoclave** / an instrument that uses pressurized steam for sterilization

**carcinogen** / a substance with the potential to produce cancer in humans or animals

**caustic** / a substance that burns or destroys skin and flesh; capable of destroying tissue

**corrosive** / a chemical agent, such as an acid, that has the ability to gradually destroy a material

**fume hood** / a device that draws contaminated air out of an area and either cleanses and recirculates it, or discharges it to the outside

**human immunodeficiency virus (HIV)** / a retrovirus that has been identified as the cause of AIDS

**material safety data sheet (MSDS)** / safety information that must be supplied by manufacturers of hazardous materials

**mutagen** / a substance with the potential to make a stable change in a gene, that is then passed on to offspring

**OSHA** / Occupational Safety and Health Administration; the federal agency that monitors the Occupational Safety and Health Act of 1971

## INTRODUCTION

Safety is a topic that should be foremost in the thoughts and actions of all health care providers, both employees and employers. The goal of health care workers should be to provide quality patient care in an environment that is safe for both workers and patients. Safety has become not just a humanitarian issue, but also a legal necessity. Increased emphasis on safety in the health care setting has come about largely because **acquired immunodeficiency syndrome (AIDS)** is contracted through contact with blood or body fluids infected with **human immunodeficiency virus (HIV)**. (See Lesson 1-6).

## THE OCCUPATIONAL SAFETY AND HEALTH ADMINISTRATION

Although laws to protect workers from biohazards have been enacted in recent years, rules to protect against physical and chemical hazards have existed for more than two decades. In 1970, Congress enacted the Occupational Safety and Health Act, which states that workers have the "right to know" about hazardous conditions present in their workplace. The Occupational Safety and Health Administration (**OSHA**) was given the power to establish rules and enforce the Act.

### Hazard Communication Rule

OSHA issued a rule to further protect workers from hazardous chemical exposure in 1983. This rule was called "Hazard Communication" and applied only to the manufacturing industry. On August 24, 1987, however, the rule was expanded to include the nonmanufacturing sector. The law places the burden on the employer to keep workers informed and protected by providing safety training, proper apparel, and a safe work environment.

## HAZARDS IN THE CLINICAL LABORATORY

Workers in the clinical laboratory may encounter three types of hazards: physical, chemical, and biological. This lesson identifies some of the physical and chemical hazards that may be present in the clinical laboratory. The lesson also outlines safety practices mandatory for safe and legal operation of a clinical laboratory. Safety procedures primarily concerned with biological hazards are addressed in Lesson 1-6.

### Physical Hazards

Physical hazards are present in ordinary equipment or surroundings. Electrical equipment, open flames, laboratory instruments, and glassware can all be hazardous if improperly used.

### Electricity

Electricity is one major source of physical hazard. All electrical equipment must be properly grounded, following the manufacturer's instructions and according to electrical codes. Even minor repairs, such as replacement of microscope light bulbs, require that the instrument be disconnected from the power supply before the work is begun. All electrical cords and plugs must be kept in good repair, with no frayed cords or exposed wires. Overloaded circuits must be avoided; they are always a potential fire hazard and can also cause equipment damage (Figure 1-5). Extension cords present several safety hazards and should not be used except in an emergency.

### Fire

Fire is another potential danger in the workplace. Fortunately, fires in the laboratory are not common and those that do occur are usually minor. Most occur where open flames, such as Bunsen burners, are in use. When open flames are in use, care must be taken to ensure that loose clothing and long hair do not catch on fire. Whenever possible, laboratory hotplates, microwave ovens, electric incinerators, and slide warmers should be used instead of open flames.

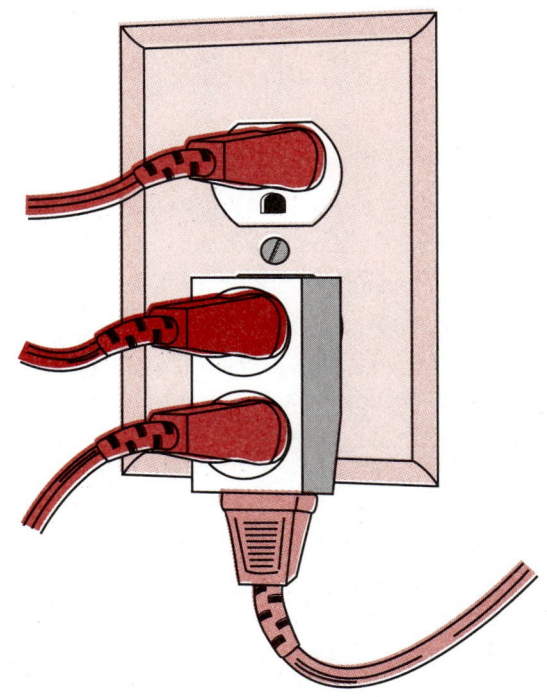

**FIGURE 1-5**   Example of an overloaded electrical circuit

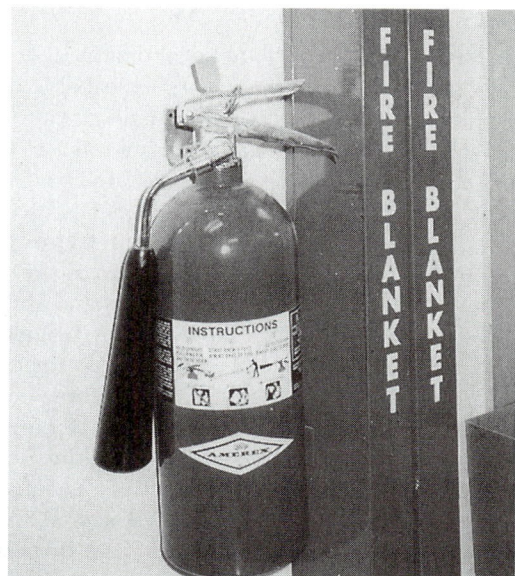

**FIGURE 1-6A** Fire extinguisher and fire blanket

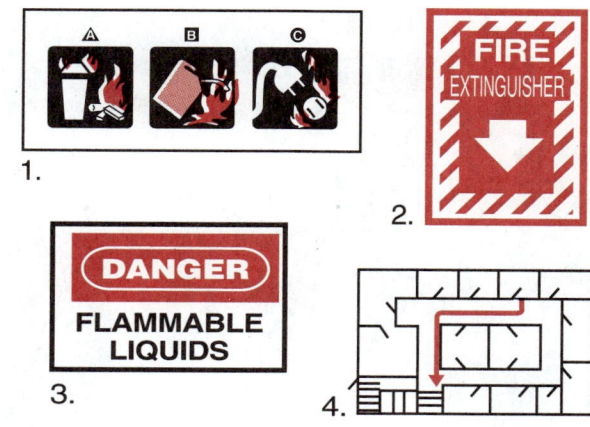

**FIGURE 1-6B** Examples of fire safety signs: (1) extinguishers for different kinds of fires, (2) fire extinguisher locator, (3) flammable liquids warning, and (4) fire escape route

Flammable chemicals should be stored in a flameproof cabinet, away from heat sources and in a well-ventilated area. A flameproof cabinet can protect flammable chemicals from flames until firefighters arrive and also allows workers more time to escape.

The correct type of fire extinguisher must be readily available. A fire blanket should be accessible in case clothing ignites. (Figure 1-6A).

Fire drills should be held frequently. Laboratory workers must know the escape route and the procedure to follow if that exit is blocked. All workers should know the locations of fire extinguishers and how to use them. Fire extinguishers must be inspected periodically and the date of inspection recorded (Figure 1-6B).

## Laboratory Equipment

Laboratory equipment must be used only as the manufacturers' instructions dictate. Any instrument that has moving parts, such as a centrifuge, must be operated with a special regard for safety. The centrifuge lid must always be latched before the instrument is turned on. When the centrifuge is turned off, the lid should not be opened until the rotor has come to a complete stop.

**Autoclaves,** which use pressurized steam to sterilize surgical instruments, glassware, and other materials, present special hazards. Manufacturers' instructions should be followed carefully to prevent explosions and burns. Insulated gloves should be worn when removing hot items from the autoclave. Lesson 1-8 contains additional information on laboratory equipment.

### Glassware

Glassware is a routine item in most laboratories, but it can cause injuries. Only glassware that is free of chips and cracks should be used. Damaged glassware is weakened and may break, resulting in injury. Broken glass should be cleaned up with a brush and dustpan, not with bare hands. Glass should not be discarded into regular trashcans, but into rigid cardboard or plastic containers specially made for this purpose (Figure 1-7). Wherever possible, plasticware should replace glass containers in the laboratory.

## Chemical Hazards

Chemicals present a variety of hazards. Chemicals may be flammable, toxic, caustic, corrosive, carcinogenic, or mutagenic. Occasionally, laboratory procedures use radioisotopes that present the hazard of potential exposure to radioactivity.

Chemicals must be labeled with hazard information. Figures 1-8A and B illustrate two different systems for identifying chemical hazards. Manufacturers are now required by law to put hazard information labels on chemical containers and to provide **Material Safety Data Sheets (MSDS)** for every potentially hazardous chemical. This information describes the hazard(s) of the chemical, the personal protective equipment required, and the body organs that could be adversely affected following exposure to the chemical. Additional information is included for first aid and further medical treatment. These MSDS papers must be kept on file in the laboratory where every employee has access to them.

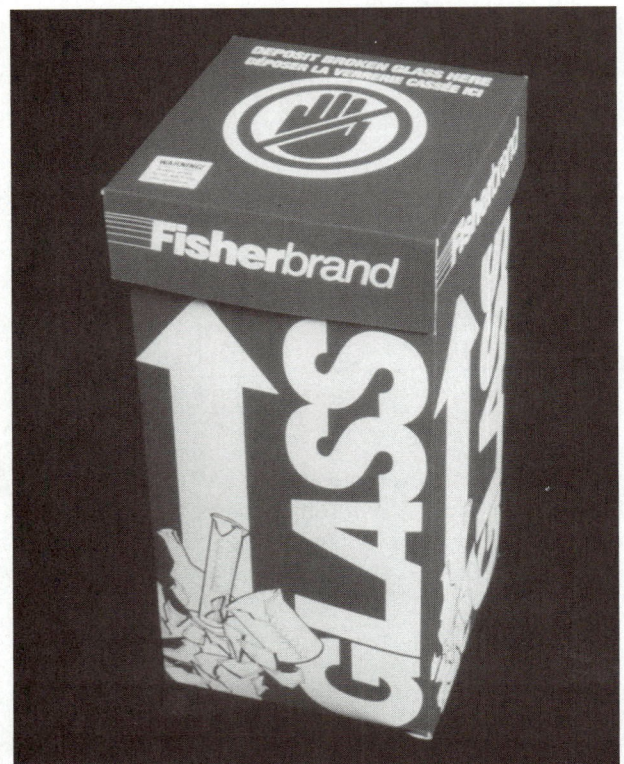

**FIGURE 1-7** Disposal box for broken glass (Photo courtesy of Fisher Scientific)

## Caustic Chemicals

Some of the chemicals used in the laboratory are **caustic**, meaning they are strong acids or bases capable of causing severe skin burns (Figure 1-9). Fumes or vapors from these chemicals can burn mucous membranes in the respiratory system. Potassium hydroxide (KOH), sodium hydroxide (NaOH), sulfuric acid ($H_2SO_4$), nitric acid ($HNO_3$), and concentrated sodium hypochlorite (concentrated bleach) are examples of caustic chemicals. These chemicals can give off fumes and should be used in a fume hood if one is available. Goggles or a face shield, gloves, and a protective apron should be worn to protect against injury from splashes and spills when working with such strong chemicals (Figure 1-10).

Any chemicals that do contact the skin should be washed off immediately with water for at least five minutes unless the container label says otherwise. A safety shower should be available in case large quantities of chemicals are spilled on a worker (Figure 1-11). An eyewash station must be accessible for workers who have chemicals splashed into their eyes (Figure 1-12).

## Toxic Chemicals

Some laboratory chemicals are toxic or poisonous either through skin contact or by respiratory exposure. When using these chemicals, the worker must follow

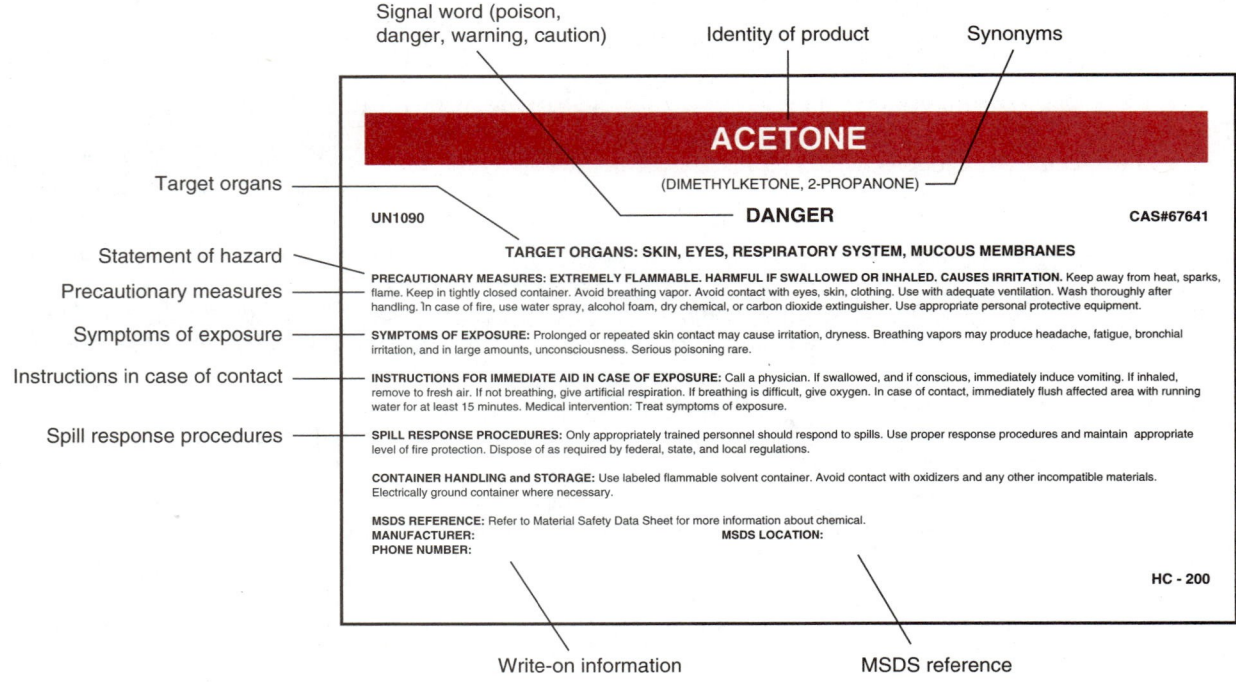

**FIGURE 1-8A** Example of hazard information on chemical labels

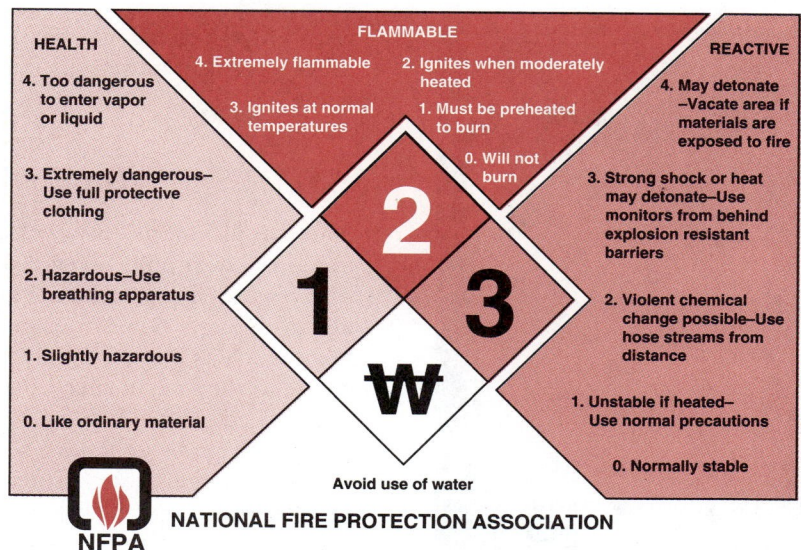

**FIGURE 1-8B** Example of hazard information on chemical labels

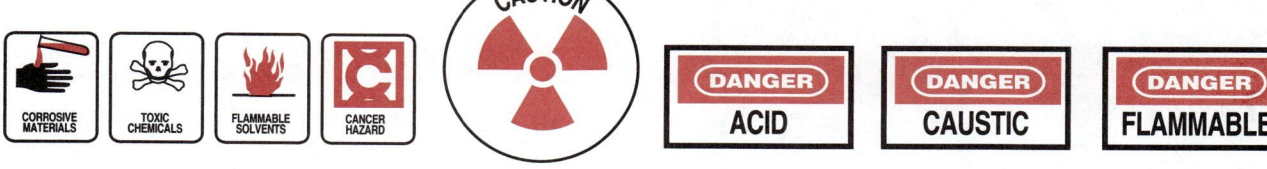

**FIGURE 1-9** Examples of symbols for chemical hazards

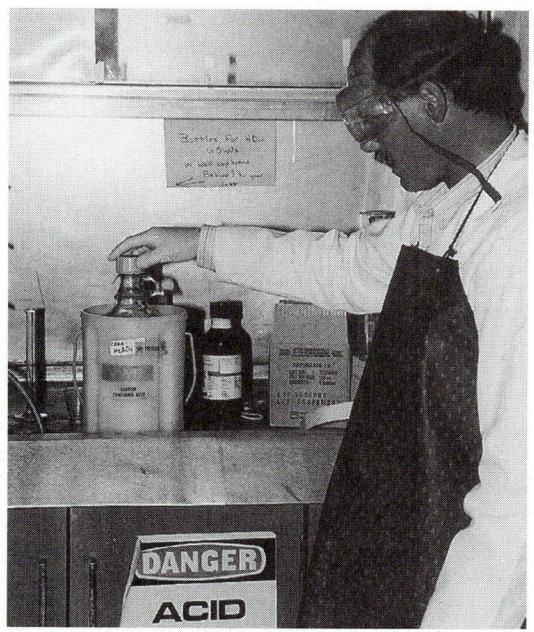

**FIGURE 1-10** Laboratory worker using a fume hood and wearing gloves, goggles, and apron (From Marshall, *Fundamental Skills for the Clinical Laboratory Professional*, p. 26)

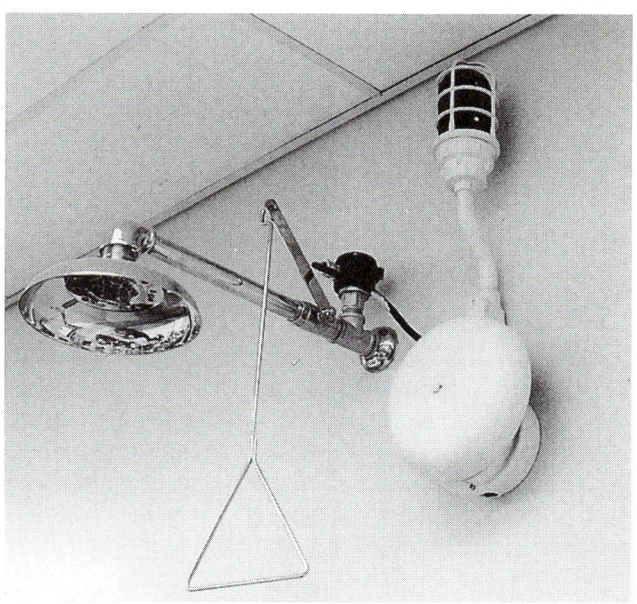

**FIGURE 1-11** Safety shower (From Marshall, *Fundamental Skills for the Clinical Laboratory Professional*, p. 25)

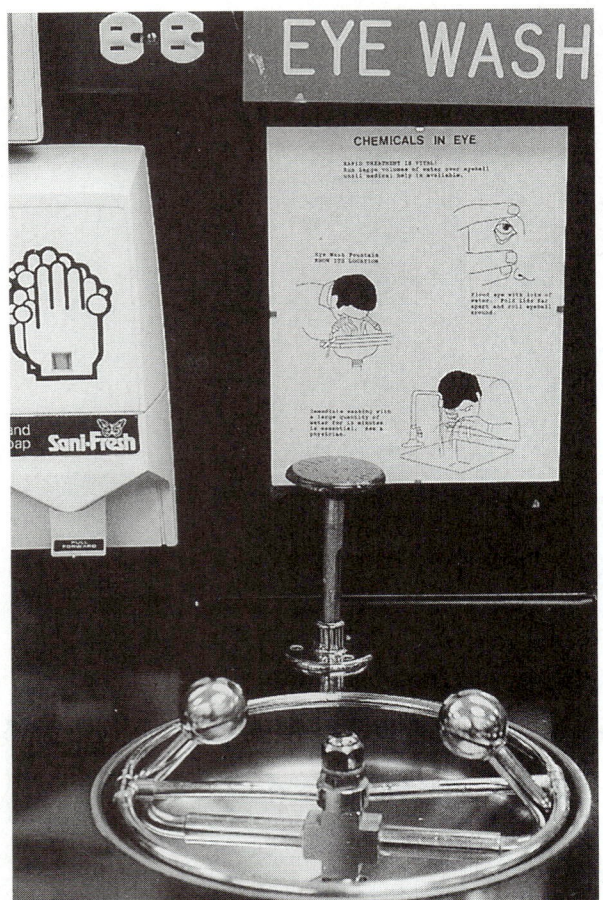

**FIGURE 1-12** Eyewash station (From Marshall, *Fundamental Skills for the Clinical Laboratory Professional*, p. 24)

safety precautions. Gloves and protective rubber or vinyl sleeves can be used to protect skin from contact. If a chemical produces harmful fumes, it should be used only in a **fume hood**, a special cabinet that draws the fumes away from the worker (see Figure 1-10).

### Carcinogens and Mutagens

Few **carcinogens** (cancer-causing substances) or **mutagens**, (substances that can cause birth defects) are used in the routine clinical laboratory. However, it is always wise to avoid direct skin contact or breathing dust containing any chemicals. Females of childbearing age should avoid exposure to mutagens such as radioisotopes (radioactive chemicals) (see Figure 1-9). Although some laboratory procedures continue to use radioisotopes for certain assays, many of these procedures have been replaced by newer and safer methods. Gloves and appropriate shields must be used when handling radioisotopes. Workers must complete special

radiation safety training before working with radioisotopes. Disposal must be according to state and federal guidelines.

## SAFE STORAGE OF CHEMICALS

Flammable liquids, concentrated acids, and concentrated bases should be stored in proper containers in safe places. Special cabinets are available for safe storage of different types of hazardous chemicals. Personal items, such as purses, should not be kept in the storage space, as they might cause a container to be overturned or knocked off the shelf.

In the past, chemicals were stored in alphabetical order to make them easier to locate. This storage method sometimes places incompatible chemicals near each other. This can be avoided by using a reliable safety guide to plan the storage of chemicals. Manufacturer color-coding of chemical container labels to indicate proper storage makes this task easier. Examples of a few incompatible chemicals are shown in Table 1-19.

## DISPOSAL OF CHEMICAL WASTES

All chemicals and reagents should be disposed of properly and according to regulations. A few laboratory chemicals can safely be poured down the drain, followed by large amounts of water to dilute them. However, many chemicals, especially those that contain heavy metals such as mercury, lead, or chromium, require special disposal by toxic waste personnel. Therefore, it is very important that the laboratory supervisor or instructor provides explicit instructions for disposal.

## LABORATORY APPAREL

Laboratory personnel must wear proper clothing when working in the laboratory. This may include a uniform, along with a buttoned, knee-length, and fluid-resistant laboratory coat to protect skin and clothing from spills and splashes of chemicals, stains, or biohazardous material. A rubberized, or other special type of apron, may be worn to protect against strong acids (Figure 1-10). If splashes are likely to occur, protective eyewear such as laboratory safety goggles must be worn (Figure 1-10, Table 1-20). Gloves made of the proper material must be worn when hazardous chemicals are handled. For example, latex gloves should not be worn when working with strong chemicals; latex allows the chemicals to penetrate to the skin. Many scientific supply catalogs contain charts to aid in selecting proper gloves.

Loose jewelry, such as long chains and bracelets, should not be worn since it may get caught in moving equipment and cause serious injury. In addition, metal

**Table 1-19.** Examples of some incompatible chemicals

| This chemical | should not be stored next to any of these: |
|---|---|
| Acetic acid | Hydroxides (NaOH, KOH), nitric acid |
| Acetone | Concentrated sulfuric or nitric acids |
| Flammable liquids | Chromic acid, hydrogen peroxide, nitric acid |
| Sodium azide | Copper (in plumbing drains) |

This is a partial listing; for details, consult a safety handbook and the labels on the chemical containers

jewelry can contact electrical parts in equipment and cause injury or death by electrical shock. Shoes should be comfortable and stable and should have closed toes to protect against spills or sharp objects. Long hair should be pulled back to prevent contact with open flames or with moving equipment parts.

## TEACHER/SUPERVISOR RESPONSIBILITY

In addition to the federal laws of 1970, 1983, and 1987, many states have enacted safety codes. These laws are designed to ensure that employers provide safe work environments. It is the responsibility of the teacher, supervisor, or employer to provide the student or worker with proper orientation and training in safety procedures. This training should be documented before the student or employee performs any work in the laboratory.

The Occupational Safety and Health Administration (OSHA) monitors adherence to the Occupational Safety and Health Act. OSHA inspectors may arrive unannounced to examine the safety conditions in a

workplace. Any failures to meet OSHA requirements are noted and fines are imposed for the infractions; the fines are levied on the managers or owners of the facility.

The laboratory procedure manual must contain safety guidelines. The manual's location must be posted so anyone can find it. The manual should include standard operating procedures (SOP); regulations for the safe handling, storage, and disposal of chemicals; and strategies to follow in case of fire. It should also provide general laboratory safety rules and guidelines for employee safety training.

Students or workers must be provided with safety equipment to protect against identified hazards in the laboratory. They must be trained to use the equipment properly. The teacher or supervisor must monitor the students or workers for adherence to the regulations. The students or workers must also comply with the laboratory's regulations.

## RESOURCES FOR SAFETY INFORMATION

Official OSHA guidelines must always be consulted to ensure the laboratory is in compliance. A copy of OSHA guidelines can be found in the *Federal Register*, available in the local library, by library loan, or on various websites. In addition, state universities or state public health laboratories often have a safety consultant who will give advice by phone or send printed information. Additional sources of information are listed in Appendix A.

### Documentation of Safety Training

Training on Hazard Communication and using safety equipment must be documented. Forms for safety training agreements can be purchased or made on the computer. When workers or students have completed the training session, they must sign the agreement which

**Table 1-20.** Measures to protect against physical and chemical hazards in the laboratory

| HAZARD | PROTECTIVE MEASURES |
|---|---|
| Spills and splashes on the skin | Wear laboratory coat, apron, gloves |
| Strong acids | Wear rubberized apron, proper gloves |
| Splashes into eyes | Use faceshield and/or ANSI* approved goggles |
| Toxic fumes | Use chemical fume hood |
| Electrical shock | Unplug equipment before repairs |

*American National Standard Institute

states that they received the training and understood the issues raised in the training. (An example of a Safety Agreement Form is included in Lesson 1-6, Figure 1-13.) Periodic continuing education reinforces the importance of safety. Each employee must receive a refresher safety training session once a year.

## GENERAL LABORATORY RULES

Despite certain safety hazards, the clinical laboratory can be a safe work environment. Each worker must be responsible, use safe work habits, and observe all safety rules.

No set of safety rules can cover every situation that might arise. Also, nothing can replace the use of good common sense when working with laboratory equipment and chemicals. Several general principles, however, should always be observed:

1. Refrain from horseplay.
2. Do not eat, drink, chew gum, or apply cosmetics in the work area.
3. Wear a laboratory apron, or buttoned laboratory coat, and closed-toe shoes.
4. Pin long hair up to prevent contact with chemicals, equipment, or flames.
5. Do not wear chains, bracelets, rings, or other loose jewelry.
6. Use gloves when handling hazardous chemicals and biological specimens.
7. Clean and disinfect the work area before and after laboratory procedures and at any other time as appropriate.
8. Wash hands before and after any laboratory procedures, after removing gloves, and at any other time as appropriate.
9. Wear safety glasses, goggles, or a faceshield or use a countertop acrylic shield when working with strong chemicals and whenever splashes are possible.
10. Wipe up spills promptly, using the appropriate procedure for the type of spill.
11. Use an appropriate mask or respirator when working with chemicals or other materials that give off dust or fumes.
12. Follow manufacturers' instructions for operating all equipment. Handle all equipment with care and store properly.
13. Report any broken or frayed electrical cords, exposed electrical wires, or damage to equipment.
14. Do not use bare hands to pick up broken glass. Use a broom or brush and a dustpan. Discard into special containers for broken glass.

15. Do not allow visitors into the work area of the laboratory unless they are properly attired and have been instructed in patient confidentiality issues and safety precautions.
16. Report any accident immediately to the supervisor.

## LESSON REVIEW

1. What are the three classifications of laboratory hazards?
2. Give two examples of physical hazards and tell how each might be avoided or corrected.
3. Give two examples of chemical hazards and tell how each might be avoided or corrected.
4. Why is it important to conduct frequent fire drills?
5. Why must safety rules be strictly observed?
6. What should be done if an accident occurs in the laboratory?
7. What type of clothing should laboratory workers wear?
8. State sixteen general laboratory safety rules and explain the importance of each.
9. What is the purpose of the safety agreement?
10. What governmental agency is responsible for enforcing safety regulations in the workplace?
11. Define acquired immunodeficiency syndrome, autoclave, carcinogen, caustic, corrosive, fume hood, human immunodeficiency virus, material safety data sheets, mutagen, and OSHA.

## STUDENT ACTIVITIES

1. Reread the information on physical and chemical hazards.
2. Review the glossary terms.
3. Make a poster warning of a laboratory hazard.
4. Use the Safety Worksheet at the end of this lesson to make a safety check of the laboratory. Check for frayed cords, exposed wires, fire extinguisher, safety posters, and posting of fire exit routes. Inspect the chemicals in the laboratory. Are they labeled with appropriate instructions? Note the procedure to follow in case of skin contact or chemical spill.
5. Practice the procedure to follow in case of fire and the use of the fire extinguisher; learn the fire escape route.

## Safety Worksheet

## LESSON 1-5 Laboratory Safety: Physical and Chemical Hazards

Name _____    Date _____

Use the worksheet to make a safety check of the laboratory. For each item listed below, determine if the conditions are satisfactory (safe), **S**, or unsatisfactory (unsafe), **U**. If unsatisfactory, recommend correction(s) in the spaces indicated.

I.  **Safety Check for Physical Hazards**

A.  Examine all electrical instruments (microscopes, spectrophotometers, etc.) for frayed wires and proper storage conditions (storage away from water and harsh chemicals, use of dust covers, etc.). Evaluate conditions and record recommendations for each instrument examined.

| Instrument | S | U | Observation/Recommendation |
|---|---|---|---|
| _____ | _____ | _____ | _____ |
| _____ | _____ | _____ | _____ |
| _____ | _____ | _____ | _____ |
| _____ | _____ | _____ | _____ |

B.  Make a fire safety check of the laboratory.

1.  Are fire extinguishers present?  _____

When was the last inspection date?  _____

Do extinguishers have instructions for their use posted with them?  _____

**Fire extinguishers:  S** _____  **U** _____

2.  Is the fire exit route posted?  _____

Is it up to date?  _____

Walk the fire exit route. Was it easy to follow?  _____

Could all exit doors be opened?  _____

**Fire exit route:    S** _____  **U** _____

Recommendation(s) for improving fire safety: _____

_____

_____

_____

## II. Safety Check for Chemical Hazards

A.  Examine the chemicals in the laboratory.

    1. Are all clearly labeled? _____

    2. Do the labels contain information on storage, disposal, and procedure in case of spills or accidental exposure? _____

    3. Are chemicals labeled "flammable" stored away from fire (Bunsen burners)? _____

    4. Where are concentrated acids and bases stored? _____

    **Chemical storage:  S** _____     **U** _____

B.  Is a fume hood present? _____

    When was it last checked for proper air flow? _____

    **Fume hood:  S** _____     **U** _____

C.  Is an eyewash station present? _____

    Are instructions for its use posted? _____

    **Eyewash station:  S** _____ **U** _____

Recommendation(s) for improving chemical safety: _____

_____

_____

_____

## III.  Laboratory Safety Policy

Inquire about the laboratory's policy regarding employee safety orientation and training.

A. Is a written Hazard Communication Program available in the laboratory? _____

B. Does the laboratory administration follow appropriate "employee right-to-know" policies in the safety orientation and training programs? _____

C. Are written records kept of employee safety training sessions? _____

D. Are all employees asked to sign safety agreement forms after safety training? _____

E. Is the location of the laboratory procedure manual posted? _____

    Does the manual contain safety guidelines and procedures? _____

F. Are MSDS sheets on file for all chemicals? _____

    Laboratory safety policy: **S** _____     **U** _____

Recommendation(s) for improving laboratory safety policy: _____

_____

_____

_____

# Laboratory Safety: Biological Hazards

## LESSON OBJECTIVES

**After studying this lesson, you should be able to:**

- *Explain the function of the Occupational Safety and Health Administration (OSHA).*
- *Explain what is meant by Bloodborne Pathogens Standard.*
- *Explain the Standard Precautions issued in 1996.*
- *Explain what is meant by exposure control plan.*
- *List the components of an exposure control plan.*
- *Explain the impact of human immunodeficiency virus (HIV) and hepatitis B virus (HBV) on safety in the health care setting.*
- *List rules that must be observed when handling biological materials.*
- *List additional safety rules necessary in the microbiology laboratory.*
- *Define the glossary terms.*

## GLOSSARY

**aerosol** / liquid in the form of a very fine mist

**alimentary tract** / the digestive tube from the mouth to the anus

**biological safety cabinet** / a special cabinet that provides protection while working with infectious microorganisms

**bloodborne pathogens** / pathogens that may be present in human blood (and blood-contaminated body fluids) that cause disease in humans

**Bloodborne Pathogens (BBP) Standard** / OSHA guidelines for preventing occupational exposure to pathogens present in human blood and body fluids, including, but not limited to, human immunodeficiency virus (HIV) and hepatitis B virus (HBV); final OSHA standard of December 6, 1991, effective March 6, 1992.

**engineering control** / using available technology and equipment to isolate the worker from hazards

**exposure incident** / an accident, such as a needlestick, in which an individual has been exposed to possible infection through contact with body substances from another individual; especially refers to bloodborne pathogens.

**hepatitis B virus (HBV)** / a virus that causes hepatitis and is transmitted by contact with infected blood or other body fluids

**hepatitis C virus (HCV)** / a virus that causes hepatitis and is transmitted by contact with infected blood or other body fluids

**OPIM** / Other Potentially Infectious Materials; any and all body fluids, tissues, organs, or other specimens from a human source

**parenteral** / any route other than the alimentary canal; intravenous, subcutaneous, intramuscular, or mucosal

**pathogenic** / capable of causing damage or injury to the host

**personal protective equipment (PPE)** / specialized clothing or equipment used by workers to protect themselves from direct exposure to blood or other potentially hazardous materials; includes, but is not limited to, gloves, laboratory apparel, eye protection, and breathing apparatus

**Standard Precautions** / a set of CDC safety procedures designed to protect patients and healthcare workers from infectious agents

**Universal Precautions** / a method of infection control in which all human blood and other body substances are treated as if known to be infectious

**work practice controls** / methods of performing tasks to reduce the worker's exposure to blood and other potentially hazardous materials

## INTRODUCTION

Safety in the clinical laboratory used to involve avoiding acid splashes onto the skin or into the eyes and avoiding fire hazards or the breathing of toxic fumes. However, with the appearance of HIV and AIDS, along with the recent increase in **hepatitis B** and **hepatitis C** infections, health care workers must be especially cautious of biological hazards as well. Many tasks formerly performed without a second thought may now require lengthy preparation and specialized safety equipment.

## THE OCCUPATIONAL SAFETY AND HEALTH ADMINISTRATION

The United States Department of Labor, the government agency charged with attending to matters that concern American workers, has developed several regulations for workers' protection. In 1970, the Department created the Occupational Safety and Health Administration (OSHA) to enforce the rules of the Occupational Safety and Health Act (OSH Act). The early regulations were concerned with preventing hazards such as falls, electrical shock, and chemical exposure.

## THE BLOODBORNE PATHOGENS STANDARD

On December 6, 1991, OSHA issued the final Standard on Occupational Exposure to Bloodborne Pathogens, which became effective on March 6, 1992. The **Bloodborne Pathogens Standard** outlines the requirements for protecting workers who may be exposed to human blood or other potentially infectious materials (**OPIM**). The standard covers employees in *all* health care facilities, as well as all other workers who may be exposed to blood or other potentially infectious material. These employees include, but are not limited to, laboratory workers, nurses, physicians, phlebotomists, and even some housekeeping and laundry employees (Table 1-21). The comprehensive standard contains several directives employers must follow. These directives are contained in each institution's exposure control plan.

## STANDARD PRECAUTIONS

**Standard Precautions** are a set of guidelines for healthcare workers developed by CDC in 1996 as an extension of the OSHA Bloodborne Pathogen (BBP) Standard. The use of Standard Precautions intensifies safety practices by requiring that every patient and every body fluid be regarded as potentially infected with bloodborne pathogens. This is important because, in addition to HIV, other bloodborne viruses such as hepatitis B and C can cause severe disease. The BBP Standard was expanded to control hospital infections, protect the patient, and protect the healthcare worker. The safety practices that must be followed using the Standard Precautions guidelines are explained in Figure 1-13. Healthcare facilities must implement Standard Precautions and insist that all workers comply with them.

**Table 1-21.** Examples of workers who may be at risk for exposure to bloodborne pathogens*

| | |
|---|---|
| Physicians | Dentists and other dental workers |
| Nurses | Laboratory and blood bank technologists |
| Pathologists | Medical technologists |
| Phlebotomists | Research laboratory scientists |
| Dialysis personnel | Emergency medical technicians |
| Some laundry workers | Funeral service personnel (morticians) |
| Medical examiners | Some maintenance personnel |
| Paramedics | Some housekeeping personnel |

*Exclusion of a job title here does not denote lack of risk.

## THE EXPOSURE CONTROL PLAN

Each employer is required to develop an **Exposure Control Plan** (infection control plan) to identify all employees with occupational exposure to human blood or OPIM. A training program must be set up to inform employees of the hazards and the training must be documented. The employer is required to update and document the training yearly. In addition, instructors may wish to develop a safety agreement form for students. An example is shown in Figure 1-14.

The exposure control guidelines deal with safe handling of specimens, contaminated sharps, contaminated laundry, and regulated waste. OSHA guidelines must be followed when the plan is written. In addition, a copy of the Bloodborne Pathogens Standard must be included in the exposure control plan. Each employee must have access to the plan; for example, a copy should be placed at each nursing station, in the laboratory, and in the housekeeping office.

The employer must provide free HBV vaccine to workers at risk and confidential medical evaluation after an **exposure incident**. The employee must have access to personal protective equipment appropriate for his or her task. Warning labels and signs must be used to identify hazards (Figure 1-15). The Exposure Control Plan should describe the control methods used to comply with the BPP standard provisions.

### STANDARD PRECAUTIONS FOR INFECTION CONTROL

**Wash Hands** (Plain soap)
Wash after touching **blood, body fluids, secretions, excretions,** and **contaminated items.** Wash immediately **after gloves are removed** and **between patient contacts.** Avoid transfer of microorganisms to other patients or environments.

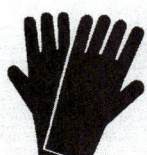

**Wear Gloves**
Wear when touching **blood, body fluids, secretions, excretions,** and **contaminated items.** Put on **clean** gloves just **before touching mucous membranes** and **nonintact skin.** Change gloves between tasks and procedures on the same patient after contact with material that may contain high concentrations of microorganisms. Remove gloves promptly after use, before touching noncontaminated items and environmental surfaces, and before going to another patient, and wash hands immediately to avoid transfer of microorganisms to other patients or environments.

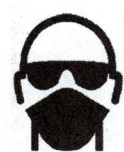

**Wear Mask and Eye Protection or Face Shield**
Protect mucous membranes of the eyes, nose and mouth during procedures and patient-care activities that are likely to generate **splashes** or **sprays** of **blood, body fluids, secretions,** or **excretions.**

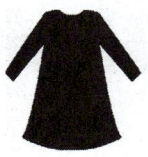

**Wear Gown**
Protect skin and prevent soiling of clothing during procedures that are likely to generate **splashes** or **sprays** of **blood, body fluids, secretions,** or **excretions.** Remove a soiled gown as promptly as possible and wash hands to avoid transfer of microorganisms to other patients or environments.

**Patient-Care Equipment**
Handle used patient-care equipment soiled with **blood, body fluids, secretions,** or **excretions** in a manner that prevents skin and mucous membrane exposures, contamination of clothing, and transfer of microorganisms to other patients and environments. Ensure that reusable equipment is not used for the care of another patient until it has been appropriately cleaned and reprocessed and single use items are properly discarded.

**FIGURE 1-13** Guide to Standard Precautions for Infection Control, issued by the CDC in 1996. (Courtesy of Brevis Corp.)

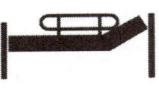

**Environmental Control**
Follow hospital procedures for routine care, cleaning, and disinfection of environmental surfaces, beds, bedrails, bedside equipment and other frequently touched surfaces.

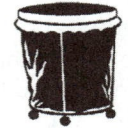

**Linen**
Handle, transport, and process used linen soiled with **blood, body fluids, secretions,** or **excretions** in a manner that prevents exposures and contamination of clothing, and avoids transfer of microorganisms to other patients and environments.

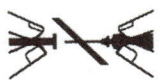

**Occupational Health and Bloodborne Pathogens**
Prevent injuries when using needles, scalpels, and other sharp instruments or devices; when handling sharp instruments after procedures; when cleaning used instruments; and when disposing of used needles.

**Never recap used needles using both hands** or any other technique that involves directing the point of a needle toward any part of the body; rather, use either a one-handed "scoop" technique or a mechanical device designed for holding the needle sheath.

Do not remove used needles from disposable syringes by hand, and do not bend, break, or otherwise manipulate used needles by hand. Place used disposable syringes and needles, scalpel blades, and other sharp items in puncture-resistant sharps containers located as close as practical to the area in which the items were used, and place reusable syringes and needles in a puncture-resistant container for transport to the reprocessing area.

**Use resuscitation devices** as an alternative to mouth-to-mouth resuscitation.

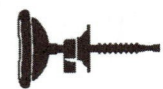

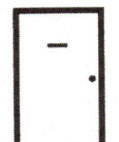

**Patient Placement**
Use a **private room** for a patient who contaminates the environment or who does not (or cannot be expected to) assist in maintaining appropriate hygiene or environmental control. Consult Infection Control if a private room is not available.

**FIGURE 1-13 (Continued)** Guide to Standard Precautions for Infection Control, issued by the CDC in 1996. (Courtesy Brevis Corp.)

---

### SAFETY AGREEMENT FORM

Please initial the items below:

____ I agree to follow all set rules and regulations as required by the instructor or supervisor.

____ I have been informed about and received training concerning the OSHA Hazard Communication.

____ I have been informed of the location of the Hazard Communication Plan and the MSDS folder.

____ I have been informed about and received training concerning the OSHA Bloodborne Pathogens Standard and Standard Precautions.

____ I understand that biological specimens and blood or blood products are potentially infectious for hepatitis viruses and the AIDS virus.

____ I understand that even though diagnostic products and reagents are screened for HIV antibodies and hepatitis B surface antigen (HBsAg), no known test can offer 100% assurance that products derived from human blood will not transmit disease.

Student Name (Please Print) _____
Student Signature _____ Date _____
Parent Signature _____ Date _____
(if student is under 18)

**FIGURE 1-14** Example of a safety agreement form

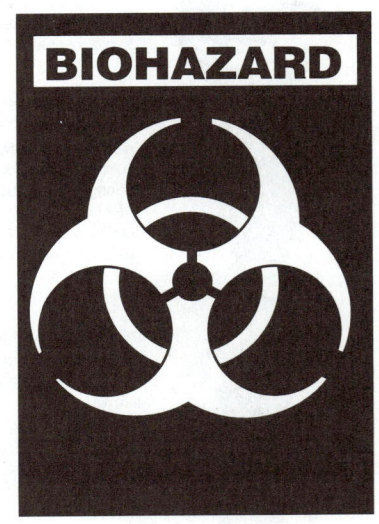

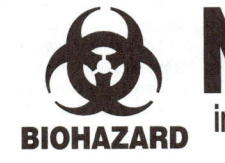

**FIGURE 1-15** Biohazard warning labels

**Table 1-22.** Examples of substances that have been recognized by the CDC as directly linked to transmission of pathogens such as HBV and HIV

| | |
|---|---|
| Blood | Synovial fluid |
| Blood products | Vaginal secretions |
| Semen | Pleural fluid |
| Peritoneal fluid | Pericardial fluid |
| Amniotic fluid | Concentrated HBV viruses |
| Cerebrospinal fluid | Concentrated HIV viruses |
| Urine | Unfixed tissue specimens |
| Organs | |
| Saliva in dental settings where bleeding occurs | |

## Identifying Employees at Risk

The written plan must identify employees who have occupational risk of exposure to blood or other potentially infectious materials (OPIM). Under this plan, workers such as laboratory technicians, nurses, and phlebotomists are not the only employees who require training. Dentists, dental technicians, dialysis personnel, some housekeeping and laundry workers, and others may all be at risk (Table 1-21).

"Blood" refers to human blood, human blood components (platelets or red cells for transfusion), and products made from human blood. Occupational exposure means "reasonably anticipated" contact with blood or other potentially infectious materials (Table 1-22). This contact may occur to the eyes, skin, mucous membranes, or through **parenteral** routes (routes other than the **alimentary tract**). An example of parenteral contact would be a stick with a needle.

## Control Methods

Control methods consist of all the components determined essential for a task to be completed safely for both the patient and the employee. These components include Universal Precautions, engineering controls, work practice controls, and personal protective equipment (Table 1-23).

### Universal Precautions

**Universal Precautions** refer to a method of infection control in which *all* human blood and other potentially infectious biological materials are treated as if known to be infected with HIV or HBV. Universal Precautions and Standard Precautions must be used *every time* a worker has contact with a specimen, even if the specimen is from a friend or a co-worker.

### Engineering Controls

**Engineering controls** are devices and technology used to isolate the worker from hazards. An example of such a device is the use of an acrylic benchtop shield to protect the worker from aerosols when a tube of blood is being uncapped (Figure 1-16A). Biohazard containers, appropriate surface and hand disinfectants, and puncture-resistant sharps containers are also engineering controls (Figure 1-16B).

### Work Practice Controls

**Work practice controls** refer to the manner in which the task is performed. These practices are actually just good, safe work habits. The use of these controls should reduce the likelihood of a worker being exposed to hazards. Examples of work practice controls include handwashing after glove removal or anytime hands are contaminated. Other examples include removal and disposal of personal protective equipment when leaving a work area or upon completion of a task, and never recapping needles (Figure 1-17).

### Personal Protective Equipment

**Personal protective equipment (PPE)** is specialized apparel, devices, or equipment used by workers to protect themselves from direct exposure to potentially infectious materials. This includes, but is not limited to, gloves, fluid-resistant gowns, face shields or masks, goggles, and safety glasses (Figure 1-18).

**Table 1-23.** Control methods required as part of an exposure control plan

| | |
|---|---|
| Universal/Standard Precautions | Treating all patients, unfixed tissue, and organ specimens as infectious |
| Engineering controls | Devices that eliminate or minimize worker exposure |
| Work practice controls | Alterations in the manner in which a task is performed to reduce the likelihood of exposure |
| Personal protective equipment | Specialized clothing or equipment used by workers to protect them from direct exposure to blood and other substances |

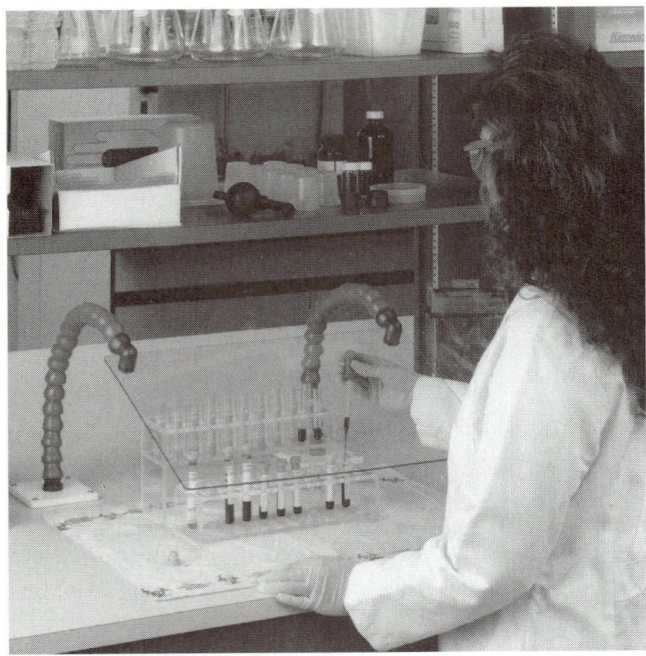

(A)

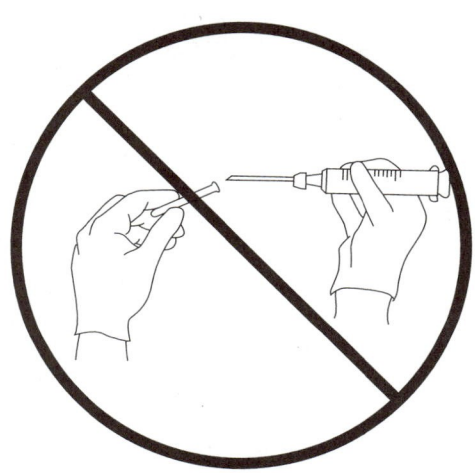

**FIGURE 1-17** Work practice control: needles must not be recapped after use

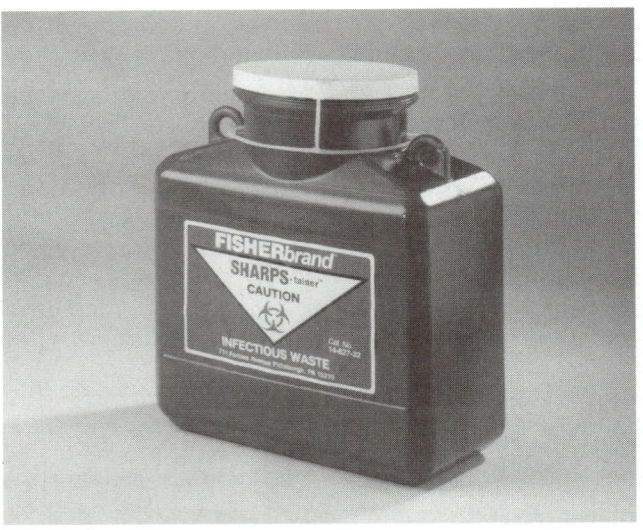

(B)

**FIGURE 1-16** (A) Engineering controls: acrylic safety shield placed between worker and biological specimens (B) Container for disposal of contaminated sharps (Top photo courtesy of ISOLAB, Inc.; bottom photo courtesy of Fisher Scientific)

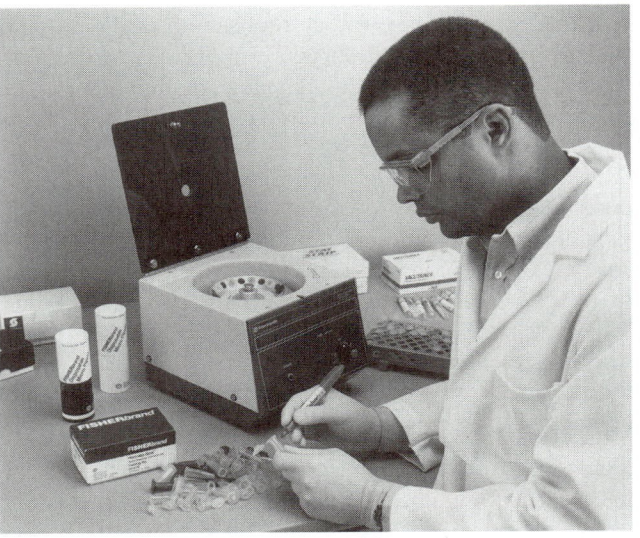

**FIGURE 1-18** Laboratory professional wearing personal protective equipment, including gloves, laboratory coat, and protective eyewear (Photo courtesy of Fisher Scientific)

## EXAMPLE OF AN EXPOSURE CONTROL PLAN

Implementation of an exposure control plan in the daily routine of the laboratory worker is not as difficult as it may seem. The example in Table 1-24 illustrates how a worker or student would use the plan while performing a venipuncture on a patient.

## ☣ BIOLOGICAL HAZARDS OTHER THAN BLOODBORNE PATHOGENS

Clinical laboratory workers are exposed to other biological hazards in addition to **bloodborne pathogens**. Clinical microbiology laboratory specimens may contain a variety of **pathogenic** microorganisms. Patient

**Table 1-24.** Example of using exposure control methods for protecting against biohazards while performing a venipuncture

| CONTROL METHOD | MECHANISM |
| --- | --- |
| Universal/Standard Precautions | Treat all patients and all specimens as infectious |
| Engineering controls | Use containers for contaminated sharps, containers for biohazardous waste, biohazard containers for contaminated reusable apparel, biohazard containers for disposable apparel, appropriate surface disinfectants |
| Work practice controls | Always wear gloves when working with blood; never recap, cut, or break needles; use a commercial device to remove needles from syringes or vacuum tube holders; immediately dispose of contaminated sharps; wash hands with hand disinfectant after removing gloves or any other time hands are contaminated |
| Personal protective equipment | Wear gloves to handle blood and body fluids; wear fluid-resistant gown or lab coat; wear eye protection if splashes are reasonably anticipated |

samples may contain bacteria, viruses, fungi, or parasites. Students or workers in the laboratory must know how to protect themselves from these hazards.

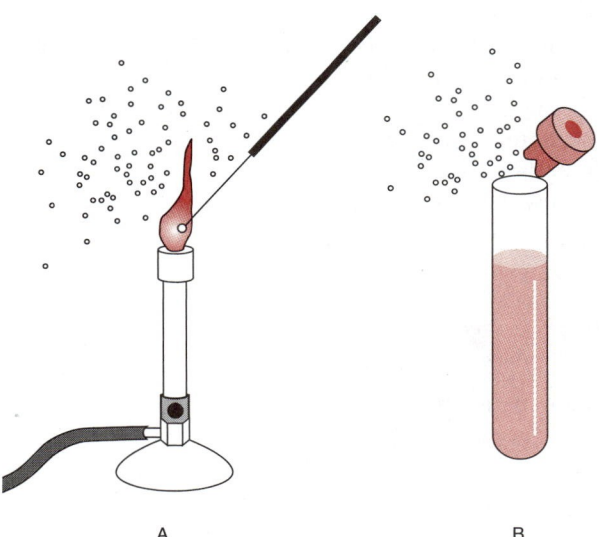

**FIGURE 1-19** Work practice control: use care to avoid the formation of aerosols when (A) sterilizing a bacteriological loop and (B) removing the cap from a tube of liquid.

## Microbiology Hazards

Workers in the microbiology laboratory can protect themselves by following the guidelines for bloodborne pathogens and Standard Precautions; however, they need to observe some additional rules. Accidents in the microbiology laboratory that can expose the worker to risk include spills of culture material, cuts on fingers and hands, and formation of **aerosols**, fine mists that can form anytime a cap is removed from a tube of liquid or when a bacteriological loop is sterilized in a flame (Figure 1-19). Culture tubes should be carried in a test tube rack to help avoid spills.

Many procedures in microbiology must be performed in a **biological safety cabinet** (Figure 1-20). Positive air pressure in the cabinet keeps infectious materials inside the cabinet. Air inside the cabinet is drawn away from the worker, into a vent or special filter. A Class II biological safety cabinet is the type most commonly used in medical laboratories.

To prevent infection from a patient's bacteriological specimen, gloves must be worn when working with the sample and hands must be washed with a disinfectant soap after the gloves are removed. When a task has been completed, work surfaces must be wiped with a disinfectant, such as a 10% solution of household (chlorine) bleach. Examples of measures that can be taken to protect workers from biological hazards are illustrated in Table 1-25.

**Table 1-25.** Measures to protect against biological hazards in the laboratory

| HAZARD | PROTECTIVE MEASURES |
|---|---|
| Blood or blood products | Wear gloves and a buttoned, fluid-resistant laboratory coat |
| Pathogenic microorganisms | Wear gloves and lab coat; use biological safety cabinet |
| Dangerous aerosols | Place acrylic benchtop shield between worker and tubes when removing stoppers; wear mask, goggles, or faceshield when pouring urine into sink |
| Contaminated work surfaces | Wipe with 10% solution of bleach (or other surface disinfectant) before and after all procedures and any other appropriate time |
| Needlesticks | Use self-sheathing needles or quick-release holders; never recap, bend, break, or cut used needles |

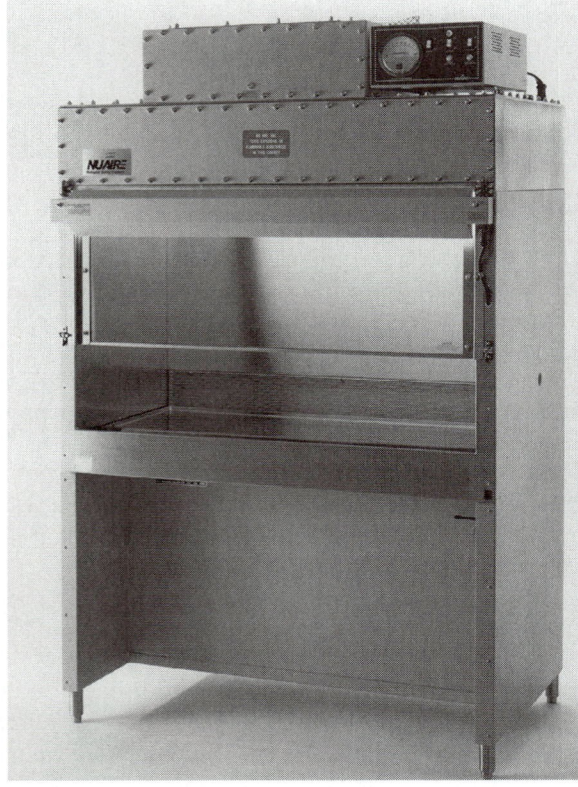

**FIGURE 1-20** Biological safety cabinet (Photo courtesy of NUAIRE)

## LESSON REVIEW

1. Why have biological safety rules become more stringent in recent years?
2. Explain the reason for the Bloodborne Pathogens Standard.

3. What is the function of the Occupational Safety and Health Administration?
4. What is meant by "exposure control plan" or "infection control plan?"
5. List the components of an exposure control plan.
6. What is meant by the terms "Universal Precautions" and "Standard Precautions?"
7. What additional safety rules and equipment are used in the microbiology laboratory?
8. What class of biological safety cabinet is most commonly used in medical laboratories?
9. Define aerosol, alimentary tract, biological safety cabinet, bloodborne pathogens, Bloodborne Pathogens Standard, engineering control, exposure incident, hepatitis B virus, hepatitis C virus, OPIM, parenteral, pathogenic, personal protective equipment, Standard Precautions, Universal Precautions, and work practice controls.

## STUDENT ACTIVITIES

1. Reread the information on biological hazards.
2. Review the glossary terms.
3. Make a poster warning of a biological hazard.
4. Design an exposure control plan for a worker who performs a capillary puncture.
5. Obtain a copy of the *Federal Register* Vol. 56, No. 235, 29 CFR Part 1910.0130 from your local library, or write to the address in the references for OSHA publications.
6. Use the worksheet at the end of this lesson to evaluate the laboratory's biological hazard safety policy.

## *Worksheet*

## **LESSON 1-6** Laboratory Safety: Biological Hazards

Name _____    Date _____

Use this worksheet to make a biological hazard safety check of the laboratory.

## SAFETY CHECK FOR BIOLOGICAL HAZARDS

### I. Examine the laboratory for biological hazards

A. Are safety rules posted? _____

B. Where are blood specimens discarded? _____

C. How are contaminated lab coats or gowns disposed of? _____

D. Where are needles and other sharps discarded? _____

   Is the container puncture-resistant? _____

E. Are all sizes of gloves available for workers? _____

F. Are eye protection devices available? _____

   faceshields _____    goggles _____    safety glasses _____

G. Are fluid-resistant gowns or coats available for tasks that might involve splashes? _____

H. Is a policy in place to require counters to be wiped at certain intervals and after every spill? _____

   Recommendation(s) for improvments: _____

   _____

   _____

   _____

### II. Laboratory Safety Policy

Inquire about the laboratory's policy regarding employee orientation and training in the safe handling of hazardous materials.

A. Does the laboratory have a written Hazard Communication Program? _____

B. Does the laboratory have Standard Precautions included in the exposure control plan? _____

C. Have all employees considered at risk of exposure to bloodborne pathogens been offered the hepatitis B vaccination series at no charge? _____

D. Are written records kept of all employee safety training sessions? _____

   Do employees sign forms acknowledging the training? _____

E. Is safety training updated yearly? _____

   Recommendations or comments concerning the laboratory's safety program: _____

   _____

   _____

   _____

# Quality Assurance in the Laboratory

**After studying this lesson, you should be able to:**

- *Explain the importance of quality assurance in the laboratory.*
- *Explain the importance of quality assurance in POCT.*
- *Discuss the use of standards and controls to ensure quality.*
- *Discuss the role of CLIA '88 in mandating quality.*
- *Explain the difference between accuracy and precision.*
- *Determine the mean value for a set of test results.*
- *Calculate the standard deviation for an analytical method.*
- *Detect a result that is out of control.*
- *Explain how to detect the development of a trend in a method.*
- *Explain coefficient of variation.*
- *Define the glossary terms.*

## GLOSSARY

**accuracy** / a measure of how close a determined value is to the true value

**average** / the sum of a set of values divided by the number of values; the mean

**coefficient of variation** / a calculated value that compares the relative variability between different sets of data

**control serum** / a serum with a known concentration of the same constituents as those being measured in the patient sample

**Gaussian curve** / a graph plotting the distribution of values around the mean; normal frequency curve

**Levey-Jennings chart** / a quality control chart used to record daily quality control values

**mean** / the sum of a set of values divided by the number of values; the average

**population** / the entire group of items or individuals from which the samples under consideration are presumed to have come

**precision** / reproducibility of results; the closeness of obtained values to each other

**random error** / error whose source cannot be definitely identified

**sample** / in statistics, a subgroup of a population

**shift** / an abrupt change from the established mean indicated by the occurrence of all control values on one side of the mean

**standard** / a chemical solution of a known concentration that can be used as a reference or calibration substance

**standard deviation** / a measure of the spread of a population of values around the mean

**statistics** / the science of collecting and classifying data to show their significance

**systematic error** / a variation that may influence results to be consistently higher or lower than the real value

**trend** / an indication of error in the analysis, detected by increasing or decreasing values in the control sample

**Westgard's rules** / a set of rules used to determine when a method is out of control

# INTRODUCTION

Quality control (QC) is an essential part of every laboratory's daily operations. It is often thought to be applicable only to testing procedures. However, a program of Quality Management or Quality Assurance (QA) should be in place to ensure quality throughout the total testing process, from ordering the test to entering the result on the patient's chart. This is called the turnaround time (TAT). Processing the samples in the laboratory, the test procedures, and procedural controls are parts of QC. Total Quality Management (TQM) is one name usually given to a program combining QC with QA. The principles and the statistics involved in QA can become quite complicated. However, the terminology and less complicated applications must be understood and used by all laboratory workers who perform tests.

Quality assurance in clinical laboratories is such an important issue because laboratory results are used to aid in diagnosing, prescribing treatment, and monitoring the progress of patients. Laboratory results must be reliable and the laboratory's QC procedures and results must be documented. Laboratory workers have the ethical and legal responsibility to ensure the work performed in the laboratory is of the highest quality. This can be guaranteed by adherence to a comprehensive quality assurance program.

# QC IN THE CLINICAL LABORATORY

Quality control is a system set up to ensure that certain limits for a test result or product are maintained. Assays of control materials and calibrating instruments are mandatory. In addition, if the laboratory performs non-waived procedures, it must subscribe to an external proficiency testing (PT) program. At regular intervals during the year, the proficiency testing agency sends the laboratory control samples for testing. The laboratory then sends its results to the agency, the values are compared to those the agency obtained in multiple analyses, and a quality assessment report is sent to the laboratory. Instrument maintenance and repair records, comparison of test methods, and reagent preparation are also part of a QC program. The laboratory director must be certain that QC guidelines are followed for compliance with CLIA '88.

Most hospital and larger laboratories have been largely unaffected by CLIA '88 because they were already following strict QC procedures. However, some smaller laboratories and those located in physician offices that may not have performed regular quality control in the past are now required to do so and document the results. The goal of CLIA '88 is to ensure that results from a small laboratory are as reliable as those from a large reference or hospital lab.

## Quality Control in Point-of-Care Testing (POCT)

POCT is regulated by CLIA '88. A large portion of the total laboratory tests performed in the United States are point-of-care tests. The test procedures are performed at point-of-care, often by non-laboratory personnel. *Waived* tests are not subject to the rigorous quality control programs required for more complex tests. However, it is required that the manufacturer's instructions for the instrument are kept on file and that their recommendations, including control procedures, are followed consistently.

Many POCT procedures are *moderately complex* and are subject to more stringent QC. Personnel performing the tests must be highly trained and their training must be documented. In addition, proficiency testing must be done and quality control records kept. The manufacturer's instructions are not sufficient for performing the tests; the procedure for each test must be written in a procedure manual.

A new subcategory under CLIA '88, in which the manufacturer must demonstrate that nonlaboratory personnel can perform an analysis accurately and precisely, is being considered. The new category, *accurate and precise technology (APT)*, would include most POCT procedures.

## Standards and Control Sera

To validate results generated in a laboratory, all analytical instruments must be calibrated and controls must be run with each set of patient samples. Calibration can be accomplished either by analyzing solutions of known composition called **standards**, by calibrating electronically, or by using a calibration strip provided by the manufacturer.

### Controls

A **control serum** is a solution that contains the same constituents as those being analyzed in the patient sample. Most laboratories use commercially produced controls made from pooled sera. The manufacturer has already analyzed each lot of serum for a variety of components; the expected range of assay values for each component is included when the controls are shipped to the laboratory. A single control serum might contain all the constituents on a certain chemistry profile and therefore be suitable to include in all the chemistry assays the laboratory performs. If it does not, the laboratory will have to purchase a combination of controls.

The control sera must be analyzed along with patient samples, using the same methods, test conditions, and reagents. At least two levels of controls must be analyzed, a normal value and an abnormal value. These must be run with each set of patient samples, at least once per shift, and any time patients' results seem questionable. Each day's results are used to construct a QC record called a **Levey-Jennings chart** (Figure 1-21). The records of the control assays must be kept for CLIA and

other inspectors. After an instrument has been repaired, the instrument must be recalibrated and controls run.

### Standards

A **standard** is a substance that has an exact known value and that, when accurately weighed or measured, can produce a solution of an exact concentration. Standards are also called reference materials. Standards are usually quite expensive and are not used on a daily basis; they are used to calibrate newly purchased instruments, to recalibrate instruments after repair, at manufacturer's recommended intervals, or if a method is out of control.

##  SAFETY

The laboratory technician can be exposed to blood-borne pathogens while using instrument calibrators and running control sera samples. Many of these samples are of human origin and, although they have been screened for certain pathogens, may be infectious. Standard Precautions must be followed while performing all control procedures, just as when working with patient samples.

## Accuracy and Precision

In any QC discussion, the terms *accuracy* and *precision* must be considered. Although accuracy and precision are sometimes used interchangeably, they do not have the same meaning.

**Accuracy** refers to the closeness of an analytical result to the actual value. Results nearer to the real value are more accurate than ones further away from the real value. For example, if the real value for an individual's glucose is 90 mg/dL, analyses that yielded results of 88, 90, or 92 mg/dL would be more accurate than analyses that yielded values of 80, 75, or 82 mg/dL.

The term **precision** refers to reproducibility of results or the closeness of obtained values to each other. An example of precision would be results of 88, 87, 92, 91, 88, and 90 on the above glucose sample; these results vary little from each other. Another way of thinking about precision is to mentally picture a target with all the arrows or bullet holes closely grouped in one area of the target.

If the values 78, 90, and 100 mg/mL are placed on the imagined target, the "arrows" will be scattered around the target, not grouped close together (Figure 1-22), indicating lack of precision.

One can have precision without accuracy; in other words, one could produce results near in value to each other, but, because of an error, the values may be inaccurate, not near the true value. The worker's goal should be to achieve both precision and accuracy in the laboratory analyses performed.

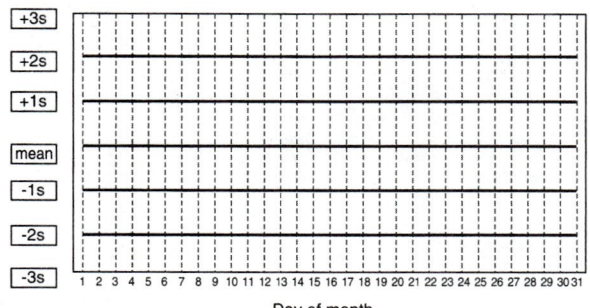

Day of month

**FIGURE 1-21** A form used to construct a Levey-Jennings chart

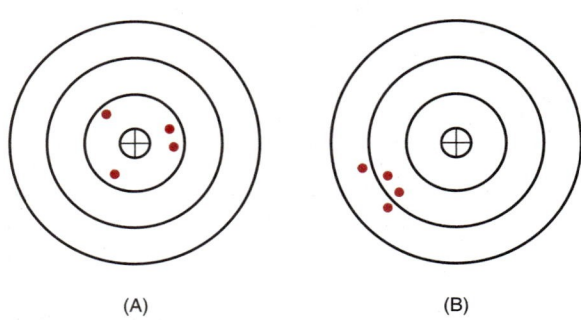

(A)                              (B)

**FIGURE 1-22**   Illustration of accuracy (A) vs. precision (B)

## BASIC STATISTICS

Quality control involves **statistics**, the science of collecting and classifying data to show their significance. The statistics involved in a good QC program can be very complicated; therefore, only the fundamentals will be covered in this lesson.

### Calculating the Mean, Variance, and Standard Deviation

In a QC program, the mean, variance, and standard deviation for analytical procedures must be calculated. The **mean** is the average of a set of values. The **standard deviation**, a measure of the scatter of the sample values around the mean, is derived from the calculation of the variance. Therefore, once the mean of a set of values has been determined, it is possible to determine the acceptable variation in the results of that analysis method.

#### Calculating the Mean

The mean is calculated by computing the sum of all the values in the set and dividing this by the number of values in the set; in other words, by calculating the **average** of a set of numbers. For example, the values obtained in repeated analyses for a glucose control serum were as follows: 82, 85, 90, 86, 91, 90, 81, 86, 94, and 89. The formula for determining the mean is:

$$\overline{X} = \frac{\Sigma X}{n}$$

where   $\overline{X}$  = the mean
$X$  = each individual value in the set
$\Sigma X$ = the sum of all the individual values
$n$  = the number of values in the set

Substituting into the formula:

$$\overline{X} = \frac{82 + 85 + 90 + 86 + 91 + 90 + 81 + 86 + 94 + 89}{10}$$

$$\overline{X}\ (mean) = \frac{874}{10} = 87.4$$

#### Calculating the Variance

The variance ($s^2$) is calculated by subtracting each value in the set from the mean, squaring this number, and calculating the sum of the squares. That sum is then divided by $n$-1, which is the number of individual values in the set *minus one*. The formula for variance is:

$$Variance\ (s^2) = \frac{\Sigma(\overline{X} - X)^2}{n - 1}$$

An example of how to find the deviation from the mean and the deviation squared is shown in Figure 1-23. The values in column two are obtained by subtracting each value in column one from the mean. Therefore, the first entry in column two is negative (–) 5.4.  This is obtained by subtracting 82, the first value in column one, from the mean, 87.4. It doesn't matter if some of the differences are negative numbers, since squaring them makes them positive numbers. From the example in Figure 1-23, the following substitutions can be made in the variance formula:

$$s^2\ (variance) = \frac{152.4}{9}$$

#### Calculating the Standard Deviation

The standard deviation is obtained by taking the square root of the variance:

$$s = \sqrt{\frac{152.4}{9}} = 4.11$$

Therefore, the standard deviation, $1s$, is 4.11, $2s$ = 8.22, and $3s$ = 12.33 for this particular control for glucose.

| Column One | Column Two | Column Three |
|---|---|---|
| Test Value (mg/dL) X | Deviation from Mean $\overline{X}-X$ | Deviation Squared $(\overline{X}-X)^2$ |
| 82 | 5.4 | 29.16 |
| 85 | 2.4 | 5.76 |
| 90 | 2.6 | 6.76 |
| 86 | 1.4 | 1.96 |
| 91 | 3.6 | 12.96 |
| 90 | 2.6 | 6.76 |
| 81 | 6.4 | 40.76 |
| 86 | 1.4 | 1.96 |
| 94 | 6.6 | 43.56 |
| 89 | 1.6 | 2.56 |
| sum = 874 | | sum = 152.4 |
| mean = $\frac{874}{10}$ = 87.4 | | |

**FIGURE 1-23**   An example of calculating the deviation from the mean and the deviation squared for a set of ten values

Even though these calculations seem complicated, most calculators have a statistics function that can be used to perform them.

## USING THE STANDARD DEVIATION IN THE LABORATORY

When a set of values with a normal distribution is plotted on a graph, the distribution of the values around the mean forms a **Gaussian curve** (Figure 1-24). This curve is also known as a normal frequency or normal distribution curve. In a normal distribution, half of the values are greater than the mean and half are less than the mean. There are also more values close to the mean than values away from the mean.

Once the standard deviation has been determined, the curve can be divided into percentage divisions as shown in Figure 1-24. This figure shows that, in a normally distributed population, 68.2% of all results obtained for this method of glucose analysis will fall between $1s$ below the mean to $1s$ above the mean. In other words, 68.2% of the values will fall between 83.29 $(87.4 - 4.11)$ and 91.51 $(87.4 + 4.11)$ in this particular example, which has a mean of 87.4. In addition, 95.4% of the values will fall between $2s$ below the mean to $2s$ above the mean, or between 79.18 $(87.4 - 8.22)$ and 95.6 $(87.4 + 8.22)$. If $3s$ is used, 99.6% of the values will be between 75.07 $(87.4 - 12.33)$ and 99.73 $(87.4 + 12.33)$.

Clinical laboratories must establish the allowable standard deviation for each analytical method, based on the component being analyzed and the method of analysis. A two-standard-deviation limit is a common choice. In this example, using a control with a mean of 87.4 mg/dL, the laboratory expects the analysis results of that control serum to be within ± $2s$ (between 79.18 and 95.62 mg/dL) each time it is analyzed along with patient samples.

## QUALITY CONTROL CHARTS

Quality control charts can be constructed based on the calculated mean and standard deviation. These **Levey-Jennings charts** demonstrate a method's precision and illustrate trends or shifts in the method.

The quality control chart shown in Figure 1-25 (top) was constructed using the mean and standard deviation calculated from the glucose data in Figure 1-23. The mean obtained was 87.4; therefore, the mean line is labeled 87.4. The lines on either side of the mean represent $1s$, $2s$, and $3s$. As control data are obtained each day, they should be entered on the chart. The chart form normally has spaces for thirty-one days, so it can be used for any month. In a hospital laboratory, every space would probably be used; in an office laboratory,

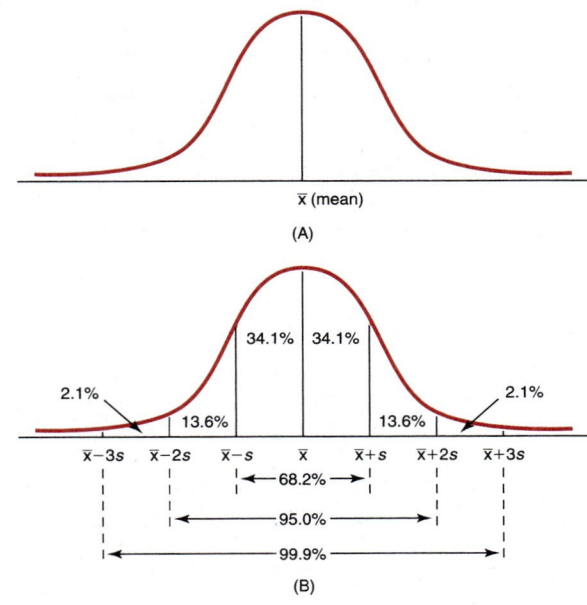

**FIGURE 1-24** Normal distribution curves. (A) Gaussian curve showing normal frequency distribution around the mean. (B) Gaussian curve showing the proportion of the population falling between the mean and ±1$s$, ±2$s$, and ±3$s$.

perhaps only five days per week would be used. Figure 1-25 (bottom) is an example of a quality control chart with control values plotted for twelve days.

### Trend

A control value can sometimes consistently increase or decrease over a period of time covered by a QC chart. This tendency can be observed after three or four values are either always high or always low. This uninterrupted rise or decline away from the mean is called a **trend** (Figure 1-25, bottom). A trend is a signal that something has gone wrong in the procedure, either in the instrument, the technique, the reagents, or the control serum itself. The laboratory worker must investigate and find the source of error and correct it. A new lot of control serum can be analyzed; if error is still present, the instrument must be recalibrated.

### Shift

A **shift** is when a majority of values fall on one side of the mean, but there are never three or four consecutively high or low (Figure 1-25, bottom). This also signals error; the reagents and the instrument must be investigated for the cause.

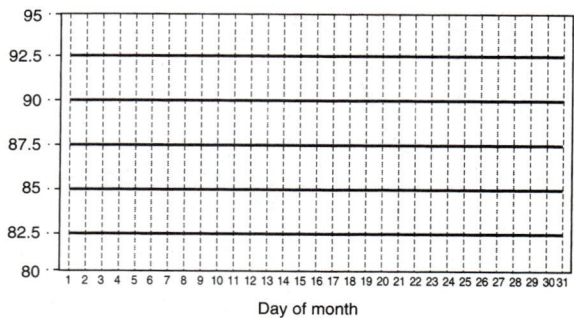

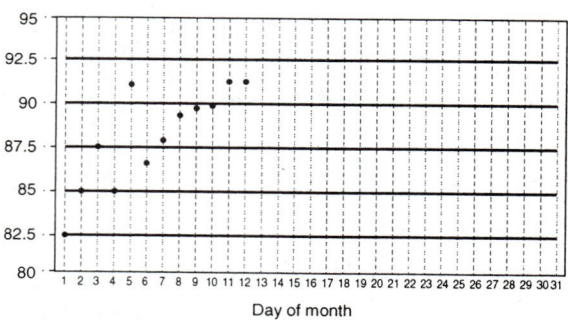

**FIGURE 1-25** QC charts. (Top) Levey-Jennings chart constructed using the mean and standard deviation obtained from glucose control values. (Bottom) plot of 12 control values, showing a normal distribution in values 1–6 and a trend and shift in values 7–12.

## Westgard's Rules

When a laboratory establishes a QC program there must be guidelines to decide whether or not a method is out of control. One set of guidelines is called **Westgard's Rules**. These rules list specific limits on how much error is acceptable in control values before patient test results are rejected. To use these rules, the laboratory must analyze two control sera of different levels (normal and abnormal) along with each set of patient samples. A "run" (set of samples) is considered out of control and the patient results must be rejected if any of the following is true:

1. both controls are outside the ±2s limit

2. the same control level (concentration) is outside the ±2s limit in two successive runs

3. controls in four consecutive runs have values greater than ±1s all in the same direction

4. ten consecutive control values fall on one side of the mean

Patient test results cannot be reported until the method is considered "in control."

## COEFFICIENT OF VARIATION

When a laboratory changes from one method of analysis to another, the precision of the new method must be compared to that of the old one. This can be done by calculating the coefficient of variation (CV) for each method. The **coefficient of variation** is a calculated value that compares the relative variability between two different sets of values by expressing each standard deviation as a percentage of the mean.

If a laboratory purchased a new instrument to perform blood glucose tests, the means and the standard deviations from the old and new methods would be used to calculate the coefficient of variation. For example, the mean glucose for one method is 98.5 mg/dL, with a standard deviation (s) of 2.5 mg/dL, and the mean glucose of a second method is 78 mg/dL with a standard deviation of 2.0 mg/dL. The CV would be calculated as shown below.

**1st method**   $CV = \dfrac{s}{\bar{x}} \times 100$

$$CV = \frac{2.5 \text{ mg/dL}}{98.5 \text{ mg/dL}} \times 100$$

$$CV = 2.5\%$$

**2nd method**  $CV = \dfrac{s}{\bar{x}} \times 100$

$$CV = \frac{2.0 \text{ mg/dL}}{78 \text{ mg/dL}} \times 100$$

$$CV = 2.6\%$$

In this case, the variations are about the same, so the precision of the methods is similar. However, if a third method had a mean of 50 mg/dL and s of 3.0 mg/dL, the CV would be calculated:

**3rd method**  $CV = \dfrac{s}{\bar{x}} \times 100$

$$CV = \frac{3.0 \text{ mg/dL}}{50 \text{ mg/dL}} \times 100$$

$$CV = 6.0\%$$

This illustrates that there is more variation between method three and methods one and two than there is between method one and method two.

## QA IN THE CLINICAL LABORATORY

Errors can occur at several points during the specimen collection, test performance, and results reporting. *Preanalytical errors* include misidentifying the patient, collecting a sample at the wrong time, and mishandling the specimen.

*Analytical errors* occur during the test procedure and may be random or systematic. **Systematic error** is defined as a variation that may make results consistently higher or lower than the actual value. Factors that may cause this type of error are deteriorated reagents, mechanical trouble in the instrument, or a peculiarity in worker methodology, such as manner of pipetting.

The source of **random error** cannot be absolutely identified. This type of error causes variations on either side of the mean. Factors that may contribute to random error include an air bubble in a reagent line, differences in technique among workers, and certain specimen characteristics.

*Postanalytical errors* also can occur. A result may be accurate but may be transferred to another patient's records by entering the wrong patient identification number in the computer. When results are transcribed by hand, the wrong value may be copied from laboratory reports to a patient's chart.

All these issues are addressed in a comprehensive QA program. The increased use of scan barcodes on request forms, patient identification bands, specimen containers, and patient charts, and interfacing laboratory computers with patient records, has eliminated many pre- and post-analytical errors.

## *Procedural Notes*

- Follow the instrument manufacturer's instructions for calibration procedures.
- Be sure to correctly insert values into the statistical formulas.
- Follow the manufacturer's instructions for reconstituting control samples received in dry form.
- Include a sufficient number of results in calculations to ensure reliability.

## *Safety Precautions*

- Observe Universal and Standard Precautions.
- Wear appropriate PPE when handling samples, calibrators, and control sera.

## SUMMARY

A good program of quality assurance (QA) is necessary if the laboratory is to perform procedures with reliable results. The Clinical Laboratory Improvements Amendments of 1988 (CLIA '88) and amendments being considered, mandate how the laboratory accomplishes this goal.

Maintaining a high standard of quality need not be a burden for the laboratory. Most manufacturers supply standards and controls for their analyzers. Instruments for large laboratories may have self-contained QC programs in which the expected values for controls are entered into the program; if the control results are not within an acceptable range, the instrument alerts the operator to investigate. As alternatives, there are many quality control software programs the laboratory may purchase.

## LESSON REVIEW

1. What is the importance of quality assurance and quality control in the laboratory?
2. Explain the use of standards and controls in the laboratory's daily operation.
3. Explain how results may be precise but not accurate.
4. How is the mean of a set of values determined?
5. Describe how to calculate the standard deviation.
6. Explain how an out-of-control result can be detected.
7. Explain how to detect a trend in a procedure.
8. How can the coefficient of variation be used to compare methods of analysis?
9. Define accuracy, average, coefficient of variation, control serum, Gaussian curve, Levey-Jennings chart, mean, population, precision, random error, sample, shift, standard, standard deviation, statistics, systematic error, trend, and Westgard's Rules.

## STUDENT ACTIVITIES

1. Reread the information on quality control.
2. Review the glossary terms.
3. Practice calculating the standard deviation using this group of numbers:  10, 9, 15, 10, 12, 11, 10, 12, 14, 12.
4. Using the results of the above calculations, construct a quality control (Levey-Jennings) chart showing the mean, $+1s$, $+2s$, $+3s$, $-1s$, $-2s$, and $-3s$.
5. Complete the quality control worksheet at the end of this lesson.

# *Worksheet*

## LESSON 1-7 Quality Assurance in the Laboratory

Name _____   Date _____

I.  **Calculating the Mean and the Standard Deviation**

Use this worksheet and the data presented below to calculate the mean and the standard deviation. The red blood cell (RBC) counts from an RBC control solution are: 3.2, 3.3, 3.5, 3.2, 3.0, 3.4, 3.8, 3.5, 3.4, and 3.3.

1.  What is the formula for finding the mean?

2.  Substitute the values into the formula.

3.  The mean of the red cell counts is: _____

4.  Following the example in Figure 1-23, calculate the deviation squared for each of the values above.

5.  What is the formula for variance?

6.  Determine the variance from the calculation in step 4.

7.  What is the formula for determining standard deviation?

8.  Substitute values from step 6 into the formula.

9.  What is the standard deviation?

What is $\pm 2s$? _____   What is $\pm 3s$? _____

## II. Constructing a Levey-Jennings Chart

1. Use the mean and standard deviation (*s*) from part A to construct a Levey-Jennings chart. Indicate the mean value, ± 1*s*, ± 2*s*, and ± 3*s* (from part A) on the appropriate lines.

2. Plot these control values obtained for days 1–10 on the chart: Day 1 = 3.2, Day 2 = 3.3, Day 3 = 3.5, Day 4 = 3.2, Day 5 = 3.0, Day 6 = 3.4, Day 7 = 3.8, Day 8 = 3.5, Day 9 = 3.4, and Day 10 = 3.3.

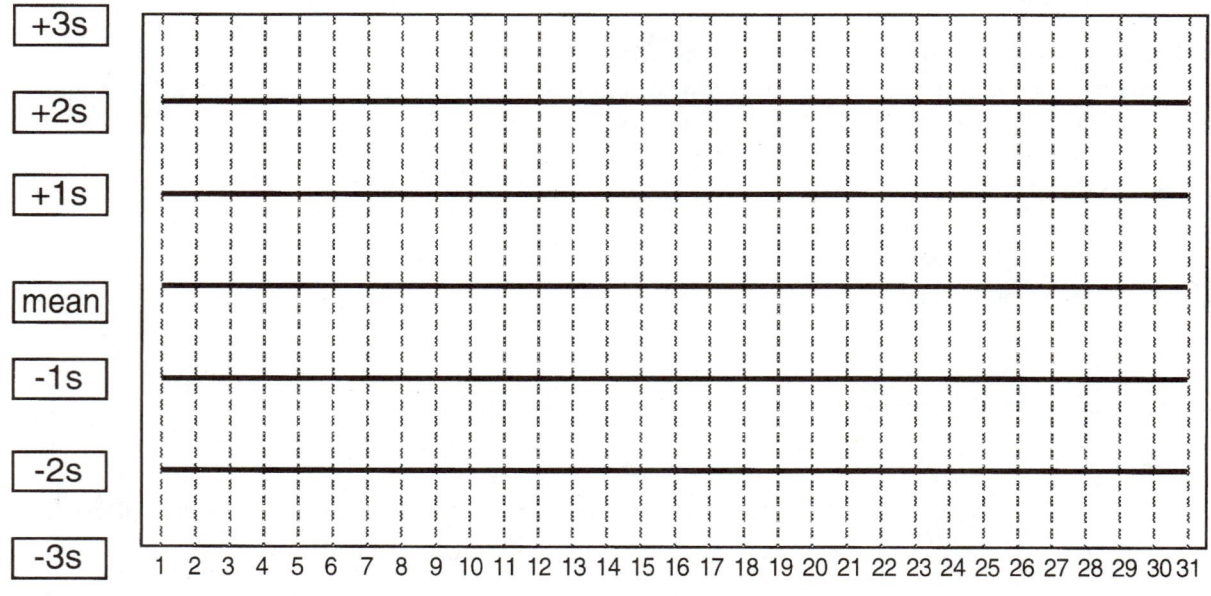

Day of month

# General Laboratory Equipment

**After studying this lesson, you should be able to:**
- *Explain and demonstrate the operation of automatic pipets.*
- *Explain the proper use of a centrifuge.*
- *Explain the function of a pH meter.*
- *Discuss the operation of an autoclave.*
- *List four rules for using a laboratory balance.*
- *Explain how distilled water and deionized water are made.*
- *Explain the importance of equipment maintenance records.*
- *Define the glossary terms.*

## GLOSSARY

**autoclave** / a device that uses pressurized steam for sterilization

**centrifuge** / an instrument that spins tubes at high speeds, forcing heavy particles in samples to the bottom of the tubes

**deionized water** / water that has had most of the mineral ions removed

**distilled water** / the condensate collected from steam after water has been boiled

**microfuge** / a centrifuge that spins microcentrifuge tubes at high rates of speed

**pH** / a measurement of the hydrogen ion concentration expressing the degree of acidity or alkalinity of a solution

**rotor** / the part of a centrifuge that holds the tubes and rotates during the operation of the centrifuge

**serofuge** / a centrifuge that spins small tubes such as those used in blood banking

## INTRODUCTION

The type of equipment required in a medical laboratory is determined by the size of the laboratory and the number and variety of tests performed. A small laboratory may have only a microscope, refrigerator, and centrifuge. However, a large laboratory will have an assortment of equipment, including instruments such as pH meters, autoclaves, balances, incubators, water baths, and blood analyzers.

For reliable test results, equipment used in the testing process must be operating correctly. Therefore, personnel must not only know how to perform a test, but also the proper care, maintenance, and, sometimes, repair of equipment used in each procedure.

This lesson introduces some general guidelines for the use, care, and maintenance of common laboratory equipment. It is imperative to consult manuals provided by the equipment manufacturer to determine the proper use of each piece of equipment and to follow general laboratory safety rules (Lessons 1-5 and 1-6). The microscope is covered in Lesson 1-10, The Microscope.

## SAFETY

The use of laboratory instruments and equipment can present hazards such as risk of exposure to BBP, moving mechanical parts, high-voltage electrical current, toxic chemicals, cuts from broken glass or sharp parts, or burns from steam or hot liquids. The hazards differ depending on the instrument in use. All instruments must be operated in a safe manner, following the manufacturers' directions. Preventive maintenance should be performed carefully, adhering to Standard Precautions and other recommended safety practices. Only trained persons should repair instruments. More specific information concerning safe equipment operation is given in each section.

### *Quality Assurance*

Laboratory procedures that use equipment and instruments are affected by equipment operation. Regular routine maintenance, calibration, and performance checks must be performed for all laboratory equipment, including refrigerators, waterbaths, centrifuges, pipetters, autoclaves, pH meters, and balances. The results of these checks must be documented and any problems detected must be corrected before the equipment is used in laboratory procedures. Each type of instrument or equipment will require performance checks specific to the instrument type. The laboratory's procedure manual will specify the frequency and type of checks that must be performed for each instrument and piece of equipment in the laboratory.

## LABORATORY EQUIPMENT

### Automatic Pipets

Glass pipets have been the standard in laboratories for many years; however, automatic pipets are now used in most laboratories (Figure 1-26). Automatic pipets draw up a preset volume when the operator depresses and releases a plunger on top of the pipet. Some automatic pipets are preset to deliver just one volume, while others are adjustable within a narrow range, such as 1-20 µL or 20-100 µL. The use of automatic pipets is usually preferable to glass pipets because there is no need for safety bulbs and other pipetting aids. Some laboratory analyzers draw up and dispense the samples automatically, thereby eliminating potential pipetting errors.

Several types of automatic pipets are available. Some use a different disposable plastic tip for each sample, while others have a reusable glass capillary tip with a teflon plunger. Since neither of these have markings to indicate the volume contained, regular scheduled calibration is very important to ensure the correct volume is delivered. All mechanical pipets should be stored vertically, tip end down, to prevent damage from liquids flowing into the working mechanism. Special pipet racks are available to hold them upright (Figure 1-26).

Another type of automatic pipet is an electric or battery-powered device used with serological and volumetric pipets of various sizes (Figure 1-27). The upper end of the pipet fits into a holder held in the operator's hand. The suction to aspirate liquids is provided by a pump; buttons on the holder control aspirating and dispensing. These devices are easy to use and allow use of pipets of various volumes.

### Quality Assurance

Improper pipetting technique is a source of error in laboratory tests. Much practice is needed to develop accu-

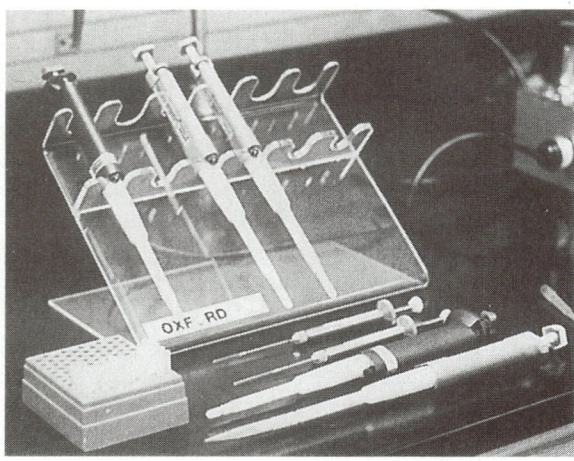

**FIGURE 1-26**  Examples of mechanical automatic pipetters (Photo courtesy of John Estridge)

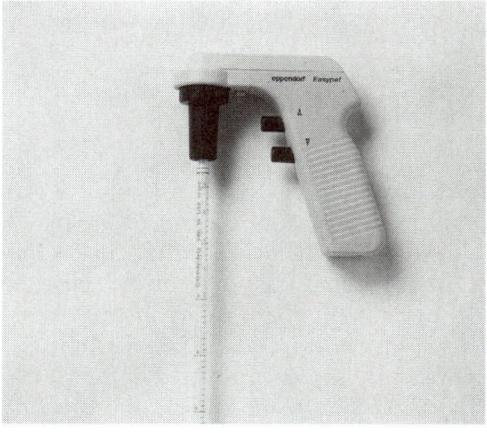

**FIGURE 1-27**  Example of automatic pipetter (Photo courtesy of Brinkman Instruments, Inc.)

racy and precision in pipetting. Instructions for the use of each type of automatic pipet must be followed. Several pipet-calibration kits and programs are provided by pipet manufacturers to keep automatic pipets working properly and accurately. A regular schedule for maintenance and calibration should be followed.

## Centrifuges

**Centrifuges** are instruments that spin samples at high speeds, forcing the heavier particles to the bottom of the container (usually a tube). The most frequent clinical laboratory use of the centrifuge is for separating the cellular components of blood from the liquid (serum or plasma) so the liquid may be used for testing.

Centrifuges vary in size, capacity, and speed capability. *Clinical centrifuge* is the name given to models that can be used for urinalysis or serum separation (Figure 1-28). These usually have a speed capacity of 0–3,000 rpm (revolutions per minute), and hold tubes ranging in size from 5 to 50 mL, depending on the adapters. A **serofuge** is a small centrifuge used in blood banking and serology to spin serological tubes (approximately 2–3 mL capacity).

Microcentrifuges, or **microfuges**, are also widely used. These spin special microtubes (0.5–1.5 mL capacity) at high speeds, usually up to 12,000–14,000 rpm. The microhematocrit centrifuge is a variation of the microfuge; it spins capillary tubes at high speeds so hematocrits can be measured.

Other types of centrifuges include high-speed refrigerated centrifuges, that have speed capabilities of 0–20,000 rpm, and ultracentrifuges that are capable of speeds over 50,000 rpm. These centrifuges are specially equipped to keep samples cool during centrifugation. Centrifuges such as these are often used in research laboratories but are not usually required for routine clinical laboratory samples. The rotation speeds and timers of centrifuges must be checked and documented at specific intervals, usually monthly or quarterly.

  Safety

Centrifuges present several safety hazards. As with other instruments, the manufacturer's instructions must always be followed when using a centrifuge. Some general rules to follow include:

1. Always operate centrifuges with the lids closed.
2. Balance the contents before turning on the centrifuge. For example, if there is only one sample to be centrifuged, a tube identical in size and volume of solution must be placed in the rotor opposite the sample tube. The **rotor** is the part of the centrifuge that holds the tubes and rotates during operation. For every sample placed in the rotor, there must be a balancing sample placed directly opposite.
3. Allow the rotor to stop spinning before opening the centrifuge lid.
4. Spin samples with lids on to avoid creating aerosols.
5. Use only tubes specified as appropriate for that particular centrifuge.

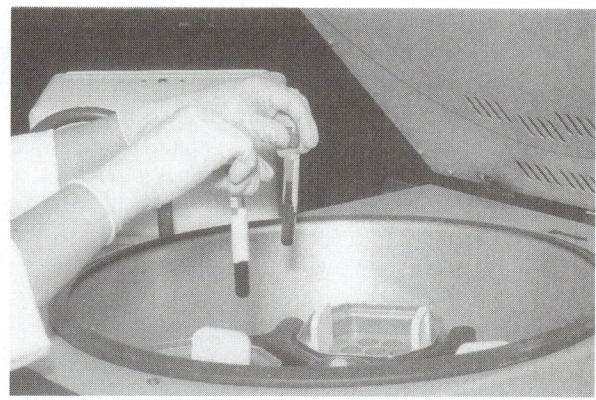

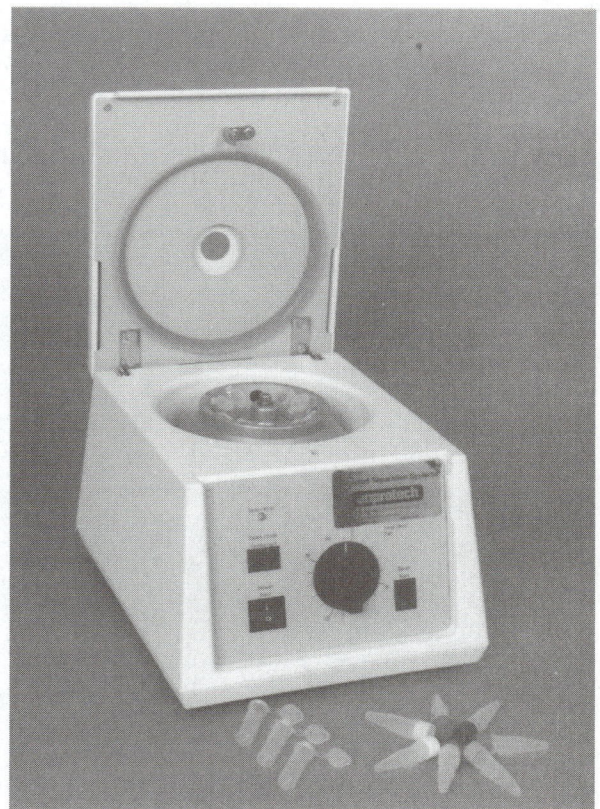

**FIGURE 1-28** Centrifuges: (top) clinical centrifuge and (bottom) microfuge (Bottom photo courtesy of Integrated Separation Systems, Division of Enprotech)

6. Clean spills with surface disinfectant immediately following incident.

## Autoclaves

**Autoclaves** are instruments that use steam under pressure to sterilize items such as gauze, dental and surgical instruments, sterile solutions, and materials to be used in microbiology (Figure 1-29). Autoclaves are also used to decontaminate materials such as blood specimens, bacterial cultures, or filled biohazard containers before disposal.

Autoclaves can range in size from very large (room size) to the size of a large cooking pot. Large autoclaves obtain steam from either an internal steam generator or a pipe connected to the facility's steam plant. Smaller ones create their own steam by heating water.

Items to be sterilized can either be placed in bags with heat-sensitive indicator strips or wrapped in paper sealed with autoclave tape that changes color to indicate the proper temperature has been reached. The items are then placed inside the autoclave on a shelf and the autoclave door is closed and locked. The temperature, length of cycle, and pounds of steam pressure are set. Typical autoclave conditions are 121°C for 15-20 minutes at fifteen pounds per square inch (psi). Steam is admitted into the chamber. Cycle timing begins when temperature and pressure have reached set levels. Autoclaves have temperature and pressure gauges, and most have a chart or digital recorder that records the temperature of each autoclave cycle. At the end of the cycle, the pressure and temperature will drop; the autoclave can be opened when the pressure gauge reads zero (0) psi.

### Safety

Because of the steam under pressure, great care must be used when operating an autoclave. The autoclave door must never be opened unless the chamber pressure is zero (0) psi. A service technician should perform regular maintenance on the autoclave.

At the end of the autoclave cycle, items must be removed from the autoclave using tongs or heat-proof gloves to prevent burns. When liquids are sterilized, they must be in loosely capped, heat-resistant containers that are no more than half full. These containers must be placed in an autoclavable tray or pan to catch overflow. Chamber pressure must be reduced slowly at the end of a "liquid run" to prevent the liquids from boiling over.

### Quality Assurance

It is important that autoclaves work properly, since non-sterile items could endanger both worker and patient or could cause problems in a test procedure that requires sterile solutions or components. There are several means to ensure that sterilization has occurred. Sterility indicator strips containing spores from the bacterium *Bacillus stearothermophilus* can be used to check the effectiveness of the steam sterilization process. The strips are autoclaved with a normal load, removed, and then incubated in a tube of bacterial growth medium. Lack of bacterial growth confirms the efficiency of sterilization; growth of bacteria indicates the sterilization method was inadequate and the items in that run are not sterile. Temperature, pressure, and time controls must then be checked to determine the cause of failure.

Daily records must be kept of sterilization times, temperatures, chamber pressures, and indicator strip results. The temperature chart recorder must be changed at specified intervals and the charts maintained in the equipment logbook.

## Laboratory Balances

Several types of balances or scales are used in the laboratory. They differ in the total amount they can accurately weigh, their sensitivities, and whether they are manual, with sliding weights on a beam balance, or electronic top-loading or cabinet balances (Figure 1-30).

Measurements that require sensitivity to 0.10 gram can be made using inexpensive double- or triple-beam

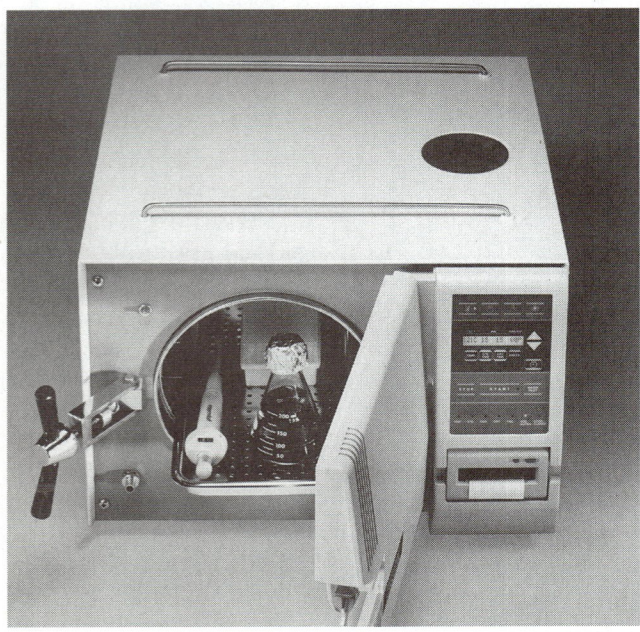

**FIGURE 1-29**    A tabletop autoclave (Photo courtesy of Brinkmann Instruments, Inc.)

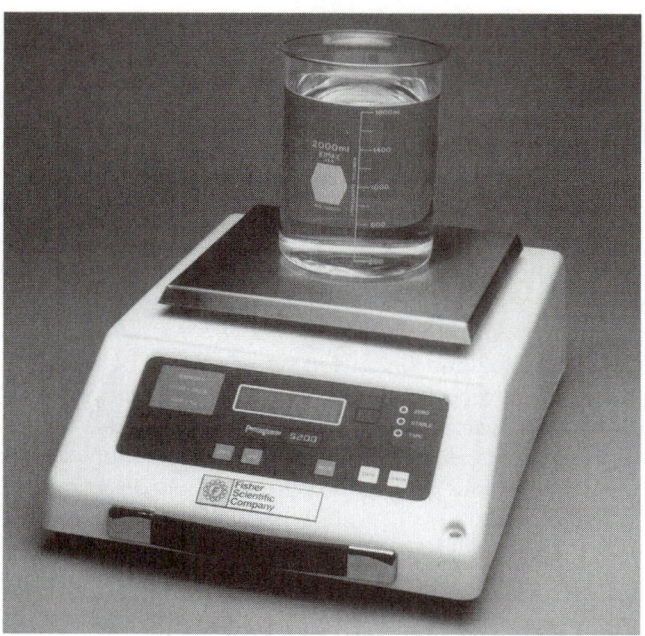

**FIGURE 1-30** Top-loading laboratory balance (Photo courtesy of Fisher Scientific)

balances. Measurements of as little as 0.0001 g ($10^{-4}$ g) or even 0.00001 g ($10^{-5}$ g) can be made using a single-pan balance with great sensitivity. However, most critical weighing is done using electronic top-loading or cabinet balances.

 Safety and Quality Assurance

Accurate measurement of chemicals is required to prepare accurate reagents. The manufacturer's instructions must be followed when using balances. Some general rules to keep in mind are:

1. Keep balances clean; wipe up any spills immediately.

2. Do not subject the balance to sudden shocks; do not move it from place to place.

3. Position the balance on a draft- and vibration-free counter. Special tables and supports are available if vibrations are a problem.

4. Respect the sensitivity of a balance; do not try to weigh 0.001 g on a balance accurate to only 0.10 g.

5. Calibrate balances on a regular schedule; perform yearly maintenance or contract to have it done.

6. Wear gloves when weighing chemicals to avoid skin exposure to chemicals.

7. Avoid breathing chemical dust by wearing a mask when weighing chemicals that are irritants.

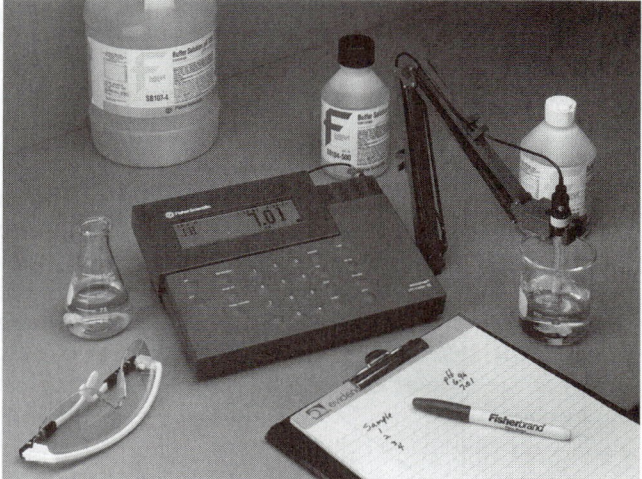

**FIGURE 1-31** pH meter (Photo courtesy of Fisher Scientific)

## Meters for pH Measurement

In most laboratory procedures, it is critical that the reagents used be of proper pH. The **pH** is a solution's degree of acidity or alkalinity. The scale for pH is 0-14. A pH of seven (7.0) is said to be neutral; values below 7.0 indicate acid solutions; values above 7.0 indicate alkaline solutions. Lemon juice, vinegar, and hydrochloric acid (HCl) are examples of acids; solutions of baking soda, sodium hydroxide (NaOH), and potassium hydroxide (KOH) are examples of alkaline solutions.

Electrodes connected to a pH meter measure the pH of a solution by measuring the hydrogen ion concentration (Figure 1-31). A reference electrode and an indicating electrode are required to measure pH. For most measurements, a single *combination* electrode is used that contains both electrodes in one probe. The electrodes measure the hydrogen ion concentration. The meter converts this information to pH and displays it on a dial or screen.

Measurement of pH may also be done using special papers treated with indicator solutions. These papers are dipped into the solution to be tested, and the color that develops is then compared to a color chart to determine the pH. This method is suitable for procedures such as measuring urine pH, but is not sensitive enough for preparing laboratory reagents.

  Safety

Care should be used when measuring chemical solutions with the pH meter. Caustic or acid solutions for adjusting pH must be used carefully. Chemical spills must be wiped up immediately. The pH meter should be disconnected from the electrical source before attempting any repair.

### Quality Assurance

Electrodes must be calibrated using solutions of known pH values, usually 4.0, 7.0, and 10.0. The electrodes are immersed in the known solutions and the meter is set to that value; the numerical pH values will appear on the dial or digital display. The meter is actually measuring the potential across a membrane inside the electrode. When an unknown solution is tested, the potential of the unknown solution is compared to the potential created by the calibration solution.

Special care must be taken in handling, maintaining, and storing the electrode so it will not dry out or be broken. The electrodes must always be rinsed with water between samples, but never stored in water. Manuals that come with the meters give detailed instructions for use.

## Temperature Control Chambers

Most test procedures and reagents require testing or storage at specific temperatures. Many reagents must be refrigerated or frozen; tests or cultures may require special incubation temperatures. Most laboratories have incubators, ovens, and water baths for controlled heat (above ambient, or room, temperature) and refrigerator/freezer units for cooling. These units should be used only for laboratory purposes, not for storing or heating food.

### Quality Assurance

All temperature-controlled units must be monitored regularly to ensure they are operating at the proper temperatures. Calibrated thermometers must be available for measuring the temperatures. Temperatures for each unit must be checked and recorded daily and before each use.

## DISTILLED AND DEIONIZED WATER

In many laboratory procedures, reagents must be reconstituted from a powder by adding a measured volume of distilled or deionized water. Tap water is not suitable to prepare most reagents because it contains impurities. **Distilled water** is the condensate collected from the steam created when water is boiled. Water that has been double distilled has most of the contaminates removed. A small distillation apparatus can be easily installed in the laboratory or distilled water may be purchased.

**Deionized water** is prepared by passing water through a purifying cartridge containing a resin bed to remove mineral salts. If charcoal is included in the bed, other contaminates will be removed. Often, water will be passed through a deionizing cartridge before distillation and the resulting water will be deionized distilled water. Good quality distilled or deionized water has a low electrical conductivity.

Distilled and deionized water should be stored in clean, dust-free containers of borosilicate glass or plastic. Stored water should be replaced frequently. Unless a procedure specifically calls for tap water, all aqueous reagents should be made using distilled or deionized distilled water.

## EQUIPMENT MAINTENANCE RECORDS

Each laboratory should have instructions in the laboratory procedure manual that outline the required maintenance and performance checks for each piece of equipment. Log sheets are used for recording maintenance, service, repair, and performance checks.

A common schedule of performance checks in a small laboratory would include:

- Monitor and record temperatures of water baths, refrigerators, and incubators daily.
- Verify and record the wavelength of spectrophotometers and perform other recommended quality control checks daily.
- Check temperature and chamber pressure record of autoclave after each use.
- Calibrate automatic pipets monthly.
- Measure rpm on centrifuge with a tachometer every three months.
- Calibrate pH meter daily and check with standard solutions before each use.

An example of an Equipment Maintenance and Performance Checklist is given at the end of this lesson.

## GENERAL GUIDELINES FOR CARE AND USE OF EQUIPMENT

Laboratory equipment is expensive and must be cared for properly. Although most equipment is sturdy, common sense should be used when operating or working near equipment. General rules to keep in mind include:

- Observe all safety rules as stated in your institution's procedure manual.
- Follow accepted safety procedures and use common sense when operating all instruments.
- Always unplug electrical instruments before attempting any repairs.
- Use care when operating instruments with moving parts. Pin long hair up and do not wear dangling jewelry.
- Wipe up all spills promptly and appropriately.
- Use equipment only according to manufacturers' instructions.
- Perform maintenance checks at proper intervals.
- Follow laboratory procedure and manufacturer's guidelines for routine equipment maintenance.
- Record all maintenance and repair of equipment.
- Report any instrument malfunction to the appropriate supervisor.

## LESSON REVIEW

1. Describe two types of automatic pipets.
2. What rules should be followed when using a laboratory balance?
3. Explain the function of a pH meter.
4. A solution with a pH of 8.5 is _____ (acidic or alkaline).
5. Give five general rules to follow when operating a centrifuge.
6. Name three types of centrifuges that may be found in a clinical laboratory.
7. Explain how autoclaves operate.
8. What type of water is used to make laboratory reagents?
9. Why is it important to be careful when using an autoclave?
10. What quality control methods are used for temperature controlled chambers?
11. Why are equipment maintenance records important?
12. List eight general safety rules for operation and care of laboratory equipment.
13. Define autoclave, centrifuge, deionized water, distilled water, microfuge, pH, rotor, and serofuge.

## STUDENT ACTIVITIES

1. Reread the information on general laboratory equipment.
2. Review the glossary terms.

Depending on which instruments are available, complete the activities in numbers 3–7. Read the instruction manual carefully before attempting to use an instrument. Then be sure to follow the instructions carefully when using that instrument.

3. If a pH meter is available, practice measuring the pH of a solution such as saline. Note how the pH changes when a few drops of 0.1% HCl or 0.1% NaOH are added to the solution. Dilute the solution by adding one part water to one part solution. Now measure the pH. Did it change? How can the result be explained?
4. If a balance is available, practice weighing a chemical or a substance such as salt or sugar. Note the capacity of the balance; what is the largest weight that can be measured? What is the smallest increment that can be read (1 g, 0.1 g, 0.01 g, etc.)?
5. If a centrifuge is available, practice centrifuging a sample. Be sure to use appropriate balance tubes. Note the speed scale; what is the maximum rpm the centrifuge can achieve? What size tubes can the centrifuge handle safely?
6. If automatic pipets are available, practice dispensing liquids using the procedure recommended by the manufacturer.
7. Use the Equipment Maintenance and Performance Checklist (at the end of this lesson) to check the performance of any available equipment.

## *Worksheet*

## **LESSON 1-8** General Laboratory Equipment

Name _____   Date _____

Use this form to record general laboratory equipment maintenance and performance. Identify each piece of equipment on the sheet. Locate instruction manuals for the equipment and find out what maintenance and/or calibration procedures are recommended and how often.

### I. Temperature-Controlled Chambers

Record the temperatures of any refrigerators, freezers, water baths, or incubators in the laboratory. In a working laboratory, this must be done at least daily. If a thermometer does not stay in the equipment, place one inside for 20-30 minutes, then record temperature. Refrigerator thermometers may be stored with the bulb immersed in water or propylene glycol in a stoppered bottle. If the temperature is not within range, make the proper adjustment and remeasure or inform the supervisor.

| Equipment I.D. | Range (°C) | Temperature Observed | Date | Comment/Sign |
|---|---|---|---|---|
| Freezer _____ | -20 ± 5 | _____ | _____ | _____ |
| Refrigerator _____ | 6 ± 2 | _____ | _____ | _____ |
| Water bath _____ | 36 ± 1 | _____ | _____ | _____ |
| Incubator _____ | 36 ± 1 | _____ | _____ | _____ |

### II. Autoclave

During or after each run of the autoclave, check to see that the proper temperature and chamber pressure were reached. Each run should be given a number.

Autoclave: Run #_____   Temp °C _____   Chamber pressure_____

### III. pH meter

Calibrate the meter before each use with two calibration solutions, one near the pH of the solution to be measured. (Commercial pH calibration solutions usually are pH 4, pH 7, and pH 10.) Check to see that the pH electrode is always stored in the appropriate solution when not in use.

| Date | Calibration Solution | Comment/Sign |
|---|---|---|
| _____ | _____ | _____ |
| _____ | _____ | _____ |
| _____ | _____ | _____ |

## IV. Centrifuges

Use a stopwatch to check the timer on the centrifuge. If available, use a tachometer to check rpm. *Do not attempt to check the speed if the centrifuge lid does not have an opening in the center or a see-through cover.*

| I.D. | Date | Timer Check | RPM Check | Comment/Sign |
|---|---|---|---|---|
| Serofuge | | | | |
| Microfuge | | | | |
| Centrifuge | | | | |

## V. Balances

Check balances to see that they are clean and placed on a stable counter in a draft-free location. If available, use standard weights to check the calibration of the balances. (Commercial services will perform maintenance and calibration on a contract basis.)

| I. D. | Date | Balance Checked | Comment/Sign |
|---|---|---|---|
| | | | |
| | | | |

# Laboratory Glassware

## LESSON OBJECTIVES

**After studying this lesson, you should be able to:**

- *Identify five basic types of containers used in the laboratory and explain the use of each.*
- *Identify heat-resistant glassware.*
- *Identify volumetric pipets and explain their proper use.*
- *Identify graduated pipets and explain their proper use.*
- *Discuss the advantages and disadvantages of using plastic containers in the laboratory.*
- *Describe the proper care of and cleaning procedures for laboratory glassware and plasticware.*
- *List precautions to be observed when using laboratory glassware and plasticware.*
- *Define the glossary terms.*

## GLOSSARY

**critical measurements** / measurements made when the accuracy of the concentration of a solution is important; measurements made using glassware manufactured to strict standards

**meniscus** / the curved upper surface of a liquid in a container

**noncritical measurements** / estimated measurements; measurements made in containers that estimate volume (such as the Erlenmeyer flask)

**reagent** / substance or solution used in laboratory analyses; substance involved in a chemical reaction

**solute** / a liquid, gas, or solid dissolved in a liquid to make a solution

**solvent** / the liquid in which substances are dissolved; a liquid that holds a solute in solution

**TC** / to contain

**TD** / to deliver

## INTRODUCTION

Most laboratory procedures require using some type of container or glassware. Basic laboratory glassware comes in many shapes and sizes. This glassware may be used in a specific test procedure or in preparing or storing **reagents**, solutions used in laboratory analysis.

In recent years, it has become common to use laboratory containers of plastic, as well as glass. Because of this, the term "labware" is sometimes used to include glassware and plasticware. Much of today's labware is designed to be used only once and then disposed of. This eliminates the possibility of contaminating solutions due to inadequate cleaning.

This lesson explains the basic types of labware (glass and plastic) and gives guidelines for its proper use, care, and cleaning.

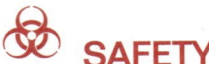 **SAFETY**

Chemical solutions must be stored in labware that cannot interact with the chemicals. Disposable labware should be used once and discarded. Reusable labware that has been used for biological fluids or specimens must be disinfected before washing by soaking the items in an appropriate disinfectant. Chipped or cracked glassware should be discarded if it cannot be repaired. Rigid, puncture-proof containers should be available for disposal of broken glass (Figure 1-7, page 40). Heavy-duty gloves and other appropriate PPE must be worn when cleaning labware.

## Heating Glassware

*Kimax* and *Pyrex* are two brands of heat-resistant glassware. Glassware marked with these brandnames may be used for boiling solutions and may be heat-sterilized. Glassware that is not manufactured to be heat-resistant must not be heated over direct heat or autoclaved.

---

### *Quality Assurance*

The quality and type of labware used can affect the outcome of test procedures. Only properly cleaned labware should be used in test procedures or for reagent storage. Pipets with chipped or broken tips are not accurate and must be discarded. Critical volume measurements, such as those required when making standard solutions, must only be made using glassware manufactured to strict standards.

---

## COMPOSITION OF LABWARE

### Glass

Glass laboratory containers are made of: (1) flint glass or (2) borosilicate glass. Flint glass has a low resistance to heat and chemicals, but is inexpensive. It is often used to make disposable containers. Borosilicate glass is usually of high thermal resistance and does not react with most chemicals. *Pyrex* and *Kimax* are brands of borosilicate glass commonly used for beakers, flasks, and other labware.

### Plastic

Plastic containers are useful because they are impact- and corrosion-resistant. Plastics do not release ions as some glass does, but may bind and release (leach)

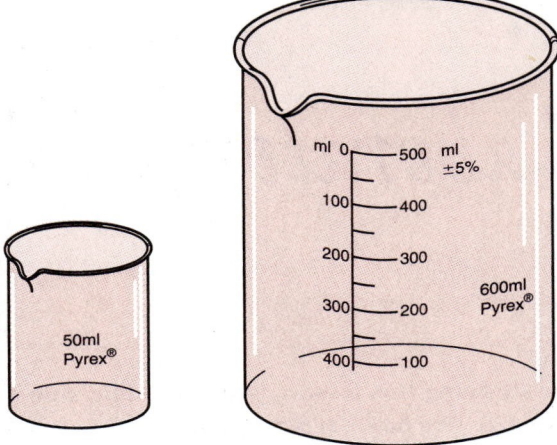

**FIGURE 1-32** Beakers with markings

solutes. Plastics are unaffected by most aqueous solutions. Two common plastics used to make labware are polyethylene, which is inexpensive and usually disposable, and polypropylene, which is sterilizable.

## GENERAL LABWARE

Basic laboratory glassware includes bottles, beakers, flasks, test tubes, graduated cylinders, and pipets.

### Bottles

Reagent bottles are available in a variety of sizes and types. Plastic bottles should be used for all reagents that do not interact with plastic. The bottle should not be much larger than the volume of reagent. Brown bottles, both glass and plastic, can be used for storing light-sensitive reagents.

### Beakers

Beakers are wide-mouthed, straight-sided containers with a pouring spout formed from the rim (Figure 1-32). They are useful for *estimating* the amount of liquids or mixing solutions, or for simply holding liquids. Each beaker is labeled to indicate the approximate capacity in milliliters (mL). Many beakers have additional markings to indicate volume increments of 10 mL to 100 mL (Figure 1-32). Beakers have many functions in a laboratory, but they must be used only for **noncritical**, or estimated, measurements.

### Flasks

Three commonly used flasks are Erlenmeyer, Florence, and volumetric (Figure 1-33). The *Erlenmeyer flask* has a flat bottom and sloping sides that gradually narrow in

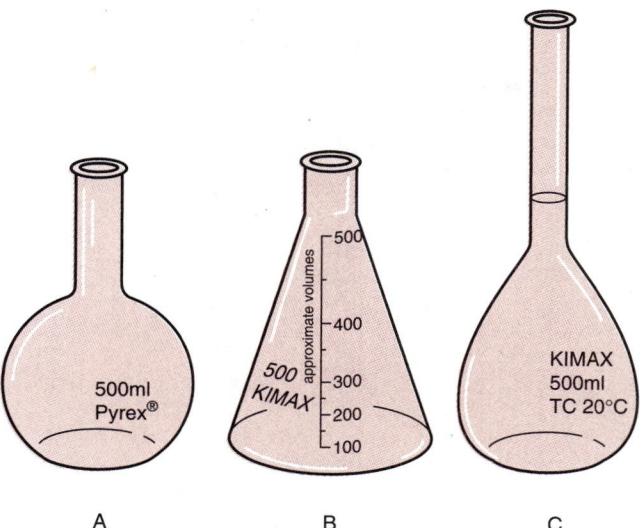

**FIGURE 1-33** (A) Florence flask, (B) Erlenmeyer flask, and (C) volumetric flask

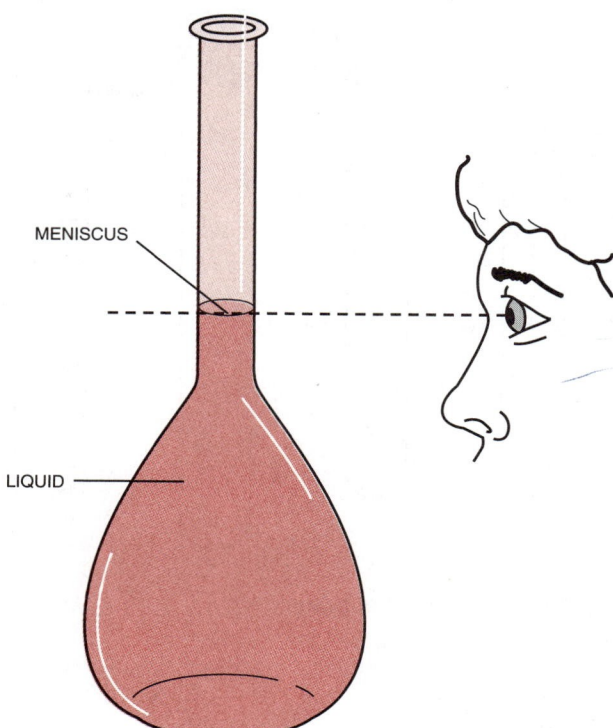

**FIGURE 1-34** Observing the meniscus at the fill line of a volumetric flask

diameter so the top opening is bottle-like. The opening may be plain, so it can be stoppered with a cork, or it may have threads for a cap. Erlenmeyer flasks range from 10 mL to 4000 mL capacity. They may be used to hold liquids, mix solutions, or measure noncritical volumes. Markings on the side indicate the capacity in mL. In addition, some also have 50 mL to 100 mL increment marks. These are called "graduated flasks" and are convenient for estimating volumes or making noncritical measurements.

The *Florence flask* has a flat bottom and rounded sides that give rise to a long cylindrical neck. The only marking is the total capacity in milliliters. These flasks usually range in size from 50 to 2000 mL capacity. The uses of the Florence flask are similar to those of beakers and Erlenmeyer flasks. Only noncritical measurements are made in a Florence flask.

The *volumetric flask* is a pear-shaped flask used for making **critical measurements**, which require accuracy. Volumetric flasks are manufactured to strict standards and guaranteed to contain a certain volume at a particular temperature. The capacity (in mL) is marked on the flask. A line is etched in the neck of the flask to indicate the appropriate fill level. Volumetric flasks are used to prepare solutions when concentration accuracy is important. Water or another **solvent** is placed in the flask. An exact amount of **solute** is measured into the flask. The remaining solvent is then added until it approaches the fill line. The last portion is added slowly until the lowest point of the **meniscus**, or curved liquid surface, is level with the fill line when viewed at eye level (Figure 1-34).

## Test Tubes

Test tubes are available in a variety of sizes and shapes and are used in many laboratory procedures (Figure 1-35). Test tubes function as containers for blood, urine, or serum. In some procedures, the analysis is performed in the test tube. Sometimes a test method requires that the contents be heated in the test tube. This should be done with caution, using only a test tube made of heat-resistant glass.

## Graduated Cylinders

A graduated cylinder is an upright, straight-sided container with a flared base that provides stability. Graduated cylinders are used to make noncritical volume measurements (Figure 1-36) and are commonly used to measure the volume of 24-hour urine specimens.

Graduated cylinders are available in capacities ranging from 5 to 2000 mL. Markings on the side indicate the total capacity and various increments in milliliters. Liquids are measured in a graduated cylinder by pouring the liquid into the cylinder until the bottom (low point) of the meniscus is level with the desired volume mark.

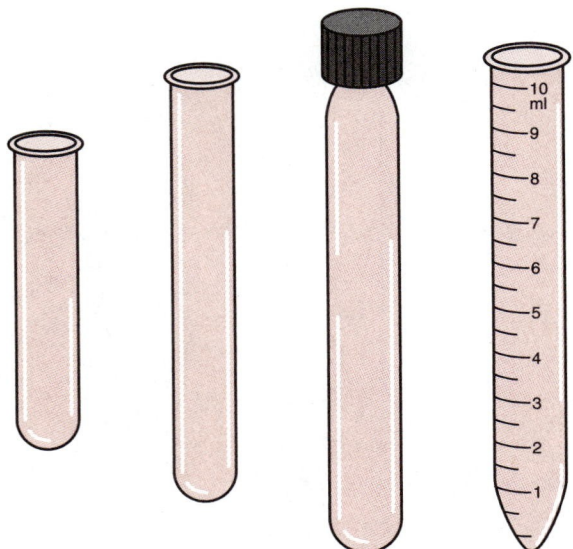

**FIGURE 1-35** Test tubes

## Pipets

Pipets are used often in laboratory work to measure and transfer liquids. Two basic types are volumetric or transfer pipets and graduated or measuring pipets (Figure 1-37).

### Volumetric Pipets

Volumetric pipets are tubes with a wide opening on the upper end, an oval bulb in the center, and a tapered tip on the other end. These are usually labeled **TD**, which indicates that they are manufactured *to deliver* a specified volume of liquid in a certain time period. They are used whenever the accuracy of a transferred volume is critical.

    To use a volumetric pipet, a pipet bulb or pipetter is attached to the upper end. The liquid is suctioned up into the pipet to the marking on the stem above the center bulb. The outside of the pipet stem is wiped dry with tissue. The pipet is held nearly vertical, and the tip is placed against the inner surface of the container into

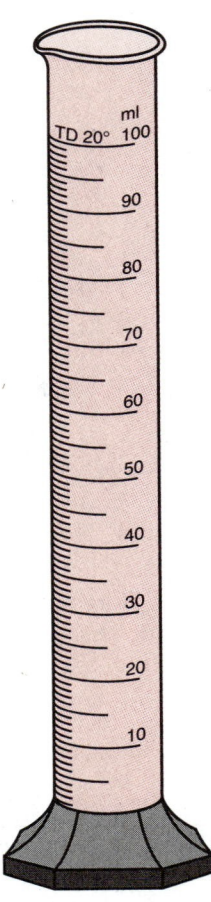

**FIGURE 1-36** Graduated cylinder with markings

which the liquid is to be transferred. The suction is released and the liquid is allowed to flow into the container. The tip is left in contact with the container surface a few seconds to completely drain the pipet. (A small drop will remain in the pipet tip.)

### Graduated Pipets

Graduated pipets are long tubes with a total capacity marking near the top. Graduated pipets are usually labeled TD. They may have a frosted band around the

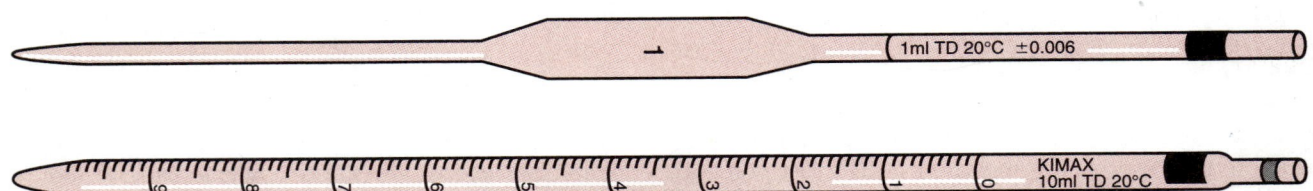

**FIGURE 1-37** Pipets: volumetric pipet (top); serological pipet (bottom)

top; this indicates that the last drop of liquid is forced out after the contents are drained. Pipets without a frosted band are used like volumetric pipets.

Graduated pipets are graduated to the tip, with markings indicating uniform increments. Graduated pipets may be used to transfer total capacity or partial volume. One commonly used graduated pipet is the serological pipet, which is usually marked TD and has a frosted band.

To use a serological pipet, a pipet bulb or pipetting device is attached (Figures 1-38 and 1-27). The liquid is suctioned up to the line as with the volumetric pipet. The pipet's outside stem is wiped dry with tissue. To deliver the total volume from the pipet, the liquid is allowed to drain out while the pipet is held almost vertically. The last remaining drops are forced out using the pipetting aid.

## Micropipets

In laboratory work, it is often necessary to accurately measure or transfer very small volumes. Micropipets, which can be calibrated for 0.5 mL or less, are available for this purpose. Micropipets may be of a semi-automated type. These can be preset to draw up and dispense a specific volume. They may also be of the manual type in which the sample is drawn up to a certain mark. Micropipets are often labeled **TC** (to contain). This means they must be rinsed to dispense the stated volume of the pipet.

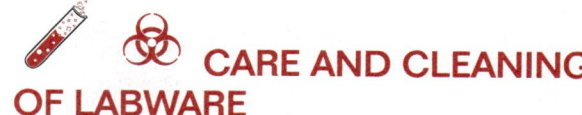

# CARE AND CLEANING OF LABWARE

Good-quality labware is expensive and must be handled with care. Clean glassware should be stored where it will be protected from dust and accidental breakage.

## Cleaning Labware

Disposable labware is intended to be used once and then discarded. Other labware must be cleaned properly after each use. For test results to be accurate, all labware must be free from chemical residues, detergents, or contaminating solutions.

The majority of cleaning problems can be avoided if labware is rinsed with water immediately after use and soaked in a mild detergent solution until it can be washed. Dried substances in containers are difficult to remove, but stubborn deposits can usually be removed by soaking the container in a laboratory detergent such as MICRO® or Cytoclean™ overnight. Before washing labware contaminated with biological fluids or specimens, it must be soaked in a disinfectant solution.

Glassware should be washed in a good laboratory detergent, using a brush if necessary, and rinsed thoroughly. Several tap-water rinses followed by two to three distilled-water rinses are sufficient in most instances.

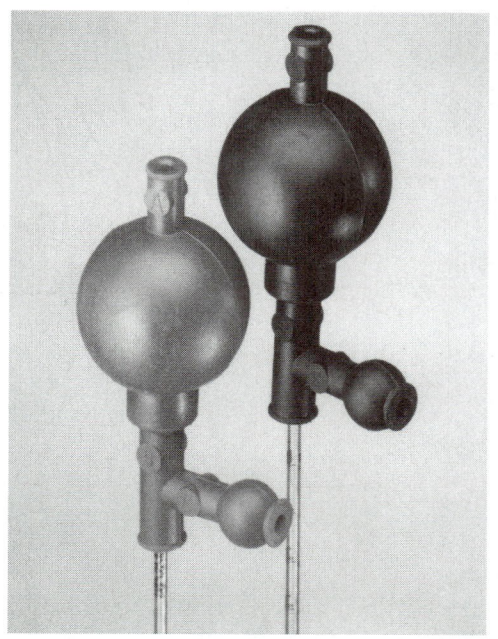 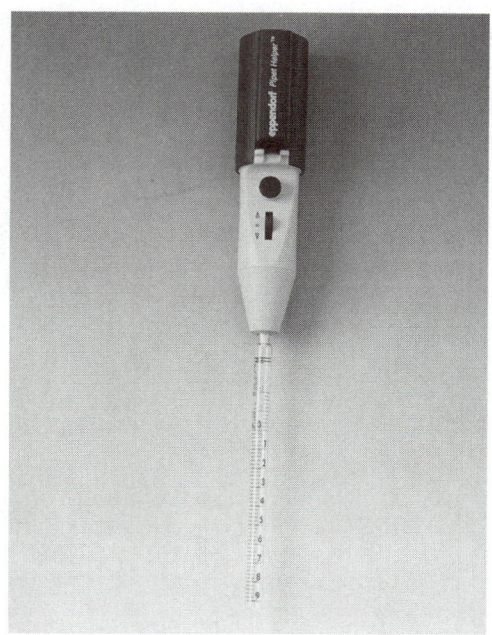

**FIGURE 1-38** Pipetting bulbs (left) and a pipetting device (right) (Photos courtesy of Fisher Scientific)

However, some sensitive test procedures require up to twelve distilled-water rinses.

Labware may be washed by hand or in an automatic dishwasher. Gloves must be worn when hand-washing labware. Pipets are best washed in a pipet washer. After washing, labware may be dried in a drying rack or a drying oven.

## Acid Cleaning

Persistent problems may require using an acid cleaning solution while wearing gloves, an apron, and a face shield. This can be a dangerous procedure and must not be attempted by a student.

### Procedural Notes

- Use the correct glassware for the task.
- Always use clean, dry glassware for measurements.
- Use a clean, dry pipet for each measurement.
- Rinse or soak glassware immediately after use.
- Do not use pipets with broken or chipped tips.

### Safety Precautions

- Wear appropriate PPE when handling labware containing blood or OPIM
- Disinfect glassware exposed to blood or OPIM before cleaning.
- Inspect beakers, flasks, and cylinders for chips and cracks before using.

## LESSON REVIEW

1. Name four types of containers used to hold liquids.
2. Name three types of laboratory flasks.
3. Which pieces of glassware are used to make critical measurements?
4. Name two types of glass pipets and explain the differences between them.
5. The last drop is forced out of which type of pipet?
6. Why is it important to immediately rinse labware after use?
7. Why must glassware be handled with care?
8. What are volumetric flasks most often used for?
9. Why is it important that labware be rinsed until it is free of detergent?
10. How do flint glass and borosilicate glass differ?
11. Define critical measurements, meniscus, noncritical measurements, reagent, solute, solvent, TC, and TD.

## STUDENT ACTIVITIES

1. Reread the information on laboratory glassware.
2. Review the glossary terms.
3. Measure 100 mL of water in a beaker and transfer it to another beaker or flask. Does it measure 100 mL in the second container?
4. Measure 100 mL of water in an Erlenmeyer flask and transfer it to a 100 mL volumetric flask. Is the volume exactly 100 mL?
5. Practice dispensing volumes from volumetric and serological pipets.
6. Practice filling a graduated cylinder to various levels and reading the meniscus.

# The Microscope

## LESSON OBJECTIVES

After studying this lesson, you should be able to:

- *Locate and name the parts of a microscope.*
- *Explain the function of each part of the microscope.*
- *Explain the use of coarse and fine adjustments.*
- *Use the low-power objective to view a specimen.*
- *Use the high-power objective to view a specimen.*
- *Use the oil-immersion objective to view a specimen.*
- *Adjust the condenser and diaphragm.*
- *Clean the oculars and objectives.*
- *Explain the proper care and storage of the microscope.*
- *Define the glossary terms.*

## GLOSSARY

**binocular** / having two oculars or eyepieces

**coarse adjustment** / control that adjusts position of microscope objectives; used to initially bring objects into focus

**condenser** / apparatus located below the microscope stage that directs light into the objective

**eyepiece** / ocular

**fine adjustment** / control that adjusts position of microscope objectives; used to sharpen focus

**iris diaphragm** / device that regulates the amount of light striking the specimen being viewed through the microscope

**lens** / a curved transparent material that spreads or focuses light

**lens paper** / a special nonabrasive material used to clean optical lenses

**microscope arm** / the portion of the microscope that connects the lenses to the base

**microscope base** / the portion of the microscope that rests on the table and supports it

**monocular** / having one ocular or eyepiece

**nosepiece** / revolving unit to which microscope objectives are attached

**objective** / magnifying lens closest to the object being viewed with a microscope

**ocular** / eyepiece of the microscope, containing a magnifying lens

**parfocal** / having objectives that may be interchanged without varying the instrument's focus

**resolving power** / the ability of a microscope to distinguish between two separate but adjacent objects; resolution

**stage** / platform that holds the object to be viewed microscopically

**working distance** / distance between the microscope objective and the microscope slide when the object is in sharp focus

## INTRODUCTION

Microscopes are used in many clinical laboratory departments to view structures or cells too small to be seen with the naked eye. The microscope is used to evaluate stained blood smears and tissue sections, perform cell counts, examine urine sediment, observe cellular reactions, and observe and interpret smears containing microorganisms.

The microscopist must be skilled in using the microscope if maximum information is to be gained from studying prepared slides. Because the microscope is a delicate, expensive instrument, special care must be taken in its use, cleaning, and storage.

## THE CLINICAL MICROSCOPE

The compound bright-field microscope is the type used in most clinical laboratories. A compound microscope has two lens systems. The **lens** system nearest the eyes is in the **ocular (eyepiece)**. The other lens system is in the **objective**, which is nearest the object being viewed. Bright-field microscopes are well suited for viewing stained specimens, such as stained blood smears.

## PARTS OF THE CLINICAL MICROSCOPE

Microscope design may differ slightly from one model to another. However, some parts are common to all microscopes. Figure 1-39 shows a monocular microscope and Figure 1-40 shows a binocular microscope with the parts labeled.

### Oculars

A microscope may be **monocular** or **binocular**. Monocular microscopes have only one eyepiece. These microscopes are inexpensive; for this reason, they are

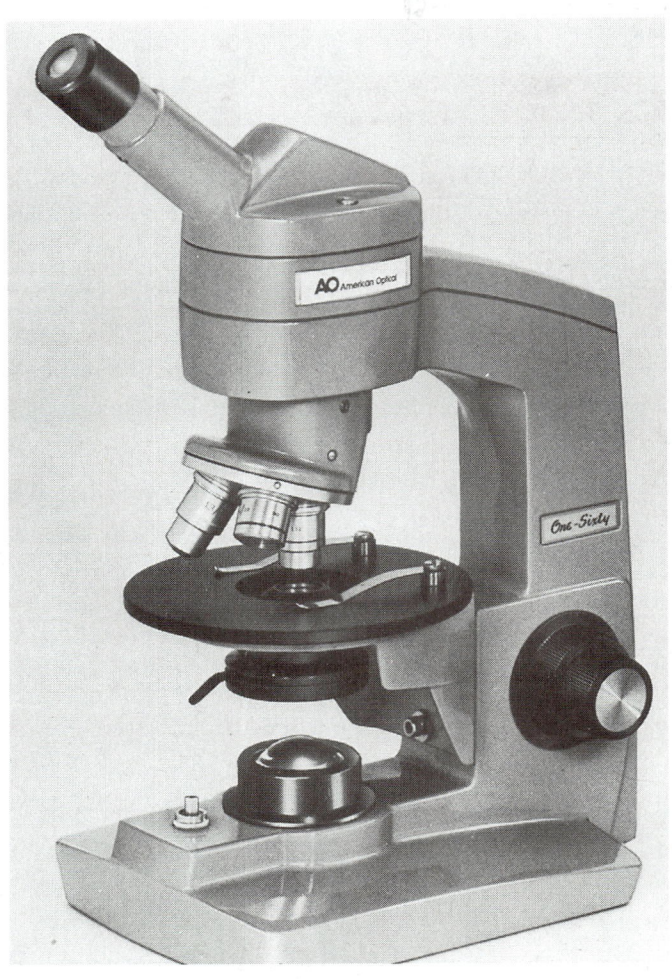

**FIGURE 1-39**  Monocular microscope (Photo courtesy of Reichert Scientific Instruments)

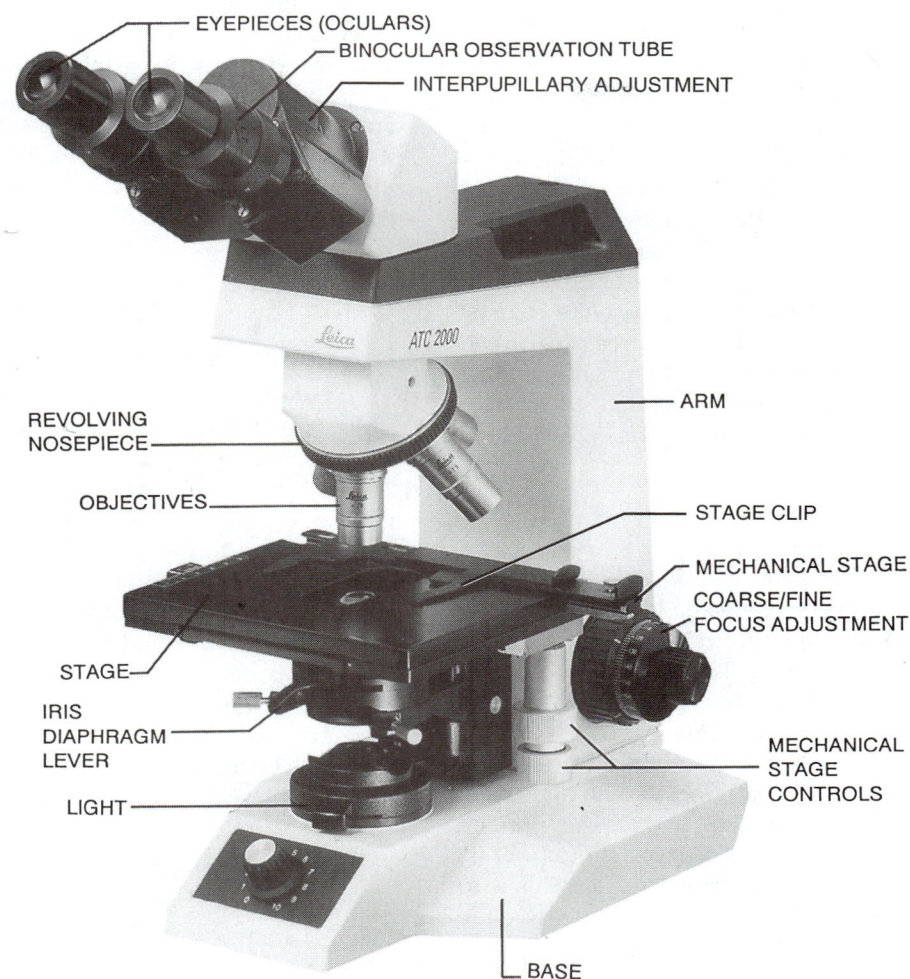

EYEPIECES (OCULARS)
BINOCULAR OBSERVATION TUBE
INTERPUPILLARY ADJUSTMENT
ARM
REVOLVING NOSEPIECE
OBJECTIVES
STAGE CLIP
MECHANICAL STAGE
COARSE/FINE FOCUS ADJUSTMENT
STAGE
IRIS DIAPHRAGM LEVER
LIGHT
MECHANICAL STAGE CONTROLS
BASE

**FIGURE 1-40** Binocular microscope with parts labeled (Photo courtesy of Leica, Inc., Buffalo, NY)

frequently used in schools. However, most people find it difficult to use them without eyestrain. Binocular microscopes have two eyepieces to allow viewing with both eyes, which results in less eyestrain.

The oculars, or eyepieces, located at the top of the microscope, are attached to a barrel or tube connected to the **microscope arm**. The oculars, through which the object is viewed, contain lenses that magnify objects. The usual magnification is ten times (10X), but oculars are also available in 15X and 20X.

## Objectives

The underside of the arm contains a revolving **nosepiece** to which the objectives are attached. Most microscopes have at least three objectives or magnifying lenses: the low-power objective, which magnifies x 10; the high-power objective, which magnifies x 40, 43, or

45; and the oil-immersion objective, which magnifies x 95, 97, or 100. Each objective is marked with color-coded bands and the power of magnification.

To determine the degree of magnification, multiply the magnification listed on the ocular (usually 10X) by the magnification listed on the objective being used. For example, an object viewed with a 10X ocular and high-power (43X) objective would be magnified 430 times (430X). An object viewed with a 10X ocular and the oil-immersion objective (97X) would be magnified 970 times. However, there is a limit to the degree of magnification that can be obtained with a microscope and still yield a clear image. The ability of a microscope to distinguish between two separate but closely spaced details in the object being viewed is called its **resolving power**. The resolving power is determined by the quality of the objective lenses.

## Light Source, Condenser, and Diaphragm

The arm of the microscope connects the objectives and eyepiece(s) to the **microscope base**, which supports the microscope. The base also contains the light or mirror, which supplies light to the object viewed. The light or mirror has a movable condenser and iris diaphragm located above it. The **condenser** focuses or directs the available light into the objective as it is raised or lowered. Lowering the condenser will increase the contrast of unstained specimens. The **iris diaphragm**, located in the condenser unit, regulates the amount of light that strikes the object being viewed (much like the shutter of a camera). The iris diaphragm may be adjusted by a movable lever.

## Coarse and Fine Adjustments

The two focusing knobs may also be located just above the base. The **coarse adjustment** is used to focus with the low-power objective only. The **fine adjustment** is used to give a sharper image after the object is brought into view with the coarse adjustment. The **working distance** is the distance between the objective and the slide when the object is in sharp focus. The higher the magnification of the objective, the shorter the working distance will be. The coarse adjustment should *not* be used when using the higher magnifications. This is to prevent the objective from accidentally striking the slide and becoming damaged.

## Stage

The stage of the microscope is supported by the arm and is located between the nosepiece and the light source. The **stage** serves as the support for the object being viewed (usually a prepared microscope slide) and has a stage clip to keep the slide stationary. Some stages can be moved by using knobs located just below the stage. These move the stage left and right or backward and forward. Other stages are fixed (immovable) so the slide must be moved manually to view different areas.

## USING THE CLINICAL MICROSCOPE

### Adjusting Oculars on Binocular Microscopes

The oculars of binocular microscopes must be adjusted for each individual's eyes. The distance between the oculars (*interpupillary distance*) should be adjusted (as

when using binoculars) so that one image is seen. The object is then brought into sharp focus with the coarse and fine adjustments, while looking through the right ocular with the right eye. The right eye is then closed and the knurled collar on the left ocular is used to bring the object into sharp focus while viewing the object through the left ocular with the left eye. This is called the *dioptic adjustment*.

## Using the Objectives

### Low-Power Objective

The low-power objective is used for initially locating objects and for viewing large objects. A slide is secured, specimen side up, on the stage with the clips. The low-power objective is rotated into position, and the microscope light is turned on. The coarse adjustment is used to bring the objective and the slide as close together as possible. Then, while looking through the ocular, the coarse adjustment is used to move the objective and slide apart until the objects on the slide come into focus. (In some microscopes, the coarse adjustment raises and lowers the objectives. In other microscopes, the stage is raised and lowered when the coarse adjustment is turned.) A clearer image is then achieved by focusing with the fine adjustment.

### High-Power Objective

The high-power (40X) objective is used when greater magnification is needed. The high-power objective is used in procedures such as cell counts and viewing urine sediments. After initial focusing with the low-power objective, the high-power objective is carefully rotated into position. The fine adjustment is used to bring the object into sharp focus. Most microscopes are **parfocal** and therefore require only slight changes in the fine adjustment. *Use only the fine adjustment when using the higher power objectives.*

### Oil-Immersion Objective

The oil-immersion objective is used to view stained blood cells, tissue sections, and stained slides containing microorganisms. This objective gives the highest magnification of all bright-field objectives. After initial focusing with low power, the objective is slightly rotated to the side. A drop of immersion oil is placed on the slide directly over the condenser. The oil-immersion objective is then carefully rotated into the drop of oil, taking care not to allow any other objective to contact the oil (the oil-immersion objective is *always* used with oil). The fine adjustment is used to focus the object. *The coarse adjustment should not be used when the oil immersion objective is in position. Immersion oil should never be used on any objective other than the one marked oil immersion.*

When the slide has been examined, the low-power objective is rotated into position and the slide is removed from the stage. All oil should be cleaned from the objective (and stage and condenser if necessary) with **lens paper**.

## Adjusting the Light

Proper light is crucial to good microscopy. The condenser and diaphragm must be adjusted according to the objective being used and the type of specimen being observed.

When viewing objects using the low-power objective, the condenser may need to be lowered somewhat to reduce the brightness of the light. The condenser should also be lowered and the iris diaphragm adjusted when viewing unstained specimens, such as urine sediments or cell dilutions to be counted, with high-power objectives. This provides more contrast between the constituents being viewed and the background.

The condenser should be raised and the diaphragm opened when viewing most stained preparations with the high-power objective. When viewing specimens such as stained blood smears with the oil-immersion objective, the condenser should be raised until it is almost touching the bottom of the slide. The diaphragm should be completely open to provide maximum light.

## OTHER TYPES OF MICROSCOPES

The clinical microscope described in this lesson uses bright-field microscopy to view objects. However, some specimens may be better viewed using other types of microscopy.

## Phase-Contrast Microscope

The phase-contrast microscope provides a way of viewing unstained cells, which are transparent. By using special objectives and a special condenser, clinical microscopes can be equipped for phase contrast. This is useful for viewing unstained specimens such as urine sediments and for performing platelet counts using the hemacytometer. In phase contrast, the background (field) appears dark and the specimen is bright.

## Epifluorescence Microscope

The epifluorescence microscope enables objects that have been stained with fluorescent dyes to be observed. When these dyes are combined with antibodies, it is possible to identify specific areas of reaction within a cell or on a cell surface. The epifluorescence microscope may be used to identify organisms such as mycobacteria and to detect the presence of antibodies in certain diseases such as syphilis and lupus erythematosus.

## Electron Microscope

The electron microscope has been used in medical research for several years, primarily in pathology and virology. The electron microscope enables objects as small as 0.001 µm (too small to be seen with light microscopes) to be viewed. The objects are visualized by using an electron beam rather than a light source. Electron microscopes are very expensive and require lengthy specimen preparation and special expertise to operate. Reference laboratories and teaching hospitals are the most likely medical locations for electron microscopes.

## CARE OF THE MICROSCOPE

### Care of Lenses

Microscope lenses should be cleaned with lens paper before and after each use. Material such as laboratory tissue should not be used because it can scratch the lenses. Lens cleaner, which is similar to a glass-cleaning solution, may be used to remove oil from objectives. It is especially important that lenses never be left with oil on them. Oil will soften the cement (glue) that holds the lens in the objective.

### Transporting the Microscope

A microscope should be left in a permanent position on a sturdy lab table where it will not get jarred. However, if the microscope must be moved, it should be held securely, with one hand supporting the base and the other holding the arm (Figure 1-41). The microscope should be placed gently to avoid jarring.

### Microscope Storage

When the microscope is not being used, it should be left with the low-power objective in position and the nosepiece in the lowest position. The stage should be centered so that it does not project from either side of the microscope. The microscope should be stored under a plastic dust cover.

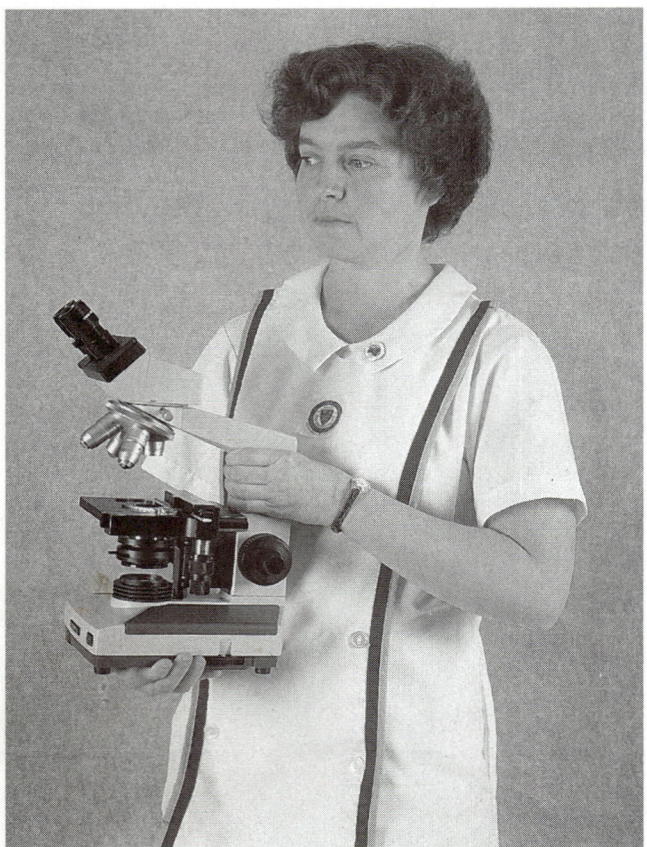

**FIGURE 1-41** Illustration of the proper way to carry a microscope

## Procedural Notes

■ Store the covered microscope in a protected area.

■ Avoid jarring or bumping the microscope.

■ Transport the microscope with one hand under the base and the other hand gripping the arm.

■ Clean all oculars and objectives with lens paper before and after each use.

■ Use the coarse adjustment with the low-power objective only.

■ Use immersion oil with the oil-immersion objective only.

## Safety Precautions

■ Use Universal and Standard Precautions when examining biological materials microscopically.

■ Clean the microscope stage with a surface disinfectant after examining fluid samples such as urine sediment.

■ Unplug the microscope before attempting to replace the bulb or perform any electrical repair.

## LESSON REVIEW

1. Explain the functions of the iris diaphragm and condenser. Supply amt of light

2. Name the three objectives commonly used on a clinical microscope. Low, high and Oil Immersion objectives

3. Explain the uses of the course and fine adjustments. Bring obj. to focus 2 to sharpen focus.

4. What is the proper method of cleaning a microscope after use? lense cleaner

5. How should a microscope be stored when not in use? low power objective, centre stage cover plastic cover.

6. When is the oil-immersion objective used? stain blood cell,

7. When is immersion oil used on a slide?

8. Explain how to adjust the interpupillary distance on a binocular microscope. individually

9. What is the purpose of making a dioptic adjustment? Explain how the adjustment is made.

10. Define binocular, coarse adjustment, condenser, eyepiece, fine adjustment, iris diaphragm, lens, lens paper, microscope arm, microscope base, monocular, nosepiece, objective, ocular, parfocal, resolving power, stage, and working distance.

## STUDENT ACTIVITIES

1. Reread the information on the microscope.

2. Review the glossary terms.

3. Locate and identify the parts of a microscope.

4. Practice using a microscope following the procedure outlined in the Student Performance Guide.

# *Student Performance Guide*

## **LESSON 1-10** The Microscope

Name _____ Date _____

### INSTRUCTIONS

1. Practice using the microscope following the step-by-step procedure.
2. Show your understanding of this lesson by:
   a. Completing a written examination successfully, and
   b. Demonstrating the proper use of the microscope satisfactorily for the instructor. All steps must be completed as listed on the instructor's Performance Check Sheet.

*Note:* Procedure will vary slightly according to microscope design. Consult operating procedure in microscope manual for specific instructions.

### MATERIALS AND EQUIPMENT

- hand disinfectant
- microscope (monocular or binocular)
- lens paper
- lens cleaner
- prepared slides (commercially available)
- immersion oil
- surface disinfectant

### PROCEDURE

Record in the comment section any problems encountered while practicing the procedure (or have a fellow student or the instructor evaluate the performance).

S = Satisfactory
U = Unsatisfactory

| You must: | S | U | Comments |
|---|---|---|---|
| 1. Wash hands | | | |
| 2. Assemble equipment and materials | | | |
| 3. Clean the ocular(s) and objectives with lens paper | | | |
| 4. Use the coarse adjustment to raise the nosepiece unit | | | |
| 5. Raise the condenser as far as possible by turning the condenser knob | | | |
| 6. Rotate the low-power (10X) objective into position, so it is directly over the opening in the stage | | | |
| 7. Turn on the microscope light. If using a mirror, position the light about ten inches in front of the microscope so it shines directly on the mirror. Adjust the mirror position so a bright light is reflected upward into the center of the condenser | | | |
| 8. Open the iris diaphragm until maximum light comes up through the condenser | | | |

| You must: | S | U | Comments |
|---|---|---|---|
| 9. Place slide on stage (specimen side up) and secure with clips. Position the condenser so it is almost touching the bottom of the slide | | | |
| 10. Locate the coarse adjustment | | | |
| 11. Look directly at the stage and low-power (10X) objective and turn the coarse adjustment until the objective is as close to the slide as it will go.  Stop turning when the objective no longer moves.<br>*Note:* Do not lower any objective toward a slide while looking through the ocular(s) | | | |
| 12. Look into the ocular(s) and slowly turn the coarse adjustment in the opposite direction (as in step 11) to raise the objective (or lower the stage) until the object on the slide comes into view | | | |
| 13. Locate the fine adjustment | | | |
| 14. Turn the fine adjustment to sharpen the image<br>*Note:* If a binocular microscope is used, the oculars must be adjusted for each individual's eyes.<br><br>a. Adjust distance between oculars so one image is seen (as when using binoculars)<br><br>b. Use coarse and fine adjustments to bring object into focus while looking through the right ocular with right eye<br><br>c. Close the right eye, look into the left ocular with left eye, and *use the knurled collar on the left ocular* to bring the object into sharp focus. (Do not turn coarse or fine adjustment at this time.)<br><br>d. Look into oculars with both eyes to observe that object is in clear focus.  If not, repeat the procedure | | | |
| 15. Scan the slide by either method:<br><br>a. Use the stage knobs to move the slide left and right and backward and forward while looking through the ocular(s), or<br><br>b. Move the slide with the fingers while looking through the ocular(s) (for microscope without movable stage) | | | |
| 16. Rotate the high-power (40X) objective into position while observing the objective and the slide to see that the objective does not strike the slide | | | |
| 17. Look through the ocular(s) to view the object on the slide; it should almost be in focus | | | |
| 18. Locate the fine adjustment | | | |
| 19. Look through the ocular(s) and turn the fine adjustment until the object is in focus.  Do not use the coarse adjustment. | | | |

| You must: | S | U | Comments |
|---|---|---|---|
| 20. Scan the slide as in step 15, using the fine adjustment if necessary to keep the object in focus | | | |
| 21. Rotate the oil-immersion objective to the side slightly (so no objective is in position) | | | |
| 22. Place one drop of immersion oil on the portion of the slide directly over the condenser | | | |
| 23. Rotate the oil-immersion objective into position, being careful not to rotate the high-power (40X) objective through the oil | | | |
| 24. Look to see that the oil-immersion objective is touching the drop of oil | | | |
| 25. Look through the ocular(s) and slowly turn the fine adjustment until the image is clear. Use only the fine adjustment to focus the oil-immersion objective | | | |
| 26. Scan the slide as in step 15 | | | |
| 27. Rotate the low-power (10X) objective into position (do not allow high-power (40X) objective to touch oil) | | | |
| 28. Remove the slide from the microscope stage and gently clean the oil from the slide with lens paper | | | |
| 29. Clean the oculars, low-power (10X) objective and high-power (40X) objective with clean lens paper | | | |
| 30. Clean the oil-immersion objective with lens paper to remove all oil | | | |
| 31. Clean any oil from the microscope stage and condenser | | | |
| 32. Turn off the microscope light and unplug the microscope | | | |
| 33. Position the nosepiece in the lowest position using the coarse adjustment | | | |
| 34. Center the stage so it does not project from either side of the microscope | | | |
| 35. Cover the microscope and return it to storage | | | |
| 36. Clean work area; return slides to storage | | | |
| 37. Wash hands | | | |

*Evaluator Comments:*

Evaluator _____ Date _____

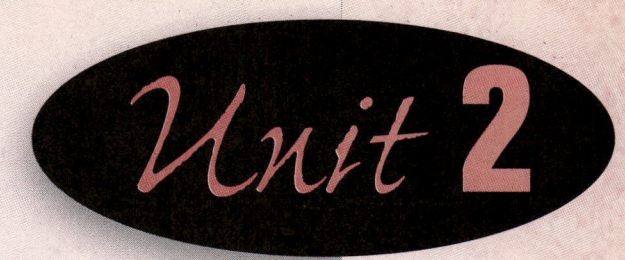

# Unit 2

# Basic Hematology

## UNIT OBJECTIVES

**After studying this unit, you should be able to:**

- *Explain the function of the hematology laboratory.*
- *Identify circulatory system components and discuss the formation of blood.*
- *Perform a capillary puncture.*
- *Perform a venipuncture.*
- *Perform a hematocrit determination.*
- *Use a hemacytometer.*
- *Perform a manual red blood cell count.*
- *Perform a manual white blood cell count.*
- *Perform a manual platelet count.*
- *Perform a hemoglobin determination.*
- *Make and stain a blood smear.*
- *Identify blood cells from a stained blood smear.*
- *Perform a differential leukocyte count.*
- *Calculate erythrocyte indices values and explain their significance.*
- *Identify selected abnormal blood cells from blood smears or from visual aids.*
- *Perform an erythrocyte sedimentation rate test.*
- *Perform a reticulocyte count.*
- *Discuss principles of hematology automation.*

## UNIT OVERVIEW

*Hematology* is the area of medicine involving the study of the cellular elements of blood and the blood-forming tissues. Unit 2 is an introduction to several basic procedures commonly performed in the hematology laboratory. The unit begins with a discussion of the discipline of hematology in Lesson 2-1, including basic information about the circulatory system, the origin of blood cells, blood composition, blood diseases, and analysis methods used in the hematology laboratory.

Lessons 2-2 and 2-3 include techniques for collecting capillary and venous blood. *Capillary puncture* is a simple procedure that can be performed when only a small blood sample is required, usually for a single test. *Venipuncture* (obtaining blood from a vein) requires more skill than capillary puncture. A properly performed venipuncture is a safe, convenient means of obtaining a blood sample from which many tests can be performed.

Information and instructions for manually performing the tests comprising the *CBC (complete blood count)*, one of the most frequently requested hematology tests, are spread over several lessons.

The CBC is a combination of tests that typically includes *hematocrit* (Lesson 2-4), *erythrocyte* and *leukocyte* counts (Lesson 2-5), *hemoglobin* (Lesson 2-7), and *leukocyte differential count* with observation of blood cell morphology (Lesson 2-9) from a stained blood smear (Lesson 2-8). Instructions for using the *hemacytometer,* a chamber for counting cells, is included in Lesson 2-5.

The *platelet* count (Lesson 2-6), although not part of the routine CBC, is included in Unit 2 following Lesson 2-5, The Hemacytometer: RBC and WBC Counts. Lesson 2-10, Morphology of Abnormal Blood Cells in Peripheral Blood, is included for those desiring more in-depth study of blood cell morphology and the causes of abnormal morphology. Lesson 2-10 also includes information on *erythrocyte indices*, calculations that estimate erythrocyte size and hemoglobin content.

The *reticulocyte* count, Lesson 2-11, is useful in evaluating the treatment and progress of anemia patients. The *reticulocyte count* gives information about the rate of red blood cell production.

The *erythrocyte sedimentation rate (ESR)*, Lesson 2-12, is a test used to follow the progress of some inflammatory disease processes. ESR results can be used with other laboratory test results to help the clinician diagnose, prescribe and evaluate treatment.

Lesson 2-13, Principles of Automated Hematology explains the theory of operating automated cell counters and hematology and coagulation analyzers. (Coagulation procedures are given in Unit 3, Basic Hemostasis.)

Examining blood in the hematology laboratory provides important information that helps in diagnosing and treating blood diseases such as anemias and leukemias. Hematology tests also help in diagnosing and managing diseases that originate in other body systems. Practice and skill are required to perform even the most basic hematology procedures in a reliable manner. The tests must be performed with accuracy, precision, and the utmost attention to proper procedure.

## SUGGESTED READINGS AND REFERENCES

Addison, L. A. & Fischer, P. M. (1990). *The office laboratory.* East Norwalk, CT: Appleton and Lange.

Brown, B. A. (6th ed.). (1993). *Hematology: Principles and procedures.* Philadelphia: Lea & Febiger.

Carr, J. H., & Rodak, B. F. (1998). *Clinical hematology atlas.* Philadelphia: W. B. Saunders Company.

Diggs, L. W., Sturm, D., & Bell, A. (5th ed.). (1988). *The morphology of human blood cells.* Abbott Park, IL: Abbott Laboratories.

Garza, D., & Becan-McBride, K. (5th ed.). (1998). *Phlebotomy handbook: Blood collection essentials.* East Norwalk, CT: Appleton and Lange.

Harmening, D. M. (Ed.). (3rd ed.). (1996). *Clinical hematology and fundamentals of hemostasis.* Philadelphia: F. A. Davis Company.

Henry, J. B. (Ed.). (19th ed.). (1996). *Clinical diagnosis & management by laboratory methods.* Philadelphia: W. B. Saunders Company.

Hoeltke, L. B. (1995). *The clinical laboratory manual series: Phlebotomy.* Albany, NY: Delmar Publishers.

Howanitz, J. H. & Howanitz, P. J. (Eds.). (1991). *Laboratory medicine test selection and interpretation.* New York: Churchill Livingstone, Inc.

Koepke, J. A. (Ed.). (1991). *Practical laboratory hematology.* New York: Churchill Livingstone Inc.

Kovanda, B. M. (1998). *Point of care testing—capillary puncture.* Albany, NY: Delmar Publishers.

Lee, R. G. et al. (10th ed.). (1998). *Wintrobe's clinical hematology.* Baltimore: Williams & Wilkins.

Lindh, W. Q., Pooler, M. S., Tamparo, C. D., & Cerrato, J. U. (1998). *Comprehensive medical assisting.* Albany, NY: Delmar Publishers.

Manufacturer's instructions, *HemoCue®,* Inc. Mission Viejo, CA.

Manufacturer's package insert, *Unopette®*, Becton Dickinson, Rutherford, NJ.

Marshall, J. (1993). *Fundamental skills for the clinical laboratory professional*. Albany, NY: Delmar Publishers.

Marshall, J. *Microbiology*. (1995). Albany, NY: Delmar Publishers.

Miale, J. B. (6th ed.). (1991). *Laboratory medicine—hematology*. St. Louis: C. V. Mosby.

Rodak, B. F. (1997). *Diagnostic hematology*. Baltimore, MD: AACC Press.

Russell, A. P. (1997). *Delmar's clinical laboratory manual series: Hematology*. Albany, NY: Delmar Publishers.

Scott, A. S. & Fong, E. (9th ed.). (1998). *Body structures & functions*. Albany, NY: Delmar Publishers.

Simmers, L. (4th ed.). (1998). *Diversified health occupations*. Albany, NY: Delmar Publishers.

Simmers, L. (4th ed.). (1998). *Diversified health occupations essentials*. Albany, NY: Delmar Publishers.

Stiene-Martin, E. A., Lotspeich-Steininger, C. A., & Koepke, J. A. (Eds.). (1998). *Clinical hematology: Principles, procedures, correlations*. Philadelphia: Lippincott-Raven Publishers.

Tilton, R. C., et al. (Eds). (1992). *Clinical laboratory medicine*. St. Louis: Mosby-Yearbook.

# Introduction to Hematology

## LESSON OBJECTIVES

**After studying this lesson, you should be able to:**

- *Discuss the origin of blood cells.*
- *Explain the differences among veins, arteries, and capillaries.*
- *List five plasma components.*
- *Name the three types of formed elements of blood and state the function of each.*
- *Name the five types of leukocytes.*
- *Name the preferred specimens for hematology tests.*
- *Explain safety precautions that must be observed in the hematology laboratory.*
- *Name the tests that make up the complete blood count (CBC).*
- *Explain how quality control (QC) in hematology differs from QC in other laboratory departments, such as clinical chemistry.*
- *Name two inherited hematological diseases.*
- *Explain what a secondary or acquired hematological disease is.*
- *Define the glossary terms.*

## GLOSSARY

**anticoagulant** / a chemical that prevents blood coagulation

**artery** / a blood vessel that carries oxygenated blood from the heart to the tissues

**capillary** / a minute blood vessel that connects the smallest arteries to the smallest veins and serves as an exchange vessel

**cardiopulmonary circulation** / the system of blood vessels that circulates blood from the heart to the lungs and back to the heart

**CBC** / complete blood count; a commonly performed group of hematological tests

**deoxyhemoglobin** / the hemoglobin formed when oxyhemoglobin releases oxygen to tissues

**EDTA** / ethylenediaminetetra-acetic acid; an anticoagulant commonly used in hematology

**erythrocyte**/ blood cell that transports oxygen ($O_2$) to tissues and carbon dioxide ($CO_2$) to the lungs; red blood cell (RBC)

**granulocyte** / a leukocyte containing granules in the cytoplasm; any of the neutrophilic, eosinophilic, or basophilic leukocytes

**hemoglobin (Hb, Hgb)** / the major functional component of red blood cells that serves as the oxygen-carrying protein

**hemopoiesis** / the process of blood cell formation and development; hematopoiesis

**hemostasis** / the process of stopping bleeding

**leukocyte** / blood cell that functions in immunity; white blood cell (WBC)

**megakaryocyte** / a large bone marrow cell from which platelets are derived

**oncologist** / a physician specializing in the study and treatment of tumors and cancers

**oxyhemoglobin** / the form of hemoglobin that binds and transports oxygen

**plasma** / the liquid portion of blood in which blood cells are suspended

**platelet** / a formed element in circulating blood that plays an important role in blood coagulation; a small disk-shaped fragment of cytoplasm derived from a megakaryocyte; a thrombocyte

**stem cell** / a primitive, undifferentiated bone marrow cell

**systemic circulation** / the system of blood vessels that carries blood from the heart to the tissues and back to the heart

**thrombocyte** / a blood platelet

**vein** /a blood vessel that carries deoxygenated blood from the tissues to the heart

## INTRODUCTION

Hematology is the branch of medicine concerned primarily with studying the formed elements of blood (blood cells) and the blood-forming tissues. The study of hemostasis, the process of stopping bleeding, is included in hematology.

The formed elements of blood are examined in the hematology laboratory. The tests may be qualitative, such as observing and recording blood cell morphology (appearance), or quantitative, such as performing leukocyte or erythrocyte counts.

Hematological tests can give important information about a patient's general well-being. The hematology laboratory also performs tests to detect and monitor treatment of anemias, leukemias, and inherited blood disorders such as hemophilia and sickle cell anemia. The effects of radiation or chemotherapy treatments for cancer can also be monitored using hematological tests.

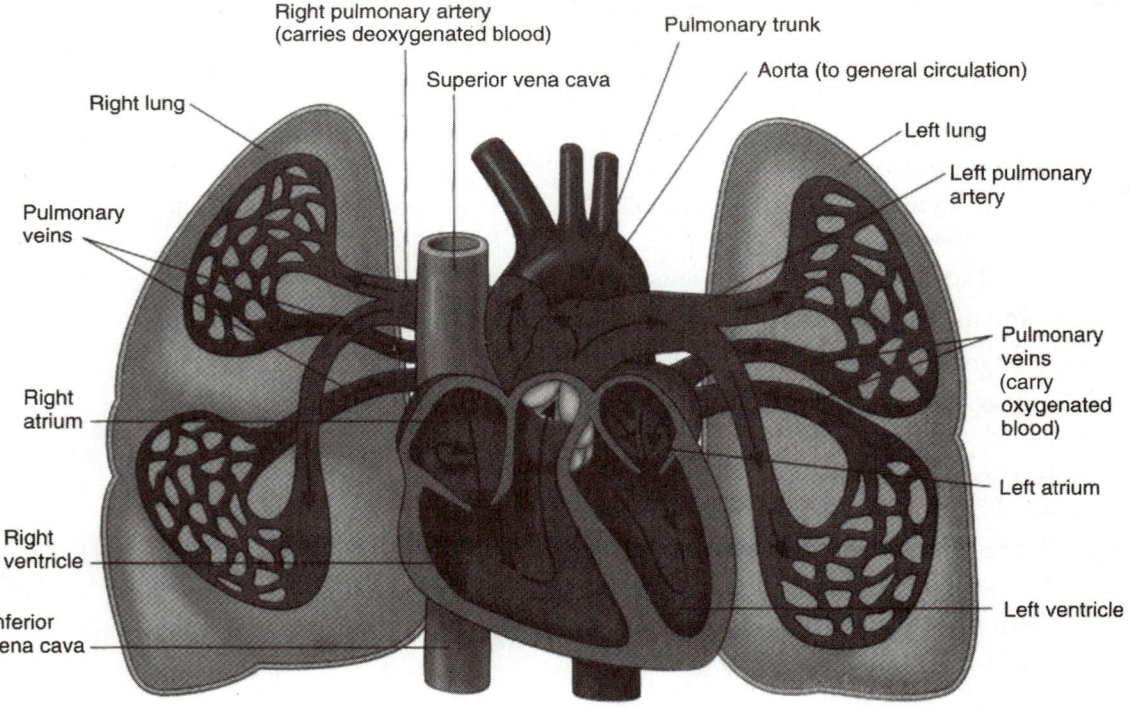

Right pulmonary artery
(carries deoxygenated blood)

Pulmonary trunk

Superior vena cava

Aorta (to general circulation)

Right lung

Left lung

Left pulmonary artery

Pulmonary veins

Pulmonary veins (carry oxygenated blood)

Right atrium

Left atrium

Right ventricle

Left ventricle

Inferior vena cava

**FIGURE 2-1** Cardiopulmonary circulation

# BLOOD VESSELS AND BLOOD CIRCULATION

## The Circulatory System

The circulatory system performs several vital functions that include delivering $O_2$, nutrients, water, and hormones to tissues and cells; removing $CO_2$ and waste products from tissues and cells; regulating body temperature; and protecting against infection. These functions are carried out by the *blood*, the fluid that circulates through the vessels of the circulatory system and bathes the tissues.

In **cardiopulmonary circulation**, blood circulates from the heart to the lungs and back to the heart. Oxygen exchange occurs in the lungs when $O_2$ is picked up by the blood and $CO_2$ is released (Figure 2-1). In **systemic circulation**, blood is carried from the heart to the tissues and back to the heart, providing $O_2$ to tissues and cells in exchange for $CO_2$, a waste product (Figure 2-2).

## Types of Blood Vessels

Blood is circulated by three major types of vessels: arteries, capillaries, and veins. There are about 60,000 miles of blood vessels in an adult human. In general, arteries carry oxygenated blood and veins carry deoxygenated blood.

**Arteries** are thick-walled, elastic, and muscular and are the strongest type of blood vessel. The aorta is the largest artery in the body. Blood flows from the heart through the aorta into a series of successively smaller arteries and arterioles (small arteries) that eventually diverge to form a network of capillaries (Figure 2-3).

**Capillaries** are the smallest of the blood vessels and connect the smallest arterioles with small veins called venules (Figure 2-3). Because capillaries have thin walls, fluid, nutrients, and wastes easily pass through these walls to or from the tissue cells.

**Veins** carry deoxygenated blood from the capillaries to the heart. Capillaries expand into venules, and then into veins that eventually converge to larger and larger vessels and form the largest vein, the vena cava. The walls of veins are not as thick, muscular, or elastic as those of arteries. Veins have valves that allow blood flow in only one direction—toward the heart.

# COMPOSITION OF BLOOD

Blood makes up 6–8% of total body weight. A normal adult's blood volume is approximately five liters, or ten times the volume of a blood donor unit. Blood is composed of cellular elements suspended in a fluid, plasma. About 50–60% of blood volume is plasma; the rest is mostly red blood cells.

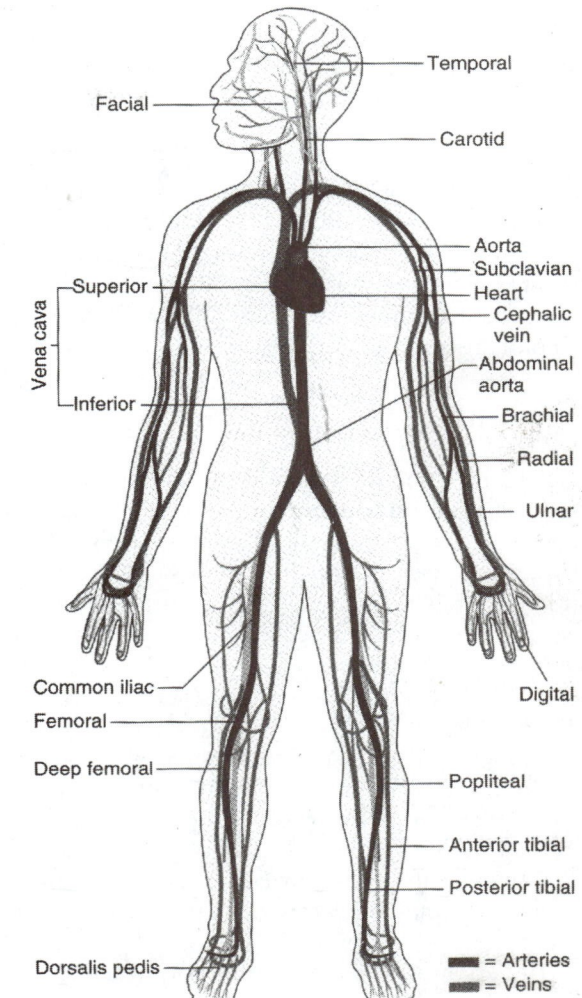

**FIGURE 2-2** Systemic circulation

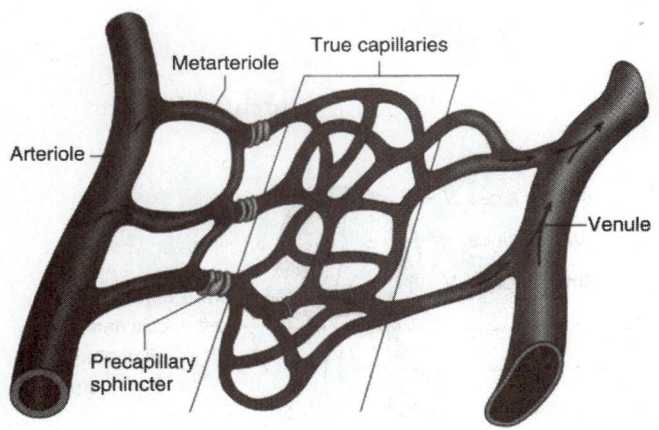

**FIGURE 2-3** Capillary bed connecting an arteriole with a venule

## Plasma

**Plasma** is a complex solution in which the blood cells are suspended. Plasma is more than 90% water; the remainder is dissolved solids such as proteins, lipids, carbohydrates, amino acids, antibodies, hormones, and electrolytes. Most of these substances are measured in the clinical chemistry department. Plasma also contains fibrinogen and the other blood-coagulation proteins. These are proenzymes that, upon activation, initiate reactions resulting in formation of a fibrin clot. Blood-coagulation proteins are necessary for normal blood clotting.

## Cellular Elements of Blood

The cellular elements of blood are commonly called blood cells. These include **erythrocytes**, or red blood cells (RBCs); **leukocytes**, or white blood cells (WBCs); and **platelets**, also called **thrombocytes** (Figure 2-4). Most hematology tests are designed to evaluate or measure a characteristic or function of one or more of the three blood cell types.

### Erythrocytes

Erythrocytes are the most numerous blood cells (Figure 2-4). Each microliter (µL) of blood contains approximately five million red blood cells; that means one drop of blood contains about 250 million red cells! Erythrocytes in the blood live an average of 120 days and remain in the circulatory system's vessels for their entire life span.

The erythrocyte's main function is to transport $O_2$ to the tissues and $CO_2$ to the lungs. This is actually performed by hemoglobin molecules, the major component of erythrocytes. Hemoglobin gives blood its red color. Arterial blood is bright red because of the **oxyhemoglobin** (hemoglobin that has bound $O_2$) and venous blood is dark red because of the presence of deoxyhemoglobin (hemoglobin that has released $O_2$).

### Leukocytes

Leukocytes are the least numerous blood cells. Approximately 5,000-10,000 leukocytes are in each microliter of blood.

Five types of leukocytes are present in normal blood: *neutrophils*, *basophils*, *eosinophils*, *lymphocytes*, and *monocytes* (Figure 2-4). The neutrophils, basophils, and eosinophils are called **granulocytes** because of granules present in the cell cytoplasm.

Leukocytes have varied life spans, from a few days to several years. Each type of leukocyte has unique functions, but all are associated with immunity or defense from infection. Leukocytes spend most of their lives, and perform their functions, in the tissues. They only use blood as a means of transport from one part of the body to another.

### Platelets

**Platelets** are not actually whole cells, but are fragments of cytoplasm that have been released into circulating blood from large cells in the bone marrow (Figure 2-4). These large bone marrow cells are called **megakaryocytes**. Platelets average about 200,000 per microliter of blood and live about ten days once they enter the bloodstream.

Platelets are important in several stages of hemostasis. They help stop bleeding by forming a plug in injured or damaged vessel walls. They also release chemicals or enzymes that are important in another stage of hemostasis, the coagulation cascade.

## ORIGIN OF BLOOD CELLS

**Hemopoiesis** (hematopoiesis) is the formation and development of blood cells. In the young fetus, blood cells are made in the fetal liver. As the fetus develops, the bone marrow begins to take over this function. In adults, most of the cellular elements of blood are produced in the bone marrow. Lymphocytes are produced not only in bone marrow but also in secondary lymphoid tissue such as the spleen and lymph nodes. After a period of development and maturation in the bone marrow, mature blood cells are released into the circulating blood, where they function in respiration (erythrocytes), immunity (leukocytes), and hemostasis (platelets).

Blood cells require the same basic growth factors for their synthesis as other cell types. In addition, because red blood cells are very specialized, they require iron, vitamin $B_{12}$, and folic acid for proper formation and maturation.

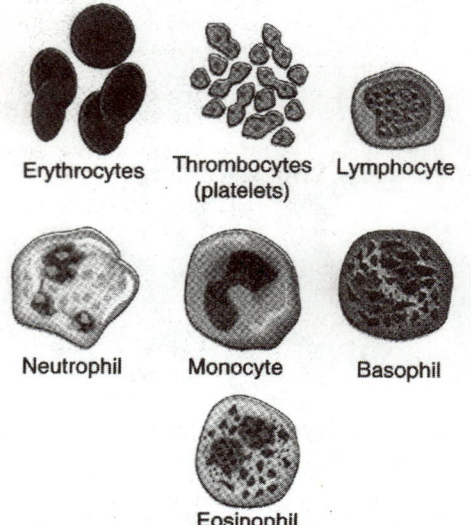

Erythrocytes  Thrombocytes (platelets)  Lymphocyte

Neutrophil  Monocyte  Basophil

Eosinophil

**FIGURE 2-4** The formed elements of blood: erythrocytes, platelets, and the five types of leukocytes

Blood cells are continuously produced throughout an individual's life. All blood cells are derived from a primitive, undifferentiated type of bone marrow cell called the *stem cell*. Stem cells continuously replicate and differentiate into all of the blood cell types.

Stem cell transplants are a valuable treatment for many disorders. Bone marrow transplants are performed in leukemia, aplastic anemia, and chemotherapy patients to give them new stem cells that will produce new normal blood cells. A few years ago, it was discovered that blood from newborns' umbilical cords is rich in these stem cells. Because cord blood is routinely collected when the umbilical cord is cut at birth, it is providing an exciting new donor source of stem cells that can be used as a substitute for bone marrow transplants.

## HEMATOLOGICAL DISEASES: DISORDERS OF ERYTHROCYTES, LEUKOCYTES, AND PLATELETS

Many diseases involve primarily the blood cells. Some of these diseases are caused by improper or insufficient production of a cell type. For instance, in *leukemia*, white cell production is out of control and too many cells are produced. In *anemia*, red cell numbers are too low, which could be due to decreased red cell production, such as might be seen when a person has an iron deficiency. Anemia can also result when blood is lost faster than the bone marrow can produce cells, as when a person has a bleeding ulcer. *Thrombocytopenia*, or low platelet count, which can be caused by viral infections or drug interactions, can result in bleeding tendencies.

Hematological diseases may also be due to defective cell function. Often, a disease may be due to a combination of improper cell production and defective function, as with most anemias and leukemias. For example, in iron-deficiency anemia, the patient has too few red blood cells which function improperly because they do not contain enough hemoglobin. This causes fatigue, pallor, and shortness of breath, typical symptoms of anemia caused by decreased $O_2$ available to the tissues. In leukemia, although the patient has many leukocytes, the cells have not matured properly and cannot provide immunity. The patient may then be highly susceptible to infections, even though the WBC count is high.

### Inherited Hematological Diseases

Some hematological diseases, such as *hemophilia*, may be inherited. Hemophiliacs have bleeding problems because they either lack one of the coagulation factors required for blood to clot or one of the coagulation factors is defective. In other inherited hematological dis-

eases, patients have abnormal hemoglobin function, such as that caused by the abnormal structure of hemoglobin in *sickle cell anemia*.

### Secondary or Acquired Hematological Diseases

Abnormalities in blood cells may also occur due to a condition or disease originating in another organ system. These are called secondary or acquired conditions. For example, abnormal-appearing red blood cells may be present in a patient with severe hypertension or renal failure because the cells become damaged as they circulate through small blood vessels. Diabetics may have "lazy leukocytes," which cause slow healing of wounds or infections because some white blood cells function improperly. Lymphocytes develop an "atypical" appearance in infectious mononucleosis, a viral disease. These lymphocytes can be observed when a stained blood smear is examined microscopically.

Blood cells may also be affected by treatments or medications. High doses of aspirin inhibit platelet function, a temporary condition that corrects itself after the drug is stopped. Chemotherapy treatments designed to stop the growth of cancer cells can also stop blood cell production. Patients receiving chemotherapy must have regular blood cell counts to be sure their blood cell concentrations do not fall to dangerous levels.

## THE HEMATOLOGY LABORATORY

### Methods of Analysis in the Hematology Laboratory

Routine hematology tests may be performed manually or using one of the many types of hematology analyzers available. Some are designed for small facilities such as physician office laboratories (POLs) and can perform only a few different tests. Others suitable for large laboratories are designed to perform several analyses on hundreds of samples daily. Lesson 2-13, Principles of Automated Hematology, describes the principles behind the design of hematology analyzers.

All laboratories that use hematology analyzers must also have backup systems for performing analyses in the event of instrument malfunction. Therefore, it is always advisable that personnel are trained in manual techniques for the most frequently requested tests.

  ### Safety in the Hematology Laboratory

Universal and Standard Precautions must be observed at all times in the hematology laboratory, as in any other laboratory section. Workers must observe the Bloodborne Pathogens Standard and use proper safety techniques to avoid body fluid spills, splatters, aerosol formation, or other potential exposure. Lesson 1-6 contains detailed laboratory biosafety information.

Many hematology departments are responsible for blood collection as well as hematology testing. Phlebotomists must wear gloves and other appropriate protective clothing such as fluid-resistant laboratory coats, goggles and masks. Safety shields can be used in the blood-collecting area, as well as the testing area, to protect against exposure from splashes. *Used venipuncture needles must not be recapped but must be discarded into puncture-proof biohazard containers for sharps or into needle-removal containers.* Using new, safer needles that automatically resheath or enclose the used needle will eliminate most needlestick hazards.

Hematology laboratory workers often have greater potential for exposure to bloodborne pathogens than workers in some other laboratory departments. A blood sample tube used to perform a CBC, differential, and sedimentation rate, three separate tests, may have to be opened three times, creating three potential exposure events. Instruments capable of sampling specimens through the tube stoppers can minimize this type of exposure potential.

## *Quality Assurance*

### Quality Control in Hematology

In clinical chemistry departments, *certified standards* for substances such as glucose or sodium are easily obtained. In hematology, however, standards are, for the most part, not available. A standard should be as close as possible to the substance being measured and ideally should be stable over a long period. This is not possible with blood cells, since they are living tissues. Hemoglobin is the only substance measured in the hematology laboratory for which certified standards are available. Other procedures, such as cell counts, must rely on commercial control solutions, suspensions of preserved or stabilized cells that are only stable for a few days or weeks. Because of this, many hematology procedures and instruments require more complex calibration and standardization than may be necessary in other laboratory departments.

## Specimens for Hematology Testing

Both capillary and venous blood are used for routine hematological procedures. Capillary blood obtained by skin puncture is good for procedures such as blood smears because no chemicals are added to the sample to alter cell appearance. However, since only a small sample volume is obtained by capillary puncture, tests usually cannot be repeated unless another sample is obtained.

When a larger sample is required, blood is obtained from a vein by venipuncture. Venous blood samples for hematology tests are usually collected in a tube containing an **anticoagulant** to prevent clotting. The anticoagulant most frequently used in the hematology laboratory is **EDTA** (ethylenediaminetetra-acetic acid).

## The Complete Blood Count (CBC)

One of the most frequently requested procedures in the hematology laboratory is the **CBC**, or complete blood count. The CBC is a combination of tests that usually includes:

■ red blood cell count

■ white blood cell count

■ hemoglobin

■ hematocrit

■ red blood cell indices

■ differential count

■ estimation of platelet numbers

■ observation of blood cell morphology

An example of a laboratory requisition form for a CBC is shown in Figure 2-5. The methods for performing these tests are explained in the remaining lessons of this unit. After completing this unit, the student should be able to perform all tests included in the CBC.

## Coagulation Tests and Special Hematology Tests

Many tests other than those included in the CBC are performed in the hematology laboratory. Some of these, such as the platelet count, erythrocyte sedimentation rate, and reticulocyte count, are included in this unit. Basic coagulation tests, such as prothrombin time and bleeding time, are explained in Unit 3, Basic Hemostasis. Other hematology tests beyond the scope of this book include special stains for blood and bone marrow cells to classify leukemias; identifying hemoglobin variants, such as the hemoglobin that causes sickle cell anemia; assessing iron status; and testing leukocyte function to help diagnose immune deficiencies.

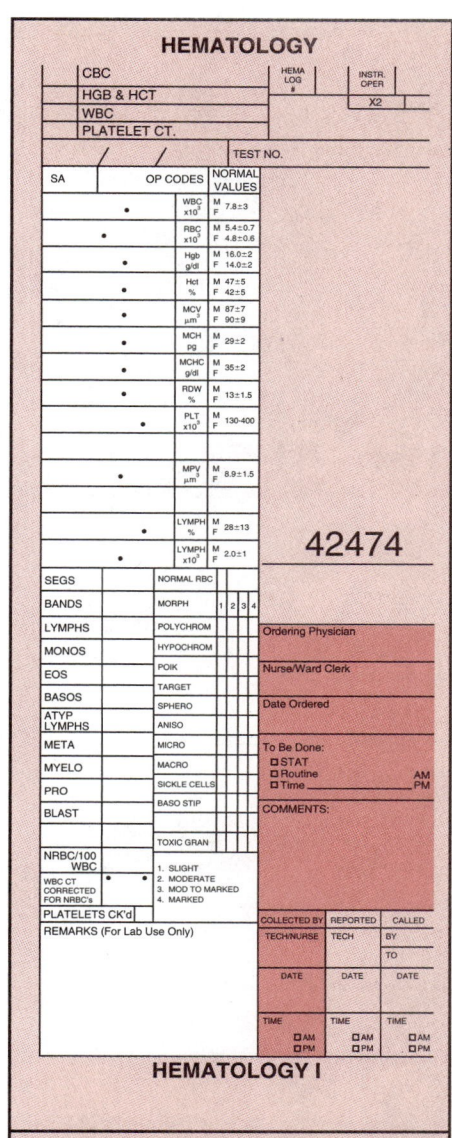

**FIGURE 2-5** Laboratory requisition form for CBC

logical disease and cell malfunctions. These technologies provide more sophisticated tests to aid in diagnosis and also have the promise of providing new treatments, such as gene therapy.

## LESSON REVIEW

1. Where are "blood cells" produced? What is the most primitive blood cell called?

2. What are the three groups of formed elements in the blood? What are the functions of each group?

3. Name the five types of leukocytes found in the blood. Which are the granulocytes?

4. Name five components of plasma.

5. What two types of blood specimens are used for most hematological tests?

6. What anticoagulant is used for most hematological tests?

7. Name the three major types of blood vessels and explain the differences among them.

8. Name three ways workers can lessen the chance of exposure to body fluids in the hematology laboratory.

9. Which blood component is responsible for oxygen exchange? *Erythrocyte*

10. Name two inherited hematological diseases. What is meant by a secondary or acquired hematological condition?

11. What is a CBC? *Cell Blood Counts*

12. Why is hematology quality control more complex than in some other laboratory departments?

13. Define anticoagulant, artery, capillary, cardiopulmonary circulation, CBC, deoxyhemoglobin, EDTA, erythrocyte, granulocyte, hemoglobin, hemopoiesis, hemostasis, leukocyte, megakaryocyte, oncologist, oxyhemoglobin, plasma, platelet, stem cell, systemic circulation, thrombocyte, and vein.

## SUMMARY

The hematology laboratory performs a wide variety of tests, some simple and some very complex. Some technicians work in hospitals or clinics, where most hematological testing is routine. Others may work in hematologists' or oncologists' laboratories and perform more specialized tests. Hematology technicians often develop close relationships with physicians and with patients who come in for frequent testing.

New technologies are being developed that allow greater understanding of the cellular basis of hemato-

## STUDENT ACTIVITIES

1. Reread the information on introduction to hematology.

2. Review the glossary terms.

3. Visit a hematology laboratory in the community. Find out what tests are performed.

4. Research a hematological disease. Report on the cause of the disease, what laboratory tests can be used for diagnosis, and what treatment would be appropriate.

# Blood Collection: Capillary Puncture

**After studying this lesson, you should be able to:**

- *Explain why a capillary puncture might be performed.*
- *Identify suitable sites for capillary punctures.*
- *Choose and prepare a site for capillary puncture.*
- *Perform a capillary puncture.*
- *Collect a blood specimen from a capillary puncture.*
- *List the safety precautions to be observed when performing a capillary puncture.*
- *Define the glossary terms.*

## GLOSSARY

**capillary** / a minute blood vessel that connects the smallest arteries to the smallest veins and serves as an exchange vessel

**capillary action** / the action by which a fluid enters a tube because of the attraction between the fluid and the tube

**capillary tube** / a glass or plastic tube of very small diameter used for laboratory procedures

**heparin** / an anticoagulant used in certain laboratory procedures

**lancet** / a sterile, sharp-pointed blade used to perform a capillary puncture

**lateral** / toward the side

## INTRODUCTION

Capillary puncture is a safe, rapid and efficient means of collecting a blood specimen. In capillary puncture, a small sterile **lancet** or blade is used to puncture the skin and **capillaries** to create a blood flow. Capillary punctures are performed when only a small amount of blood is required, when obtaining blood from infants, or when the patient has a condition that makes venipuncture difficult.

For many years, laboratories preferred venous blood for testing and used capillary blood only in special situations, because of the small sample volume available and clotting of the sample before it reached the laboratory. However, the development of small, portable, easy-to-use instruments, such as blood glucose meters, that require only a drop or two of blood, has made capillary blood the specimen of choice for these analyzers. The rapid increase in use of these instruments in bedside testing, POLs, and other point-of-care testing (POCT) sites has increased the need to train a variety of medical personnel in correct capillary puncture techniques.

## THE CAPILLARY PUNCTURE

### Capillary Puncture Sites

The usual site for capillary puncture in adults and children is the fingertip (Figure 2-6). In adults, the ring finger is often selected because it usually is not calloused. The ear lobe also may be used as a puncture site.

In infants, usually the **lateral**, or side, portion of the heel pad is used (Figure 2-6). Special pediatric lancets are available that limit the depth of puncture. If possible, recent puncture sites should always be avoided.

### Capillary Puncture Equipment

#### Puncture Devices

Several types of lancets are available for capillary puncture. These vary in length and design of the blades. Lancet holders that make punctures of uniform depth at the touch of a button are available for most lancet types (Figure 2-7). Other lancets come in single-use, disposable units.

#### Capillary Collection Containers and Devices

Capillary blood is often collected in **capillary tubes**, slender glass or plastic tubes about 7 cm long and 1 mm in diameter. Several types of capillary tubes are avail-able: plain, heparinized, calibrated, flexible, and self-sealing. Tubes coated with the anticoagulant **heparin** should be used when collecting capillary blood samples to prevent clotting of the blood. Heparinized tubes have a red ring on one end. Pre-calibrated tubes are usually heparinized. Uncoated (non-heparinized) capillary tubes with a blue ring on one end are used when a test is being performed on venous blood that has been previously collected in an anticoagulant.

Capillary tubes are made of glass, flexible plastic, or glass sheathed in plastic. In 1999, a joint advisory issued by FDA, NIOSH, and OSHA recommended that glass tubes not be used unless sheathed in puncture-resistant film. It was also recommended that sealing putty not be used for sealing tubes to be centrifuged for hematocrit. To minimize exposure risk from potential tube breakage, glass-tube alternatives such as CLAY ADAMS® Sure Prep capillary tubes, which have a protective mylar

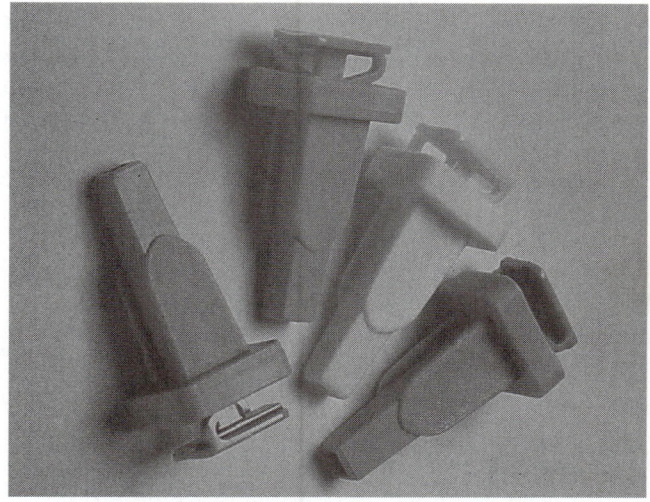

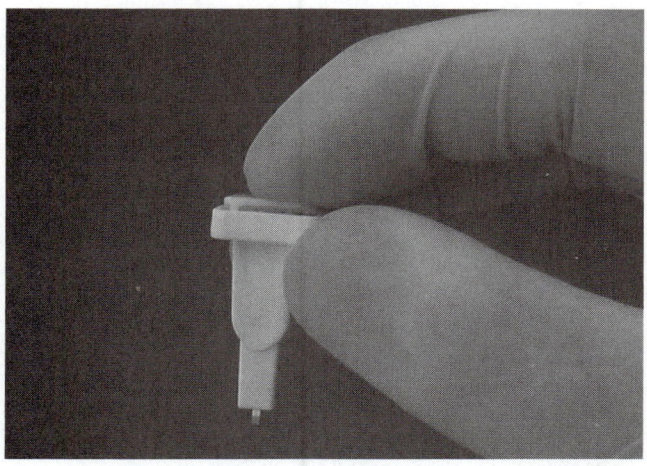

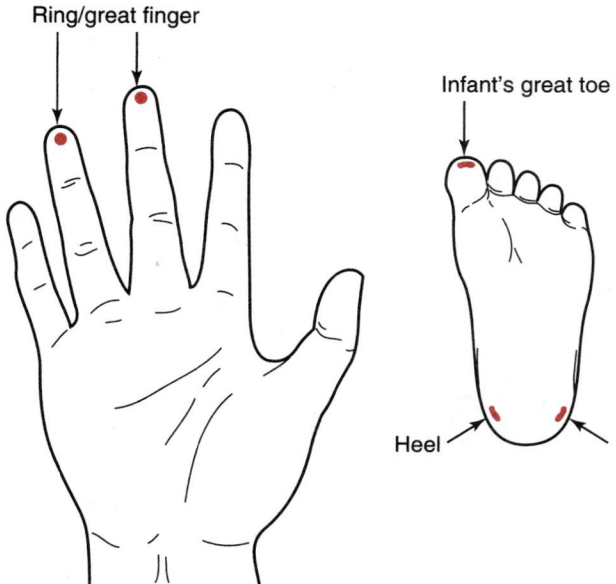

**FIGURE 2-6** Capillary blood collection sites

**FIGURE 2-7** Single-use lancets for capillary puncture (Photos courtesy of Becton Dickson and Co.)

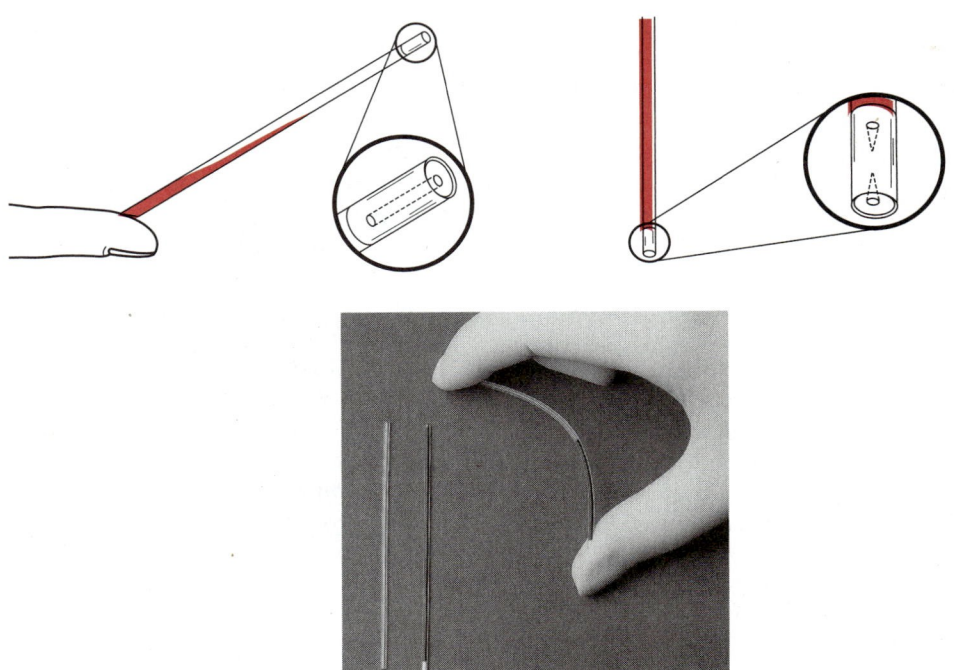

**FIGURE 2–8** Hematocrit tubes with improved safety features. Self-sealing mylar-wrapped capillary tubes. Top left, plug has channel that allows air to escape while tube is being filled; Top right, channel seals automatically when blood touches the plug. Bottom, flexible hematocrit tubes (Courtesy of StatSpin, Inc. Norwood, MA)

wrapping and self-sealing plugs that eliminate the need for sealing clay, should be used whenever possible (Figure 2-8).

When blood is required for tests other than hematocrit, the sample may be collected in special vials containing a capillary extension that directs the blood into the vial (Figure 2-9).

### Procedures that Use Capillary Blood

Several hematology procedures, such as blood cell counts, hemoglobin, hematocrit, and the blood smear, can be performed using capillary blood. Small handheld analyzers are available that can test a parameter using only a drop or two of capillary blood. These are widely used in POCT sites for hemoglobin, glucose, coagulation, serology, and electrolyte testing.

## PERFORMING A CAPILLARY PUNCTURE

 **Safety**

Universal and Standard Precautions must be observed in collecting capillary blood. Gloves and other appropriate protective clothing must be worn by the technician. The puncture may be performed behind an acrylic safety shield if face protection is not available. Plastic- or mylar-sheathed tubes should be used to minimize risk of injury and exposure to bloodborne pathogens due to tube breakage. Contaminated lancets and tubes must be discarded into puncture-proof biohazard containers for sharps.

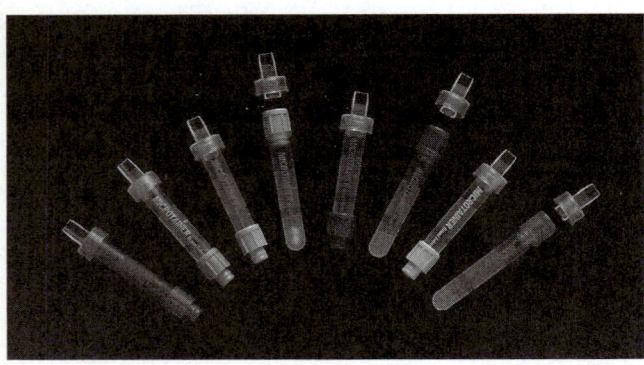

**FIGURE 2–9** Capillary collection vials

*Quality Assurance*

Personnel responsible for procedures involving capillary puncture must be adequately trained in the correct procedure for capillary blood sampling. Good sampling technique is the first step toward obtaining reliable test results.

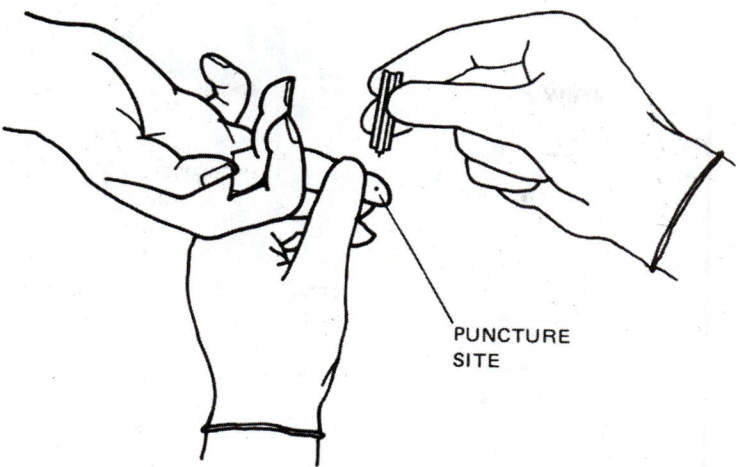

**FIGURE 2-10** Illustration of the proper position for the patient's and phlebotomist's hands during capillary puncture

## Selecting the Puncture Site

The capillary puncture procedure should be explained to the patient. The puncture site should not be calloused and should have good circulation. Warm skin indicates adequate circulation; cool skin indicates decreased circulation. A patient's hands may be gently massaged or placed in warm water for a few minutes to enhance circulation.

## Preparing the Puncture Site

Alcohol-soaked gauze or cotton should be used to cleanse and disinfect the puncture site. The site should then be allowed to air-dry or should be wiped dry with sterile gauze. A well-rounded drop of blood will not form on moist skin.

## Performing the Puncture

The patient's hand and finger should be held so the puncture site is readily accessible (Figure 2-10). Using a lancet, the puncture is made at the tip of the fleshy pad and slightly to the side (Figure 2-11). If the tips of the fingers are heavily calloused or thickened, a special lancet with a longer point may be used. The puncture should be performed in one quick steady motion.

## Collecting the Blood Sample

The first drop of blood is wiped away with dry, sterile gauze because it contains tissue fluid, which dilutes the

blood drop and can also activate clotting. The second and following drops of blood are used for the test samples. Depending on the tests to be performed, the blood may be collected in capillary tubes, other capillary collecting devices, or directly onto a reagent test strip or cartridge. Capillary blood should be collected as quickly as possible following puncture, to avoid blood clotting.

It may be necessary to massage the finger to increase blood flow. It is best to massage the whole hand, taking care not to apply excessive pressure near the puncture site. Squeezing the fingertip should be avoided; this forces tissue fluid into the blood sample and dilutes it.

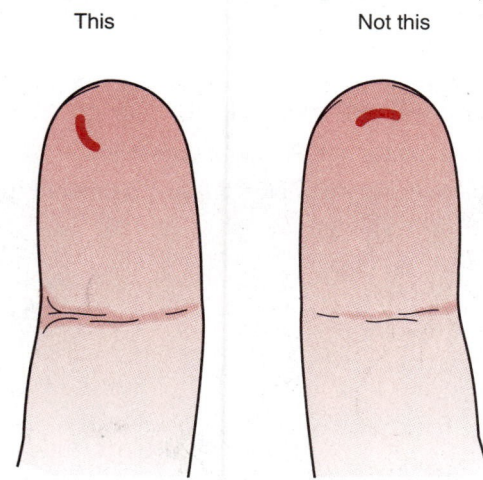

This        Not this

**FIGURE 2-11** The correct direction of capillary puncture

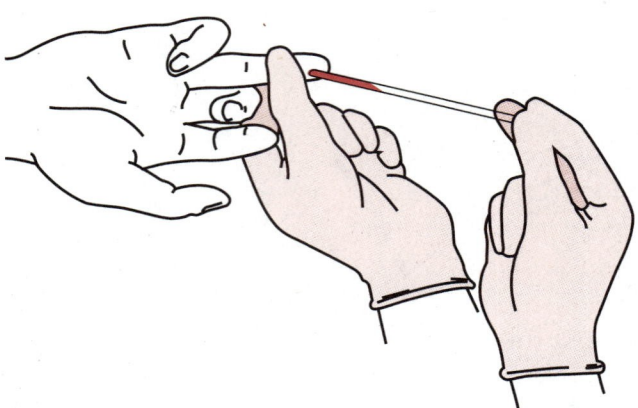

**FIGURE 2–12** Collecting capillary blood into a capillary tube

The capillary tube or collecting device should be held in an almost horizontal position, or tilted slightly downward. When the tip of the capillary tube is touched to the drop of blood, blood will enter the tube by **capillary action** because of the attraction between the liquid and the tube (Figure 2-12). Tubes should be filled two-thirds to three-quarters full. Usually, two to three tubes are filled from a capillary puncture.

## Caring for the Puncture Site

After the blood has been collected, sterile gauze or a cotton ball should be placed on the site and pressure

### Procedural Notes

■ Select a puncture site with adequate circulation.
■ Clean the puncture site thoroughly before puncture.
■ Dry the puncture site before puncture to get a well-formed drop of blood.
■ Do not squeeze the finger excessively.
■ Collect capillary samples quickly to prevent the blood from clotting.

### Safety Precautions

■ Use Universal and Standard Precautions when collecting capillary blood.
■ Wear gloves when performing capillary puncture.
■ Use an acrylic safety shield to avoid exposure.
■ Use plastic- or mylar-sheathed capillary tubes to minimize risk of breakage, subsequent injury, and potential exposure to pathogens.

should be applied until bleeding stops. It is usually not necessary to bandage the site.

## LESSON REVIEW

1. What is a capillary puncture? *is a safe, faster means of blood collection*
2. Why would a capillary puncture be performed? *for small amount of blood*
3. What are the usual puncture sites for adults; for infants? *Adult = ring finger, infant = heel pad*
4. How is a capillary puncture site prepared? *clean & warm*
5. What is the procedure if the patient has cold hands? *Wash hand in warm water*
6. Why is the first drop of blood wiped away? *has tissue fluid*
7. List the safety precautions that must be observed when performing a capillary puncture.
8. When is a capillary tube with a blue band used? When is a tube with a red band used?
9. Why should the blood from capillary puncture be used quickly? *avoid coagulation = clotting*
10. What is the advantage of using plastic capillary tubes? *Minimise risk of breakage*
11. Define capillary, capillary action, capillary tube, heparin, lancet, and lateral.

## STUDENT ACTIVITIES

1. Reread the information on capillary puncture.
2. Review the glossary terms.
3. Practice performing a capillary puncture as outlined in the Student Performance Guide.

# Student Performance Guide

## LESSON 2-2 Blood Collection: Capillary Puncture

Name _____   Date _____

### INSTRUCTIONS

1. Practice the procedure for performing a capillary puncture following the step-by-step procedure.
2. Demonstrate your understanding of this lesson by:
   a. Completing a written examination successfully, and
   b. Performing the procedure for capillary puncture satisfactorily for the instructor. All steps must be completed as listed on the instructor's Performance Check Sheet.

*Note:* Follow manufacturer's instructions for the type of capillary tubes used.

### MATERIALS AND EQUIPMENT

■ acrylic safety shield or protective face shield
■ gloves
■ hand disinfectant
■ lancets (sterile, disposable)
■ sterile cotton balls or gauze squares
■ 70 % alcohol or alcohol swabs
■ Mylar-coated capillary tubes (heparinized and plain, self-sealing)
■ precalibrated capillary tubes (optional)
■ surface disinfectant or 10% chlorine bleach solution
■ biohazard container
■ puncture-proof biohazard container for sharps

### PROCEDURE

Record in the comment section any problems encountered while practicing the procedure (or have a fellow student or the instructor evaluate your performance).

S  = Satisfactory
U = Unsatisfactory

| You must: | S | U | Comments |
|---|---|---|---|
| 1. Wash hands and put on gloves and protective facewear (use safety shield if facewear is not available) | | | |
| 2. Assemble equipment and materials | | | |
| 3. Explain the procedure to the patient | | | |
| 4. Select and warm the puncture site | | | |
| 5. Cleanse the puncture site with alcohol-soaked gauze or cotton | | | |
| 6. Allow the site to air-dry or wipe with dry sterile gauze or cotton | | | |
| 7. Position the puncture site, holding the skin taut with one hand and holding the lancet in the other hand | | | |
| 8. Perform the capillary puncture, using a quick, firm stab | | | |
| 9. Wipe the first drop of blood away with sterile gauze or cotton | | | |

| You must: | S | U | Comments |
|---|---|---|---|
| 10.  Massage the finger gently to produce the second drop of blood | | | |
| 11.  Collect the blood specimen:<br><br>    a.  For hematocrit test:<br><br>        1. Fill a capillary tube two-thirds to three-quarters full using the second and subsequent drops of blood (fill to the line if using pre-calibrated tubes).  Follow manufacturer's directions for the type of tube used<br><br>        2. Fill a second tube and seal the tubes<br><br>    b.  For other POCT:<br><br>        1. Apply a free-flowing drop of blood to test strip, slide, or cartridge<br><br>        2. Follow directions with instrument to complete the analysis | | | |
| 12.  Apply pressure to the puncture site by pressing with dry sterile gauze or cotton.  Instruct patient to continue applying pressure | | | |
| 13.  Place used lancet into a puncture-proof biohazard container for sharp objects | | | |
| 14.  Discard used gauze or cotton into biohazard container | | | |
| 15.  Clean and return equipment to proper storage | | | |
| 16.  Clean work area with surface disinfectant | | | |
| 17.  Remove and discard gloves into biohazard container.  Wash hands with hand disinfectant | | | |

*Evaluator Comments:*

Evaluator _____   Date _____

# Blood Collection: Venipuncture

## LESSON OBJECTIVES

After studying this lesson, you should be able to:

- ■ *Explain the venipuncture procedure to a patient.*
- ■ *Select the equipment necessary to perform a venipuncture.*
- ■ *Apply a tourniquet.*
- ■ *Select a proper venipuncture site.*
- ■ *Perform a venipuncture.*
- ■ *List the safety precautions to be observed when performing a venipuncture.*
- ■ *Explain the use of vacuum tubes.*
- ■ *Name three common anticoagulants and state why they are used.*
- ■ *Define the glossary terms.*

## GLOSSARY

**artery** / a blood vessel that carries oxygenated blood from the heart to the tissues

**cephalic vein** / a superficial vein of the arm commonly used for venipuncture

**gauge** / a measure of the diameter of a needle

**hematoma** / the swelling of tissue around a vessel due to leakage of blood into the tissue

**hypodermic needle** / a hollow needle used for injections or for obtaining fluid specimens

**lumen** / the open space within a tubular organ or tissue

**median cubital vein** / a superficial vein located in the bend of the elbow (cubital fossa) that connects the cephalic vein to the basilic vein

**palpate** / to examine by touch

**phlebotomy** / venipuncture; entry of a vein with a needle

**syringe** / a hollow, tube-like container with a plunger, used for injecting or withdrawing fluids

**tourniquet** / a band used to constrict blood flow

**vein** / a blood vessel that carries deoxygenated blood from the tissues to the heart

**venipuncture** / entry of a vein with a needle; a phlebotomy

## INTRODUCTION

The most common method of obtaining blood for laboratory examination is by **venipuncture**. The venipuncture is a quick way to obtain a large sample of blood on which many different analyses can be performed. In a venipuncture, also called a **phlebotomy**, a superficial **vein** is punctured with a **hypodermic needle** and blood is collected into a **syringe** or tube.

Performing a venipuncture involves several important steps that must be thoroughly understood before the procedure is attempted:

- observing safety precautions throughout procedure
- selecting the proper equipment
- preparing the patient for venipuncture
- applying the tourniquet
- selecting and preparing the puncture site
- obtaining the blood
- caring for the puncture site and observing the patient for adverse reaction

The venipuncture is a safe procedure when performed correctly by a skilled worker. The procedure must be performed carefully to preserve the condition of the vein. Much observation and practice is required to become skilled and self-confident in the art of venipuncture.

## THE VENIPUNCTURE

 **Safety**

Universal and Standard Precautions must be observed and gloves must be worn by the phlebotomist when performing all venipunctures. It is best to use gloves without talc to avoid contaminating collection tubes. The phlebotomist should wear PPE such as a buttoned, fluid-resistant laboratory coat and face protection.

Students learning to perform venipunctures must be supervised by a qualified instructor.

Care must be taken to avoid inadvertent needlesticks. Used needles must not be recapped but must be discarded using a needle-disposal device (Figure 2-13) or in a needle-disposal container. Whenever possible, safety needles must be used to reduce the risk of accidental needlesticks and transmission of bloodborne pathogens. Venipuncture products with enhanced safety designs are rapidly becoming available. Several types of safety needles are available that have sleeves or covers that slide over the used needle (Figure 2-14). Regulatory agencies began requiring the use of these improved needles in 1999.

### *Quality Assurance*

For laboratory tests that require a blood specimen, collection of the specimen is the first step in ensuring quality test results. The venipuncturist must properly identify the patient, select the proper tubes for blood collection, and deliver the specimen to the testing site within the specified time limits. Some test procedures require specialized collection and handling, such as immediate placement of the blood specimen on ice. Specimen-collection parameters for each laboratory test are described in the laboratory procedure manual and must be followed.

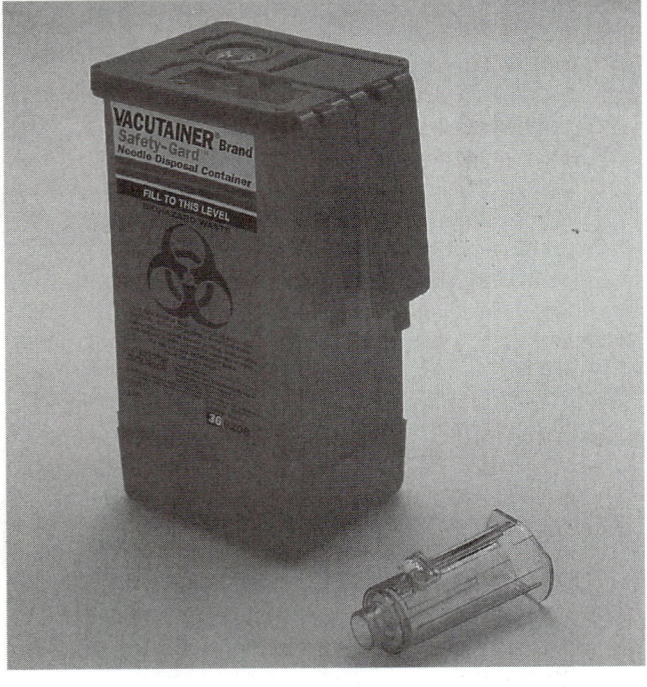
(A)

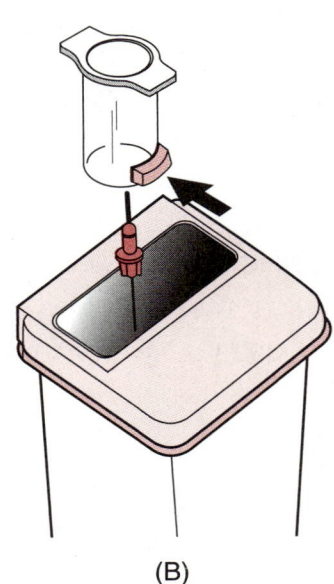
(B)

**FIGURE 2-13** Needle-disposal devices. (A) needle-disposal container; (B) DROP-IT™ quick-release needle holder

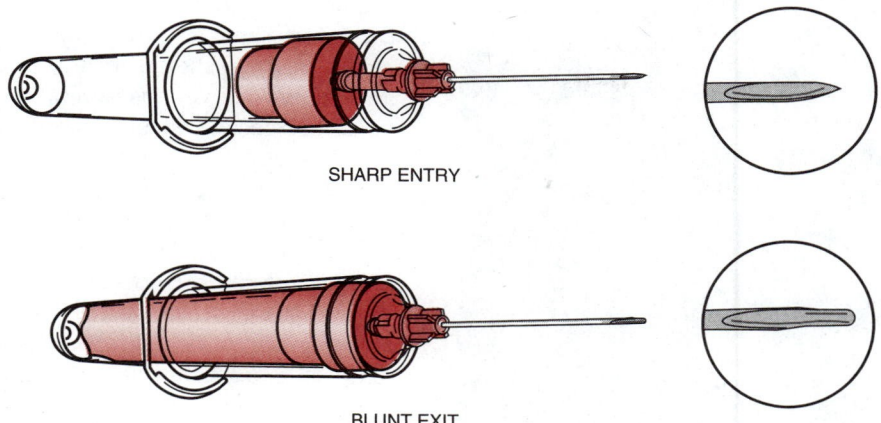

SHARP ENTRY

BLUNT EXIT

**FIGURE 2-14** Safety needles for venipuncture.  Top, needle with sharp entry; bottom, needle that blunts on exit from puncture.

## Materials and the Equipment for Venipuncture

Venipuncture may be performed using needle and syringe (Figure 2-15), a vacuum tube system (Figure 2-16), or butterfly devices (Figure 2-17). Materials required for the syringe method include a sterile disposable syringe and needle, 70% alcohol swab, sterile gauze, tourniquet, and a blood-collecting tube. Materials required for the vacuum tube method include needle and holder (Figure 2-16), 70% alcohol swab, sterile gauze, tourniquet, and vacuum collecting tube.

### Needles

The length and **gauge** (diameter) of the needle used varies according to the procedure or preference of the phlebotomist. Needles of 20 to 22 gauge are used for routine venipuncture. (The higher the gauge, the smaller the needle diameter.) Larger diameter needles are required for collecting blood donor units. Butterfly devices similar to those used for intravenous fluids are available that connect to syringes or vacuum tube holders (Figure 2-17). These are used for patients who have small, delicate veins that make routine venipuncture difficult.

### Vacuum Tubes and Anticoagulants

Vacuum tubes are available in a variety of types and sizes. Tubes may be sterile or non-sterile, glass or plastic.

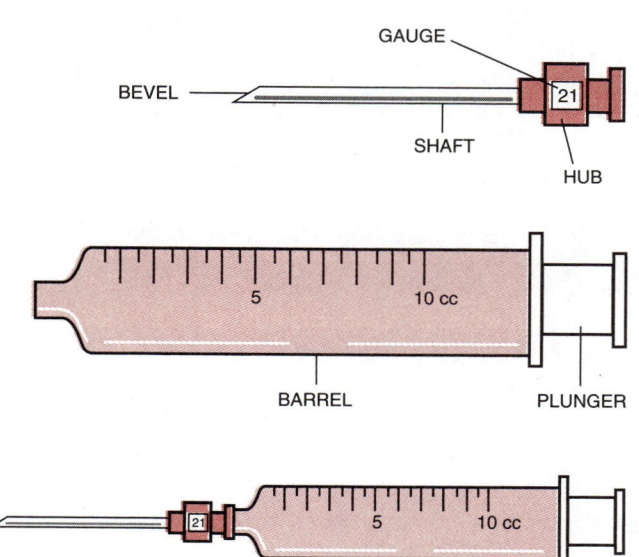

GAUGE

BEVEL

SHAFT

HUB

21

BARREL  PLUNGER

21  5  10 cc

**FIGURE 2-15** Needle (top), syringe (center), and syringe and needle assembled (bottom)

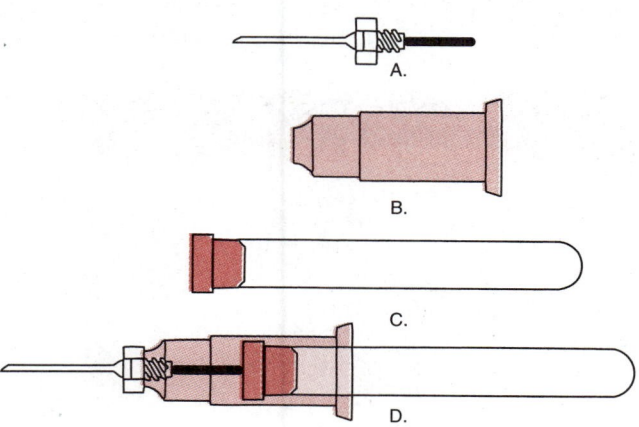

A.

B.

C.

D.

**FIGURE 2-16** Vacuum tube blood-collecting system: (A) needle, (B) needle holder, (C) vacuum tube, and (D) assembled unit

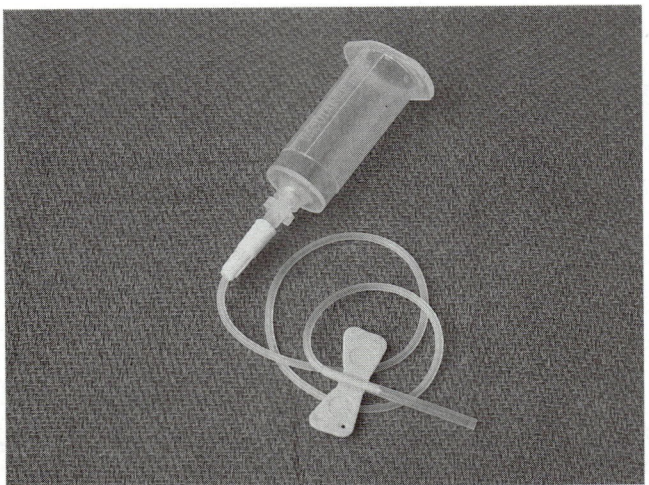

**FIGURE 2-17** Butterfly needle (Photo courtesy of Becton Dickinson Vacutainer Systems, Rutherford, NJ)

Color-coded stoppers note which, if any, anticoagulant is present in the tube (Table 2-1).

Laboratory procedures performed on plasma usually require that blood be collected with a specific anticoagulant. For example, tubes with lavender stoppers contain EDTA, which is the anticoagulant used for most hematology studies, such as cell and differential counts. For coagulation tests such as prothrombin time, a blue-stoppered tube containing sodium citrate is commonly used. Tubes with green stoppers contain heparin, which is used for some special tests in chemistry and hematology, but should not be used if stained blood smears are to be prepared. Gray-stoppered tubes contain potassium oxalate and sodium fluoride and are used for certain glucose tests. Red-stoppered tubes contain no anticoagulant and are used for tests that require serum, such as most blood chemistries. Special tubes are also available with agents such as clotting activators or serum separators. These tubes shorten the time required for obtaining serum from the tube and keep the serum separated from the clot. The laboratory procedure manual should include a list of tests performed and the type of venous sample required. Table 2-1 is a guide to selecting vacuum tubes.

Vacuum tubes are available in a variety of sizes; each size draws a specific volume of blood. Sizes commonly used are 3 mL, 5 mL, 7 mL, 10 mL, and 15 mL. The tubes contain the proper amount of anticoagulant for the volume of blood that the tube will draw. It is important that tubes be filled to their stated capacities since an improper ratio of anticoagulant to blood may alter cell morphology and interfere with test results.

## PERFORMING A VENIPUNCTURE USING A SYRINGE

### Selecting the Equipment

All materials should be placed within easy reach of the venipuncturist. Gloves must be worn while performing venipuncture. The syringe and needle should be assembled to maintain sterility.

The needle should be positioned firmly on the syringe so the bevel and graduations of the syringe face in the same direction. The syringe plunger should be pushed up and down to see that it moves freely. It should then be left pushed completely into the barrel so no air remains in the syringe.

### Preparing the Patient

The venipuncturist (phlebotomist) must always identify the patient by name and by checking the laboratory request form. If the patient is hospitalized, the patient identification wristband must be checked. For some procedures, such as collecting blood for typing and crossmatching, the phlebotomist may place an addition-

| **STOPPER COLOR** | **ANTICOAGULANT IN TUBE** | **EXAMPLES OF USE** |
|---|---|---|
| Red | None | Tests that require serum, such as most blood chemistries and serology tests |
| Red/gray | None | Serum-separator tube; used for tests that require serum |
| Lavender | EDTA | Most hematological tests, blood-typing |
| Green | Heparin | Some special chemistry tests, certain lymphocyte studies, lupus erythematosus test |
| Light blue | Sodium citrate | Most coagulation studies |
| Gray | Sodium fluoride | Certain glucose tests |
| Black | Buffered sodium citrate | Westergren ESR |

**Table 2-1.** Guide for selecting vacuum tubes

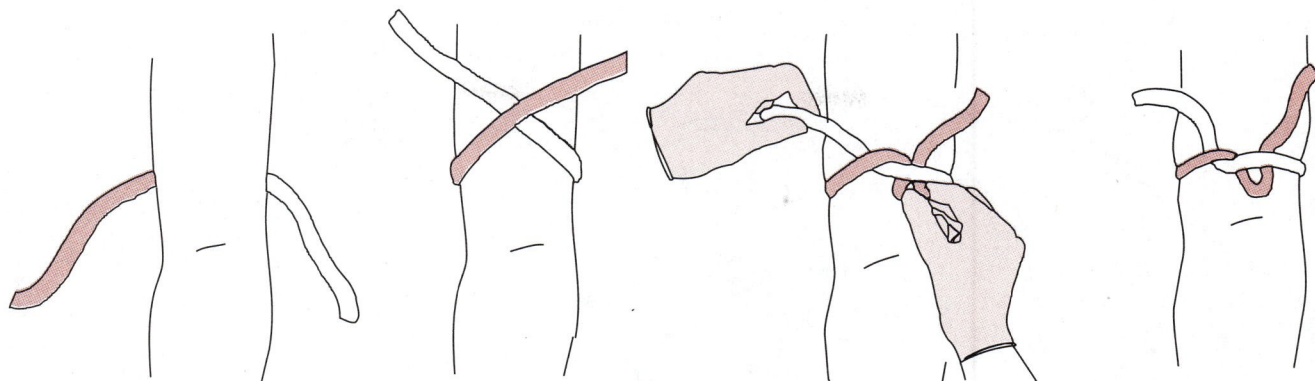

**FIGURE 2-18** Steps in tying a tourniquet

al identification wristband on the patient that is coded to the blood-collection tubes.

The venipuncture procedure should be explained to the patient to minimize apprehension. The patient should be lying down or seated in a chair with arm supports. The patient's arm must be fully extended and firmly supported during the venipuncture. The phlebotomist should be trained to administer first aid to be prepared for the occasional patient who may faint.

## Applying the Tourniquet

A **tourniquet** is applied to the arm to slow blood flow and make the veins more prominent. Disposable tourniquets are preferred.

The tourniquet is placed under the arm above the elbow and the two ends are stretched and crossed over the top of the arm. While tension is maintained on the

ends, one side is looped and pulled halfway through in a slipknot (Figure 2-18). If the tourniquet is tied in this manner, it will release easily with a gentle pull on one end (Figure 2-19).

The tourniquet should be applied while the puncture site is being selected. It should then be released while the site is cleansed, and retied before the puncture is performed. *A tourniquet should never be tied tight enough to restrict blood flow in the artery.* The tourniquet should be left in place for no more than two minutes, to avoid hemoconcentration. Once the vein is entered and blood flow is obtained, the tourniquet may be released while the blood is collected. *After the venipuncture has been completed, the tourniquet is always released before the needle is withdrawn from the vein, to prevent hematoma at the venipuncture site.*

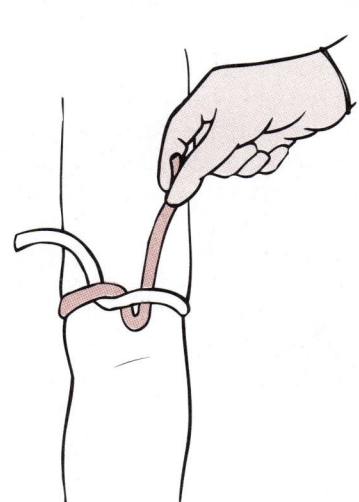

**FIGURE 2-19** Releasing the tourniquet

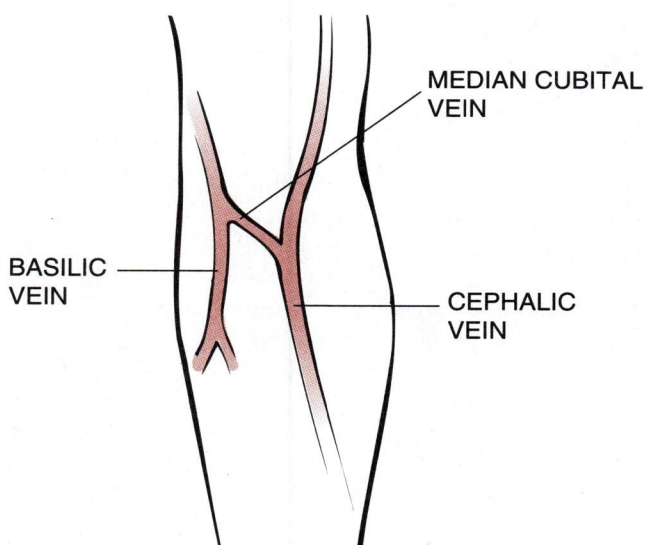

MEDIAN CUBITAL VEIN

BASILIC VEIN

CEPHALIC VEIN

**FIGURE 2-20** Veins commonly used for venipuncture (left arm shown)

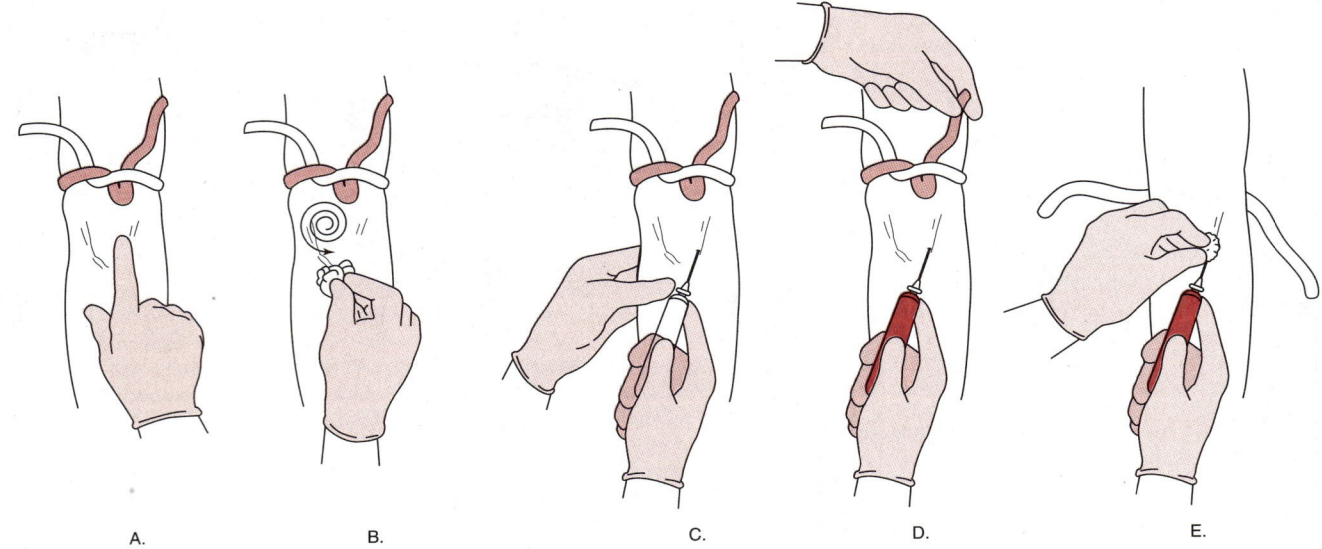

A.      B.      C.      D.      E.

**FIGURE 2-21** Palpating a vein with fingertip

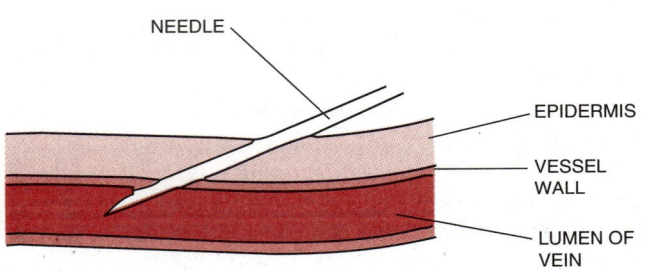

NEEDLE

EPIDERMIS

VESSEL WALL

LUMEN OF VEIN

**FIGURE 2-22** Expanded view of needle positioned in lumen of vein

## Selecting and Preparing the Venipuncture Site

The puncture site should be selected after inspecting both arms to locate the best vein. The veins most frequently used are the **median cubital vein** or the **cephalic vein** of the forearm (Figure 2-20). The phlebotomist should gently **palpate** the vein to determine its direction and estimate its size and depth (Figure 2-21). The vein will feel like an elastic tube.

The area around the puncture site should be cleansed thoroughly in a circular motion from the inside out with 70% alcohol and sterile gauze (Figure 2-21). The site may then be dried using dry sterile gauze, or it may be allowed to air-dry. Once the site is cleansed, it should not be touched again except to enter the vein with the sterile needle. If the vein is palpated again, the skin must be recleansed.

## Performing the Venipuncture

When the puncture site has been cleansed, the tourniquet should be reapplied to the arm; it should not touch the cleansed area. The syringe should be held in one hand at a 15–30° angle to the surface of the arm. The bevel should be up, and the needle should point in the same direction as the vein (Figure 2-22). When the sheath is removed from the needle, the needle should be inspected to be sure there are no visible burrs or defects, and that the point is intact.

The thumb should be placed about one inch below the point of entry, and the skin pressed and pulled toward the venipuncturist (Figure 2-21) to anchor the vein and lessen the needle's pull on the skin. The skin and vein should be entered in one smooth motion until the needle is in the **lumen** of the vein (Figure 2-22). Penetrating the vein at the proper angle will prevent penetrating both vessel walls.

Once the vein has been entered, the syringe and needle should be steadied with one hand while the other hand gently pulls back on the plunger to draw blood into the syringe. The needle should be observed while the syringe is filling to be sure it is not pulled out of the vein.

When the desired amount of blood has been obtained, the tourniquet should be released. The needle can then be withdrawn from the vein while gauze is placed over the puncture site and pressure is applied (Figure 2-21). The blood can be transferred to a vacuum tube by inserting the needle into the stopper of the tube and allowing the tube to fill by vacuum. The tube must be in a secure rack, *not* held in the hand. The syringe-needle unit can then be discarded in a biohazard sharps container. Used needles should not be recapped.

The tube should be labeled with the date, patient's name, identification number, time of collection, and initials of the venipuncturist. Tubes should not be prelabeled; this prevents the possibility of using a prelabeled tube for the wrong patient.

## Caring for the Venipuncture Site

The patient should be instructed to press the gauze on the puncture site for two to five minutes with the arm extended to ensure that bleeding stops and a **hematoma**, or swelling, does not form. The venipuncturist should check the site to see that it has stopped bleeding before leaving the patient and should apply a bandage if necessary.

## PERFORMING A VENIPUNCTURE USING A VACUUM-TUBE SYSTEM

The most widely used method of collecting venous blood is by using a vacuum-tube system such as VACU-TAINER® or VENOJECT®. Vacuum-tube systems consist of a special disposable needle; a needle holder or adapter; and vacuum tubes, blood-collecting tubes from which most of the air has been evacuated (Figure 2-16). The needle used has two sharp ends. The short end, which is enclosed in a retractable rubber sheath, is fit-

### Procedural Notes

- Identify patient by asking his or her name and checking armband.
- Be sure patient's arm is firmly supported before performing venipuncture.
- Do not allow tourniquet to remain on the arm for more than two minutes.
- Always release the tourniquet before removing the needle from the vein.
- If a hematoma or swelling begins to form, release tourniquet immediately, withdraw needle, and apply pressure to puncture site with gauze.
- Label filled tubes as soon as the venipuncture is completed, and before leaving the patient.

### Safety Precautions

- Observe Universal and Standard Precautions when performing venipuncture.
- Never reuse needles or syringes.
- Do not recap needles; discard in appropriate needle-disposal container.
- Use safety devices such as self-sheathing needles or quick-release needle holders whenever possible.

ted into the needle adapter. The longer end is used to puncture the vein.

To perform a venipuncture using a vacuum-tube system, the puncture site is selected and prepared as in the syringe method. After the vein is entered with the needle, the collecting tube is pushed onto the short sheathed needle in the adapter and blood is drawn into the tube by vacuum. When the tube is full, it is removed from the needle and replaced with another tube. The rubber sheath on the needle prevents leakage of blood from the needle between changes in tubes. In this manner, several tubes of blood can be collected, using a variety of types of vacuum tubes.

When more than one vacuum tube is to be filled, the "clot tube" (red top) must be filled first and tubes containing anticoagulant should be filled last. Tubes containing anticoagulant should be inverted gently a few times immediately after they are filled to mix the blood with the anticoagulant.

When the venipuncture has been completed, the needle must not be recapped or removed from the needle holder by hand. Instead, the needle should be discarded using a special needle-disposal device. Safety needles should be used whenever possible to reduce the phlebotomist's risk of exposure to bloodborne pathogens through accidental needlesticks (Figures 2-13 and 2-14).

## LESSON REVIEW

1. Why is a venipuncture performed?
2. What is the purpose of a tourniquet? *to slow blood flow & make veins prominent when many tests require*
3. Name five precautions that must be observed when performing a venipuncture.
4. What are the steps in performing a venipuncture?
5. Where is the most common venipuncture site?
6. Why must the tourniquet be removed before taking the needle out of the vein?

7. How should the puncture site be treated after the needle is removed?

8. Explain briefly the vacuum system of obtaining venous blood.

9. What precautions should the phlebotomist take when performing a venipuncture to avoid exposure to blood?

10. Name three anticoagulants used in collecting blood. Which one is most commonly used in hematology?

11. Why is it important to verify patient identification before performing a venipuncture?

12. Define artery, cephalic vein, gauge, hematoma, hypodermic needle, lumen, median cubital vein, palpate, phlebotomy, syringe, tourniquet, vein, and venipuncture.

## STUDENT ACTIVITIES

1. Reread the information on venipuncture.

2. Review the glossary terms.

3. Practice applying a tourniquet and locating suitable veins for venipuncture.

4. Practice performing a venipuncture as outlined in the Student Performance Guide.

## *Student Performance Guide*

## **LESSON 2-3** Blood Collection: Venipuncture—Syringe Method

Name _____ Date _____

### ☣ INSTRUCTIONS

1. Practice performing a venipuncture using a syringe and following the step-by-step procedure.
2. Demonstrate your understanding of this lesson by:
   a. Completing a written examination successfully, and
   b. Performing a venipuncture using a syringe satisfactorily for the instructor. All steps must be completed as listed on the instructor's Performance Check Sheet.

### MATERIALS AND EQUIPMENT

- acrylic safety shield
- gloves
- hand disinfectant
- tourniquet
- sterile gauze or cotton
- 70% alcohol or alcohol swabs
- sterile disposable 20 to 22 gauge safety needle
- sterile syringe
- collection tubes
- test tube rack
- needle-disposal container (sharps container)
- surface disinfectant (10% chlorine bleach solution)
- biohazard container

### PROCEDURE

Record in the comment section any problems encountered while practicing the procedure (or have a fellow student or the instructor evaluate your performance).

S = Satisfactory
U = Unsatisfactory

| You must: | S | U | Comments |
|---|---|---|---|
| 1. Wash hands and put on gloves | | | |
| 2. Assemble equipment and materials | | | |
| 3. Place venipuncture equipment and clean gauze within easy reach | | | |
| 4. Identify patient | | | |
| 5. Explain venipuncture procedure to, and position, patient | | | |
| 6. Attach the capped needle to the syringe, maintaining sterility | | | |
| 7. Slide the plunger up and down in the barrel of the syringe to be sure it moves freely | | | |
| 8. Push the plunger to the bottom of the barrel so no air remains in the syringe | | | |

| You must: | S | U | Comments |
|---|---|---|---|
| 9. Place the tourniquet around the patient's arm two to three inches above the elbow.  It should be just tight enough so venous circulation is restricted, but not so tight that arterial circulation is stopped.<br>*Caution:* Do not allow the tourniquet to remain on for more than two minutes | | | |
| 10. Instruct the patient to open and close his/her fist a few times to increase circulation and make the veins more noticeable | | | |
| 11. Inspect the bend of the elbow to locate a suitable vein | | | |
| 12. Palpate the vein with the fingertip(s) to determine its direction, and estimate its size and depth.  *Note:* The vein most frequently used is the median cubital vein of the forearm | | | |
| 13. Release the tourniquet | | | |
| 14. Cleanse the puncture site in a circular motion from the inside out using an alcohol-soaked gauze | | | |
| 15. Allow alcohol to dry | | | |
| 16. Retie the tourniquet, being careful not to touch the cleansed puncture site | | | |
| 17. Instruct the patient to straighten his/her arm and make a fist | | | |
| 18. Uncap the needle and hold the syringe so the graduations on the syringe and the bevel of the needle are in full view (facing toward the ceiling).  With thumb of the other hand, hold skin taut below puncture site, anchoring the vein | | | |
| 19. Inspect the needle to see that the point is smooth and sharp | | | |
| 20. Hold the needle at a 15–30° angle to the arm and insert it into the vein.  Watch for blood flow into the syringe | | | |
| 21. Instruct the patient to open his/her fist as soon as the vein has been entered | | | |
| 22. Pull the plunger back slowly with one hand to withdraw the blood, while steadying the syringe and needle with the other hand | | | |
| 23. Release the tourniquet when the desired amount of blood is obtained | | | |
| 24. Place a dry, sterile gauze over the puncture site and withdraw the needle from the vein (do not press down on the needle) | | | |
| 25. Instruct the patient to press the sterile gauze over the wound for three to five minutes with the arm extended | | | |
| 26. Fill blood-collecting tube:<br>a. Place tube in rack; insert needle into stopper of vacuum tube and allow tube to fill by vacuum, or<br>b. Discard needle into needle-disposal container (do not recap), place tube in rack, and fill collecting tube with safety shield placed between blood and worker (to avoid exposure to aerosols)<br>*Caution:* Do not hold tube in hand to fill | | | |

| You must: | S | U | Comments |
|---|---|---|---|
| 27. Label the tube properly | | | |
| 28. Discard used syringe into biohazard sharps container | | | |
| 29. Check patient to be sure bleeding has stopped; apply bandage, if necessary | | | |
| 30. Clean and return equipment to storage | | | |
| 31. Clean work area with surface disinfectant | | | |
| 32. Remove and discard gloves in biohazard container | | | |
| 33. Wash hands with hand disinfectant | | | |

*Evaluator Comments:*

Evaluator _____ Date _____

## Student Performance Guide

**LESSON 2-3** Blood Collection: Venipuncture—Vacuum-Tube Method

Name _____ Date _____

### ☣ INSTRUCTIONS

1. Practice performing a venipuncture using a vacuum-tube system and following the step-by-step procedure.
2. Demonstrate your understanding of this lesson by:
   a. Completing a written examination successfully, and
   b. Performing a venipuncture using a vacuum-tube system satisfactorily for the instructor. All steps must be completed as listed on the instructor's Performance Check Sheet.

### MATERIALS AND EQUIPMENT

- acrylic safety shield
- gloves
- hand disinfectant
- tourniquet
- sterile gauze or cotton
- 70% alcohol or alcohol swabs
- vacuum-tube safety needle and holder
- evacuated blood-collection tubes
- needle-disposal container
- 10% chlorine bleach solution
- biohazard container

### PROCEDURE

Record in the comment section any problems encountered while practicing the procedure (or have a fellow student or the instructor evaluate your performance).

S = Satisfactory
U = Unsatisfactory

| You must: | S | U | Comments |
|---|---|---|---|
| 1. Wash hands and put on gloves | | | |
| 2. Assemble equipment and materials | | | |
| 3. Place venipuncture equipment and clean gauze within easy reach | | | |
| 4. Identify patient | | | |
| 5. Explain venipuncture procedure to, and position, the patient | | | |
| 6. Attach the sterile capped needle to the needle holder | | | |
| 7. Insert vacuum-collection tube into needle holder, but do not pierce stopper with needle | | | |

| You must: | S | U | Comments |
|---|---|---|---|
| 8. Place the tourniquet around the patient's arm two to three inches above the elbow. It should be just tight enough so venous circulation is restricted, but not so tight that arterial circulation is stopped.<br>*Caution:* Do not allow the tourniquet to remain on for more than two minutes | | | |
| 9. Instruct the patient to open and close his/her fist a few times to increase circulation and make the veins more noticeable | | | |
| 10. Inspect the bend of the elbow to locate a suitable vein | | | |
| 11. Palpate the vein with the fingertips to determine its direction, and estimate its size and depth. *Note:* The vein most frequently used is the median cubital vein of the forearm | | | |
| 12. Release the tourniquet | | | |
| 13. Cleanse the puncture site in a circular motion from the inside out using an alcohol-soaked gauze | | | |
| 14. Allow alcohol to dry | | | |
| 15. Retie the tourniquet, being careful not to touch the sterile puncture site | | | |
| 16. Instruct the patient to straighten his/her arm and make a fist | | | |
| 17. Uncap the needle and hold the needle holder and tube assembly so the bevel of the needle is facing upward (toward ceiling). With the thumb of your other hand, hold the skin below puncture site taut | | | |
| 18. Inspect the needle to see that the point is smooth and sharp | | | |
| 19. Hold the needle at a 15–30° angle to the arm and insert it into the vein. | | | |
| 20. Push the vacuum tube gently onto the inner needle in the holder while steadying the needle holder with the other hand. Watch for blood flow into the tube | | | |
| 21. Instruct the patient to open his/her fist as soon as the vein has been entered | | | |
| 22. Release the tourniquet when the desired amount of blood is obtained | | | |
| 23. Remove the vacuum tube from the needle holder | | | |
| 24. Place a dry, sterile gauze over the puncture site and withdraw the needle from the vein (do not press down on the needle) | | | |
| 25. Instruct the patient to press the sterile gauze over the wound for three to five minutes with his/her arm extended | | | |

| You must: | S | U | Comments |
|---|---|---|---|
| 26. Discard the needle into the needle-disposal container. DO NOT RECAP | | | |
| 27. Label the collecting tube properly | | | |
| 28. Discard used materials as indicated by the instructor | | | |
| 29. Check patient to be sure bleeding has stopped; apply bandage, if necessary | | | |
| 30. Clean and return equipment to storage | | | |
| 31. Clean work area with surface disinfectant | | | |
| 32. Remove and discard gloves in biohazard container | | | |
| 33. Wash hands with hand disinfectant | | | |

*Evaluator Comments:*




Evaluator _____ Date _____

# Hematocrit

## LESSON OBJECTIVES

**After studying this lesson, you should be able to:**

- *Explain what the hematocrit measures.*
- *List the reference values for the hematocrit.*
- *List conditions that affect the hematocrit value.*
- *Prepare a hematocrit sample.*
- *Centrifuge a hematocrit sample.*
- *Determine the hematocrit value.*
- *List safety precautions that should be observed in performing the hematocrit.*
- *Define the glossary terms.*

## GLOSSARY

**buffy coat** / a light-colored layer of leukocytes and platelets that forms on top of the red blood cell layer when a sample of blood is centrifuged or allowed to stand undisturbed

**hematocrit** / the volume of erythrocytes packed by centrifugation in a given volume of blood and expressed as a percentage; abbreviated "crit" or Hct

**microhematocrit** / a hematocrit performed in capillary tubes using a small quantity of blood

**microhematocrit centrifuge** / an instrument that spins capillary tubes at a high speed to rapidly separate liquid from cellular components

**packed cell column** / the layers of blood cells that form when a tube of whole blood is centrifuged

## INTRODUCTION

The hematocrit is a commonly performed test that provides the clinician with an estimate of the patient's red cell volume and, thus, the blood's oxygen-carrying capacity. The hematocrit measurement is useful in screening for anemia, evaluating anemia therapies, estimating blood loss following hemorrhage or trauma, and screening potential blood donors.

There are two methods of determining the hematocrit. The hematocrit can be performed manually using a centrifuge, a "spun hematocrit." This manual method is sometimes called a microhematocrit because only a small volume of blood is required. It is a simple procedure in which whole blood is centrifuged in narrow capillary microhematocrit tubes. The spun hematocrit is a CLIA-waived test.

Another method of determining hematocrit is by using a hematology analyzer that includes the hematocrit as part of the complete blood count (CBC). The hematocrit is electronically calculated (using the red cell count and volume) by hematology analyzers. Measurements made using hematology analyzers are called hematocrits, while those made using the centrifuge are called microhematocrits. However, the terms are interchangeable, and both methods provide rapid, reliable results.

# PRINCIPLE OF THE MANUAL HEMATOCRIT TEST

The hematocrit test is based on the principle of separating the cellular elements of blood from the plasma by centrifugation. After the blood is centrifuged in a slender tube, the red cells will be at the bottom of the tube, the white cells and platelets will form a thin layer on top of the red cells, and the plasma will be at the top (Figure 2-23). This layered arrangement following centrifugation is called the **packed cell column**. (Another term sometimes used for hematocrit is *packed cell volume*, or *PCV*). The layer containing white cells and platelets has a whitish-tan appearance and is commonly referred to as the **buffy coat** (Figure 2-23).

The hematocrit is determined by comparing the volume of red cells to the total volume of the whole blood sample. This is commonly reported as a percentage. Laboratory personnel often refer to a hematocrit as a "crit" or abbreviate it with the letters "Hct."

## Materials and Equipment

### Hematocrit Centrifuges

Several types of centrifuges are available for performing manual hematocrits. Some centrifuges, such as the CritSpin® (Figure 2-24) are used only for microhematocrits, and will spin only capillary tubes. Other centrifuges are multifunctional and can spin samples for urinalysis, coagulation, and blood chemistry as well as microhematocrit tubes. Hematocrit centrifuges may have built-in hematocrit readers that require the use of precalibrated capillary tubes. For other centrifuges, a separate hematocrit reader that can accept both uncalibrated and precalibrated tubes is used.

The STAT-CRIT®, a small, portable instrument from Wampole Laboratories, assays blood hemoglobin and hematocrit in 30 seconds. The test is performed by collecting the second drop of blood from a capillary puncture into a disposable blood-sample carrier. The carrier is inserted in the front of the instrument for analysis and the result is displayed digitally.

### Hematocrit Tubes

Several types of capillary tubes are available for manual hematocrit determinations. Heparinized tubes, with a red ring, are used for capillary blood; unheparinized tubes are used for venous blood that already has had anticoagulant added. Mylar-wrapped glass tubes or flexible plastic capillary tubes should be used whenever possible, since they are less likely to break than unwrapped glass tubes. Self-sealing tubes are available that eliminate the need for sealing clay. Lesson 2-2 on capillary puncture contains additional information about capillary tubes.

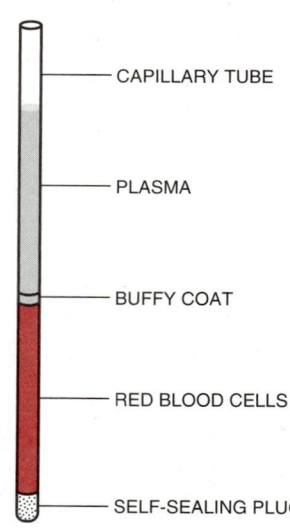

CAPILLARY TUBE

PLASMA

BUFFY COAT

RED BLOOD CELLS

SELF-SEALING PLUG

**FIGURE 2-23** Diagram of packed cell column in a microhematocrit tube

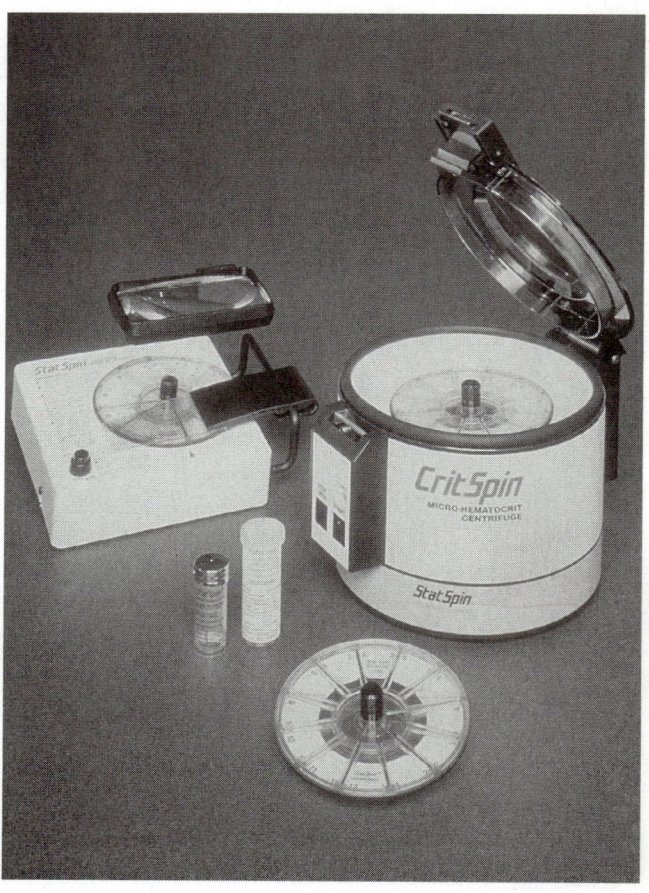

**FIGURE 2-24** Microhematocrit centrifuge with built-in reader (Photo courtesy of Clay Adams Division of Becton Dickinson & Co.)

# HEMATOCRIT REFERENCE VALUES

The normal hematocrit value varies with the gender and age of the patient and with the test method (Table 2-2). The values range from a low of 32% for a one-year-old to a high of 60% for a newborn. Hematocrits for females are usually lower than for males. The System of International Units (SI) value for the hematocrit can be obtained by multiplying the hematocrit percentage by a factor of 0.01.

## Factors That Influence Hematocrit Values

The values obtained for hematocrits can be influenced by physiological and pathological factors, and by the way the specimen is handled during the test procedure (Table 2-3). A low hematocrit value can indicate anemia or the presence of bleeding in a patient. An increased value may be caused by dehydration in the patient or a condition such as polycythemia.

Improper blood collection or the use of inadequately mixed blood can cause unreliable results. The speed of the centrifuge and the length of centrifugation also affect hematocrit values. Increased speed or increased centrifugation time will falsely decrease the hematocrit reading. Decreased speed or time will falsely increase values.

## PERFORMING THE MANUAL HEMATOCRIT TEST

### Safety

Universal and Standard Precautions must be observed when performing hematocrit measurements. Plastic or mylar-coated self-sealing tubes must be used.

Special care must be taken when operating the centrifuge. Centrifuges for hematocrits operate at more than 10,000 rpm (revolutions per minute). Internal locking lids, as well as outer lids, are used to keep tubes in position during high-speed centrifugations. It is unsafe to operate these instruments unless all lids are secured. Lids should never be opened until the rotor has come to a complete stop.

### Quality Assurance

Reliable hematocrit tests require proper specimen collection and test setup, accurate centrifuges, and careful reading and reporting of hematocrit values. Manual hematocrits require few quality control measures. Hematology controls should be run daily and the results charted. Hematocrit tubes should be filled from well-mixed specimens. Each patient sample should be run in duplicate and should agree within ±1%. If they do not, the sample should be thoroughly mixed and the test repeated if it is a venous anticoagulated sample, or recollected and repeated if it is capillary blood.

The centrifuge speed and accuracy of the timer must be checked at designated intervals and the results documented. Periodic preventive maintenance must be performed and documented.

### Obtaining and Preparing the Specimen

The blood sample for a microhematocrit may be obtained from a capillary puncture or from a tube of

**TABLE 2-2.** Hematocrit reference values

| | AVERAGE | | RANGE | |
|---|---|---|---|---|
| | Percent | SI Units | Percent | SI Units |
| Adults | | | | |
| Males | 47 | 0.47 | 42–52 | 0.42–0.52 |
| Females | 42 | 0.42 | 36–48 | 0.36–0.48 |
| Children | | | | |
| Newborn | 56 | 0.56 | 51–61 | 0.51–0.61 |
| 1 year | 35 | 0.35 | 32–38 | 0.32–0.38 |
| 6 years | 38 | 0.38 | 34–42 | 0.34–0.42 |

**TABLE 2-3.** Factors affecting hematocrit values

| CONDITION | EFFECT ON HEMATOCRIT VALUE |
|---|---|
| Age | |
| Newborns | Increased |
| Children | Less than adult value |
| Older adults | Decreased from adult value |
| Gender | Adult female value less than adult male value |
| Severe dehydration | Increased |
| Anemias | Decreased |
| Polycythemia | Increased |
| Leukemias | Decreased |
| Residence at high altitudes | Increased |

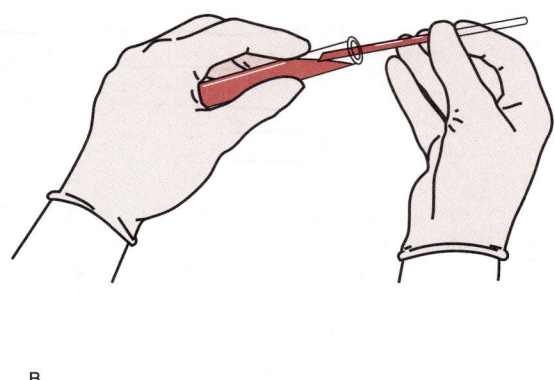

A.                                                                B.

**FIGURE 2-25**  (A) Filling a capillary tube from a capillary puncture  (B) Filling a capillary tube from a tube of blood

venous blood to which the anticoagulant EDTA has been added (Figure 2-25). Before sampling from tubes of venous anticoagulated blood, the blood must be gently mixed by either inverting the tube approximately sixty times, or placing it on a mechanical mixer for a minimum of two minutes (Figure 2-26).

The blood is drawn by capillary action into capillary tubes (Figure 2-25), which are then sealed.  Self-sealing tubes should be used.  These have a dry plug in one end that expands to form a seal when blood contacts it.

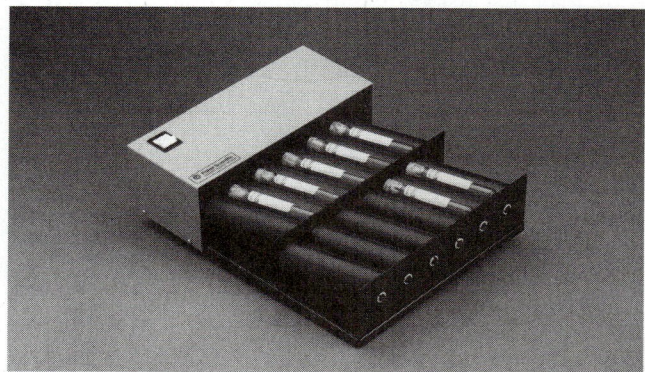

**FIGURE 2-26**  Mixer for hematology specimens (Courtesy of Fisher Scientific)

## Centrifuging the Samples

The sealed tubes are placed in a special **microhematocrit centrifuge** (Figure 2-24). The sealed ends of the tubes are placed against the rubber gasket and the open ends toward the center (Figure 2-27). The lids to the centrifuge are secured and the tubes are centrifuged for a prescribed time, usually two to five minutes.

## Determining the Hematocrit Value

The hematocrit percentage is determined by placing the tubes on a special hematocrit reader (Figure 2-28). Some centrifuges, such as the Clay Adams Readacrit, have a built-in reading scale. Special precalibrated capillary tubes must be used with this type of centrifuge.

Hematocrits should be performed in duplicate on each specimen. The two values should not vary by more than ±1%. The average of the two results is reported.

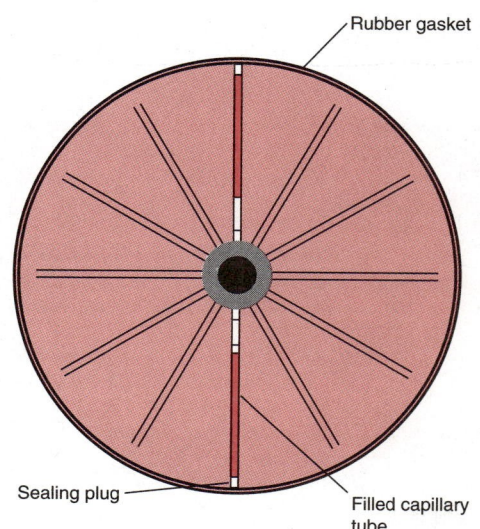

Rubber gasket

Sealing plug

Filled capillary tube

**FIGURE 2-27**  Illustration showing proper placement of sealed capillary tubes in microhematocrit centrifuge

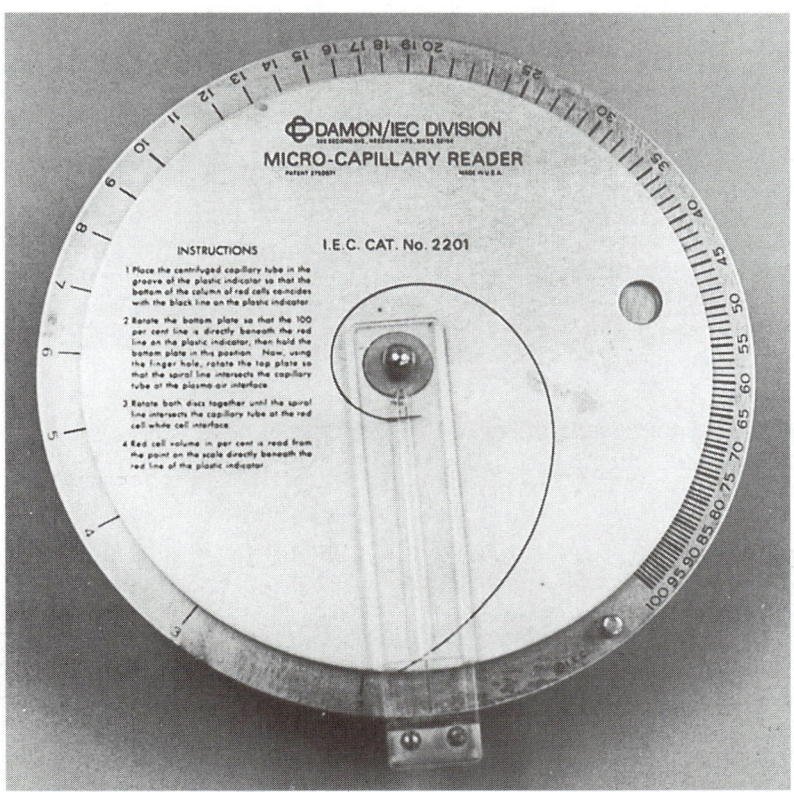

**FIGURE 2-28** Hematocrit reader (Photo courtesy of International Equipment, Division of Damon)

## Procedural Notes

- Follow time recommendations for the centrifuge being used.
- Run duplicate tubes for each patient specimen.
- Read the hematocrit value at the top of the red cell layer, not at the top of the buffy coat.
- Mix venous anticoagulated blood well before filling capillary tubes.

## Safety Precautions

- Observe Universal and Standard Precautions when performing hematocrits.
- Use plastic or mylar-coated self-sealing tubes.
- Check that capillary tubes are completely sealed before centrifugation.
- Place the sealed end of the capillary tubes against the rubber gasket in the centrifuge.
- Close both centrifuge lids securely before operating the centrifuge.
- Never try to open a centrifuge until the rotor has come to a complete stop.

## LESSON REVIEW

1. What does the hematocrit measure? *RBC Volume*
2. Give the hematocrit reference values for males, females, and newborns.
   *Male = 47-57*
   *Female = 37-47*
   *N. Born = 50-60*

3. Name a condition that could cause a decreased hematocrit value. *increase in speed & time Centrifuge*
4. Explain the hematocrit procedure.
5. Blood enters the capillary tube by what action?
6. Why must the capillary tube be sealed securely? *to avoid blood split*

7. What is the usual length of time for centrifugation of the hematocrit tubes? *2-5 mines*

8. What precautions should be observed when performing a hematocrit? *no Coagulation, proper collection*

9. Define buffy coat, hematocrit, microhematocrit, microhematocrit centrifuge, and packed cell column. *buffy coat > wbc, Platelet*
   *Hematocrit = RBC volume*
   *MIC V   = method*

## STUDENT ACTIVITIES

1. Reread the information on hematocrit.

2. Review the glossary terms.

3. Practice performing an hematocrit test on several blood samples as outlined in the Student Performance Guide.

4. Repeat the hematocrit procedure on a blood sample, lengthening or shortening the centrifugation time. Record the results and give the reason for the different values obtained from the previous hematocrit.

5. Demonstrate the importance of using well-mixed blood: perform a hematocrit on a well-mixed sample; allow the sample tube to stand upright five to ten minutes and perform another hematocrit without remixing the blood. Compare the results and explain the difference.

## *Student Performance Guide*

## LESSON 2-4 Hematocrit

Name _____ Date _____

  ### INSTRUCTIONS

1. Practice the hematocrit procedure following the step-by-step instructions.

2. Demonstrate your understanding of this lesson by:

   a. Completing a written examination successfully, and

   b. Performing the procedure for the hematocrit satisfactorily for the instructor. All steps must be completed as listed on the instructor's Performance Check Sheet.

*Note:* Consult the instruction manual for the centrifuge being used. Refer to the specific procedure being performed.

## MATERIALS AND EQUIPMENT

- gloves
- acrylic safety shield
- hand disinfectant
- self-sealing capillary tubes, Mylar-coated, heparinized, and plain
- precalibrated capillary tubes (optional)
- microhematocrit centrifuge and reader
- tube of anticoagulated venous blood (or commercially available simulated blood)
- paper towels or soft laboratory tissue
- 70% alcohol or alcohol swabs
- gauze or cotton balls, sterile
- blood lancets, sterile, disposable
- surface disinfectant or 10% chlorine bleach solution
- biohazard container
- puncture-proof biohazard container for sharps

## PROCEDURE

Record in the comment section any problems encountered while practicing the procedure (or have a fellow student or the instructor evaluate your performance).

S = Satisfactory
U = Unsatisfactory

| You must: | S | U | Comments |
|---|---|---|---|
| 1. Wash hands and put on gloves | | | |
| 2. Assemble equipment and materials for capillary puncture and hematocrit; place acrylic safety shield into position | | | |
| 3. Fill two capillary tubes from a capillary puncture: | | | |
|    a. Perform a capillary puncture | | | |
|    b. Wipe away the first drop of blood | | | |
|    c. Touch one end of a heparinized capillary tube to the second drop of blood | | | |
|    d. Allow the tube to fill three-quarters full by capillary action. A slight downward angle of the tube may be necessary. If using precalibrated tubes, fill to the line | | | |

| You must: | S | U | Comments |
|---|---|---|---|
| e. Fill a second tube in the same manner | | | |
| f. Wipe the outside of the filled capillary tube with soft tissue, if necessary, to remove excess blood | | | |
| g. Seal the capillary tube. Check to see that the plug has expanded | | | |
| 4. Fill two capillary tubes using a tube of EDTA anticoagulated blood (If not available, proceed to step 5): | | | |
|    a. Mix the tube of blood thoroughly by gently rocking tube from end to end a minimum of two minutes by mechanical mixer or fifty to sixty times by hand | | | |
|    b. Remove cap from tube (with an acrylic safety shield placed between worker and tube) | | | |
|    c. Tilt the tube so the blood is very near the top edge of the tube | | | |
|    d. Insert the tip of a plain capillary tube into the blood and fill three-quarters full by capillary action. If using precalibrated tubes, fill to the line<br>*Note:*  Wipe the outside of the filled capillary tube with tissue, if necessary, to remove excess blood | | | |
|    e. Seal the tube. Check to see that plug expanded | | | |
|    f. Fill a second tube in the same manner | | | |
| 5. Place tubes into the hematocrit centrifuge with sealed ends securely against the gasket. Balance the load by placing the tubes directly opposite each other | | | |
| 6. Fasten both lids securely | | | |
| 7. Set the timer and adjust the speed if necessary | | | |
| 8. Centrifuge for the prescribed time | | | |
| 9. Allow centrifuge to come to a complete stop and unlock lid(s) | | | |
| 10. Determine the hematocrit values using one of the following methods: | | | |
|    A. A centrifuge that requires calibrated tubes and has a built-in scale: | | | |
|       (1) Position the tubes as directed by the manufacturer's instructions | | | |
|       (2) Read the hematocrit value | | | |
|    B. A centrifuge without a built-in reader: | | | |
|       (1) Remove capillary tubes from centrifuge carefully | | | |
|       (2) Place tubes on the hematocrit reader provided | | | |
|       (3) Follow instructions on the reader to obtain the hematocrit value | | | |

| You must: | S | U | Comments |
|---|---|---|---|
| 11. Average the values from the two tubes and record the hematocrit. (The values must agree within ±1%) | | | |
| 12. Discard capillary tubes and used lancets in a puncture-proof biohazard container for sharps | | | |
| 13. Clean and return equipment to proper storage | | | |
| 14. Clean the work area with surface disinfectant | | | |
| 15. Remove gloves, discard in biohazard container, and wash hands with hand disinfectant | | | |

*Evaluator Comments:*

Evaluator _____ Date _____

# The Hemacytometer: WBC and RBC Counts

## LESSON OBJECTIVES

**After studying this lesson, you should be able to:**

- *Identify the parts of a hemacytometer.*
- *Use the microscope to identify the hemacytometer areas where RBCs and WBCs are counted.*
- *Fill the hemacytometer using a micropipetter or capillary tube.*
- *Write the general formula for calculating cell counts using a hemacytometer.*
- *List the RBC count reference values for adult males, adult females, and newborns.*
- *List the WBC count reference values for adults, children, and newborn infants.*
- *Perform a manual RBC count and calculate the results.*
- *Perform a manual WBC count and calculate the results.*
- *Name a condition or disease associated with an increased RBC count and one associated with a decreased RBC count.*
- *Name a condition that causes leukocytosis and one that causes leukopenia.*
- *State the important properties of RBC diluting fluids and of WBC diluting fluids.*
- *List the safety precautions to observe when performing manual blood cell counts.*
- *Define the glossary terms.*

## GLOSSARY

**anemia** / decrease below normal in the red blood cell count or in the blood hemoglobin level

**aperture** / an opening

**cell diluting fluid** / a solution used to dilute blood for cell counts

**erythrocytosis** / an excess of red blood cells in the peripheral blood; sometimes called polycythemia

**hemacytometer** / a heavy glass slide made to precise specifications and used to count cells microscopically; a counting chamber

**hemacytometer coverglass** / a special coverglass of uniform thickness used with a hemacytometer

**hemolysis** / the destruction of red blood cells resulting in the release of hemoglobin from the cells

**immunity** / resistance to disease or infection

**isotonic solution** / a solution that has the same concentration of dissolved particles as the solution or cell with which it is compared

**leukocytosis** / increase above normal in the number of leukocytes (white blood cells) in the blood

**leukopenia** / decrease below normal in the number of leukocytes (white blood cells) in the blood; leukocytopenia

**micropipet** / a pipet that measures or holds volumes less than 1 mL

## INTRODUCTION

Red blood cell (RBC) and white blood cell (WBC) counts are commonly performed hematology tests that are usually part of the complete blood count (CBC). The RBC count approximates the number of circulating red blood cells and is helpful in diagnosing and treating many diseases, especially anemias. The WBC count gives information about a patient's immune response, since WBCs play important roles in our resistance to disease.

Manual cell counts are performed microscopically using the hemacytometer, a special glass counting chamber. Hemacytometers are manufactured to meet the specifications of the National Institute of Standards and Technology (NIST).

This lesson explains the proper use of the hemacytometer and methods of calculating cell counts using the hemacytometer. Procedures for performing WBC and RBC counts using UNOPETTES® systems are outlined. In addition, the use of automated cell counters in hematology is briefly discussed.

## THE HEMACYTOMETER

The hemacytometer is a heavy, precision-made glass slide with two counting areas. The hemacytometer must be used with a hemacytometer coverglass of uniform thickness (0.4 mm) which has been manufactured to meet NIST specifications. The hemacytometer is used to perform manual cell counts of peripheral blood, semen, and cerebrospinal fluid.

## General Features of the Hemacytometer

When viewed from the top, the hemacytometer has two polished raised platforms surrounded by depressions on three sides (Figure 2-29). The depressions surrounding these platforms are called "moats" and form an "H." Each raised surface contains a ruled counting area marked off by precise lines (rules) etched into the glass. Most hematology laboratories use hemacytometers with Neubauer type rulings.

The hemacytometer coverglass is positioned so it covers both ruled areas of the hemacytometer (Figures 2-29 and 2-30). The coverglass creates a chamber, confines the fluid when the chamber is filled, and regulates the depth of the fluid. The chamber depth in the Neubauer-type hemacytometer is 0.1 mm with the coverglass in place.

## Hemacytometer Counting Areas

The hemacytometer contains two identical ruled areas composed of etched lines that define squares of specific dimensions. In the Neubauer counting chamber, each ruled area consists of a large square, 3 mm x 3 mm,

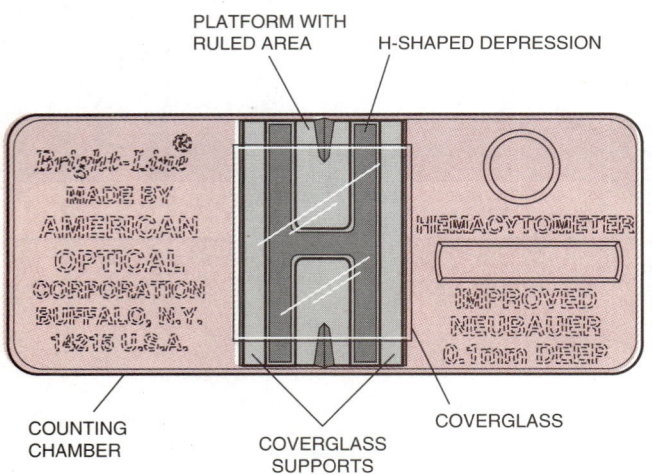

PLATFORM WITH RULED AREA · H-SHAPED DEPRESSION

*Bright-Line* ® MADE BY AMERICAN OPTICAL CORPORATION BUFFALO, N.Y. 14215 U.S.A.

HEMACYTOMETER IMPROVED NEUBAUER 0.1mm DEEP

COUNTING CHAMBER · COVERGLASS SUPPORTS · COVERGLASS

**FIGURE 2-29** Hemacytometer with coverglass in place

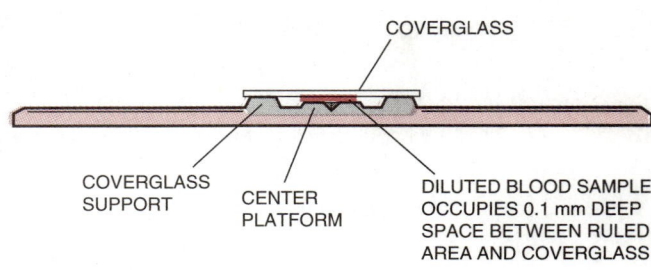

COVERGLASS

COVERGLASS SUPPORT · CENTER PLATFORM · DILUTED BLOOD SAMPLE OCCUPIES 0.1 mm DEEP SPACE BETWEEN RULED AREA AND COVERGLASS

**FIGURE 2-30** Side view of hemacytometer with coverglass in place

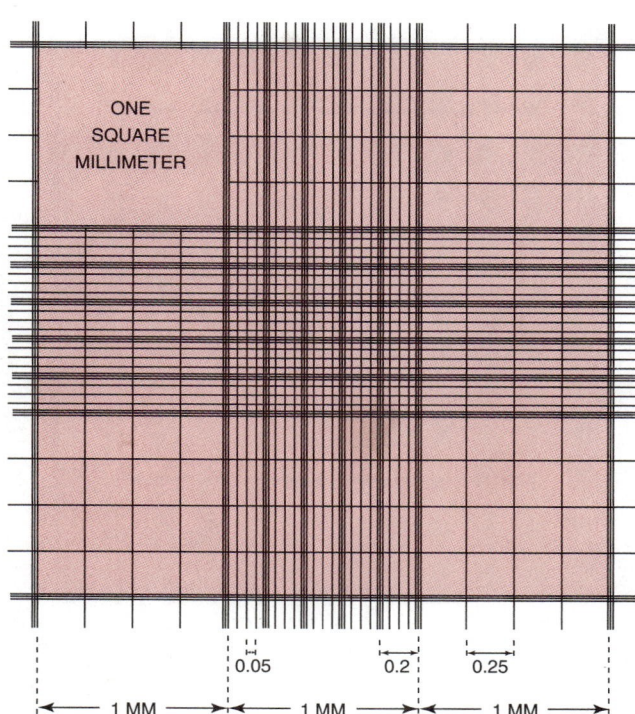

**FIGURE 2-31**  Ruled area of hemacytometer showing dimensions

divided into nine equal squares (Figure 2-31), each 1 mm square (mm$^2$). The total area of the large square is 9 mm$^2$.

## WBC Counting Area

The WBC counting area using the UNOPETTE® method consists of all nine large squares (Figure 2-32).

## RBC Counting Area

The large center square is used for RBC counts. This center square is subdivided into 25 smaller squares, which in turn are each divided into 16 squares. Of the 25 squares, only the four corner squares and the center square within the large center square are used to perform RBC counts (Figure 2-33).

## Platelet Counting Area

The large center square is used to count platelets. Platelets in all 25 squares within the large center square are counted (Figures 2-31 and 2-33).

# USING THE HEMACYTOMETER

## Filling the Hemacytometer

A clean hemacytometer coverglass should be positioned so it covers both ruled areas of a clean hemacytometer. Then, the hemacytometer is filled or charged.

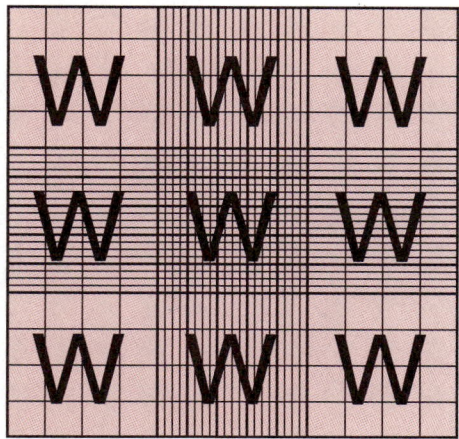

**FIGURE 2-32**  WBC counting area using UNOPETTE® method.  All nine large squares of the hemacytometer grid are used to count WBCs

This is done by touching the tip of a micropipet or capillary pipet to the point on one side where the coverglass and the raised platform meet (Figure 2-34). The fluid from the pipet is allowed to flow by capillary action into one side of the hemacytometer, using one-half to one drop of fluid (approximately 10 µL). The opposite side of the hemacytometer is then filled in the same manner. (Some hemacytometers have a V-shaped trough on each raised platform to guide the placement of the pipet tip when filling, as in Figure 2-29.)

The fluid should flow into the chamber in a smooth, unbroken stream. *It should not be allowed to overflow into the depressions or moats*. After the hemacytometer has been correctly filled, it should then stand for two minutes to allow the cells to settle.

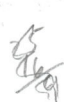

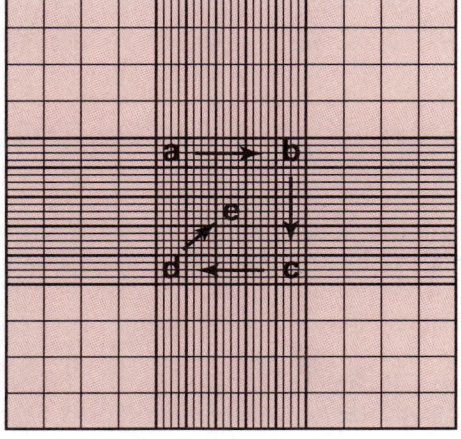

**FIGURE 2-33**  RBC counting area.  The four corner squares and center square (labeled a-e) within the large center square are used to count RBCs

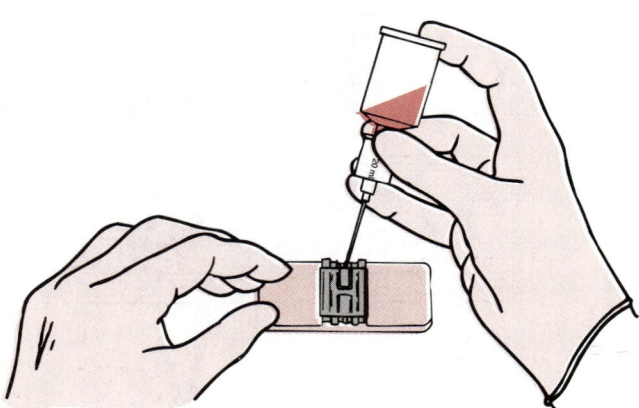

**FIGURE 2-34**   Filling the hemacytometer using a UNOPETTE® capillary

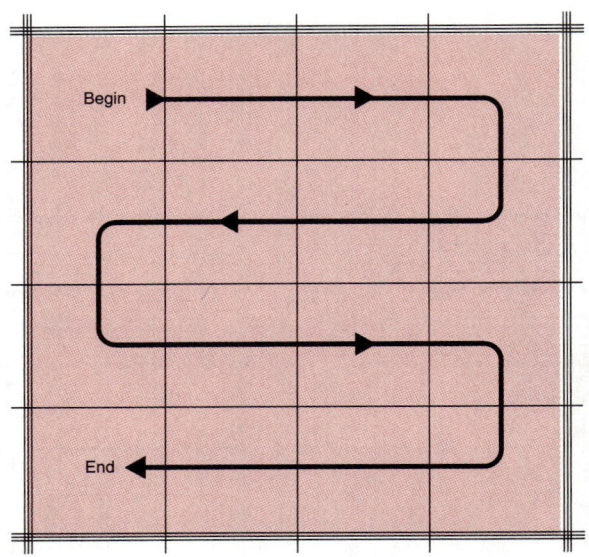

**FIGURE 2-35**   Left-to-right, right-to-left counting pattern (shown here in one of the large corner squares of the hematocytometer grid)

## Viewing the Ruled Areas

The hemacytometer should be placed on the microscope stage with the low-power (10X) objective in place so that one of the ruled areas is located over the light source. The coarse adjustment knob should be used to move the hemacytometer and objective close together until the objective is almost touching the coverglass. *This must be done carefully, since some microscopes do not have a stop.* The coarse adjustment knob is then used to increase the distance between the objective and the hemacytometer while looking through the oculars. This is continued until the etched lines come into view. The fine adjustment knob is then used to bring the etched lines into sharp focus. The etched lines are more easily viewed when the condenser is lowered and light intensity is reduced.

When the ruled area is in sharp focus, the WBC counting area (all nine large squares) is located by moving the stage (or moving the hemacytometer carefully if the microscope does not have a mechanical stage). After the WBC counting area has been observed, the central square used for the RBC counts should be located. The high power (40X) objective should be carefully rotated into place. (If the microscope is parfocal, the ruled area will be brought into focus with only a slight rotation of the fine adjustment.) The center square used for platelet counts and the five small squares used in an RBC count should be located (Figure 2-33).

Once all parts of the ruled area of one side have been located, the hemacytometer should be carefully moved so the second ruled area can be viewed. When moving the hemacytometer, the low-power objective should be in position. *The oil-immersion objective is never used with a hemacytometer.*

## The Counting Pattern

A counting pattern of left-to-right, right-to-left must be used to ensure that cells are counted only once. The count should begin in the upper left corner of a square and proceed in a serpentine manner (Figure 2-35).

Squares are divided by boundary lines, which may be single, double, or triple. When triple lines are present, the center line is considered the boundary. When double lines are present, the outer line is considered the boundary. All cells that are within a square, touch the left boundary of the square, or touch the top boundary of the square are counted. Cells that touch the right boundary of a square and cells that touch the lower boundary (see Figure 2-35) of a square should not be counted in that square even though they may lie within the square.

The cells in the designated squares should be counted on both sides of the chamber. The results for each side should be recorded. The counts for the two sides are then totaled and the average is calculated.

## CALCULATING THE CELL COUNTS

The total number of cells per microliter (μL) of sample can be calculated from the average number of cells counted. This is because the ruled areas of the hemacytometer contain an exact volume of diluted sample. Since only a small volume of diluted sample is counted, a general formula must be used to convert the count into the number of cells/μL: (Note: 1 mm³ = 1 μL)

$$C/\mu L = \frac{Avg \times D \,(mm) \times DF}{A \,(mm^2)}$$

Where:  C/µL   =   Final cell count/µL
      Avg   =   Average # of cells counted
  D (mm)   =   Depth factor in mm
      DF   =   Dilution factor
  A (mm$^2$)   =   Area counted (mm$^2$)

The dilution factor used in the formula is determined by the blood dilution used in the cell count. The depth factor used in the formula is always 10 (the counting chamber is 0.1 mm deep; the depth is converted to 1 mm by multiplying by 10). The area counted will vary for each type of cell count and is calculated using the dimensions of the ruled area.

## Care of the Hemacytometer

The hemacytometer is an expensive piece of equipment that must be handled carefully. It should be held by the sides and bottom only, to avoid getting fingerprints on the raised ruled areas.

Before each use, the raised surfaces should be wiped with lens paper dipped in 70% or 95% alcohol. The hemacytometer should then be immediately dried and polished gently with lens paper. The coverglass should be handled by the edges, and both sides cleaned in the same manner as the hemacytometer.

After use, the hemacytometer should be disinfected by soaking in 10% chlorine bleach for at least 10 minutes before washing. The hemacytometer should be stored in a container to keep dirt and dust off the surface and to protect the ruled areas from scratches. When transporting the hemacytometer, hold it carefully and place it gently on a secure surface.

## UNOPETTE® SYSTEMS

Manual blood cell counts were formerly performed by making blood dilutions using a glass pipet called the Thoma pipet, loading the dilution in the hemacytometer and counting the cells. Now, the most acceptable manual method of counting blood cells is using self-filling, self-diluting systems such as the UNOPETTE® marketed by Becton Dickinson (Figure 2-36). These systems provide acceptable accuracy and have disposable components. UNOPETTE® systems are available for RBC, WBC, and platelet counts, as well as for hemoglobin determinations and more specialized tests such as erythrocyte osmotic fragility.

## Components of a UNOPETTE® System

Each UNOPETTE® system for cell counts includes a sealed reservoir containing a pre-measured volume of diluting fluid and a pipet assembly that includes a calibrated capillary pipet and a pipet shield (Figure 2-36). The shield protects the pipet and is used to puncture the diaphragm that seals the reservoir.

 ## SAFETY

Universal and Standard Precautions must be observed when using UNOPETTE® systems. Special care must be taken to avoid creating aerosols or breaking capillary tubes. When making blood dilutions, workers must wear gloves and suitable protective clothing, and either wear a face shield or work behind a safety shield. All contaminated materials must be disposed of in appropriate biohazard containers.

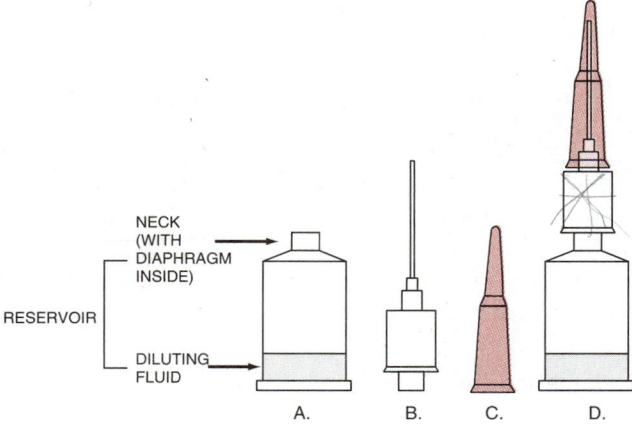

**FIGURE 2-36** Parts of a UNOPETTE® disposable blood diluting unit: (A) prefilled reservoir containing premeasured diluting fluid and sealed at the neck with a diaphragm, (B) capillary pipet with overflow chamber and capacity marking, (C) pipet shield, and (D) assembled unit

### Quality Assurance

Since there are no blood cell standards available in hematology, quality assurance for hemacytometer counts is primarily concerned with specimen collection and preparation, counting techniques, and calculations. These are all areas where good technique is very important. Care must be taken to avoid overloading the counting chamber, which would allow the fluid to flow into the moat and alter the cell distribution in the counting chamber. Large variations among squares counted or between counts from the two hemacytometer sides are signals that the count should be repeated.

## Cell Counts Using UNOPETTE® Systems

A different UNOPETTE® system is used for each type of cell count. Each type of UNOPETTE® system is designed to provide a particular dilution of the blood; therefore, different counting methods and calculations are required for each system.

### RBC Counts

The UNOPETTE® system for RBC counts contains 1.99 ml of red cell diluting fluid consisting of a physiological saline (0.85%) solution plus a preservative. The RBC diluting fluid is an **isotonic solution.** This is necessary to prevent **hemolysis,** or destruction, of the osmotically sensitive red cells. The capillary pipet for measuring the blood sample is made to contain 10 µL (0.01 mL). When the 10 µL is added to the 1.99 mL of diluting fluid, the blood is diluted 1 part blood plus 199 parts diluting fluid. This equals a 1:200 dilution (1 part blood in a total of 200 parts).

### WBC Counts

The UNOPETTE® system for WBC counts consists of a sealed reservoir containing 1.98 mL of WBC diluting fluid and a 20 µL (0.02 mL) capillary. The WBC diluting fluid is a 3% acetic acid solution which lyses (destroys) the RBCs so the WBCs are more easily seen using the microscope. When the 20 µL of blood is added to the 1.98 mL of diluting fluid, the blood is diluted 1 part blood plus 99 parts diluting fluid (a 1:100 dilution).

## PERFORMING RBC AND WBC COUNTS

### Performing a Manual RBC Count Using the UNOPETTE® System

#### Preparing the UNOPETTE®

A UNOPETTE® RBC system is selected. The pipet shield is used to puncture the diaphragm in the neck of the reservoir, making an opening large enough to accept the capillary pipet.

#### Diluting the Blood Sample

The UNOPETTE® 10 µL capillary is filled with blood from a capillary puncture or from a tube of well-mixed EDTA blood. The filled capillary pipet is inserted into the reservoir, allowing the blood to mix with the diluting fluid. The resulting blood dilution is 1:200. This blood and diluting fluid mixture is stable for up to six hours, but can be used immediately.

### Loading the Hemacytometer

A clean coverglass is positioned on a clean hemacytometer to cover both counting areas. The capillary pipet is removed from the reservoir and re-inserted in the reservoir with the pipet extending upward. The reservoir is swirled to mix the contents and a few drops are expelled from the pipet tip and discarded. The tip of the pipet is touched to the edge of the coverglass, and one side of the chamber is allowed to fill by capillary action. The opposite side is then filled in the same manner. If the fluid overflows into the depression around the platforms, or if air bubbles occur, the chamber must be cleaned and refilled.

### Counting the Cells

The cells are allowed to settle for two to three minutes and the hemacytometer is placed carefully on the microscope stage. The RBC ruled area is located using the low-power (10X) objective. The high-power (40X) objective is then carefully rotated into place to perform the count. Color plate 7 illustrates the RBC appearance on the hemacytometer using the 40X objective.

The RBC count is performed using the center square of the ruled area as shown in Figure 2-33. Within the center square are twenty-five smaller squares. Of these twenty-five squares, the four corner ones and the center square (marked a, b, c, d, and e in Figure 2-33) are used for the count. Each of these five squares in turn contains four rows of squares. All cells within each of the small squares are counted using the left-to-right, right-to-left counting pattern. The cells touching either the top or left boundaries of the squares are included in the count. The cells touching the right boundary and the cells touching the lower boundary of each square are not counted. Cells lying beyond these boundaries are *not* counted (Figure 2-37).

A hand tally counter is used to tabulate the red cells in the designated squares. The numbers for each of the squares are recorded and totaled. A count is then performed in the five squares of the second side of the chamber in the same manner. In an RBC count, if the number of cells in a square varies from any other square on the same side of the hemacytometer by more than twenty-five cells, the count must be repeated, after remixing the sample and reloading the hemacytometer.

### Calculating the RBC Count

The general formula to use for the hemacytometer is:

$$\text{cells/µL} = \frac{\text{Avg} \times \text{D(mm)} \times \text{DF}}{\text{A (mm}^2)}$$

To calculate an RBC count using the UNOPETTE® method, the formula is used in the following manner:

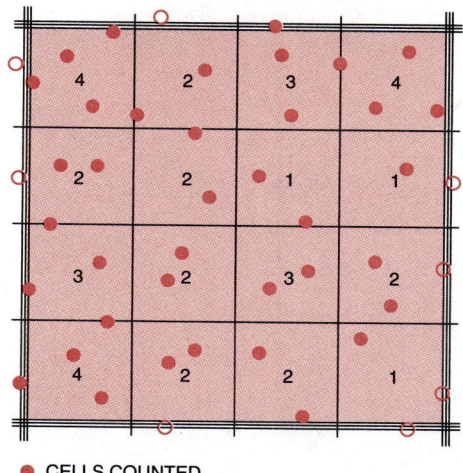

● CELLS COUNTED
○ CELLS NOT COUNTED

**FIGURE 2-37** Illustration of a sample RBC count, showing which cells are to be counted in a square, using the boundary rule. The numbers shown denote the number of cells counted in each of the small squares.

1. The average number of cells is obtained by totaling the counts for the five squares on each side of the chamber and dividing the total by two. This gives the average cell count.
2. The depth factor (mm) is always ten. (The depth of the chamber is 0.1 mm which, when multiplied by ten, is one.)
3. The dilution using the RBC UNOPETTE® system is 1:200. Therefore, the dilution factor is 200.
4. The area counted is 0.20 mm². (Each square, a to e, has a length of 0.2 mm and a width of 0.2 mm. This

gives each square an area of 0.04 mm². Since five squares are counted, the area is 5 x 0.04 mm² or 0.20 mm².) Substitute these numbers into the formula as shown:

$$RBC/\mu L = \frac{Average \times 10 \times 200}{0.20}$$

$$= Average \text{ # cells} \times 10,000$$

When an RBC count is performed this way, the count/μL may be calculated by simply adding four zeroes to the average number of cells counted (or multiplying by 10,000). A sample calculation is shown in Figure 2-38.

### Reference Values for RBC Counts

The reference values for RBC counts range from approximately four million per microliter of blood (4.0 x 10⁶/μL) to six million per microliter (6.0 x 10⁶/μL). Males usually have slightly higher RBC counts than females (Table 2-4). Newborns have an elevated RBC count that slowly declines during childhood, only to increase to adult levels at puberty.

Red blood cell counts may be reported as the number of cells per cubic microliter (μL), or liter (L) of blood. For example, a count of 5.6 x 10⁶ RBC/μL would be reported as 5.6 x 10¹² RBC/L.

### Conditions Associated with Changes in RBC Counts

Since RBCs carry oxygen, a reduction in their number results in decreased oxygen available to body tissues. This condition is called **anemia**. The symptoms of anemia include fatigue, weakness, headache, and pallor. Extreme anemia causes increased heart rate. Iron deficiency and sickle cell are two different types of anemia.

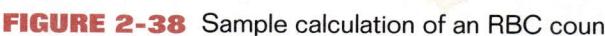

**FIGURE 2-38** Sample calculation of an RBC count

*Erythrocytosis ↑ RBC count*
*Polycythemia Vera ↑ by disease*

**TABLE 2-4.** Reference ranges for RBC counts

| AGE/GENDER | REFERENCE RANGE | |
|---|---|---|
| | Conventional Units | SI Units |
| Adult male | $4.5–6.0 \times 10^6/\mu L$ | $4.5–6.0 \times 10^{12}/L$ |
| Adult female | $4.0–5.5 \times 10^6/\mu L$ | $4.0–5.5 \times 10^{12}/L$ |
| Newborn | $5.0–6.3 \times 10^6/\mu L$ | $5.0–6.3 \times 10^{12}/L$ |

Some anemias may be due to deficiencies of vitamins such as $B_{12}$ or folic acid (Table 2-5).

An increased RBC count is called **erythrocytosis**. People who live at very high altitudes have erythrocytosis because the lower oxygen content of the air stimulates RBC production. Polycythemia vera is a disease in which the RBC count is greatly increased.

## Performing a Manual WBC Count Using the UNOPETTE® System

The five types of WBCs are neutrophils, eosinophils, basophils, monocytes, and lymphocytes. WBCs (leukocytes) are not as numerous in the blood as the RBCs, but they have many functions.

All WBCs play important roles in our resistance to disease. The number of lymphocytes may increase in response to a viral infection. Lymphocytes also have important functions in **immunity**, or resistance to infection and disease. Neutrophils provide defense from infections by directly attacking the invading organisms and may increase in response to bacterial infections.

The WBC count is part of the complete blood count (CBC). The WBC count is also often ordered separately to follow the recovery of a patient being treated for an infection.

### Preparing the UNOPETTE®

A UNOPETTE® WBC system is selected. The pipet shield is used to puncture the diaphragm in the neck of the reservoir, making an opening large enough to accept the capillary pipet.

### Diluting the Blood Sample

The tip of the capillary pipet is inserted into a drop of capillary blood or into a tube of well-mixed EDTA blood, and 20 µL (0.02 mL) is automatically drawn up. While pressing lightly on the sides of the reservoir, the filled capillary pipet is inserted into the reservoir, allowing the blood to mix with the diluting fluid, but not to overflow from the top of the capillary. The 20 µL of

**TABLE 2-5.** Examples of conditions affecting RBC counts

| CONDITION | EFFECT ON RBC COUNT |
|---|---|
| Anemias | Decreased |
|    Iron deficiency | |
|    Sickle cell | |
|    $B_{12}$ deficiency | |
|    Folic acid deficiency | |
| Erythrocytosis | Increased |
| Polycythemia vera | Increased |

*1:100 dilut. fluid*

blood is mixed with the 1.98 mL of diluting fluid, making a blood dilution of 1:100. The blood-and-fluid mixture must stand for at least ten minutes before loading the hemacytometer to allow the RBCs to be destroyed.

### Loading the Hemacytometer

After 10 minutes, the reservoir is swirled to mix the contents and the pipet assembly is removed and re-inserted in the reservoir with the pipet extending upward. A few drops are expelled from the pipet tip and the hemacytometer is then filled on both sides.

### Counting the Cells

When the cells have settled, the hemacytometer is placed securely onto the microscope stage for counting. The low-power objective (10X) is used to locate the ruled grid. The WBCs will be more distinct if the microscope's light level is reduced. This can be accomplished by lowering the condenser and partially closing the iris diaphragm.

Cells in all nine of the large ruled areas are counted, as shown in Figure 2-32, using the 10X objective (100X magnification). The WBCs will appear as refractile round objects with a definite outline (Color Plate 8). The WBCs lying within each of the nine squares are counted using the left-to-right, right-to-left pattern (Figure 2-35). All cells touching either the upper or left boundary of the square are counted. Cells touching the lower or right boundary of the square are not counted (Figure 2-39). The results from side 1 are recorded and the procedure is repeated for side 2. The results are added together and divided by two to obtain the average.

## Calculating the WBC Count

The total number of WBCs per microliter of blood can be calculated using the average number of cells counted, the depth of the counting chamber, the area counted, and the dilution. The dilution made with the WBC UNOPETTE® system is 1:100. The total volume counted is 0.9 µL (depth x area = volume; 0.1 mm x 9 mm² = 0.9 mm³ = 0.9 µL). However, the WBC count is reported as cells per 1.0 µL (or cells/L). To correct for this, the following formula is used:

$$\frac{WBC}{\mu L} = \text{average counted} + (0.1 \times \text{average counted}) \times 100$$

A sample WBC calculation is shown in Figure 2-40.

## Reference Values for the WBC Count

The normal (reference) WBC count varies according to the age of the individual (Table 2-6). Newborn infants usually have a WBC count of 9,000-30,000/µL. Within a few weeks after birth, the count drops rapidly and approaches the children's normal of 6,000-14,000/µL. By adulthood, the normal count is in the range of 4,500-11,000/µL.

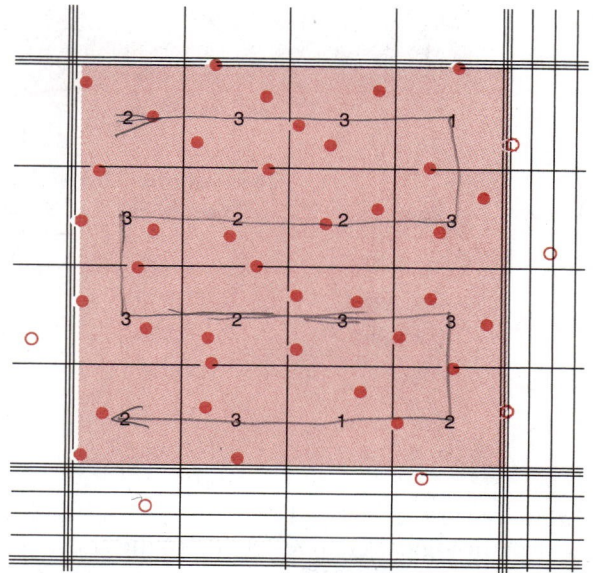

**FIGURE 2-39** Sample WBC count in large corner square on one side of chamber. The numbers shown denote the number of cells counted in each small square.

## Factors Influencing WBC Counts

Many factors can increase or decrease the WBC count. Stress, exercise, and anesthesia may cause temporary increases in the WBC count; these are called physiological increases. Changes in the WBC count due to disease

1. **Count the cells:**

| Square | Side 1 Cells counted | Side 2 Cells counted |
|---|---|---|
| 1 | 8 | 9 |
| 2 | 9 | 9 |
| 3 | 10 | 7 |
| 4 | 9 | 10 |
| 5 | 7 | 8 |
| 6 | 9 | 7 |
| 7 | 9 | 7 |
| 8 | 10 | 9 |
| 9 | 7 | 10 |
| Total | 78 | Total 76 |

2. **Compute the average:**

$$\frac{78 + 76}{2} = 77$$

3. **Calculate the count:**

| | |
|---|---|
| WBC/µL = | [Average counted + (0.1 × average counted)] × 100 |
| WBC/µL = | [77 + (.10) 77] × 100 |
| WBC/µL = | (77 + 7.7) × 100 |
| WBC/µL = | (77 + 8) × 100 |
| WBC/µL = | 85 × 100 |
| WBC/µL = | 8500 (8.5 × 10³) |
| WBC/L = | 8.5 × 10⁹ |

**FIGURE 2-40** Sample calculation of a WBC count using a 1:100 dilution UNOPETTE® system

**TABLE 2-6.** Reference values for WBC counts

| Age | AVERAGE | | RANGE | |
| | Conventional Units (cells/µL) | SI Units (cells/L) | Conventional Units (cells/µL) | SI Units (cells/L) |
|---|---|---|---|---|
| Newborn | 18,000 | $1.8 \times 10^{10}$ | 9,000–30,000 | $9.0–30.0 \times 10^9$ |
| One year | 11,000 | $1.1 \times 10^{10}$ | 6,000–14,000 | $6.0–14.0 \times 10^9$ |
| Six years | 8,000 | $8.0 \times 10^9$ | 4,500–12,000 | $4.5–12.0 \times 10^9$ |
| Adult | 7,400 | $7.4 \times 10^9$ | 4,500–11,000 | $4.5–11.0 \times 10^9$ |

continue until the illness is under control; these are called pathological changes. Usually the increase or decrease in the total WBC count is due to a change in only one type of cell.

An increase above normal in the total number of WBCs is called **leukocytosis**. Conditions that may cause leukocytosis include infections and certain diseases such as leukemias.

A decrease below normal in the total number of WBCs is called **leukopenia** (leukocytopenia). Leukopenia may be caused by viral infections, exposure to ionizing radiation, certain chemicals, and chemotherapy drugs. Infection by the human immunodeficiency virus (HIV) is an example of a disease that causes a decrease in the WBC count (Table 2-7).

## AUTOMATED CELL COUNTS

The majority of blood cell counts are performed by automation, using instruments that range from relatively simple, inexpensive cell counters, to very elaborate and expensive hematology analyzers. Small analyzers may be used in a physician office laboratory (POL) or a small hospital. More elaborate equipment may be found in large hospitals and reference laboratories. Some instruments perform only RBC and WBC counts, and hemoglobin and hematocrit tests. Other more complex models also perform platelet counts, the RBC indices, and automated WBC differentials. Most hematology analyzers can complete a cell count in less than one minute.

Automated cell counters operate on one of two principles. In some instruments, the cells to be counted are diluted in a fluid that conducts an electrical current. The cells are aspirated through a special narrow opening called an **aperture**. As the cells are aspirated, they interrupt the flow of the current across the opening. Each interruption is recorded and counted as a cell.

In another type of instrument, the diluted blood sample is aspirated into a special channel that is so narrow only one cell can pass through at a time. As the cells pass through the channel, they interrupt a laser beam. Each interruption of the beam is counted as a cell. Lesson 2-13 discusses in more detail the principles on which some of these instruments are based.

Use of automated cell counters has improved the cell count accuracy and laboratory efficiency. Although automated cell counters are essential in most laboratories, there are times when manual counts are required. If an automated cell counter malfunctions and a backup instrument is not available, manual counts must be done. At other times, a manual count may be required if the patient has a very low WBC or platelet count that cannot be read by instruments. Therefore, it is important to keep supplies stocked for manual counts and to have trained employees who can perform the procedures.

**TABLE 2-7.** Causes of leukocytosis and leukocytopenia

| CAUSES OF LEUKOCYTOSIS | CAUSES OF LEUKOCYTOPENIA |
|---|---|
| **Pathological** | **Pathological** |
| Infection | Some viral infections, including HIV |
| Leukemias | Ionizing radiation |
| Polycythemia | Certain chemicals |
| | Chemotherapy drugs |
| **Physiological** | |
| Exercise | |
| Exposure to sunlight | |
| Obstetric labor | |
| Stress | |
| Anesthesia | |

## Procedural Notes

- Clean and polish the hemacytometer and coverglass before use to be sure the surfaces are free of debris and oil.

- Do not allow the microscope objectives to touch the coverglass when viewing the hemacytometer ruled areas.

- Do not allow the fluid to overflow the counting chamber when filling the hemacytometer; this changes the cell distribution.

- Follow proper counting and calculation methods as directed by the package insert.

- Repeat the count if there is large variation from one square to another.

- Store and handle the hemacytometer and coverglass carefully to avoid scratching the surfaces.

## Safety Precautions

- Observe Universal and Standard Precautions when using the hemacytometer and performing cell counts.

- Clean all spills with surface disinfectant.

- Disinfect the hemacytometer and coverglass after each use.

- Use only gentle pressure on the UNOPETTE® reservoir when mixing the blood and diluent to avoid accidentally expelling the mixture through the top.

## LESSON REVIEW

1. Diagram the hemacytometer and its parts. Show which areas are counted for a WBC count and for an RBC count.

2. Explain how to fill a hemacytometer using a capillary tube.

3. What is the proper procedure for disinfecting and cleaning the hemacytometer and coverglass?

4. What is the general formula used to calculate cell counts when using the hemacytometer?

5. What is the normal RBC count for a male; a female; a newborn?

6. What are the reference WBC values for newborns, children, and adults?

7. Name three diseases or conditions in which the RBC count is usually abnormal.

8. What is one requirement of an RBC diluting fluid?

9. Name three causes of leukocytosis.

10. Name three factors that may cause leukopenia.

11. Describe how the UNOPETTE® systems for RBC and WBC counts differ.

12. What are the functions of the WBC diluting fluid?

13. Explain why it is important to know how to perform manual blood cell counts.

14. Define anemia, aperture, cell-diluting fluid, erythrocytosis, hemacytometer, hemacytometer coverglass, hemolysis, immunity, isotonic solution, leukocytosis, leukopenia, and micropipet.

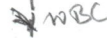

## STUDENT ACTIVITIES

1. Reread the information on the hemacytometer and RBC and WBC counts.

2. Review the glossary terms.

3. Practice loading the hemacytometer and microscopically viewing the counting areas using the Student Performance Guide.

4. Practice performing and calculating RBC counts as outlined in the Student Performance Guide, using the worksheet.

5. Practice performing and calculating WBC counts as outlined in the Student Performance Guide.

6. Calculate the total WBC counts when the average number of cells counted is: 71, 141, and 49.

7. Experiment to see what happens when RBCs are exposed to 0.1 N hydrochloric acid (0.1 N HCl) or to water.

# *Student Performance Guide*

## **LESSON 2-5** The Hemacytometer

Name _____ Date _____

### ☣ INSTRUCTIONS

1. Practice using the hemacytometer following the step-by-step procedure.
2. Demonstrate your understanding of this lesson by:
   a. Completing a written examination successfully, and
   b. Demonstrating the procedure for using the hemacytometer satisfactorily for the instructor. All steps must be completed as listed on the instructor's Performance Check Sheet.

### MATERIALS AND EQUIPMENT

- gloves
- hand disinfectant
- hemacytometer
- 10% chlorine bleach solution
- hemacytometer coverglass
- lens paper
- 70% ethyl or isopropyl alcohol
- micropipet (10–20 µL capacity)
- pipet tips for micropipet
- microscope
- paper towels or gauze
- laboratory detergent
- distilled water
- soft tissue
- biohazard container
- puncture-proof sharps container

### PROCEDURE

Record in the comment section any problems encountered while practicing the procedure (or have a fellow student or the instructor evaluate your performance).

S = Satisfactory
U = Unsatisfactory

| You must: | S | U | Comments |
|---|---|---|---|
| 1. Assemble equipment and materials | | | |
| 2. Use lens paper and alcohol to carefully clean hemacytometer and coverglass | | | |
| 3. Place the coverglass carefully over the ruled areas (chamber) of the hemacytometer | | | |
| 4. Wash hands and put on gloves | | | |
| 5. Draw distilled water into the micropipet (approximately 10 µL will be needed for each side of the chamber) | | | |
| 6. Wipe excess fluid from the tip of the pipet using soft tissue | | | |

| You must: | S | U | Comments |
|---|---|---|---|
| 7. Hold the pipet at a 45° angle and touch the tip to the point where the coverglass and the hemacytometer meet (do not move coverglass) | | | |
| 8. Allow fluid to flow into one side of the chamber by capillary action (the chamber should fill in one smooth flow without flooding over into the depressions) | | | |
| 9. Fill the other side of the chamber in the same manner | | | |
| 10. Position the low-power (10X) objective in place | | | |
| 11. Place the hemacytometer on the microscope stage securely with one ruled area over the light source | | | |
| 12. Look *directly at the hemacytometer* (not through microscope eyepiece) and turn the coarse-adjustment knob to bring the microscope objective and the hemacytometer close together, continuing until the objective is almost touching the coverglass. *Note:* Use coarse-adjustment knob with care | | | |
| 13. Look into the eyepiece and slowly turn the coarse-adjustment knob in the opposite direction until the etched lines come into view | | | |
| 14. Rotate the fine-adjustment knob until the lines are in clear focus | | | |
| 15. Find all nine squares used for the WBC count on one side of the chamber by moving the stage or the hemacytometer | | | |
| 16. Scan squares using left-to-right, right-to-left counting pattern and note boundary lines | | | |
| 17. Locate the center square used for the RBC count | | | |
| 18. Rotate the high-power (40X) objective carefully into position and adjust focus using the fine-adjustment knob until the etched lines appear distinct | | | |
| 19. Locate the four small corner squares and the center square (within the large center square) used for the RBC count | | | |
| 20. Scan counting area using left-to-right, right-to-left pattern and note boundary lines | | | |
| 21. View the second ruled area, repeating steps 15–20 | | | |
| 22. Rotate the low-power objective into position | | | |
| 23. Remove the hemacytometer carefully from the microscope stage (Place hemacytometer and coverglass into chlorine bleach solution to disinfect, if blood was used) | | | |
| 24. Clean the hemacytometer and the coverglass carefully using alcohol and lens paper | | | |
| 25. Dry the hemacytometer and coverglass with lens paper | | | |

| You must: | S | U | Comments |
|---|---|---|---|
| 26. Clean and return all equipment to proper storage | | | |
| 27. Clean work area with surface disinfectant | | | |
| 28. Remove and discard gloves in biohazard container | | | |
| 29. Wash hands with hand disinfectant | | | |

*Evaluator Comments:*

Evaluator _____  Date _____

*Student Performance Guide*

## LESSON 2-5 The Hemacytometer: Red Blood Cell Count

Name _____    Date _____

  ### INSTRUCTIONS

1. Practice performing and calculating an RBC count using the RBC UNOPETTE® system and following the step-by-step procedure.

2. Demonstrate your understanding of this lesson by:

   a. Completing a written examination successfully, and

   b. Performing the RBC count procedure satisfactorily for the instructor. All steps must be completed as listed on the instructor's Performance Check Sheet.

*Note:* The following is a general procedure for using a UNOPETTE® system. Consult the package insert for specific instructions.

### MATERIALS AND EQUIPMENT

- gloves
- hand disinfectant
- materials for capillary puncture, or blood sample, anticoagulated with EDTA
- gauze or paper towel
- hemacytometer with coverglass
- test tube rack or beaker to hold blood sample
- UNOPETTE® RBC system (reservoir and pipet assembly)
- microscope
- lens paper
- alcohol (70% ethanol)
- hand tally counter
- surface disinfectant or 10% chlorine bleach solution
- biohazard container
- biohazard container for sharps
- acrylic safety shield

### PROCEDURE

Record in the comment section any problems encountered while practicing the procedure (or have a fellow student or the instructor evaluate your performance).

S = Satisfactory
U = Unsatisfactory

| You must: | S | U | Comments |
|---|---|---|---|
| 1. Assemble equipment and materials. Set up acrylic safety shield | | | |
| 2. Place a clean hemacytometer coverglass over a clean hemacytometer | | | |
| 3. Wash hands and put on gloves | | | |
| 4. Puncture the diaphragm of the UNOPETTE® reservoir. Hold the reservoir firmly on a flat surface with one hand and use the tip of the pipet shield to puncture the diaphragm. *Note:* The opening must be made large enough to easily accommodate the pipet | | | |

| You must: | S | U | Comments |
|---|---|---|---|
| 5.  Remove the shield from the pipet assembly | | | |
| 6.  Fill the capillary pipet from a capillary puncture or from a tube of well-mixed EDTA anticoagulated blood.  The pipet will fill by capillary action and will stop filling automatically.<br>*Note:*  Keep pipet horizontal or at a slight (5°) upward angle to avoid overfilling | | | |
| 7.  Wipe excess blood from the outside of the capillary pipet with soft laboratory tissue.<br>*Note:*  Do not allow tissue to touch pipet tip | | | |
| 8.  Squeeze the reservoir slightly, being careful not to expel any of the liquid | | | |
| 9.  Maintain the pressure on the reservoir and insert the capillary pipet into the reservoir, seating the pipet firmly in the neck of the reservoir.  Do not expel any of the liquid | | | |
| 10.  Release the pressure on the reservoir, drawing the blood out of the capillary pipet into the diluent | | | |
| 11.  Squeeze the reservoir gently three to four times to rinse the remaining blood from the capillary pipet.<br>*Note:*  Do not allow the blood-diluent mixture to flow out the top | | | |
| 12.  Mix the contents of the reservoir thoroughly by gently swirling the reservoir or turning it side to side | | | |
| 13.  Withdraw the capillary pipet from the reservoir and insert it in the neck of the reservoir in reverse position (the pipet tip should now project upward from the reservoir) | | | |
| 14.  Mix the contents of the reservoir thoroughly.  Invert the reservoir and gently squeeze to discard four to five drops onto gauze or paper towel | | | |
| 15.  Fill both sides of the hemacytometer | | | |
| 16.  Place the hemacytometer on the microscope stage carefully and securely | | | |
| 17.  Use the low-power (10X) objective to bring the ruled area into focus | | | |
| 18.  Locate the large central square | | | |
| 19.  Rotate the high-power (40X) objective into position carefully and focus with the fine-adjustment knob until lines are clear | | | |
| 20.  Adjust the light or condenser so RBCs are visible | | | |
| 21.  Count the cells in the four corner squares and one center square within the larger center square of the counting area, using the left-to-right, right-to-left counting pattern | | | |

| You must: | S | U | Comments |
|---|---|---|---|
| 22. Record the results for each of the five squares (four corners and one center) | | | |
| 23. Repeat the count using the other side of the hemacytometer | | | |
| 24. Use the worksheet to calculate the RBC count | | | |
| 25. Record the result | | | |
| 26. Disinfect the hemacytometer and coverglass using 10% chlorine bleach solution | | | |
| 27. Discard the specimen and disposable materials appropriately | | | |
| 28. Return the equipment to proper storage | | | |
| 29. Clean work area with surface disinfectant | | | |
| 30. Remove and discard gloves in biohazard container and wash hands with hand disinfectant | | | |

*Evaluator Comments:*

Evaluator _____ Date _____

## *Worksheet*

## **LESSON 2-5** The Hemacytometer: Red Cell Count

Name _____ Date _____

| **SIDE 1** | **NUMBER OF CELLS COUNTED** |
|---|---|
| Square a | _____ |
| Square b | _____ |
| Square c | _____ |
| Square d | _____ |
| Square e | _____ |
| Total cells counted side 1 = | _____ |

| **SIDE 2** | **NUMBER OF CELLS COUNTED** |
|---|---|
| Square a | _____ |
| Square b | _____ |
| Square c | _____ |
| Square d | _____ |
| Square e | _____ |
| Total cells counted side 2 = | _____ |
| Total of sides 1 and 2 = | _____ |
| Average of two sides (total divided by two) = | _____ |
| Multiply average number of cells by 10,000 | _____ = RBC/μL |
| Convert to SI units (RBC/L) by multiplying above number by $10^6$ | _____ = RBC/L |

## *Student Performance Guide*

### LESSON 2-5  The Hemacytometer: White Blood Cell Count

Name _____   Date _____

 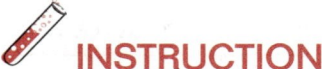 INSTRUCTIONS

1. Practice performing and calculating a WBC count following the step-by-step procedure.

2. Demonstrate your understanding of this lesson by:

   a. Completing a written examination successfully, and

   b. Performing the WBC count procedure satisfactorily for the instructor. All steps must be completed as listed on the instructor's Performance Check Sheet.

*Note:*   The following is a general procedure for using the UNOPETTE® system. Consult the package insert for specific instructions.

## MATERIALS AND EQUIPMENT

- gloves
- surface disinfectant (10% chlorine bleach solution)
- gauze or paper towel
- tube of EDTA blood or supplies for a capillary puncture
- hand disinfectant
- UNOPETTE® WBC or WBC/Platelet system
- hemacytometer with coverglass
- hand tally counter
- 70% alcohol
- microscope
- lens paper
- acrylic safety shield
- biohazard container
- biohazard container for sharps

## PROCEDURE

Record in the comment section any problems encountered while practicing the procedure (or have a fellow student or the instructor evaluate your performance).

S = Satisfactory
U = Unsatisfactory

| You must: | S | U | Comments |
|---|---|---|---|
| 1. Assemble equipment and materials; obtain a UNOPETTE® system for WBC or WBC/platelet count | | | |
| 2. Place a clean hemacytometer coverglass on a clean hemacytometer | | | |
| 3. Pierce the diaphragm of the UNOPETTE® reservoir with the pipet shield | | | |
| 4. Set up acrylic safety shield | | | |
| 5. Wash hands and put on gloves | | | |

| You must: | S | U | Comments |
|---|---|---|---|
| 6. Remove the shield from the pipet assembly (Perform steps 7–14 with acrylic safety shield between you and the blood or blood solution) | | | |
| 7. Fill the UNOPETTE® capillary pipet from a capillary puncture or from a tube of well-mixed EDTA blood | | | |
| 8. Allow the blood to flow into the capillary until it automatically stops | | | |
| 9. Wipe any excess blood from the outside of the pipet, being careful not to touch the tip with the tissue | | | |
| 10. Squeeze the reservoir lightly, being careful not to expel any of the liquid | | | |
| 11. Maintain pressure on the reservoir and insert the capillary pipet into the reservoir, seating the pipet firmly in the neck of the reservoir. Do not expel any of the liquid | | | |
| 12. Release the pressure on the reservoir, drawing the blood out of the capillary into the diluent | | | |
| 13. Squeeze the reservoir gently three to four times to rinse the remaining blood from the capillary pipet. *Note:* Do not allow the blood-diluent mixture to flow out the top | | | |
| 14. Mix contents of the reservoir by gently swirling the reservoir or tilting it from side to side | | | |
| 15. Let the reservoir sit for ten minutes (but no longer than an hour) to destroy the red blood cells | | | |
| 16. Remove the pipet from the reservoir and insert it in the neck of the reservoir so the pipet tip extends *upward* from the reservoir | | | |
| 17. Mix the contents of the reservoir thoroughly. Invert the reservoir and gently squeeze to discard four or five drops onto paper towel or gauze | | | |
| 18. Touch the tip of the pipet to the edge of the coverglass and hemacytometer. Fill both sides of the hemacytometer | | | |
| 19. Place the hemacytometer on the microscope stage carefully and secure it | | | |
| 20. Use the low-power (10X) objective to bring the ruled area into focus. Identify the nine white blood cell squares | | | |
| 21. Count the WBCs lying within all nine squares, using the boundary rule | | | |
| 22. Record the results | | | |
| 23. Repeat the count, using the other side of the hemacytometer, and record the results | | | |

| You must: | S | U | Comments |
|---|---|---|---|
| 24. Obtain the average count by adding the results from the two sides together and dividing by two | | | |
| 25. Calculate 10% of the average and add that to the average. Then multiply that total by 100 to get the number of white blood cells per µL | | | |
| 26. Place hemacytometer and coverglass into bleach solution for ten minutes, then rinse with water. Dry carefully with lens paper | | | |
| 27. Discard any sharps into a puncture-proof biohazard container | | | |
| 28. Return tube of blood to storage area or discard into biohazard waste. Discard UNOPETTE® assembly in biohazard sharps container | | | |
| 29. Return equipment to proper storage | | | |
| 30. Clean work area with surface disinfectant | | | |
| 31. Remove and discard gloves in biohazard container | | | |
| 32. Wash hands with hand disinfectant | | | |

*Evaluator Comments:*

Evaluator _____ Date _____

# Platelet Count

## LESSON OBJECTIVES

**After studying this lesson, you should be able to:**
- *Discuss the functions of platelets.*
- *Name two pathological conditions in which the platelet counts may be abnormal.*
- *Perform a platelet count using the UNOPETTE® system.*
- *Calculate the results of a platelet count.*
- *List three precautions that must be observed when performing a platelet count.*
- *Define the glossary terms.*

## GLOSSARY

**hemostasis** / the process of stopping bleeding

**Petri dish** / a shallow, covered dish made of plastic or glass

**thrombocytopenia** / abnormal decrease in the number of platelets in the blood

**thrombocytosis** / abnormal increase in the number of platelets in the blood

## INTRODUCTION

Platelets are the smallest of the formed elements in the blood. They play an important role in **hemostasis**, the process of stopping bleeding. The platelet count is an important test used to investigate bleeding disorders and assess clotting ability. Since the number of platelets in circulation is affected by drugs that affect bone marrow cells, the platelet count is often used to monitor toxic effects of drug and radiation treatments. Because platelets form clumps or aggregates, accurate platelet counting requires good technique. More comprehensive information about the function of platelets is in Lesson 3-1, Principles of Hemostasis.

## REFERENCE VALUES FOR PLATELET COUNT

The normal platelet count is 150,000 to 400,000 platelets per microliter (µL) of blood. Platelets control bleeding by forming a sticky plug that seals damaged vessel walls. They also help initiate a series of enzymatic reactions that result in formation of the fibrin clot. Increases or decreases in the numbers of platelets can interfere with these mechanisms and cause either excessive clotting or bleeding.

**Thrombocytosis**, an increase in the number of platelets, may occur in conditions such as polycythemia or hemolytic anemia, or after splenectomy. **Thrombocytopenia**, a decrease in platelets, may occur in some anemias and leukemias, and following chemotherapy and radiation therapy. Table 2-8 gives examples of conditions that cause thrombocytosis and thrombocytopenia.

## PERFORMING A MANUAL PLATELET COUNT

The most acceptable manual method of counting platelets is to use self-filling, self-diluting systems such as the UNOPETTE® system. UNOPETTE® systems consist of a sealed reservoir containing premeasured diluting fluid, a capillary pipet, and a pipet shield. The

**TABLE 2–8** Conditions that may cause thrombo-cytopenia or thrombocytosis

**Thrombocytopenia**
Bone marrow damage
Sequestration by enlarged spleen
Disseminated intravascular coagulation (DIC)
Chronic alcoholism
Idiopathic thrombocytopenic purpura (ITP)

**Thrombocytosis**
Polycythemia vera
Bleeding disorders
Hemolytic anemias
Inflammatory reactions
Chronic granulocytic leukemia

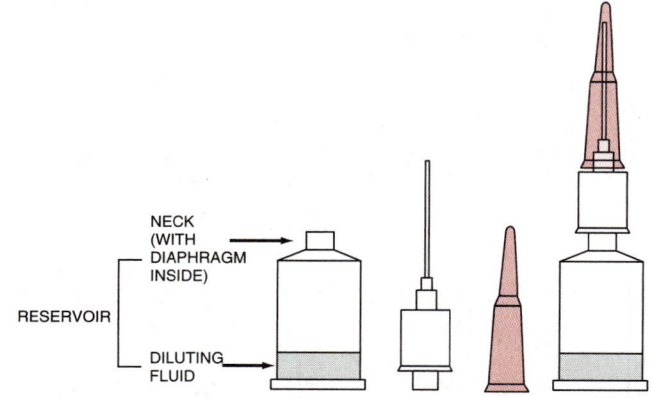

**FIGURE 2-41** UNOPETTE® microcollection system

UNOPETTE® system for platelet counts uses a 20 µL capillary pipet to measure the sample and contains 1.98 µL of ammonium oxalate diluting fluid in the reservoir (Figure 2-41).

  **Safety**

Universal and Standard Precautions must be observed when performing all hematology procedures. The worker must wear gloves and a buttoned, fluid-resistant laboratory coat. In addition, the worker should wear protective face wear or work behind an acrylic safety shield when opening vacutainer tubes and pipetting blood. All spills must be wiped up with surface disinfectant. Contaminated equipment, such as the hemacytometer and coverglass, must be soaked in disinfectant and then washed with laboratory detergent.

*Quality Assurance*

Careful attention must be paid to maintaining good technique when performing hemacytometer counts. Since platelets are so small, the hemacytometer must be clean to avoid mistaking dirt particles for platelets. Care must be taken to avoid overloading the chamber, which would allow the fluid to flow into the moat and alter the cell distribution in the counting chamber.

Because of the tendency of platelets to clump, attention must be paid to distribution of the platelets in the counting chamber. If clumping is seen, the hemacytometer should be cleaned and reloaded. If clumping is still seen, the blood sample should be recollected.

After the hemacytometer is loaded, the cells must be allowed to settle before performing the count. Otherwise, the cell count may be inaccurate. If cell counts vary by more than 10% between the two sides of the hemacytometer, the count should be repeated. An estimation of platelet numbers may be made by examining a stained blood smear prepared at the time of the platelet count (see Lesson 2-9).

## Collecting the Blood Specimen

Blood collected in EDTA is the preferred specimen for platelet counts. Capillary blood may also be used for platelet counts, but venous anticoagulated blood gives better results, because platelets tend to clump rapidly in a capillary sample.

## Diluting the Blood Specimen

Using a UNOPETTE® system for platelet counts, the diaphragm in the neck of the reservoir is pierced with the pipet shield, making a hole large enough for the capillary pipet. Working behind an acrylic safety shield, the pipet tip is inserted into a drop of capillary blood (from a capillary puncture) or into a tube of well-mixed EDTA blood, and 20 µL (0.02 mL) is automatically drawn up. The capillary pipet is inserted in the reservoir and the blood is drawn into the diluting fluid. The 20 µL of blood mixed with the 1.98 mL of diluting fluid makes

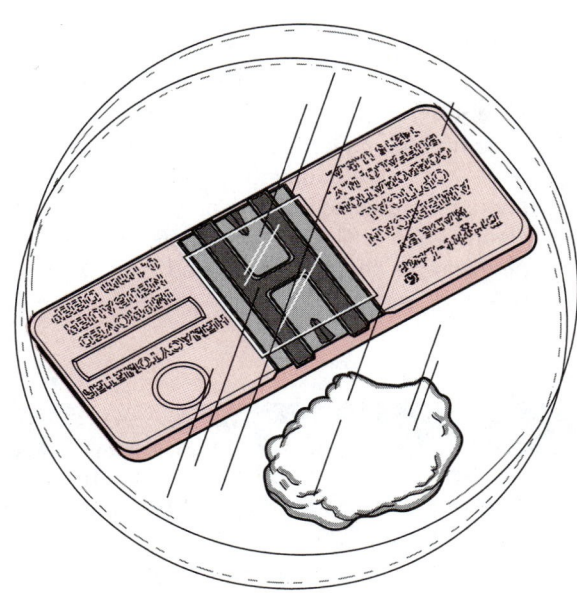

**FIGURE 2-42** Hemacytometer in moist chamber (covered Petri dish containing moistened cotton)

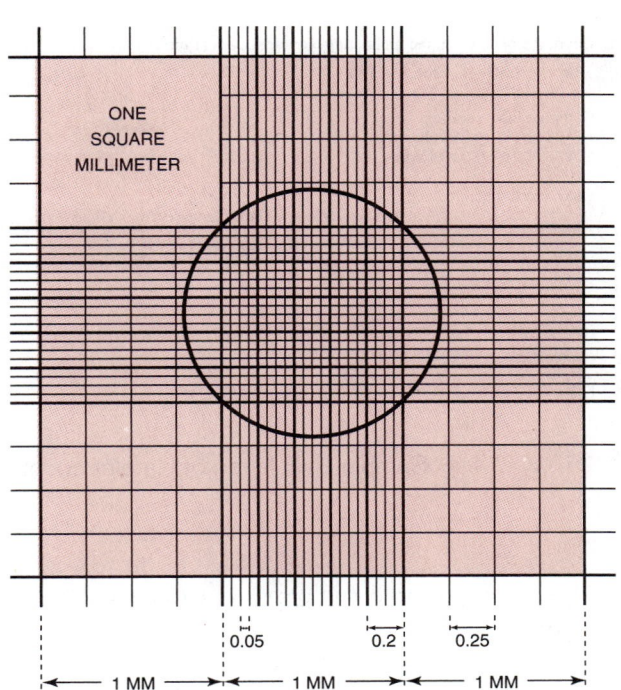

**FIGURE 2-43** Platelet counting area. Count the cells in the 25 squares inside the large center square (circled)

a blood dilution of 1:100. The fluid is swirled to mix, and then is allowed to stand for at least 10 minutes, but no longer than three hours, to allow the red blood cells to be lysed (destroyed). After 10 minutes, the reservoir is again swirled to mix the contents and the pipet assembly is removed and reinserted in the reservoir with the pipet extending upward.

## Filling the Hemacytometer Chamber

A clean hemacytometer coverglass is placed on a clean hemacytometer so both sides of the chamber are covered by the coverglass. A few drops are expelled and discarded from the well-mixed diluted sample through the capillary pipet. Both sides of the hemacytometer are filled.

The filled hemacytometer is placed into a covered petri dish with a moist cotton ball for 10 minutes (Figure 2-42). This provides a moist chamber to prevent evaporation of the solution in the counting chamber while allowing time for the platelets to settle so they may be more accurately counted.

## Counting the Platelets

To perform the platelet count, the hemacytometer is removed from the moist chamber and placed on the microscope stage. The low-power (10X) objective is used to locate the counting area. In a platelet count, the entire center square (1 mm²) is counted (Figure 2-43) using the high-power (40X) objective.

Manual platelet counts are best performed using a phase-contrast microscope. If a brightfield microscope is used, the platelets may be seen more easily if the condenser is lowered and the light is decreased (by adjusting the iris diaphragm). The platelets will appear as shiny refractile objects that darken when the fine-adjustment knob is rotated (see Color Plate 9). The platelets in *all 25 small squares of the large central square* are counted. The count is performed on both sides of the chamber and the average of the two sides is calculated.

## Calculating the Platelet Count

The number of platelets per mm³ of blood is calculated using the general formula:

$$C/\mu L = \frac{Avg \times D \ (mm) \times DF}{A \ (mm)^2}$$

To simplify, use the following figures:

1. The platelet average is computed using counts from both sides of the chamber.
2. The depth factor (D) is 10.
3. The dilution factor (DF) is 100.
4. The area (A) counted is 1 mm².

These numbers are substituted into the formula as follows:

1. Count the platelets in the entire large center square (1 mm²):

    Side 1 = 166        Side 2 = 170

2. Compute the average:
    A. 166 + 170 = 336 platelets
    B. 336 ÷ 2 = 168 average

3. Calculate the count:

$$\text{Platelets/}\mu\text{L} = \frac{\text{Average \# platelets} \times \text{Depth factor (mm)} \times \text{Dilution factor}}{\text{Area counted (mm}^2)}$$

$$\text{Platelets/}\mu\text{L} = \frac{168 \times 10 \times 100}{1}$$

$$\text{Platelets/}\mu\text{L} = 168 \times 1000$$

$$\text{Platelets/}\mu\text{L} = 168{,}000 \ (\text{or } 1.68 \times 10^5)$$

$$\text{Platelets/L} = 1.68 \times 10^{11}$$

**FIGURE 2-44** Sample calculation of platelet count

$$\frac{\text{Platelets}}{\mu\text{L}} = \frac{\text{Average \# of platelets} \times 10 \times 100}{1}$$

$$\frac{\text{Platelets}}{\mu\text{L}} = \text{Average \# of platelets} \times 1000$$

Therefore, the platelet count can be determined by simply multiplying the average number of platelets by 1000 (or by adding three zeroes). A sample calculation of a platelet count is shown in Figure 2-44.

## AUTOMATED PLATELET COUNTS

Although manual platelet counts are still performed in some laboratories, instruments that perform platelet counts have been in use for several years. The platelet counter may be part of an analyzer that performs several other procedures, such as cell counts and hemoglobin measurements, or it may perform only platelet counts. Lesson 2-13 contains more information on hematology automation.

### Procedural Notes

■ The platelet count must be performed within three hours of diluting the sample.

■ The hemacytometer must be free of dirt and debris before the sample is loaded.

■ The cotton ball in the moist chamber must not touch the coverglass or the fluid in the hemacytometer.

■ The high-power (40X) objective must be used to count platelets.

■ The microscope condenser, iris diaphragm, and light intensity must be adjusted to provide good contrast when observing and counting platelets.

■ If clumps or uneven distribution of platelets are observed in the counting chamber, the sample should be remixed and the chamber should be cleaned and refilled. If clumps are still present, a new sample should be obtained.

### Safety Precaution

■ Universal and Standard Precautions must be observed when performing platelet counts by the UNOPETTE® method.

■ The worker should wear protective face wear or work behind an acrylic safety shield.

■ The hemacytometer and coverglass must be disinfected by soaking in a 10% chlorine bleach solution.

## LESSON REVIEW

1. Explain the function of platelets. *depend infection*
2. Name a condition in which thrombocytosis may occur. *inflammation, Polycytomia*
3. Name a cause of thrombocytopenia. *Leukemia, decrease in Polycyte platelet*
4. Why is it important to thoroughly clean the coverglass and hemacytometer before performing the platelet count? *for acurate test result*
5. What is the purpose of the moist chamber? *to prevent evaporation*
6. What area of the hemacytometer is used to count platelets? *Centre 25 squares*
7. State the formula for calculating a platelet count.
8. What blood dilution is used for a platelet count using the UNOPETTE® system? *EDTA*
9. What personal protective equipment (PPE) must be worn while performing manual platelet counts?
10. Define hemostasis, Petri dish, thrombocytopenia, and thrombocytosis. *High platelet count* *Low platelet count*

## STUDENT ACTIVITIES

1. Reread the information on platelet counts.
2. Review the glossary terms.
3. Practice performing a platelet count as outlined on the Student Performance Guide, using the worksheet.

## Student Performance Guide

## LESSON 2-6 Platelet Count

Name _____ Date _____

### INSTRUCTIONS

1. Practice performing a platelet count following the step-by-step procedure.
2. Demonstrate your understanding of this lesson by:
   a. Completing a written examination successfully, and
   b. Performing a platelet count satisfactorily for the instructor. All steps must be completed as listed on the instructor's Performance Check Sheet.

*Note:* The following is a general procedure for the use of the UNOPETTE® system. Consult the package insert for specific instructions.

### MATERIALS AND EQUIPMENT

- gloves
- hand disinfectant
- blood sample, anticoagulated with EDTA
- acrylic safety shield or face shield
- hemacytometer with coverglass
- test-tube rack or beaker to hold blood sample
- UNOPETTE® for platelet count (reservoir and pipet assembly)
- microscope
- Petri dish
- cotton ball (moistened slightly with water)
- lens paper
- alcohol (70% ethanol)
- hand tally counter
- surface disinfectant (10% chlorine bleach solution)
- biohazard container
- puncture-proof container for sharps

### PROCEDURE

Record in the comment section any problems encountered while practicing the procedure (or have a fellow student or the instructor evaluate your performance).

S = Satisfactory
U = Unsatisfactory

| You must: | S | U | Comments |
|---|---|---|---|
| 1. Wash hands and put on gloves | | | |
| 2. Assemble equipment and materials | | | |
| 3. Place a clean hemacytometer coverglass over a clean hemacytometer | | | |
| 4. Puncture the diaphragm of the UNOPETTE® reservoir. Hold the reservoir firmly on a flat surface with one hand and use the tip of the pipet shield to puncture the diaphragm. Remove the shield from the pipet assembly<br>*Note:* The opening must be made large enough to easily accommodate the pipet | | | |

| You must: | S | U | Comments |
|---|---|---|---|
| 5. Work behind safety shield or wear face shield | | | |
| 6. Fill the capillary pipet from a capillary puncture or from a tube of well-mixed EDTA anticoagulated blood. The pipet will fill by capillary action and will stop filling automatically<br>*Note:* Keep pipet horizontal or at a slight (5°) upward angle to avoid overfilling | | | |
| 7. Wipe excess blood from the outside of the capillary pipet with soft laboratory tissue.<br>*Note:* Do not allow tissue to touch pipet tip | | | |
| 8. Squeeze the reservoir lightly, being careful not to expel any of the liquid | | | |
| 9. Maintain the pressure on the reservoir and insert the capillary pipet into the reservoir, seating the pipet firmly in the neck of the reservoir. Do not expel any of the liquid | | | |
| 10. Release the pressure on the reservoir, drawing the blood out of the capillary pipet into the diluent | | | |
| 11. Squeeze the reservoir gently three to four times to rinse the remaining blood from the capillary pipet.<br>*Note:* Do not allow the blood-diluent mixture to flow out the top | | | |
| 12. Mix the contents of the reservoir thoroughly by gently swirling the reservoir or tilting it from side to side | | | |
| 13. Let reservoir stand at least 10 minutes<br>*Note:* Do not allow to stand longer than three hours | | | |
| 14. Prepare a moist chamber: Place a slightly moist cotton ball into a Petri dish, leaving enough space for the hemacytometer | | | |
| 15. Withdraw the capillary pipet from the reservoir and place it in the neck of the reservoir in reverse position (the pipet tip should now project upward from the reservoir) | | | |
| 16. Mix the contents of the reservoir thoroughly. Invert the reservoir and gently squeeze to discard four to five drops onto gauze or paper towel | | | |
| 17. Fill both sides of the hemacytometer using the capillary pipet | | | |
| 18. Place the hemacytometer in the Petri dish. Do not allow the cotton ball to touch the hemacytometer | | | |
| 19. Place the cover on the Petri dish and allow the preparation to stand 10 minutes (this permits the platelets to settle in the chamber). Do not wait longer than 30 minutes to complete the platelet count | | | |
| 20. Place the hemacytometer on the microscope stage carefully and securely | | | |

| You must: | S | U | Comments |
|---|---|---|---|
| 21. Use the low-power (10X) objective to bring the ruled area into focus | | | |
| 22. Locate the large central square | | | |
| 23. Rotate the high-power (40X) objective into position carefully and focus with the fine-adjustment knob until the ruled lines are clear | | | |
| 24. Lower the condenser and reduce the light by partially closing the diaphragm for best contrast. Platelets should appear as round or oval particles that are refractile and smaller than RBCs | | | |
| 25. Count the platelets in the entire center square of the ruled area (all 25 small squares) using the left-to-right, right-to-left counting pattern and record results | | | |
| 26. Repeat the count on the other side of the hemacytometer | | | |
| 27. Average the results from the two sides | | | |
| 28. Calculate the platelet count: $$\text{platelets/}\mu L = \frac{\text{Avg x D (mm) x DF}}{\text{A (mm}^2)}$$ or platelets/µL = average # platelets x 1000 | | | |
| 29. Record the results | | | |
| 30. Disinfect hemacytometer and coverglass with 10% chlorine bleach solution and then wash them | | | |
| 31. Discard specimen and UNOPETTE® assembly into sharps container | | | |
| 32. Return equipment to proper storage | | | |
| 33. Clean work area with surface disinfectant | | | |
| 34. Remove and discard gloves in biohazard container | | | |
| 35. Wash hands with hand disinfectant | | | |

*Evaluator Comments:*




Evaluator _____ Date _____

# Hemoglobin Determination

## LESSON OBJECTIVES

After studying this lesson, you should be able to:

- List the two main components of hemoglobin.
- State the function of hemoglobin.
- Explain the manual and automated methods for determining hemoglobin.
- List the hemoglobin reference values for children and adults.
- Perform a hemoglobin determination using a hemoglobinometer.
- List the precautions to be observed when performing a hemoglobin determination.
- Define the glossary terms.

## GLOSSARY

**cyanmethemoglobin** / a stable colored compound formed when hemoglobin is reacted with Drabkin's reagent; hemiglobincyanide (HiCN)

**Drabkin's reagent** / a hemoglobin diluting reagent that contains iron, potassium, cyanide, and sodium bicarbonate

**globin** / the protein portion of the hemoglobin molecule

**heme** / the iron-containing portion of the hemoglobin molecule

**hemiglobincyanide (HiCN)** / cyanmethemoglobin

**hemoglobin (Hb, Hgb)** / the major functional component of RBCs that serves as the oxygen-carrying molecule

## INTRODUCTION

The measurement of blood hemoglobin is one of the most common clinical laboratory tests. The hemoglobin test is used to indirectly evaluate the oxygen-carrying capacity of the blood. This makes it an important aid in detecting and evaluating blood loss and diagnosing and treating anemia.

The hemoglobin determination may be performed using either capillary or venous blood. It may be requested as an individual test or as part of a complete blood count (CBC). The hemoglobin test is precise, simple to perform, and easily standardized. It may be performed manually or by using analyzers.

## CHARACTERISTICS OF HEMOGLOBIN

**Hemoglobin (Hb** or **Hgb)** is the main constituent of RBCs, making up over 98% of RBC protein content. This molecule gives the characteristic red color to erythrocytes and to the blood. The primary function of hemoglobin is to transport oxygen ($O_2$) from the lungs to the tissue cells of the body and to carry carbon dioxide ($CO_2$) from the tissues to the lungs to be expelled.

## Hemoglobin Structure

The hemoglobin molecule is composed of two parts, heme and globin. The **globin** portion of a hemoglobin molecule contains four protein chains. Hemoglobins are named according to the structure of the protein chains. For example, the hemoglobin present in sickle cell anemia (Hb S) has a different globin structure than the normal adult hemoglobin (Hb A).

The **heme** portion of hemoglobin molecules contains iron; more than two-thirds of the body's iron is contained in hemoglobin and a muscle protein, myoglobin. Therefore, iron is required for hemoglobin synthesis. If sufficient iron is not available in the body, hemoglobin production will decrease, causing the RBCs to be deficient in hemoglobin. When this happens, the oxygen-carrying capacity of the blood is decreased, and the individual will develop symptoms of anemia, such as fatigue and pallor. In situations involving excessive blood loss, such as a bleeding ulcer, anemia may develop because the loss of iron (in the blood lost) exceeds the intake of dietary iron.

## Hemoglobin Reference Values

The hemoglobin value at birth is normally 16–23 g/dL. In early childhood, the value declines and 10–14 g/dL is considered normal. When children begin the rapid growth associated with adolescence, hemoglobin values increase until adult levels are reached.

Adult males usually have hemoglobin values in the range of 13–17 g/dL and females have values of 12–16 g/dL. Hemoglobin reference values are listed in Table 2-9.

A rule-of-thumb is that the hemoglobin value should be approximately one-third the hematocrit value. Therefore, a person with an hematocrit of 45% would be expected to have a hemoglobin of approximately 15 g/dL.

| TABLE 2–9. Hemoglobin reference values | |
|---|---|
| **AGE/GENDER** | **HEMOGLOBIN RANGE (g/dL)** |
| Newborn | 16–23 |
| Children | 10–14 |
| Adult males | 13–17 |
| Adult females | 12–16 |

## Factors Affecting Hemoglobin Levels

The blood hemoglobin concentration is affected by factors such as diet, age, and gender. The diet must contain adequate amounts of iron for the RBCs to make hemoglobin. Some foods are higher in iron than others; for example, red meat has more iron than cow's milk. If the diet is deficient in iron, iron deficiency anemia may develop.

The hemoglobin value is affected by the age and gender of the individual. Normally, males have higher hemoglobin values than females. Newborns have higher values than both children and adults.

People who live at very high altitudes have higher hemoglobin values (and RBC counts) than people who live at lower altitudes. This is because more RBCs are necessary to carry sufficient oxygen, since the oxygen pressure is lower in "thin air" than it is at sea level.

## PRINCIPLES OF HEMOGLOBIN DETERMINATION

Various methods of determining hemoglobin have been used throughout the years. Current methods in use include the specific gravity technique, the cyanmethemoglobin method, and methods that use discrete analyzers. Some of these analyzers are described in Lesson 2-13.

## Specific Gravity Technique

The specific gravity method of measuring hemoglobin gives only an estimate of hemoglobin concentration and requires no special instrument. A drop of blood is dropped into a copper sulfate ($CuSO_4$) solution of a particular density (specific gravity). If the drop falls through the solution rapidly, the specific gravity of the blood is greater than the specific gravity of the copper sulfate. Blood with the normal amount of hemoglobin falls rapidly; blood with a low hemoglobin concentration does not fall rapidly or may float (not drop at all).

The specific gravity technique of estimating hemoglobin has primarily been performed in the United States in recent years as a hemoglobin-screening method for potential blood donors. Many blood donation centers measure hemoglobin by hemoglobinometer or estimate hemoglobin indirectly by performing an hematocrit.

## Cyanmethemoglobin/ Hemiglobincyanide Method

Measurement of cyanmethemoglobin is the most widely used method of determining blood hemoglobin. In this method, blood is reacted with **Drabkin's reagent**, which contains iron, potassium, cyanide, and sodium bicarbonate. The Drabkin's and the hemoglobin combine to form a very stable colored end-product, **cyanmethemoglobin**, also called **hemiglobincyanide (HiCN)**

# METHODS OF HEMOGLOBIN DETERMINATION

The cyanmethemoglobin method of hemoglobin determination can be performed manually, but is usually done using a hematology analyzer or hemoglobinometer.

  **Safety**

Universal and Standard Precautions must be observed when performing hemoglobin measurements. In addition, because most hemoglobin reagents contain hazardous chemicals such as cyanide or azide, care must be taken when performing the tests and handling the reagents. Precautions include wearing gloves, working in a well-ventilated area, properly disposing of used reagents, wiping up all spills, and handwashing after completion of the procedure.

---

### *Quality Assurance*

The use of Drabkin's reagent to form the stable compound cyanmethemoglobin was an important advancement in hematology because it made reliable hemoglobin standards available for the first time. A hemoglobin solution made with Drabkin's is stable for at least six months and provides laboratories a reliable standard to use for standardizing hemoglobin assays.

Spectrophotometers and hemoglobin analyzers used for hemoglobin assays must be calibrated at regular intervals as specified by the manufacturer. Appropriate control solutions must be run at least daily or when patient samples are run, control results must be recorded, and the records must be maintained. Each instrument used will have its own particular checks that must be performed and documented.

---

## Manual Method

Manual methods of measuring hemoglobin concentration are based on converting the hemoglobin to a stable oxidized form (methemoglobin) by adding chemicals such as Drabkin's reagent (to form cyanmethemoglobin). These methods require the use of a spectrophotometer and an understanding of spectrophotometry principles.

### UNOHEME Method

UNOHEME, a trademark of Becton Dickinson and Company, is a manual system for measuring hemoglobin that consists of a reservoir containing a modified Drabkin's solution and a 20 μL capillary pipet. It is used like other UNOPETTE® systems except that the hemoglobin concentration in the diluted blood sample is measured spectrophotometrically.

## Hemoglobinometers

Several small analyzers are available that include hemoglobin measurements in their array of tests. There are also hemoglobin meters that test only hemoglobin. These are sometimes called "dedicated hemoglobinometers." Hemoglobinometers are available that are inexpensive, easy to use, accurate, and have been granted waived status under CLIA.

### HemoCue®

Hemoglobin determination using the HemoCue® is a CLIA-waived procedure, which makes it a good choice for use in POLs, POCT, and public health settings. The HemoCue® B-Hemoglobin Analyzer is designed specifically to measure blood hemoglobin (Figure 2-45). It is small, portable, simple to use, and performs measurements on capillary or venous blood.

In the HemoCue®, blood is drawn up directly into special self-filling cuvettes that contain the hemoglobin reagent (Figure 2-46). The reagent in the cuvette reacts with the blood hemoglobin to form azidemethemiglobin, which has a stable color for 10 minutes. The filled cuvettes are inserted into the photometer and the hemoglobin concentration is displayed in g/dL in less than one minute. Calibration is verified with a control cuvette provided by the manufacturer and the photometer autozeroes itself after each measurement.

## Automated Methods/Discrete Analyzers

Most hematology analyzers, such as cell counters, also perform hemoglobin determinations. In many of these, the sample is aspirated from the capped tube by a probe that penetrates the stopper, offering convenience and safety for the worker.

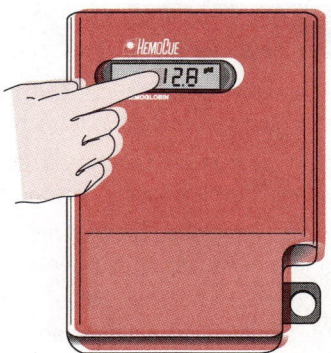

**FIGURE 2-45** HemoCue® hemoglobin photometer.

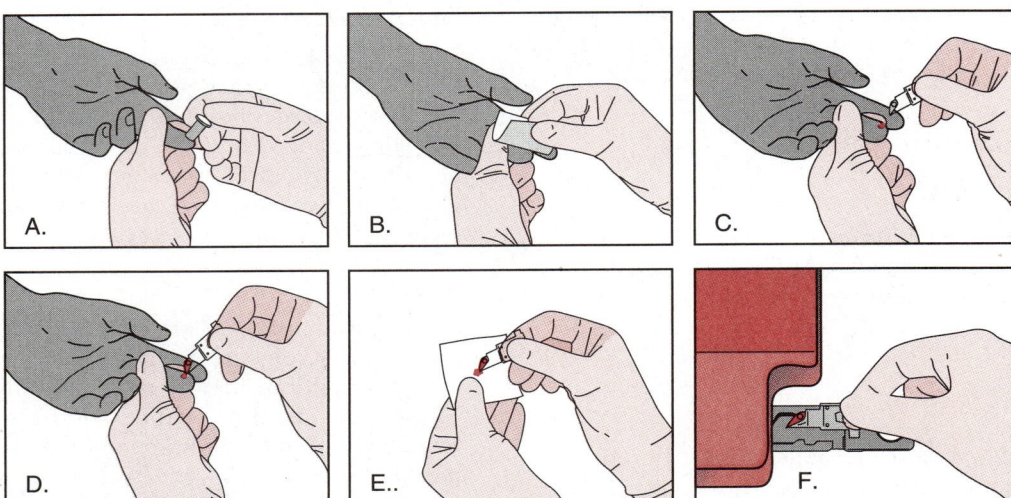

**FIGURE 2-46** Sample collection for HemoCue®

Several clinical chemistry analyzers also are capable of performing hemoglobin assays. Some of the instruments use solid-phase or centrifugal analysis technology, described in Lesson 6-4. (The mention of instruments in this text does not constitute endorsement of the instrument, just as omission of (an) instrument(s) does not imply lack of endorsement.)

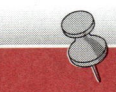

## Procedural Notes

- ■ Use appropriate controls and standards when performing hemoglobin determinations.
- ■ Store reagent strips, cuvettes, and cartridges as recommended by the manufacturer.
- ■ Do not use reagents beyond the expiration date.

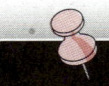

## Safety Precautions

- ■ Observe Universal and Standard Precautions when performing hemoglobin determinations.
- ■ Wear gloves, protective face wear, and a buttoned, fluid-resistent laboratory coat.
- ■ Work in a well-ventilated area and wear gloves when handling hemoglobin reagents containing cyanide.
- ■ Dispose of cyanide-containing reagents properly.

## LESSON REVIEW

1. What are the two main components of hemoglobin?

2. Explain the function of hemoglobin. *transport oxygen & co2*

3. What was the significance of the development of the cyanmethemoglobin method?

4. Explain the principle of the specific gravity technique of estimating hemoglobin concentration.

5. Explain the principle of the cyanmethemoglobin method.

6. Give hemoglobin reference values for children and adults. *12 - 16 g/dL*

7. List safety precautions to be observed when measuring hemoglobin using Drabkin's reagent.

8. Define cyanmethemoglobin, Drabkin's reagent, globin, heme, hemiglobincyanide, and hemoglobin.

## STUDENT ACTIVITIES

1. Reread the information on hemoglobin determination.

2. Review the glossary terms.

3. Inquire at physician offices, blood donation centers, or anemia screening clinics in the community to find out what methods of hemoglobin determination are used.

4. Practice the procedures for determining hemoglobin as listed in the Student Performance Guide.

# *Student Performance Guide*

## LESSON 2-7 Hemoglobin Determination: Hemoglobin Analyzer

Name _____ Date _____

### INSTRUCTIONS

1. Practice the procedure for determining blood hemoglobin concentration using a hemoglobin analyzer and following the step-by-step procedure.

2. Demonstrate your understanding of this lesson by:

   a. Completing a written examination successfully, and

   b. Performing a hemoglobin determination using a hemoglobin analyzer satisfactorily for the instructor. All steps must be completed as listed on the instructor's Performance Check Sheet.

*Note:* Consult manufacturer's instructions for specific procedure.

### MATERIALS AND EQUIPMENT

- acrylic safety shield or protective facewear
- gloves
- hand disinfectant
- 10% chlorine bleach solution
- capillary puncture equipment or blood samples collected in EDTA
- HemoCue® System, or other hemoglobin analyzer with supplies appropriate for the analyzer
- biohazard container
- puncture-proof biohazard container for sharps
- hemoglobin control solution

## PROCEDURE

Record in the comment section any problems encountered while practicing the procedure (or have a fellow student or the instructor evaluate your performance).

S = Satisfactory
U = Unsatisfactory

| You must: | S | U | Comments |
|---|---|---|---|
| 1. Wash hands and put on gloves | | | |
| 2. Assemble equipment and materials for HemoCue® B-Hemoglobin analyzer or go to step 14 for other analyzer | | | |
| 3. Turn on instrument to warm up. The display screen should read "Hb" | | | |
| 4. Pull out the slide arm that holds the cuvette to the first stop. Within 2–6 seconds, the screen should read "Ready", with three flashing dashes | | | |
| 5. Place the control cuvette into the holder and push the holder completely in. The screen should read "Measuring" | | | |

| You must: | S | U | Comments |
|---|---|---|---|
| 6. Record the value of the reading that appears after 10–15 seconds; the value should be within ±0.3 g/dL of the assigned value. If the value is not within the acceptable range, contact the manufacturer | | | |
| 7. Remove a cuvette from the vial. Immediately replace the cap tightly to prevent humidity damage to cuvettes | | | |
| 8. Perform a capillary puncture observing Standard Precautions. Wipe away the first drop or two of blood with a tissue or sterile cotton ball | | | |
| 9. Touch the pointed tip of the cuvette to a well-rounded drop of blood and allow the cuvette to fill in one continuous motion. A partially filled cuvette must be discarded and the collection repeated using a new cuvette | | | |
| 10. Wipe excess blood from the outside of the cuvette, being careful not to touch the open end of the curved edge | | | |
| 11. Insert the filled cuvette into the holder of the HemoCue® photometer within 10 minutes of filling the cuvette | | | |
| 12. Push the holder into the analyzer to the "measuring" position | | | |
| 13. Read the hemoglobin value from the display and record | | | |
| 14. If using another hemoglobin analyzer, follow the manufacturer's instructions for performing a hemoglobin determination | | | |
| 15. Discard all contaminated materials in biohazard containers | | | |
| 16. Turn off the instrument, wipe up any spills, and return all equipment to proper storage | | | |
| 17. Wipe counters with surface disinfectant | | | |
| 18. Remove and discard gloves in appropriate biohazard container | | | |
| 19. Wash hands with hand disinfectant | | | |

*Evaluator Comments:*




Evaluator _____ Date _____

# Preparing and Staining a Blood Smear

## LESSON OBJECTIVES

**After studying this lesson, you should be able to:**

- *Explain the purpose of staining blood smears.*
- *Explain what information can be obtained from a stained blood smear.*
- *List the blood components that may be observed in a stained normal blood smear.*
- *Prepare a blood smear.*
- *Preserve a blood smear.*
- *Stain a blood smear.*
- *List five features of a properly prepared blood smear.*
- *List the safety precautions to observe when preparing and staining a blood smear.*
- *Define the glossary terms.*

## GLOSSARY

**buffer** / a substance that lessens change in the pH of a solution when acid or base (alkali) is added

**cytoplasm** / the fluid portion of the cell surrounding the nucleus

**eosin** / a red-orange stain or dye

**fixative** / preservative; a chemical that prevents deterioration of cells or tissues

**methylene blue** / a blue stain or dye

**morphology** / the form and structure of cells, tissues, and organs

**nucleus (pl. nuclei)** / the central structure of a cell that contains DNA and controls cell growth and function

**polychromatic** / having many colors

## INTRODUCTION

The examination of a stained blood smear is a routine part of the CBC, or complete blood count. Stains are applied to blood smears so the formed elements—RBCs, WBCs, and platelets—may be viewed, identified, and evaluated using the microscope, as in the differential count.

A properly prepared blood smear enables the technologist to view the cellular components of blood in as natural a state as possible. The **morphology**, or structure, of the cellular components can be studied. Careful examination of a well-prepared stained blood smear can provide valuable information to the physician for diagnosing and treating many diseases, including infectious mononucleosis, leukemia, sickle cell anemia, and malaria.

Information gained during routine evaluation of blood smears may lead the physician to order special blood stains for further study. These special stains may be used to identify specific components of cells such as iron granules or nucleic acids. Bone marrow smears may be examined to evaluate blood cell production.

 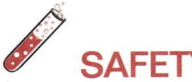 **SAFETY**

Universal and Standard Precautions must be observed when preparing and staining blood smears. Gloves, protective face wear, and a fluid-resistent laboratory coat must be worn when making and staining smears. Since most blood stains contain methanol, care should be taken to avoid skin exposure or inhalation of fumes. Slides should be handled with care to prevent accidental cuts. Used slides should not be cleaned and reused, but must be discarded in puncture-proof sharps containers.

## *Quality Assurance*

Blood smears must be prepared in a manner that alters relative distribution and morphology of cells as little as possible. Attention must be paid to specimen collection and handling. Anticoagulated blood must be well mixed before smears are made. Smears must be made within two hours of blood collection. Anticoagulants other than EDTA should not be used, since they may alter the morphology or staining characteristics of the cells.

# PREPARING A BLOOD SMEAR

## Cleaning the Slides

Slides used for blood smears must be free of grease and dust. Slides may be purchased precleaned or may be washed with soap and water, rinsed thoroughly in hot water and then distilled water, dipped in 95% ethanol, and polished with a clean, lint-free cloth. Clean slides may be stored in 95% ethanol and should be handled by the edges only. Slides with frosted ends are preferred because they can be easily labeled.

## Collecting the Blood Specimen

The preferred specimen for blood smears is capillary blood that has no added anticoagulant. Capillary blood can be applied directly to the slide from the puncture site or can be collected in capillary tubes and then dispensed onto the slides.

A satisfactory smear may also be made from venous blood which has the anticoagulant EDTA added to it, provided the smear is made within two hours of collection. Tubes of anticoagulated blood must be mixed for at least two minutes by mechanical mixer or inverted gently sixty times by hand before the sample is taken. Devices such as DIFF•SAFE® by Alpha Scientific eliminate the need to remove the stopper from a tube of blood to make a blood smear (Figure 2-47). When used properly, the dispenser deposits an appropriately sized drop of blood onto the slide, without the necessity of opening the blood-collection tube.

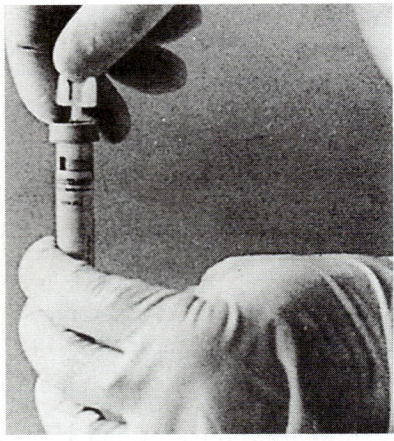 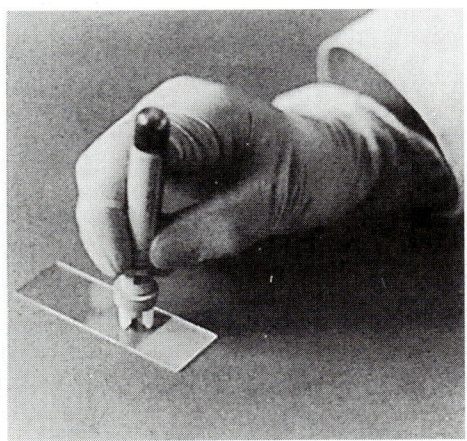 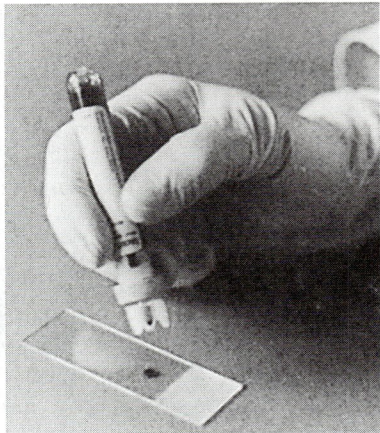

**FIGURE 2-47** Illustration of the use of DIFF•SAFE® blood-dispensing device: (left) cannula is inserted through rubber stopper; (center) tube is inverted and pressed against slide; and (right) drop of blood is dispensed onto slide (Courtesy of Alpha Scientific Corporation, Southeastern, PA)

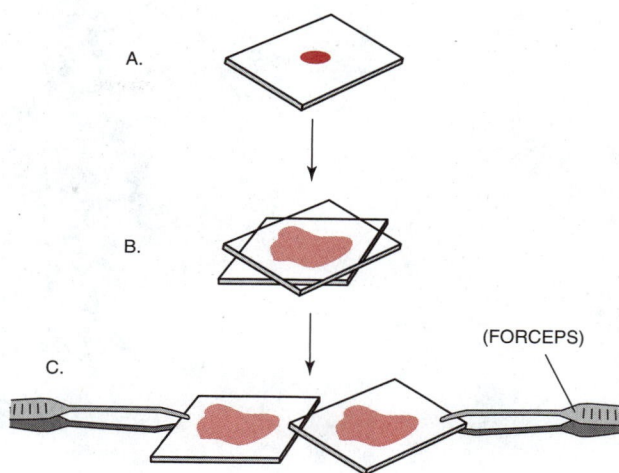

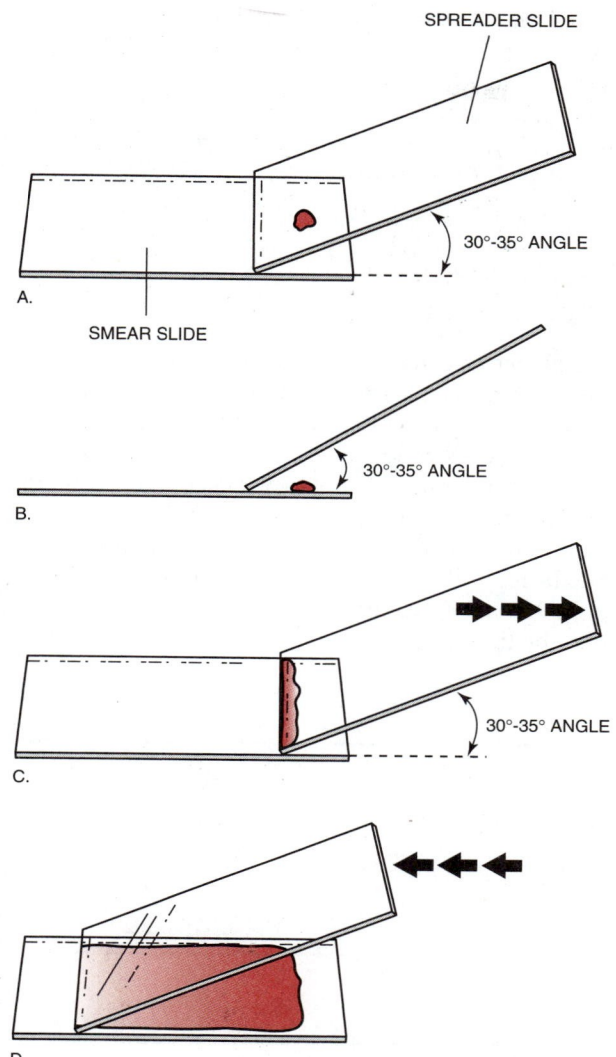

**FIGURE 2-49** Making a blood smear using the coverglass method: (A) place a small drop of blood on coverglass, (B) place a clean coverglass over drop of blood, and (C) when blood drop has spread between the coverglasses, slide them apart parallel to each other.

**FIGURE 2-48** Making a bloodsmear. Position the spreader slide in front of the drop of blood: (A) top view; (B) side view. (C) Spread the blood with a spreader slide. Gently bring the back edge of the spreader slide into contact with the drop of blood and (D) push the spreader slide forward to spread the blood.

at a 30–35° angle in front of the drop of blood (Figure 2-48). The spreader is then brought back into the drop of blood until the drop spreads along three-quarters of the edge of the spreader slide. This should be performed in a smooth, quick sliding motion. As soon as the blood spreads along the edge of the spreader, the spreader is pushed to the left (right for left-handed) with a quick, steady motion (avoiding pressure on the slide) to spread the blood into a thin film (Figure 2-48). Each end of the spreader slide should be used only once and then the slide should be discarded in a biohazard container for sharps. The smear is placed in a slide-drying rack and allowed to air-dry as quickly as possible. It is then ready for staining or preserving.

### Coverglass Method

A small drop of blood (venous or capillary) is placed on a clean 22 mm square coverglass. A clean coverglass is placed on the drop of blood crosswise so the coverglasses form an eight-pointed star (Figure 2-49). The blood will spread between the two coverglasses. As soon as it has stopped spreading, forceps are used to slide the two coverglasses apart parallel to each other. Blood smears will be on both coverglasses, but the cell distribution is usually more uniform on one coverglass than the other. The smears are air-dried and then may be stained or fixed.

### DiffSpin™ Method

The DiffSpin™ Slide Spinner is a centrifuge that produces uniform, monolayer blood smears that can be stained for differential counts (Figure 2-50). This

## Making the Smear

Several methods of spreading blood on a slide result in good smears. Each individual needs to find the technique that is least awkward and provides good results.

### Two-Slide Method (Wedge Method)

The blood smear can be prepared by placing a small drop of well-mixed blood about one-half to three-quarters of an inch from the right end (left end for left-handed) of a precleaned slide placed on a flat surface. The end of a second "spreader" slide is brought to rest

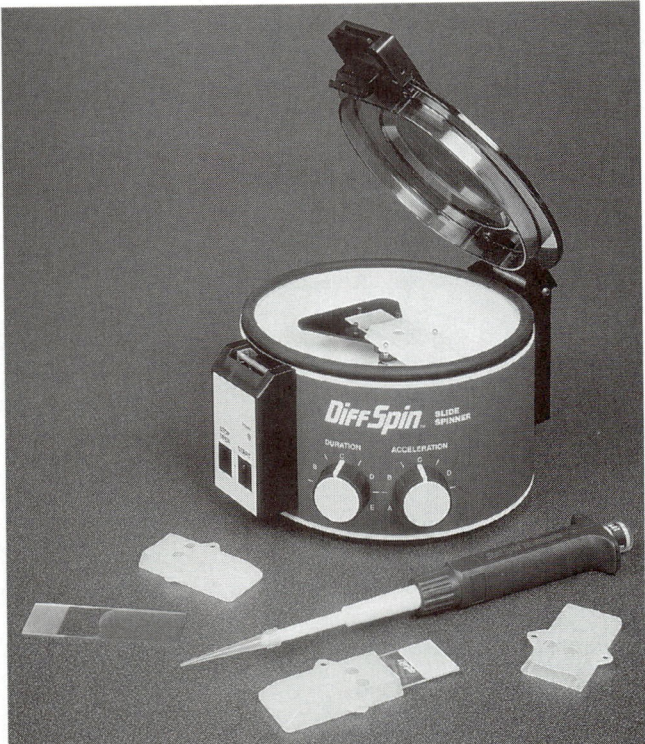

**FIGURE 2-50** DiffSpin® Slide Spinner produces a monolayer blood smear in seconds (Photo courtesy of StatSpin, Inc., Norwood, MA)

method eliminates differences in smear quality due to technique and allows all personnel to make quality smears. Because the cells on these smears are uniformly distributed, cell distribution may be slightly different from that obtained when making smears using the two-slide (wedge) technique.

## Preserving and Staining the Smear

Dried smears should be stained immediately. If this is not possible, the dried smear may be immersed in methanol for 30-60 seconds and then allowed to air-dry. It may then be stained at a later date. The methanol is a **fixative**, or preservative, that prevents changes or deterioration of the cellular components.

## Features of a Good Blood Smear

A well-prepared smear is illustrated in Figure 2-51. The smear should cover about one-half to three-fourths of the slide and should show a gradual transition from thick to thin. It should have a smooth appearance, with no holes or ridges, and should have a feathered edge (about 1.5 cm long) at the thin end. When the smear is examined microscopically, the cells should be distributed evenly. There should be an area at the thin end where cells are not overlapping.

## Factors Affecting Blood Smear Quality

Several factors can affect the quality of the blood smear (Table 2-10). The length and thickness of the smear are affected by the size of the drop of blood and the angle at which the spreader slide is held. Thick smears occur when the angle of the spreader is too high or the drop of blood is too large. Thin smears occur when the drop is too small or the angle is too low. Thin, uneven smears may also occur when too much pressure is applied to the spreader. The faster the spreading procedure, the thinner the smear.

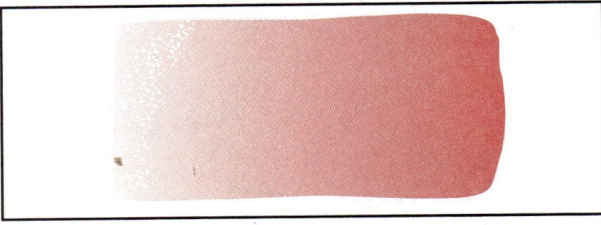

A.

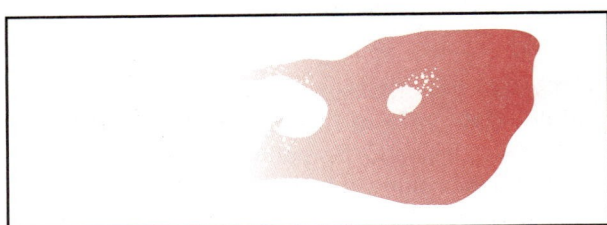

B.

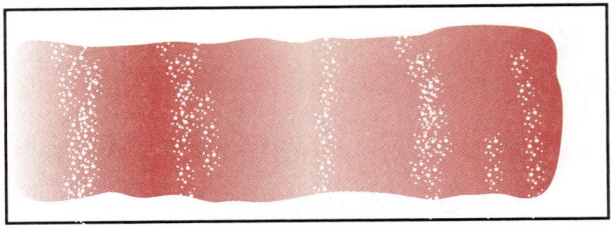

C.

**FIGURE 2-51** Properly prepared smear (A) vs. improper smears (B and C)

**TABLE 2-10.** Common problems encountered in preparing blood smears and the possible causes

| PROBLEM | POSSIBLE CAUSE(S) |
|---|---|
| Smear too thin or too long | Drop of blood too small<br>Spreader slide at too low an angle<br>Improper speed in making smear |
| Smear too thick or too short | Drop of blood too large<br>Spreader slide at too high an angle<br>Improper speed in making smear |
| Ridges or waves in smear | Uneven pressure on spreader slide<br>Hesitation in pushing spreader slide |
| Holes in smear | Slides not clean<br>Uneven or dirty edge of spreader slide |
| Uneven cell distribution | Uneven pressure during spread of blood<br>Delay in spreading blood<br>Uneven or dirty edge of spreader slide |
| Artifacts or unusual cell morphology | Smear dried too slowly<br>Smear not fixed within one hour after preparation<br>High humidity |

Drying time may affect the appearance of the cellular elements. If high humidity causes slow drying, the cells may appear abnormal. For example, the RBCs may appear moth-eaten.

## STAINING A BLOOD SMEAR

### Types of Blood Stains

The stains commonly used for the routine microscopic examination of blood are **polychromatic** stains. These stains contain dyes that stain various cell components different colors. Most polychromatic blood stains contain combinations of **methylene blue**, a basic dye that gives a blue stain, and **eosin**, an acid dye that gives a red-orange stain. Methyl alcohol, a fixative, may also be in the stain.

Some structures, such as cell nuclei, attract the basic dyes and stain blue or purple. Other cell structures may attract the acid dyes and stain pink-red. The cells and structures are thus more easily visualized and differentiated (hence the name differential count). The two most commonly used blood stains in the United States are Wright stain and Giemsa stain.

## Staining Procedures

Smears may be stained by a two-step method, a quick-step method, or an automatic stainer. A quick-stain is adequate for most routine work, but the two-step method (or automatic stainer) should be used to evaluate cell abnormalities and bone marrow cells.

### Quick Stains

Quick stains are available in kits from several companies. These stains are modified Wright or Wright-Giemsa stains. The stains contain three components: a fixative, a red dye such as eosin, and a blue dye such as methylene blue.

To perform a quick stain, the smear is dipped into the staining solution(s) and then rinsed and dried (Figure 2-52). The entire quick-staining method takes only two to five minutes. It may be easier for the inexperienced technician to obtain an adequate stain with quick methods, but experienced technicians can achieve superior results using the two-step method.

### Two-Step Method

In a two-step method, a smear is placed on a staining rack and flooded with Wright stain (Figure 2-52). Fixation occurs in this step because of the methyl alcohol in the stain. After approximately one to three minutes, an equal volume of **buffer** is added dropwise to the stain, mixing the stain and buffer together. A buffer is a substance that prevents changes in the pH of a solution when acid or alkali is added. A green metallic sheen appears when the solutions mix, usually within two to four minutes. Times may vary according to the stain and buffer used. The slide is rinsed gently, allowed to air-dry, and can then be examined using the microscope.

### Automatic Stainers

There are two basic types of automatic slide stainers. In one type of stainer, the slides are placed on a moving belt, which carries them through the staining reagents. Another type of stainer is the "basket" or "batch" type, in which baskets of slides are taken stepwise through the staining process. One basket of slides is fixed, then dipped into the stain solution, and so on. This is continued throughout the complete staining process.

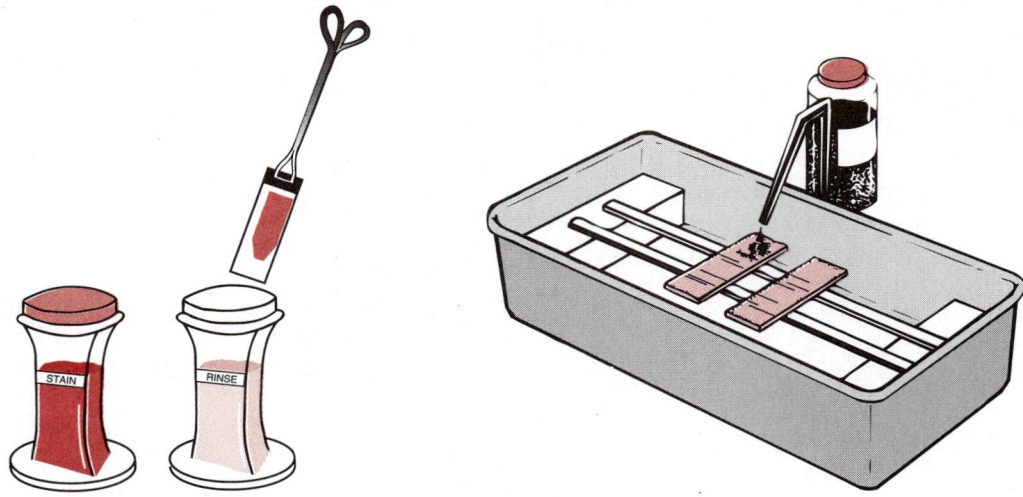

**FIGURE 2-52** Illustration of Coplin staining jars (left) and slide-staining rack (right)

Automatic stainers are helpful when large numbers of slides must be stained or staining must be performed frequently during a workday. A disadvantage of automatic stainers is that if the stain solutions are not working correctly, many slides may be processed before the worker becomes aware of the problem.

## Evaluating Stain Quality

A properly stained smear should appear somewhat pink to the naked eye. When viewed microscopically, the RBCs should appear pink-tan. The **nucleus**, or central structure, of the leukocytes should appear purple. The leukocyte **cytoplasm**, or area surrounding the nucleus, may vary from pink to blue or blue-gray, depending on the cell type (Figure 2-53). Variations in color intensities may be due to pH, timing, or characteristics of the stain or buffer. Colors are best evaluated using the oil-immersion objective.

- Slides that are too pink may be due to the stain time being too short, the wash time being too long, or the pH of the stain or buffer being too acidic.

- Slides that are too blue may be due to overstaining, wash or buffering time being too short, or the pH of the stain or buffer being too alkaline.

## Storage of Blood Smears

Stained (or preserved) smears should be stored in the dark in a dust-free slide box or container. If protected from light, stained smears will last for years, with little fading. The smear may be protected from scratches by mounting a permanent coverglass over it. For routine work, however, this is not necessary.

A. ERYTHROCYTE

CENTRAL AREA OF PALLOR (NO NUCLEUS)

B. NEUTROPHIL

NUCLEUS (LOBED)

CYTOPLASM

CYTOPLASMIC GRANULES

C. LYMPHOCYTE

CYTOPLASMIC GRANULES

CYTOPLASM

NUCLEUS

**FIGURE 2-53** Stained blood cells: (A) erythrocyte, (B) segmented neutrophil, and (C) lymphocyte

## Procedural Notes

■ Use a spreader slide with a clean, polished end.

■ Use the proper size drop of blood to make the slide.

■ Spread capillary blood immediately to avoid clotting.

■ Avoid hesitation or jerky motion when spreading the blood.

■ Preserve or stain smears within one to two hours after preparation.

■ Store stains tightly capped to prevent evaporation or absorption of moisture.

■ Do not allow stain to dry on the slide before rinsing.

■ Rinse slides thoroughly after staining.

■ Observe proper staining and/or buffering times.

## Safety Precautions

■ Observe Universal and Standard Precautions when preparing and handling blood smears.

■ Handle products containing methanol with care; it is poisonous; do not inhale fumes or allow skin contact.

■ Wear gloves and fluid-resistant laboratory coat and handle slides with forceps.

■ Handle glass slides and coverglasses carefully to prevent accidental cuts.

## LESSON REVIEW

1. What is the purpose of staining blood smears?
2. What specimen(s) may be used to prepare blood smears?
3. What blood components can be viewed on a stained smear?
4. Explain the two-slide method for making a blood smear.
5. Describe the coverglass method of making a blood smear.
6. What are some of the errors to avoid when making a blood smear?
7. Describe and diagram the appearance of a properly prepared blood smear.
8. How may unstained blood smears be preserved?
9. Explain what is meant by polychromatic stains.
10. Name two commonly used blood stains.
11. How should a properly stained smear appear?
12. What is the proper method of storing preserved or stained slides?
13. Name three factors that can affect staining results.
14. Define buffer, cytoplasm, eosin, fixative, methylene blue, morphology, nucleus, and polychromatic.

## STUDENT ACTIVITIES

1. Reread the information on preparing and staining a blood smear.
2. Review the glossary terms.
3. Practice preparing and staining blood smears by the two-step or quick-stain method as outlined in the Student Performance Guide.
4. Compare smears stained by the two-step and quick-stain methods. Which method produced the most desired effect?
5. Experiment with variations in staining and buffering times using the two-step method. Explain the results.

# Student Performance Guide

## LESSON 2-8 Preparing and Staining a Blood Smear

Name _____ Date _____

## INSTRUCTIONS

1. Practice preparing and staining a blood smear following the step-by-step procedure.
2. Demonstrate your understanding of this lesson by:
   a. Completing a written examination successfully, and
   b. Demonstrating the procedure for preparing and staining a blood smear satisfactorily for the instructor. All steps must be completed as listed on the instructor's Performance Check Sheet.

*Note:* Stain characteristics may vary with stain lot. Follow manufacturer's instructions for best results.

## MATERIALS AND EQUIPMENT

- gloves
- hand disinfectant
- slide storage box
- pencil
- microscope slides (1" x 3"), frosted end optional
- 95% ethyl alcohol
- laboratory tissue
- plastic or mylar-sheathed capillary tubes (plain and heparinized)
- slide-drying rack
- hot water
- detergent
- distilled water
- methanol in covered staining (Coplin) jar
- EDTA anticoagulated blood specimen (fresh)
- materials for capillary puncture
- surface disinfectant or 10% chlorine bleach solution
- biohazard container
- puncture-proof container for sharp objects
- glass-etching pen
- Blood stain reagents: Wright stain and buffer, or commercial blood stain kit (quick stain)
- staining rack
- immersion oil
- microscope
- lens paper
- lens cleaner
- forceps
- laboratory tissue
- lab apron or lab coat
- staining jars for quick stains

## PROCEDURE

Record in the comment section any problems encountered while practicing the procedure (or have a fellow student or the instructor evaluate your performance).

S = Satisfactory
U = Unsatisfactory

| You must: | S | U | Comments |
|---|---|---|---|
| **A. Prepare blood smears** | | | |
| 1. Assemble equipment and materials | | | |
| 2. Prepare several clean slides:<br>a. Use precleaned slides, or<br>b. Clean slides with soap, rinse with hot water followed by distilled water, dip in 95% ethyl alcohol, and polish dry with clean lint-free cloth | | | |

| You must: | S | U | Comments |
|---|---|---|---|
| 3. Place a clean slide on a flat surface (be sure to touch only the edges of the slide with fingers). Write patient identification on the frosted area with a pencil or etch I.D. on slide using etching pen | | | |
| 4. Wash hands and put on gloves | | | |
| 5. Obtain an anticoagulated blood sample (provided by the instructor) | | | |
| 6. Mix blood well and fill a plain capillary tube with blood | | | |
| 7. Dispense a small drop of blood from the capillary tube onto the slide about one-half to three-quarters of an inch from the right end (if left-handed, reverse instructions) | | | |
| 8. Place the end of a clean, polished unchipped spreader slide in front of the drop of blood at a 30–35° angle. Spreader should be lightly balanced with fingertips | | | |
| 9. Pull the spreader slide back into the drop of blood by sliding it gently along the slide until the blood spreads along three-fourths of the width of the spreader | | | |
| 10. Push the spreader slide forward with a quick steady motion (use other hand to keep slide from moving while spreader is pushed) | | | |
| 11. Examine the smear to see if it is satisfactory | | | |
| 12. Repeat the procedure until two satisfactory smears are obtained | | | |
| 13. Allow the smear(s) to air-dry quickly (stand slide on end in slide-drying rack) and label the slide | | | |
| 14. Place the dried smears in absolute methanol for 30–60 seconds to preserve the smear | | | |
| 15. Remove the slides from the methanol and allow to air-dry | | | |
| 16. Store slides for staining | | | |
| 17. Perform a capillary puncture, wipe away the first drop of blood, and fill one or two capillary tubes | | | |
| 18. Prepare two blood smears from capillary blood, repeating steps 7–16 | | | |
| 19. Discard blood specimens appropriately or store for later use. Place contaminated materials in biohazard or sharps container | | | |
| **B. Stain blood smears:** | | | |
| 1. Stain a blood smear by one of the following methods:<br>a. Two-step method<br>  (1) Place the dried smear on the staining rack, blood side up<br>  (2) Flood the smear with Wright stain, but do not let stain overflow the sides of the slide<br>  (3) Leave stain on slide one to three minutes (get exact time from instructor)<br>  (4) Add buffer drop by drop to the stain until buffer volume is about equal to that of the stain<br>  (5) A green metallic sheen should appear on the surface | | | |

| You must: | S | U | Comments |
|---|---|---|---|
|     (6) Allow buffer to remain on slide for two to four minutes (do not allow mixture to run off slide); get exact time from instructor<br>    (7) Rinse thoroughly and continuously with a gentle stream of tap or distilled water<br>    (8) Drain water from slide<br>    (9) Wipe the *back* of the slide with a wet gauze to remove excess stain<br>    (10) Stand smear on end to dry<br>        or | | | |
|   b. Quick stain<br>    (1) Dip dry smear into solutions as directed by manufacturer's instructions (do not allow slide to dry between solutions)<br>    (2) Rinse slide (if instructed to do so)<br>    (3) Remove excess stain from the *back* of the slide with wet gauze<br>    (4) Allow slide to air-dry by standing on end | | | |
| 2. Place thoroughly dried slide on microscope stage, stain side up | | | |
| 3. Focus with low-power (10X) objective | | | |
| 4. Scan slide to find area where cells are barely touching each other (in feathered edge of smear) | | | |
| 5. Place a drop of immersion oil on the slide | | | |
| 6. Rotate oil-immersion lens carefully into position | | | |
| 7. Focus with fine-adjustment knob only | | | |
| 8. Observe erythrocytes; color should be pink-tan | | | |
| 9. Observe leukocytes; nuclei should be purple; neutrophil granules should be pink-lavender | | | |
| 10. Observe platelets; they should appear purple and granular | | | |
| 11. Rotate the low-power (10X) objective into position | | | |
| 12. Remove slide from microscope stage | | | |
| 13. Clean oil objective thoroughly with lens paper | | | |
| 14. Wipe oil from slide gently with soft tissue | | | |
| 15. Clean equipment and return to proper storage | | | |
| 16. Discard slides as instructed or store in slide box for use in Lesson 2-9 | | | |
| 17. Clean work area with surface disinfectant | | | |
| 18. Remove and discard gloves in biohazard container and wash hands with hand disinfectant | | | |

*Evaluator Comments:*


Evaluator _____   Date _____

# Blood Cell Morphology and Differential Count

## LESSON OBJECTIVES

**After studying this lesson, you should be able to:**

- *State the importance of blood cell identification.*
- *List three features of cells that are evaluated during blood cell identification.*
- *Use the microscope to identify five types of leukocytes from a stained, normal blood smear.*
- *Identify platelets microscopically.*
- *Identify erythrocytes microscopically.*
- *Explain the purpose of a differential count.*
- *List the reference ranges for differential counts.*
- *Perform a differential count and report the results.*
- *Evaluate and report the morphology of the erythrocytes from a stained blood smear.*
- *Evaluate the morphology of platelets and estimate their numbers from a stained blood smear.*
- *List five precautions that should be observed when performing a differential count.*
- *Define the glossary terms.*

## GLOSSARY

**anisocytosis** / marked variation in the sizes of erythrocytes when observed on a peripheral blood smear

**band cell** / an immature granulocyte with a nonsegmented nucleus; a "stab cell"

**basophil** / a leukocyte containing basophilic-staining granules in the cytoplasm

**basophilic** / blue in color; having affinity for the basic stain

**differential count** / a determination of the relative numbers of each type of leukocyte in a stained blood smear

**eosinophil** / a leukocyte containing eosinophilic granules in the cytoplasm

**hypochromic** / having reduced color or hemoglobin content

**lymphocyte** / a small basophilic-staining leukocyte having a round or oval nucleus and playing a vital role in the immune process

**macrocytic** / having a larger-than-normal cell size

**microcytic** / having a smaller-than-normal cell size

**monocyte** / a large leukocyte usually characterized by a convoluted or horseshoe-shaped nucleus

**neutrophil** / a neutral-staining leukocyte, usually the first line of defense against infection

**normochromic** / having normal color

**normocytic** / having a normal cell size

**poikilocytosis** / significant variation in the shape of erythrocytes

**vacuole** / in cell cytoplasm, a clear compartment filled with fluid or air

# INTRODUCTION

Much useful information can be gained from the microscopic examination of a stained blood smear. Many situations arise in which the physician requires more knowledge than is provided by a cell count alone. By viewing a blood smear microscopically, the technologist or physician can identify blood cells and evaluate any abnormalities present. Many hematologists (blood specialists) believe that more information is obtained from a blood smear than any other single laboratory test.

Examination of the leukocytes and classification of cells into different types is a **differential count**. The "diff," as it is often called, is usually a part of a complete blood count (CBC). However, the "WBC count and diff" combination is also a common laboratory request.

The differential count can be used to diagnose and monitor the treatment of leukemias, anemias, and other diseases. For example, the viral infection causing infectious mononucleosis produces a characteristic leukocyte differential. Iron deficiency anemia produces a characteristic RBC morphology, with small RBCs that have a reduced amount of hemoglobin.

# THE DIFFERENTIAL COUNT

The differential procedure involves counting 100–200 WBCs on a stained blood smear and recording how many of each of the five types of WBCs are seen. Information is also obtained concerning the RBCs and platelets. The RBCs are evaluated for morphology and hemoglobin content. The platelets are evaluated for morphology and an estimation of platelet numbers.

## Examining the Stained Blood Smear

A well-prepared Wright's stained blood smear, along with a good blood cell atlas, is used to learn cell identification. The smear should always be examined using immersion oil on the slide and the oil-immersion objective (97X or 100X).

The condenser of the microscope should be raised until it almost touches the bottom of the slide being observed. With the microscope diaphragm open, the light should be bright enough so the stained cell features can easily be seen.

The area of the smear to be examined is called the feathered edge, where the cells do not overlap each other (Figure 2-54). The RBCs should be barely touching each other. Cells are easiest to identify in this area of the smear because of their slightly flattened shape, which allows better viewing of cell structures.

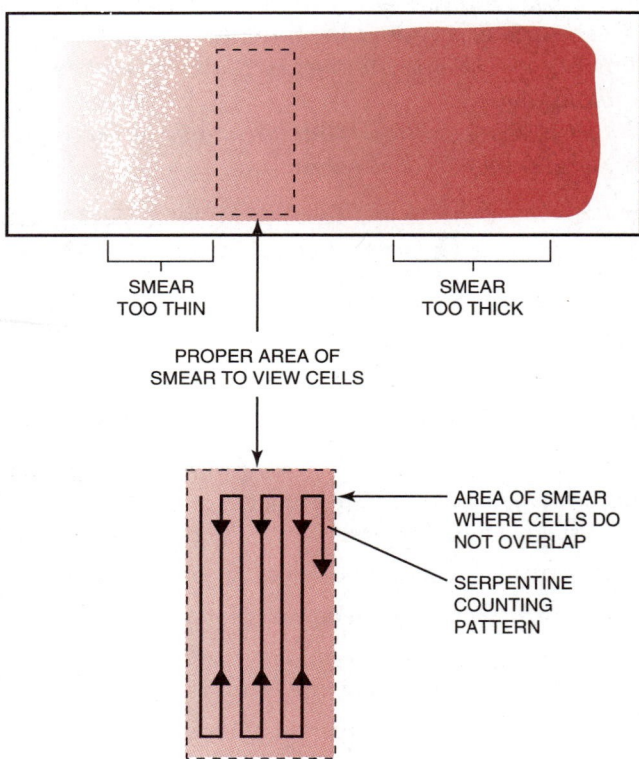

SMEAR TOO THIN          SMEAR TOO THICK

PROPER AREA OF SMEAR TO VIEW CELLS

AREA OF SMEAR WHERE CELLS DO NOT OVERLAP

SERPENTINE COUNTING PATTERN

**FIGURE 2-54** Proper area of a blood smear to view for the differential count and illustration of counting pattern

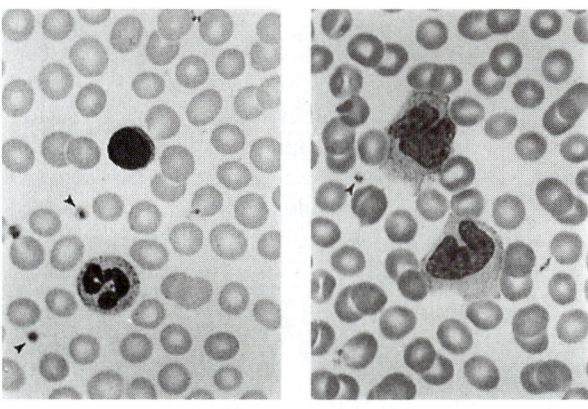

**FIGURE 2-55** Photmicrographs of stained peripheral blood smears showing erythrocytes, leukocytes, and platelets. Left, lymphocyte (top) and neutrophil (bottom); right, two monocytes. Arrowheads denote platelets. (Photos courtesy of F. A. Davis Company)

## Cellular Features Evaluated in Identification

The WBC features that must be observed and evaluated are: (1) cell size, (2) nuclear characteristics, and (3) cytoplasmic characteristics. The size of cells can be estimated by comparing them with RBCs. The nucleus must be observed for shape, size, structure, and color. The cytoplasm is evaluated by noting the color, amount, and type of inclusions. When the information from these three observations is combined, most cells can be identified.

Beginners will find it necessary to consciously consider each of the cell properties. As experience is gained, the process becomes almost automatic, for normal cells. Much practice is required to be able to recognize and classify abnormal cells that may be seen in various disease states.

## IDENTIFICATION OF BLOOD CELLS IN A NORMAL BLOOD SMEAR

The cells usually seen in a normal blood smear are described below. The descriptions are for cells as they would appear in Wright stained smears (Figure 2-55). A leukocyte identification guide with abbreviated descriptions is given in Figure 2-56, and Color Plates 1–6, 10, and 12 depict typical appearances of stained cells.

### Erythrocytes

Erythrocytes (red blood cells) are the most numerous of the blood cells. Normal mature RBCs stain pink-tan,

| | Neutrophilic Series | | Eosinophil | Basophil | Lymphocyte | Monocyte |
|---|---|---|---|---|---|---|
| | Segmented (mature) | Band or Stab (immature) | | | | |
| Cell Size (μm) | 10–15 | 10–15 | 10–15 | 10–15 | 8–15 | 12–20 |
| **Nucleus** | | | | | | |
| Shape | 2–5 lobes | Sausage or U-shaped | Bilobed | Segmented | Round, oval | Horseshoe |
| Structure | Coarse | Coarse | Coarse | Difficult to see | Smudged (smoothly stained) | Folded, convoluted |
| **Cytoplasm** | | | | | | |
| Amount | Abundant | Abundant | Abundant | Abundant | Scant | Abundant |
| Color | Pale pink-tan | Pale pink-tan | Pale pink-tan | Pale pink-tan | Clear blue | Opaque, blue-gray |
| Inclusions | Small, lilac granules | Small, lilac granules | Coarse, orange-red granules | Coarse, blue-black granules | Occasional red-purple granules | Ground-glass appearance |

**FIGURE 2-56** Leukocyte identification guide

have no nuclei, and are 6–8 μm in diameter. The pink-tan color is due to the staining of hemoglobin within the cells. RBCs are shaped like biconcave discs. Because they are thin in the center, the central area of the cell stains less than the margins. This is called the "central area of pallor."

## Platelets

Platelets (thrombocytes) are the smallest of the stained blood elements. They are usually 2-3 μm in diameter, or one-third the diameter of an RBC. No nucleus is present because the platelet is simply a fragment of cytoplasm from a large bone marrow cell called a megakaryocyte. The platelet cytoplasm stains bluish and usually contains small reddish-purple granules (Color Plates 1 and 12). Platelets may be round, oval, or have spiny projections.

## Leukocytes

Leukocytes (WBCs) are the largest of the normal blood components. Their sizes range from slightly larger than an RBC to more than twice the diameter of an RBC. Each of the five types of WBCs has a characteristic appearance.

The granular leukocytes—neutrophil, eosinophil, and basophil—contain many distinctive cytoplasmic granules, and may have segmented nuclei. The lymphocyte and monocyte have few, if any, easily visible cytoplasmic granules and have nonsegmented nuclei.

### Neutrophil

The granular leukocyte that stains a neutral color is called the **neutrophil.** The neutrophil nucleus is usually segmented into two to five lobes, each connected by a strand or filament. The nucleus stains a dark purple and has a coarse appearance. The cytoplasm is pale pink to tan and contains fine pink or lilac granules. The neutrophil is about twice the diameter of an RBC and is the most numerous of the WBCs in normal adult blood. Other names for the neutrophil are PMN (polymorphonuclear neutrophil), "poly," or "seg." (Color Plates 1, 2, and 10)

### Band Cell

The younger (more immature) stage of the neutrophil is called a **band cell.** The staining characteristics are like the neutrophil. However, the nucleus is not segmented, but is shaped like a curved sausage. (Color Plates 4 and 10)

### Eosinophil

The **eosinophil** is the WBC with granules that have an affinity for the eosin portion of the stain. The nucleus of the eosinophil is usually divided into two or three lobes and stains purple. The cytoplasm is pink-tan, but may be difficult to see because it is filled with large red-orange (eosinophilic) granules. Eosinophils are approximately the size of neutrophils, but are much less numerous. (Color Plates 5 and 10)

### Basophil

The **basophil** is the WBC with granules that have an affinity for the basic portion of the stain. The nucleus of the basophil is segmented and stains light purple. The nuclear shape is often difficult to see because numerous coarse blue-black granules often obscure the nucleus and cytoplasm. Basophils are seen only occasionally in normal smears. (Color Plates 6 and 10)

### Lymphocyte

The **lymphocytes** are the smallest of the WBCs. Most lymphocytes are only slightly larger than an RBC. The nucleus is usually rather smooth, has a round or oval shape, and stains purple. The cytoplasm is **basophilic** (blue) and varies in amount. Occasionally, a few red-purple granules may be present in the cytoplasm. (Color Plates 2 and 3)

### Monocyte

The **monocyte** is the largest circulating WBC. The nucleus may be oval, indented, or horseshoe-shaped and may have brain-like convolutions or folds. The cytoplasm is a dull gray-blue and may have an irregular outline. Very fine granules are distributed throughout the cytoplasm, giving it a ground-glass appearance. **Vacuoles** that appear as a clear space may also be present in the cytoplasm. (Color Plates 2 and 12)

## REFERENCE VALUES FOR THE DIFFERENTIAL COUNT

The reference ranges for the differential count vary with age. Normal values for adults and children are listed in Table 2-11. In a normal differential count, neutrophils and lymphocytes comprise 85-95% of cells, with monocytes, eosinophils, and basophils making up the remaining 5–15%. Children normally have a higher percentage of lymphocytes than adults.

**TABLE 2–11.** Reference ranges for the differential count

| TYPE OF CELL | REFERENCE VALUES | | | |
|---|---|---|---|---|
| **White Cell** | **1-month-old** | **6-year-old** | **12-year-old** | **Adult** |
| Neutrophil (seg) | 15–35% | 45–50% | 45–50% | 50–65% |
| Neutrophil (band) | 7–13% | 0–7% | 6–8% | 0–7% |
| Eosinophil | 1–3% | 1–3% | 1–3% | 1–3% |
| Basophil | 0–1% | 0–1% | 0–1% | 0–1% |
| Monocyte | 5–8% | 4–8% | 3–8% | 3–9% |
| Lymphocyte | 40–70% | 40–45% | 35–40% | 25–40% |
| **Platelets** | An average of 7–20 platelets per oil immersion field is considered normal | | | |

## Factors Affecting the WBC Percentages

Many disease states can change the percentages of the different types of WBCs (Table 2-12). Bacterial infections usually cause an increase in the bands and segmented neutrophils. Viral infections can increase the number of lymphocytes or change their morphology, causing them to appear atypical. The number of eosinophils is increased in parasitic infections and allergies. The number of monocytes is usually not affected by infections, but occasionally will increase in tuberculosis. In leukemias, there is usually an increase and abnormality in one type of cell. The leukemia is named according to the predominant cell present. For example, an increased ratio of lymphocytes is found in lymphocytic leukemias.

**TABLE 2–12.** Factors affecting WBC percentages

| CONDITION | EFFECT ON WBCS |
|---|---|
| Bacterial infections | Increased total WBCs, increased percentage of neutrophils |
| Viral infections | Decreased total WBCs, increased percentage of lymphocytes |
| Infectious mononucleosis | Increased total WBCs, increased lymphs, increased "atypical" (reactive) lymphs |
| Parasitic infections, allergic reactions | Increased eosinophils |
| Leukemias | Total WBCs usually increased, increase in type of leukocyte involved |
| Newborns, children | Increased lymphocytes |

## Factors Affecting Red Blood Cells

Normal production and development of RBCs requires certain factors such as vitamins and minerals. Iron deficiency is one cause of microcytic, hypochromic RBCs. Deficiencies of vitamins such as $B_{12}$ and folic acid cause the cells to be macrocytic. —large size

## Factors Affecting Platelets

The platelets can be affected by several factors. In some leukemias, the number of platelets is below normal. Exposure to chemicals, radiation, or drugs used in cancer therapy can also reduce platelets. If there is a delay in making a smear from a capillary puncture, the platelet distribution may be uneven; this may cause the platelet estimate to be erroneous.

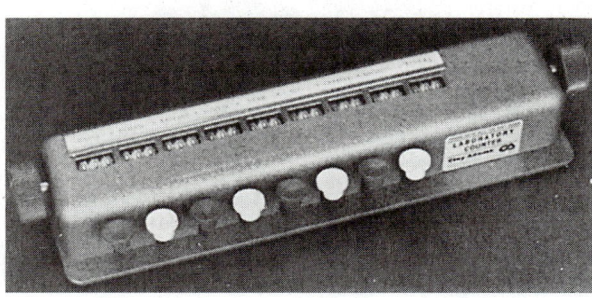 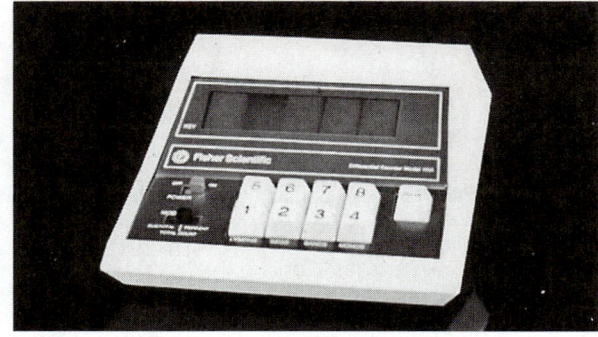

**FIGURE 2-57** Differential cell counters: (Left) manual counter (Courtesy of Clay Adams Division, Becton Dickinson); (right) counter with digital display (Photo courtesy of Fisher Scientific)

# PERFORMING THE DIFFERENTIAL COUNT

## Quality Assurance

The differential report can give rise to a variety of actions, treatments, and further testing. Therefore, it is imperative that great care and thoroughness are used when examining the cells and making the report.

The staining procedure must be carefully followed so cell components are properly stained. In addition, the area of observation must be where the RBCs are just touching, but not overlapping, each other when viewed microscopically (Figure 2-54). The proper area should be located by looking through the low-power (10X) objective; the oil-immersion (97X) objective is used to perform the differential count.

## White Blood Cell Observations

When an area of the slide has been located in which the stain appears satisfactory and the cells are not crowded or distorted, 100 WBCs are counted. A definite pattern, such as the one shown in Figure 2-54, must be followed to avoid counting the same cells twice. The numbers of each type of WBC observed are recorded using a differential counter (Figure 2-57) or a tally counter. Any abnormalities of the cells are also noted.

## Red Blood Cell Observations

After the differential count has been completed, the stained RBCs and platelets are observed and evaluated. With some experience, one may estimate the RBC size as **normocytic** (normal), **microcytic** (small), or **macrocytic** (large). The condition in which markedly different sizes of RBCs are present in a smear is called **anisocytosis**.

The hemoglobin content of the RBCs can also be estimated. A RBC with the normal amount of hemoglobin is called **normochromic**. It stains evenly, with only a small pale area in the center of the cell. A **hypochromic** RBC is one that has less than the normal amount of hemoglobin, with only a ring of hemoglobin around the outer edge and a large pale area in the center. Normal RBCs are round or slightly oval. The condition in which there is a significant variation in the shape of RBCs is called **poikilocytosis**. Table 2-13 lists some conditions that affect RBC morphology.

## Platelet Observations

Platelets are also observed for any abnormalities in their morphology. The total number of platelets counted in 10 oil-immersion fields is divided by 10 to give the average number per field. Seven to 20 platelets per oil-immersion field indicates a normal platelet count.

## Automated Differentials

Almost all hematology blood cell counters, even the smaller units for POCT, can be used to perform automated differentials. The automated differential may be either a three-part or five-part. In a three-part differen-

**TABLE 2–13.** Conditions that affect RBC morphology

| CELL MORPHOLOGY | CONDITIONS |
| --- | --- |
| **Size** | |
| Normocytic | Normal |
| Microcytic | Iron deficiency anemia, thalassemias |
| Macrocytic | Vitamin $B_{12}$ deficiency, folate deficiency |
| **Shape** | |
| Round, biconcave disk | Normal |
| Sickle (drepanocyte) | Sickle cell disease |
| Sphere | Hereditary spherocytosis |
| **Hemoglobin Content** | |
| Normochromic | Normal |
| Hypochromic | Iron deficiency anemia |
| Hyperchromic | Appearance caused by thickness of cells in spherocytosis |

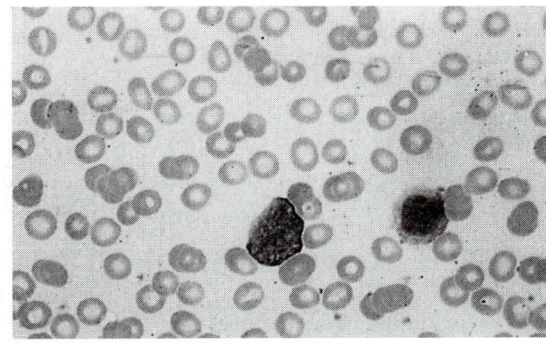

**FIGURE 2-58** Photomicrograph showing two reactive (atypical) lymphocytes

technologist is allowed to report such cells, but all smears with abnormal cells reported are later reviewed by the supervisor or pathologist.

In performing a differential count, it is important to learn what is normal so well that it becomes easy to recognize something abnormal. If suspicious cells are seen, the differential can be repeated, counting 500 cells to increase the chances of finding more abnormal cells. Whenever there is doubt about identification of a cell, more experienced personnel should be consulted.

tial, the blood is subjected to a special reagent that shrinks the cytoplasm of each type of WBC in a specific way. The analyzer then sorts the cells by size and classifies them as either lymphocytes, granulocytes, or mononuclear cells. Five-part differentials in which neutrophils, lymphocytes, eosinophils, basophils, and monocytes are classified and counted, are available on most of the mid-size and large hematology analyzers. The majority of these instruments use impedance technology (electrical interruption) or a combination of impedance, cell conductivity, and light scatter to classify cells. Details about automation are found in Lesson 2-13, Principles of Automated Hematology.

## ABNORMAL OR ATYPICAL CELLS

Recognition and identification of atypical or abnormal WBCs requires much study and practice. The reporting of such cells should be left to the hematology supervisor or the pathologist. One exception to this is the "atypical" or "reactive" lymphocyte found in infectious mononucleosis (Figure 2-58). In most laboratories the

### Procedural Notes

■ Observe and count cells in an area of the smear where cells are just touching.

■ Avoid counting near the edges and ends of the smear.

■ Raise the microscope condenser and open the iris diaphragm.

■ Consult a more experienced technologist or hematology supervisor if there is difficulty in identifying cells.

### Safety Precautions

■ Observe Universal and Standard Precautions.

■ Handle slides carefully to avoid cuts.

## LESSON REVIEW

1. Why is it important to identify blood cells?
2. What three features of cells are evaluated during cell identification?
3. List the five types of WBCs.
4. What is the source of platelets? *bone marrow megakaryo*
5. Describe the area of the smear used to perform a differential count.
6. Describe the microscopic appearance of stained RBCs.
7. List the reference ranges for WBCs in a differential count.
8. What features of platelets should be noted during the differential?
9. What color granules are present in neutrophils? *dark purple* Eosinophils? Basophils? *blue* *black* *red*
10. Explain what the technician should do if the WBCs appear abnormal or difficult to identify. *Call consultant*
11. Define anisocytosis, band cell, basophil, basophilic, differential count, eosinophil, hypochromic, lymphocyte, macrocytic, microcytic, monocyte, neutrophil, normochromic, normocytic, poikilocytosis, and vacuole. *immature smallest large size small size larger size normal color normal size variable size contain air or fluid*

## STUDENT ACTIVITIES

1. Reread the information on blood cell morphology and the differential count.
2. Review the glossary terms.
3. Practice blood cell identification as outlined in the Student Performance Guide.
4. Practice identifying blood cells in additional stained smears or from unlabeled colored illustrations of cells.
5. Practice performing a differential count as outlined in the Student Performance Guide, using the worksheet.
6. Perform differential counts on additional smears provided by the instructor.
7. If an automated cell counter is available to perform differentials, compare the results of a manual differential count with the instrument result.

# *Student Performance Guide*

## **LESSON 2-9** Blood Cell Morphology and Differential Count

Name _____ Date _____

### ☣ INSTRUCTIONS

1. Practice identification of erythrocytes, leukocytes, and platelets from a stained smear.
2. Practice the procedure for performing the differential count following the step-by-step procedure.
3. Demonstrate your understanding of this lesson by:
   a. Completing a written examination successfully, and
   b. Performing the differential count satisfactorily for the instructor. Identify erythrocytes, five types of leukocytes, and platelets satisfactorily for the instructor. All steps must be completed as listed on the instructor's Performance Check Sheet.

### MATERIALS AND EQUIPMENT

- gloves
- hand disinfectant
- stained normal blood smears
- microscope with oil-immersion objective
- immersion oil
- lens paper and lens cleaner
- soft tissue or soft paper towels
- blood cell atlas; drawings or photographs and descriptions of stained blood cells
- tally counter or differential counter
- worksheet
- puncture-proof container for contaminated sharps
- surface disinfectant or 10% chlorine bleach solution

## PROCEDURE

Record in the comment section any problems encountered while practicing the procedure (or have a fellow student or the instructor evaluate your performance).

S = Satisfactory
U = Unsatisfactory

| You must: | S | U | Comments |
|---|---|---|---|
| 1. Wash hands and put on gloves | | | |
| 2. Assemble materials and equipment | | | |
| 3. Place stained blood smear on microscope stage and secure with clips | | | |
| 4. Use the low-power (10X) objective to locate the feathered edge of the smear | | | |
| 5. Bring the cells into focus using the 10X objective and coarse adjustment | | | |
| 6. Scan the smear to find an area where the RBCs are barely touching | | | |
| 7. Place one drop of immersion oil on the smear | | | |
| 8. Rotate the oil-immersion objective (97X or 100X) carefully into position | | | |

| You must: | S | U | Comments |
|---|---|---|---|
| 9. Focus, using the fine adjustment, until cells can clearly be seen | | | |
| 10. Raise the condenser and open the iris diaphragm to allow maximum light into the objective | | | |
| 11. Scan the slide to observe the leukocytes | | | |
| 12. Study the smear; try to find and identify all five types of WBCs | | | |
| 13. Scan the smear to find platelets | | | |
| 14. Scan the smear to observe RBCs | | | |
| 15. Repeat steps 3–14 until cells can readily be identified | | | |
| 16. Repeat steps 1–10 using the same smear or a different one | | | |
| 17. Count 100 consecutive WBCs, moving the slide so that consecutive microscopic fields are viewed; use the counting pattern illustrated in Figure 2-54 | | | |
| 18. Record on the worksheet how many WBCs of each type are seen | | | |
| 19. Observe the RBCs in at least 10 fields. Note the hemoglobin content; record as normochromic or hypochromic | | | |
| 20. Observe the RBC size. Record as normocytic, microcytic, or macrocytic. If present, estimate number of microcytic or macrocytic RBCs by using a grading system of 1+ to 4+, or small, medium, large numbers present | | | |
| 21. Observe platelets in at least 10 fields:<br>a. Note morphology<br>b. Estimate the number of platelets per oil-immersion field: record as adequate, decreased, or increased, using the guide on the worksheet | | | |
| 22. Rotate the low-power (10X) objective into place | | | |
| 23. Remove the slide from the stage | | | |
| 24. Clean the oil-immersion objective thoroughly, using lens paper | | | |
| 25. Check the microscope stage and condenser for oil and clean with soft tissue if necessary | | | |
| 26. Place the slide on its edge in plastic slide box or discard slides as instructed | | | |
| 27. Clean remaining equipment and return it to proper storage | | | |
| 28. Wipe work counter with surface disinfectant | | | |
| 29. Remove and discard gloves in biohazard container and wash hands with hand disinfectant | | | |

*Evaluator Comments:*

Evaluator _____   Date _____

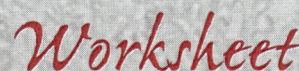

## *Worksheet*

## LESSON 2-9 Differential Count

Name _____  Date _____

Specimen I.D.  _____

| | | | REFERENCE VALUES (ADULT) |
|---|---|---|---|
| Segmented Neutrophils | _____ % | | 50–65% |
| Lymphocytes | _____ % | | 25–40% |
| Monocytes | _____ % | | 3–9% |
| Eosinophils | _____ % | | 1–3% |
| Basophils | _____ % | | 0–1% |
| Bands | _____ % | | 0–7% |
| Other | _____ | | |

Platelet Estimate: ❏ appear adequate                                          7–20/oil-immersion field

❏ appear decreased (<7/oil-immersion field)

❏ appear increased (>20/oil-immersion field)

RBC Morphology:

Cell size:   ❏ normocytic

❏ microcytic                                    normocytic (6–8 µm)

❏ macrocytic

Cell color:   ❏ normochromic                                    normochromic

❏ hypochromic

Comments: _____

_____

_____

_____

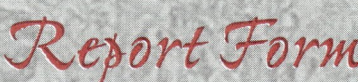

*Report Form*

## LESSON 2-9 Hematology CBC Report Form

Name _____  Date _____

Specimen I.D.  _____

| | | **REFERENCE VALUES (ADULT)** |
|---|---|---|
| WBC/L | _____ | 4.5–11.0 x 10⁹/L |

WBC/L      _____

RBC/L      _____

Hgb (g/dL)      _____

Hct %      _____

MCV (fL)      _____

MCH (pg)      _____

MCHC (%)      _____

**REFERENCE VALUES (ADULT)**

4.5–11.0 x 10⁹/L

4.5–6.0 x 10¹²/L male

4.0–5.5 x 10¹²/L female

13–17 g/dL male

12–16 g/dL female

42–52% male

36–48% female

80–100 fL

27–32 pg

32–37%

**Differential Count:**

_____ %  segmented neutrophils      50–65%

_____ %  lymphocytes      25–40%

_____ %  monocytes      3–9%

_____ %  eosinophils      1–3%

_____ %  basophils      0–1%

_____ %  bands      0–7%

_____ %  other

RBC Morphology:

   Cell size:       ❐ normocytic

                 ❐ microcytic      normocytic

                 ❐ macrocytic

   Cell color:       ❐ normochromic      normochromic

                 ❐ hypochromic

Platelet      ❐ appear adequate      7–20/oil-immersion field

Estimate:      ❐ appear decreased <7/oil-immersion field

                 ❐ appear increased >20/oil-immersion field

Comments:  _____

                       _____

# Morphology of Abnormal Blood Cells in Peripheral Blood

## LESSON OBJECTIVES

**After studying this lesson, you should be able to:**

- *State the importance of differentiating between normal and abnormal blood cells on a peripheral blood smear.*
- *List two conditions in which anisocytosis is found.*
- *List two conditions in which poikilocytosis is found.*
- *List two conditions in which hypochromic erythrocytes may be found.*
- *Discuss the relationship of the erythrocyte indices to the morphology of the erythrocytes.*
- *Discuss the significance of RBC inclusions.*
- *List two causes of leukopenia.*
- *List two causes of leukocytosis.*
- *Discuss neutrophilia and a shift to the left.*
- *Discuss the characteristics of leukemias.*
- *List conditions in which abnormal thrombocytes may be found.*
- *Define the glossary terms.*

## GLOSSARY

**basophilic stippling** / fine granular remnants of RNA and other basophilic nuclear material remaining inside the erythrocyte after the nucleus is lost from the cell

**blast cell** / an immature blood cell normally found only in the bone marrow

**femtoliter (fL)** / a unit of volume; $10^{-15}$L

**folic acid** / a member of the B vitamin complex

**Howell-Jolly body** / nuclear remnant remaining in RBCs after the nucleus is lost; common in pernicious anemia and hemolytic anemias

**indices** / plural of index; erythrocyte indices are values that compare RBCs in a blood sample to standard values

**leukemia** / a chronic or acute disease involving unrestrained growth of leukocytes in the bone marrow and peripheral blood

**mean corpuscular hemoglobin (MCH)** / mean cell hemoglobin; average RBC hemoglobin, expressed in picograms (pg)

**mean corpuscular hemoglobin concentration (MCHC)** / mean cell hemoglobin concentration; comparison of the weight of hemoglobin in an RBC to the size of the RBC, expressed in percentage or g/dL

**mean corpuscular volume (MCV)** / mean cell volume; average RBC volume; an estimate of RBC volume in a blood sample, expressed in femtoliters (fL) or cubic microns ($\mu^3$)

**picogram (pg)** / micromicrogram; $1 \times 10^{-12}$ gram

**reactive lymphocyte** / lymphocyte that occurs in response to viral infections; common in infectious mononucleosis; atypical lymph

**shift to the left** / the appearance of an increased number of immature neutrophil forms in the peripheral blood; occurs in response to bacterial infections

**thalassemia** / a genetic condition in which abnormal hemoglobin is produced, resulting in anemia

**vitamin B$_{12}$** / a vitamin essential to the proper maturation of blood and other cells in the body

## INTRODUCTION

The information gained from a complete blood count (CBC) with a differential count can be very valuable to the physician in making or confirming a diagnosis. Several conditions can be indicated by the presence of abnormal red or white blood cells observed while performing a differential. Such conditions as iron deficiency anemia, folic acid or vitamin B$_{12}$ deficiencies, and sickle cell anemia have distinctive RBC morphology that can be seen on a peripheral blood smear. Abnormal WBCs can signal the presence of conditions such as bacterial or viral infections and leukemias. Abnormalities in the number or morphology of platelets can also indicate disease.

Evaluation of RBC and WBC morphology is an important part of the differential count. Correct identification of cells and accurate evaluation of RBC, WBC, and platelet morphology requires much knowledge and practice. The technician must realize that the results may determine diagnosis or treatment of disease and must be proficient in identifying cells before studying abnormal morphology.

 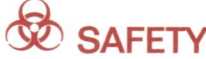 **SAFETY**

Standard and Universal Precautions must be observed if blood smears are being prepared and stained. Microscope slides should be handled carefully to avoid cuts to the hands and fingers.

### *Quality Assurance*

All differential counts must be performed using standardized technique and with attention paid to WBC, RBC, and platelet morphology. A smear may contain abnormal cells, even though the patient seems "normal." Technicians performing differential counts should be experienced and conscientious. A more experienced worker or the laboratory director should be consulted if there are any questions.

## ABNORMAL ERYTHROCYTE MORPHOLOGY

Disorders that affect the RBCs may cause *poikilocytosis*, variations in their shape, or *anisocytosis*, variations in their size. Increase (erythrocytosis) or decrease (anemia) of the RBC numbers from the normal reference range and changes in the hemoglobin content of RBCs can also occur (Table 2-14). Normal development of the RBC line is shown in Figure 2-59.

### Anisocytosis

Red blood cells of normal size, 6–8 micrometers in diameter, are said to be normocytic. Red blood cells that are smaller than six micrometers in diameter are microcytic (Fig. 2-60). Patients who have conditions

**Table 2-14.** Conditions that affect red blood cell morphology

| CELL MORPHOLOGY | CONDITIONS |
| --- | --- |
| **Size** | |
| Normocytic | Normal |
| Microcytic | Iron deficiency anemia, thalassemias |
| Macrocytic | Vitamin B$^{12}$ deficiency, folate deficiency |
| **Shape** | |
| Round, biconcave disk | Normal |
| Sickle | Sickle cell disease |
| Sphere | Hereditary spherocytosis |
| **Hemoglobin Content** | |
| Normochromic | Normal |
| Hypochromic | Iron deficiency anemia |
| Hyperchromic | Appearance caused by thickness of cells in spherocytosis |

This is only an introduction to red blood cell morphology; a good hematology reference book should be consulted for more complete descriptions.

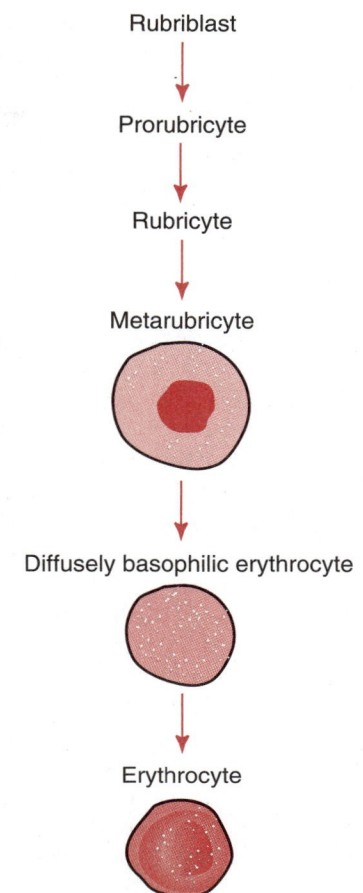

**FIGURE 2-59** Development of erythrocytes (red blood cells)

such as iron deficiency anemia and those who have inherited a **thalassemia** have microcytic RBCs. Iron deficiency anemia can result from either inadequate intake of dietary iron, an increased iron demand in pregnancy, or chronic blood loss. Thalassemias are caused by genetic defects in the synthesis of the globin portion of the hemoglobin molecule. The RBCs produced are smaller than normal and have insufficient hemoglobin (Table 2-14).

RBCs with a diameter greater than eight microns are macrocytes, also called megalocytes. Macrocytes are produced in deficiencies of vitamin B$_{12}$ or folic acid (folate) and in liver disease (Color Plate 14). Deficiency of either or both vitamin B$_{12}$ or folic acid prevents proper maturation of blood cells in the bone marrow and other cells in the body; therefore, they remain larger than normal. B$_{12}$ deficiency was formerly known as pernicious anemia because it was a fatal disease until its cause and treatment were found about 50 years ago.

## Poikilocytosis

Many conditions can cause variations in the shape of RBCs. Sickle cell disease is a genetic condition in which an abnormal hemoglobin causes the RBCs to have a

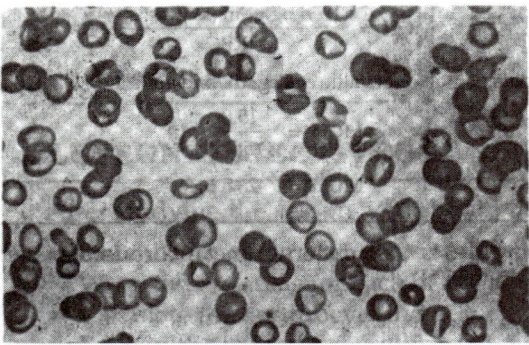

**FIGURE 2-60** Photomicrograph of hypochromic, microcytic erythrocytes as might be seen in iron deficiency anemia

characteristic "sickle" shape (*drepanocyte*) when exposed to decreased levels of oxygen (Figure 2-61A and Color Plate 15). Because of their abnormal shape, they "dam up" the smaller blood vessels, cutting off oxygen to tissues in that area. The lowered oxygen level then causes more RBCs to change to the sickle shape. This is called a "crisis," a serious and painful event for the patient because of damage to vital organs.

In hereditary spherocytosis, the RBCs are thicker than normal and have lost their biconcave shape (Figure 2-61B). Anemia develops because the spleen recognizes these cells as abnormal and destroys them prematurely.

*Elliptocytes*, elongated RBCs, are found in small numbers on most normal smears (Figure 2-61). However, in hereditary elliptocytosis the patient has large numbers of these abnormal cells. Anemia develops because the spleen destroys these RBCs and only a small number of normal RBCs remain.

Red blood cells with a linear area of pallor through the center are called *stomatocytes*, because the pale area is shaped like a mouth. These cells occur in the condition known as hereditary stomatocytosis.

In thalassemia, sickle cell disease, and other hemoglobin abnormalities, RBCs called *codocytes* are produced. They are also called "target cells" because they stain dark in the center and around the edge, with a pale area in between (Figure 2-61D).

Fragmented RBCs are called either keratocytes or schizocytes. The *keratocytes* are RBCs that have been deformed by some mechanical trauma, such as passing through an artificial heart valve or being cut by a fibrin strand in a blood clot (Figure 2-61F and Color Plate 13). When cells are actually sheared into fragments, as may happen in severe burn patients, they are called *schizocytes*.

*Crenated* RBCs have bumpy projections on the cell surface (Figure 2-61E). These are caused by prolonged exposure to anticoagulant or incorrect blood-to-anticoagulant proportions and should not be confused with pathological conditions. When using anticoagulated blood, it is important to make blood smears within two to four hours of the blood being drawn to prevent alterations in blood cell morphology.

## Variations in Hemoglobin Content

Red blood cells containing the correct amount of hemoglobin for their size are normochromic (Color Plate 1). A deficiency of hemoglobin, due to lack of iron or another condition, causes the RBCs to have a large central area of pallor with only a small outer rim of hemoglobin; these cells are hypochromic (Figure 2-60). Red blood cells that appear to be completely filled with hemoglobin are called hyperchromic.

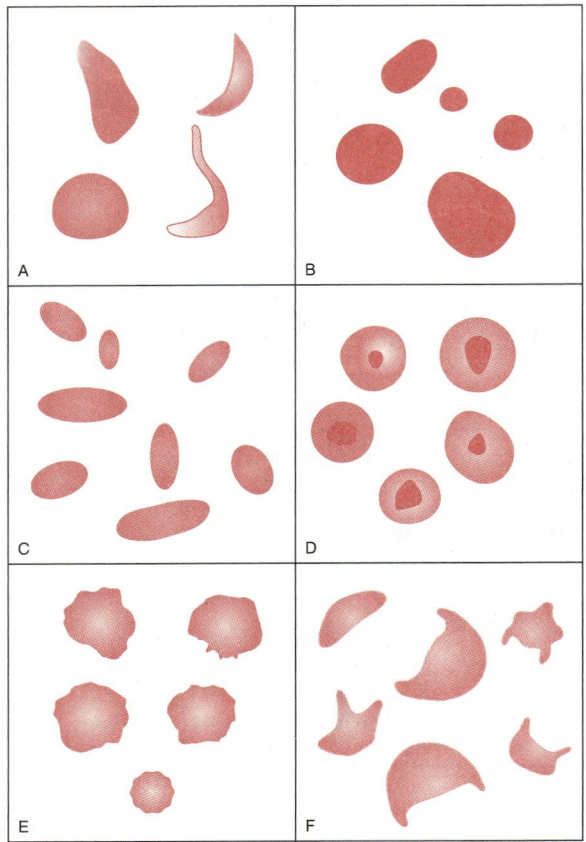

**FIGURE 2-61** Morphology of selected abnormal RBCs: (A) drepanocytes (sickle cells), (B) spherocytes, (C) elliptocytes, (D) codocytes (target cells) (E) crenated cells, (F) keratocytes including helmet cells

## Red Blood Cell Inclusions

**Basophilic stippling** is caused by the fine granular remnants of RNA and other basophilic substances left inside the RBC when it loses its nucleus. These RBCs are also known as reticulocytes when stained with a vital stain. On a Wright stained smear, the RNA remnants cause cells to have a diffuse blue color (diffuse basophilia), orange and blue mottled appearance (polychromatophilia), or punctate fine and coarse granules (basophilic stippling.) Normally, only an occasional stippled cell will be present. An increased number on the peripheral blood smear can indicate certain toxic conditions such as lead poisoning. The stippled cells are also elevated in response to increased production of RBCs due to acute hemorrhage, or after treatment for iron, $B_{12}$, or folate deficiency.

**Howell-Jolly bodies** are nuclear remnants in the RBC after the nucleus is lost. They appear on Wright stained smears as intense dark blue-purple bodies

$$MCV = \frac{\text{Hematocrit (percent)}}{RBC} \times 10$$

Using a hematocrit of 36% and an RBC of $4.0 \times 10^{12}/L$:

$$MCV = \frac{36}{4.0} \times 10$$

$$MCV = 90 \text{ fL (or } \mu^3)$$

**FIGURE 2-62** Calculation of mean corpuscular volume (MCV).

$$MCH = \frac{\text{Hemoglobin (grams)}}{RBC} \times 10$$

Using a hemoglobin value of 15 g/dL and an RBC of $5.2 \times 10^{12}/L$:

$$MCH = \frac{15.0}{5.2} \times 10$$

$$MCH = 28.8 \text{ pg}$$

**FIGURE 2-63** Calculation of mean corpuscular hemoglobin (MCH)

inside the cell and are common in pernicious anemia and hemolytic anemias.

*Cabot rings* are found in RBCs in certain anemias and in lead poisoning. They appear as dark blue-purple ring-like structures.

Nucleated red blood cells (NRBCs), normally found only in bone marrow, can be seen in peripheral blood in severe anemia. The *metarubricyte* is the form most commonly seen (Figure 2-59). These cells are also present in small numbers in the peripheral blood of normal newborns.

$$MCHC = \frac{\text{Hemoglobin (grams)}}{\text{Hematocrit (percent)}} \times 100$$

Using a hemoglobin value of 15 g/dL and a hematocrit of 44%:

$$MCHC = \frac{15}{44} \times 100$$

$$MCHC = 34\%$$

**FIGURE 2-64** Calculation of mean corpuscular hemoglobin concentration (MCHC)

## THE ERYTHROCYTE INDICES

The erythrocyte **indices** are values obtained by calculations using the RBC count, the hemoglobin value, and the hematocrit (Figures 2-62, 2-63, and 2-64). The indices are also known as the mean corpuscular values or the mean cell values. The indices consist of the mean corpuscular volume (MCV), the mean corpuscular hemoglobin (MCH), and the mean corpuscular hemoglobin content (MCHC).

### Mean Corpuscular Volume

The **mean corpuscular volume (MCV)** is the volume of an average erythrocyte in a blood sample. The MCV is calculated by using the hematocrit value and the RBC count (Figure 2-62). It is reported in **femtoliters (fL)**. The MCV was formerly reported in cubic microns. The normal reference range for MCV is given in Table 2-15. An elevated MCV indicates macrocytes; a decreased value indicates microcytes.

### Mean Corpuscular Hemoglobin

The **mean corpuscular hemoglobin (MCH)** estimates the average weight of hemoglobin in an RBC. The unit of weight is the **picogram (pg)**, which is equiva-

lent to $10^{-12}$ gram. The calculation for MCH involves the hemoglobin value in grams/dL and the RBC count (Figure 2-63). The normal reference range is given in Table 2-15. Since the result is obtained without using the hematocrit, it is not useful in classifying anemias.

### Mean Corpuscular Hemoglobin Concentration

The **mean corpuscular hemoglobin concentration (MCHC)** expresses the concentration of hemoglobin in the RBCs in relation to their size and volume. The MCHC is obtained from calculations involving the

**Table 2-15.** Reference ranges for erythrocyte indices

| METHOD | REFERENCE RANGE |
| --- | --- |
| MCV | 80–100 fL |
| MCH | 27–32 pg |
| MCHC | 32–37% |

hemoglobin and the hematocrit (Figure 2-64). The result is expressed in percentage. A value within the reference range (Table 2-15) indicates normochromia while a decreased value indicates hypochromia. Hyperchromia is usually considered not possible, except in spherocytes.

The indices results can be used to classify anemias. However, the results obtained when calculating the indices depend on the accuracy of the RBC count, the hemoglobin, and the hematocrit. Laboratories with automated cell counters rely on the instrument to automatically calculate the indices. There may be certain occasions when the indices must be calculated manually, such as in a smaller laboratory or in research.

## WBC DISORDERS

Diseases or conditions affecting the WBC can be detected from the presence of abnormal WBCs on the peripheral blood smear or from the total WBC count (Table 2-16). A WBC count increased above the normal range is called *leukocytosis*; a decrease below the normal range is called *leukopenia*. The total WBC count and the types of cells present are usually very specific for a particular condition.

### Leukopenia

Leukopenia is usually defined as a reduction below 4 x $10^9$ WBCs/L in peripheral blood. A reduction in all WBC types is called balanced leukopenia; however, in most cases, only one WBC type is involved. *Neutropenia*, a reduced number of neutrophils, may be inherited or may be caused by certain infections, antibiotics, sulfa drugs, and chemotherapy treatments. *Lymphopenia*, a reduced number of lymphocytes, can be caused by exposure to radiation, or by conditions such as lupus erythematosus, cardiac failure, or even stress.

### Leukocytosis

Many factors can cause an increase in circulating WBCs (leukocytosis). A leukemoid reaction is an excessive response of the WBCs in which their count may be 50 x $10^9$/L or higher. It is not leukemic and the reason for the heightened response is not understood.

In leukemias, the increase is almost always an increase in percentage and total number of just one cell line, such as lymphocytes or granulocytes. Bacterial infections, exercise, anxiety, or pain usually cause leukocytosis and neutrophilia. Lymphocytosis occurs in viral infections, particularly infectious mononucleosis ("mono"). See Table 2-16.

**Table 2-16.** Factors affecting WBC percentages

| CONDITION | EFFECT ON WBCS |
| --- | --- |
| Bacterial infections | Increased total WBCs increased percentage of neutrophils |
| Viral infections | Decreased total WBCs increased percentage of lymphocytes |
| Infectious mononucleosis | Increased total WBCs increased lymphs, increased "atypical" (reactive) lymphs |
| Parasitic infections, allergic reactions | Increased eosinophils |
| Leukemias | Total WBCs usually increased, increase in type of leukocyte involved |
| Newborns, children | Increased lymphocytes |

### Neutrophilia

Bacterial infection is the most common cause of neutrophilia. In acute infections, the neutrophilia is accompanied by an increase in immature neutrophils in the peripheral blood. This is called a **shift to the left**, in which immature forms known as bands, metamyelocytes (juveniles), or myelocytes enter the peripheral blood prematurely to help fight the infection (Figure 2-65). The reference values for these in normal adult peripheral blood is one to five bands and zero metamyelocytes and myelocytes (Table 2-17). In mild infections, only the band cells may be elevated; however, in more severe infections, the WBC count and the neutrophil count may increase or more bands and metamyelocytes may appear in the peripheral blood. Vacuoles may be present in the cytoplasm of the neutrophils and indicates a serious infection; toxic granulation in the cytoplasm also indicates infection.

### Lymphocytosis

The total lymphocyte count is normally higher in infants and young children than in adults. In adolescents and adults, an increase may be due to acute viral infection, especially infectious mononucleosis, or lymphocytic leukemia. The prominent cell in infectious mononucleosis is the **reactive lymphocyte**, also called an atypical

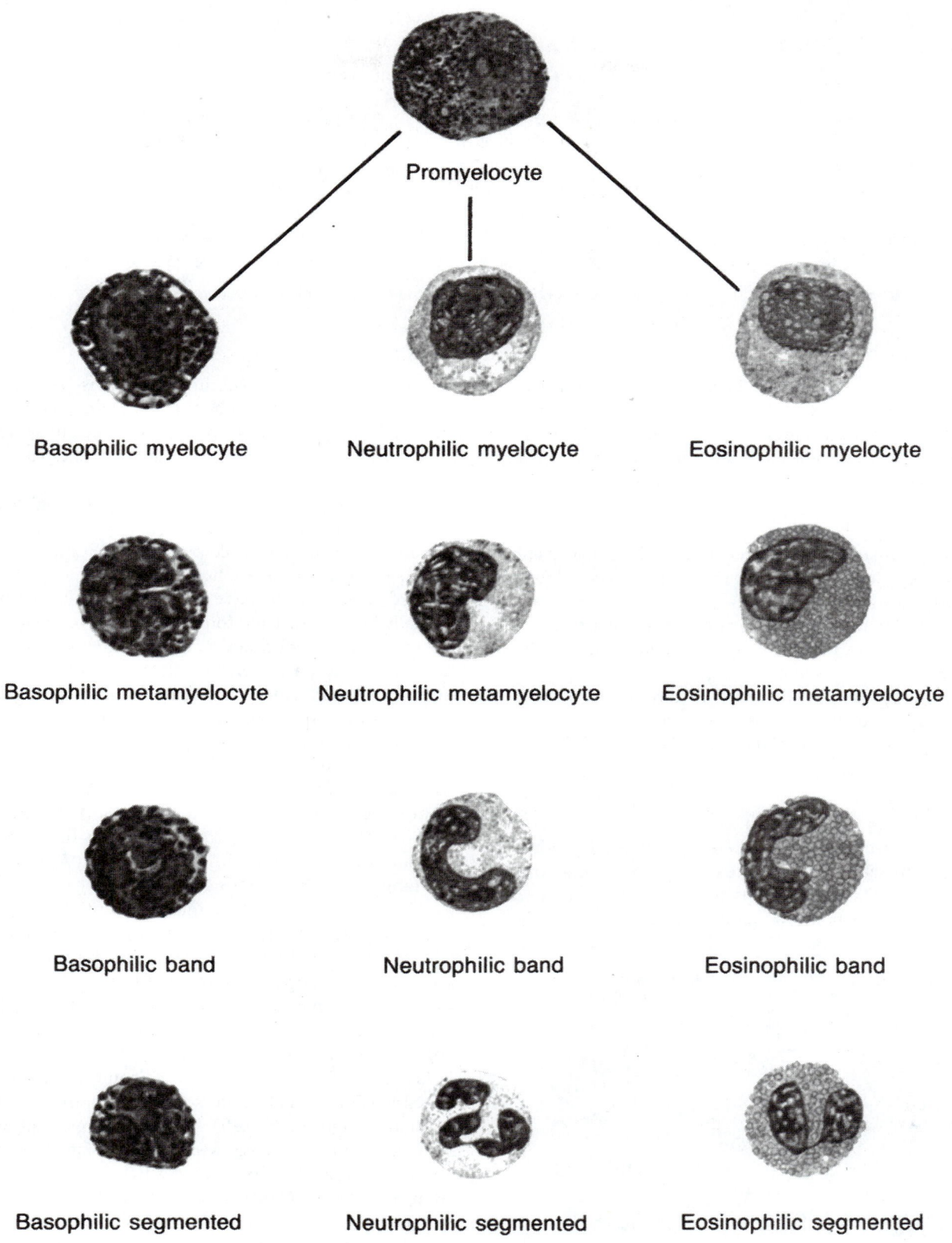

**FIGURE 2-65** Origin and development of the granulocytic (myeloid) blood cells (Courtesy of Abbott Laboratories, Inc.)

| Table 2-17. Reference ranges for the differential count | | | | |
|---|---|---|---|---|
| **TYPE OF CELL** | **REFERENCE VALUES** | | | |
| | **1 month** | **6-year-old** | **12-year-old** | **Adult** |
| Neutrophil (seg) | 15-35% | 45-50% | 45-50% | 50-65% |
| Neutrophil (band) | 7-13% | 0-7% | 6-8% | 0-7% |
| Eosinophil | 1-3% | 1-3% | 1-3% | 1-3% |
| Basophil | 0-1% | 0-1% | 0-1% | 0-1% |
| Monocyte | 5-8% | 4-8% | 3-8% | 3-9% |
| Lymphocyte | 40-70% | 40-45% | 35-40% | 25-40% |
| **Platelets** | An average of 7–20 platelets per oil-immersion field is considered normal | | | |

lymphocyte (Table 2-16 and Figure 2-66). The reactive lymphocyte is characterized by a large amount of sky-blue cytoplasm easily indented by RBCs; the indentations may cause it to assume a "holly leaf" shape. The nucleus is usually large and appears immature.

### Increases in Other WBCs

Eosinophils increase in allergic conditions and parasitic infections. Certain skin diseases may also cause eosinophilia.

Basophilia is a rare occurrence, usually associated with an increase in all the granulocytes, such as in chronic myelogenous leukemia.

Monocytosis, an increase in circulating monocytes, is rare but may occur in tuberculosis, subacute bacterial endocarditis, typhus, and rickettsial infections.

### Leukemias

**Leukemias** are distinguished by unrestrained production and growth of leukocytes in the bone marrow, causing red cells and platelets to be literally "crowded out" by the overwhelming numbers of leukemic WBCs.

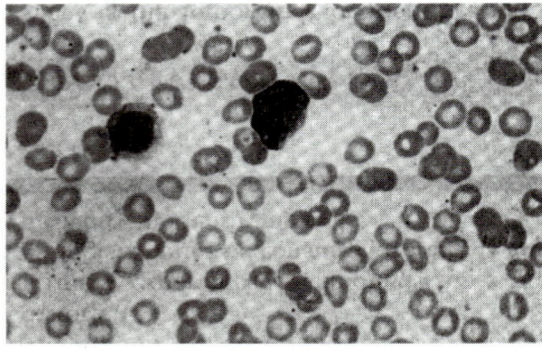

**FIGURE 2-66** Photomicrograph showing two reactive (atypical) lymphocytes.

The patient develops bleeding problems because of decreased platelets and fatigue from the anemia. Leukemias may be classified as chronic or acute. In general, the survival rates are better for chronic leukemias than for acute leukemias.

Diagnosing leukemias is a task for pathologists and hematology specialists. However, many cases are first noticed by a technician while performing a differential or because an automated hematology analyzer has "flagged" a sample to have a peripheral blood smear manually evaluated. Therefore, it is critical for the technician to carefully perform every differential and to closely examine all the characteristics of any cells that appear "different." Sometimes it may be necessary to count 200-500 leukocytes to find more of the abnormal cells.

Acute myelocytic leukemia (AML) and chronic myelocytic leukemia (CML) are two forms that affect the granulocytes. In AML, the predominant leukocyte on the peripheral blood smear is the **blast cell**, the earliest precursor (Figure 2-67, right). In CML, less than 10% of the leukocytes are "blasts," but the total WBC count may range from 50 to 300 x $10^9$/L.

Two lymphocytic leukemias are acute lymphocytic leukemia (ALL) and chronic lymphocytic leukemia (CLL). In ALL, the leukocyte count may be three times normal, with a large number of "blasts." The disease occurs predominantly in children and responds well to treatment, with more than 80% surviving five years or longer. When the disease occurs in adults, the prognosis is poorer than for children. Chronic lymphocytic leukemia (CLL) usually occurs in later life, from middle to old age (Figure 2-67, left). The onset is gradual, with the major symptoms being weakness and fatigue due to the anemia that develops. The WBC count is usually about 50 x $10^9$/L. The patient may live up to 20 years after diagnosis.

Other rarer conditions also involve uncontrolled growth of one or more types of bone marrow or blood cells. Approximately 10–15% of all leukemias are either

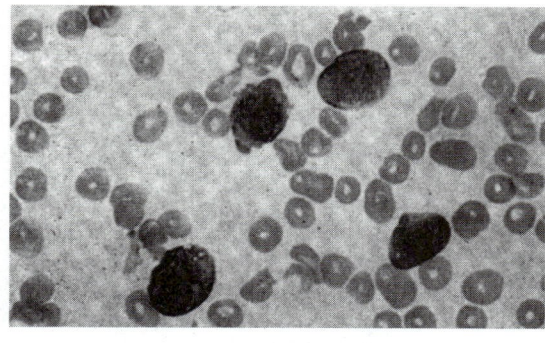

(A)

(B)

**FIGURE 2-67**   Photomicrographs of stained blood cells: (A) chronic lymphocytic leukemia; (B) acute myelocytic leukemia (Photos courtesy of Marshall, *Fundamental Skills for the Clinical Laboratory Professional*, Delmar Publishers, Inc.)

acute or chronic monocytic, which usually occurs after middle age. In a few leukemias, the predominant cell is the primitive stem cell. This disease usually occurs only in children. Plasma cell leukemia, hairy cell leukemia, and erythroleukemia also affect the WBCs. In erythroleukemia, early forms of erythrocytes appear first and then myeloblasts; the final stage is conversion to myeloblastic leukemia.

## PLATELET DISORDERS

Platelets may be abnormal in number or in function. In *thrombocytopenia*, platelet numbers fall below the normal reference range. Many factors can cause decreased platelets including radiation exposure, certain drugs, chronic alcoholism, platelet destruction by the spleen, and the effect of diseases like leukemia on bone marrow.

Elevation of platelet numbers above the normal reference range is called *thrombocytosis*. Some causes of thrombocytosis include a reaction to inflammatory conditions, a secondary reaction to other blood disorders, and removal of the spleen (Table 2-18 and Color Plate 12). Thrombasthenia is a condition in which normal numbers of platelets are produced, but do not function normally.

**Table 2-18.** Conditions that may cause thrombocytopenia or thrombocytosis

**Thrombocytopenia**
Bone marrow damage
Sequestration by enlarged spleen
Disseminated intravascular coagulation (DIC)
Chronic alcoholism
Idiopathic thrombocytopenic purpura (ITP)

**Thrombocytosis**
Polycythemia vera
Bleeding disorders
Hemolytic anemias
Inflammatory reactions
Chronic granulocytic leukemia

ential. A more experienced and knowledgeable technician or the lab director must be consulted before certain types of abnormal cells are reported. (This depends on the particular healthcare facility's policy.)

## SUMMARY

The technician must remember that any smear being examined may contain abnormal blood cells even though the patient seems in good health. The peripheral blood smear must be properly prepared and stained to obtain an accurate picture of the blood. The technician must be very familiar with normal and abnormal blood cell morphology to accurately identify and evaluate the morphology of cells observed during the differ-

## LESSON REVIEW

1. Why is it important to recognize an abnormal blood cell?
2. List three conditions in which abnormal RBC morphology may be found.
3. Why is it important to report RBC inclusions?
4. How can erythrocyte indices be used to classify anemias?
5. List three conditions in which abnormal leukocyte morphology may be found.

6. What is leukemia?

7. Discuss the differences between acute and chronic leukemias.

8. Why do leukemia patients develop anemia?

9. List one cause of thrombocytosis and one cause of thrombocytopenia.

10. Define basophilic stippling, blast cell, femtoliter, folic acid, Howell-Jolly bodies, indices, leukemia, mean corpuscular hemoglobin, mean corpuscular hemoglobin concentration, mean corpuscular volume, picogram, reactive lymphocyte, shift to the left, thalassemia, and vitamin $B_{12}$.

## STUDENT ACTIVITIES

1. Reread the information on morphology of abnormal blood cells in peripheral blood.

2. Review the glossary terms.

3. Prepare a short report on current treatments for leukemia.

4. Practice calculating the erythrocyte indices, using the worksheet.

5. Practice recognizing and identifying abnormal blood cells as outlined on the Student Performance Guide.

# *Student Performance Guide*

## **LESSON 2-10** Morphology of Abnormal Blood Cells in Peripheral Blood

Name _____   Date _____

## INSTRUCTIONS

1. Practice calculating the erythrocyte indices, identifying abnormal blood cells, and using the worksheet.
2. Demonstrate your understanding of this lesson by:
   a. Completing a written examination successfully, and
   b. Recognizing and identifying abnormal blood cells on peripheral smears or other visual learning aids. All steps must be completed as listed on the instructor's Performance Check Sheet.

## MATERIALS AND EQUIPMENT

- gloves
- hand disinfectant
- worksheet for erythrocyte indices
- microscope with oil-immersion objective
- microscope immersion oil
- microscope slides of various blood disorders: iron deficiency anemia, $B_{12}$ or folate deficiency, infectious mononucleosis, leukocytosis, more common leukemias, and sickle cell disease are especially recommended
- blood cell atlas

## PROCEDURE

Record in the comment section any problems encountered while practicing the procedure or have a fellow student or the instructor evaluate your performance.

S = Satisfactory
U = Unsatisfactory

| You must: | S | U | Comments |
|---|---|---|---|
| 1. Wash hands and put on gloves | | | |
| 2. Assemble appropriate equipment and materials to view blood smears using the microscope. | | | |
| 3. Observe the slide or visual aid of iron deficiency anemia. Look in several oil-immersion fields and identify microcytic RBCs | | | |
| 4. Observe the slide or visual aid of $B_{12}$ or folate deficiency:<br>a. Look in several oil-immersion fields and locate macrocytic RBCs<br>b. Observe the WBCs and identify any that are larger than normal | | | |
| 5. Observe the slide or visual aid of infectious mononucleosis or other viral infection:<br>a. Scan the differential counting area of the smear. Observe the WBCs for an increase in total number of lymphocytes | | | |

| You must: | S | U | Comments |
|---|---|---|---|
| b. Locate several reactive lymphocytes and note the characteristics of the cytoplasm and the nucleus | | | |
| 6. Observe the slide or visual aid of sickle cell disease:<br>a. Identify any sickled RBCs present<br>b. Identify microcytic RBCs<br>c. Look in several fields; identify codocytes | | | |
| 7. Observe the leukemia slide:<br>a. Locate and identify the predominant WBC type present<br>b. Observe the RBC morphology<br>c. Observe the platelets for an increase or decrease in number | | | |
| 8. Wipe the immersion oil from the slides and replace them in their storage containers or return visual aids to storage | | | |
| 9. Clean the microscope objectives and return the microscope to proper storage | | | |
| 10. Remove and dispose of gloves in biohazard container | | | |
| 11. Wash hands with hand disinfectant | | | |

*Evaluator Comments:*

Evaluator _____ Date _____

# Reticulocyte Count

**After studying this lesson, you should be able to:**

- *Explain the purpose of performing a reticulocyte count.*
- *Prepare a reticulocyte smear.*
- *Perform a reticulocyte count.*
- *Calculate a reticulocyte percentage.*
- *Name two dyes that may be used in the reticulocyte procedure.*
- *Name two conditions in which the reticulocyte count would be low.*
- *Name two conditions in which the reticulocyte count would be elevated.*
- *List the normal reticulocyte count for an adult and a newborn.*
- *Define the glossary terms.*

## GLOSSARY

**reticulocyte** / an immature erythrocyte that has retained RNA in the cytoplasm

**reticulocytopenia** / a decrease below the normal number of reticulocytes

**reticulocytosis** / an increase above the normal number of reticulocytes in the circulating blood

**reticulum** / a network

**RNA** / a nucleic acid found in all living cells and that is important in protein synthesis; ribonucleic acid

**supravital stain** / a dye that stains living cells or tissues

## INTRODUCTION

The reticulocyte count is a method of estimating the number of immature RBCs in the circulating blood; therefore, it is an indirect method of estimating the rate of RBC production. The test is most commonly used to determine the cause of a low RBC count, or anemia. It is also used to monitor the course of treatment for anemia.

## PRINCIPLE OF THE RETICULOCYTE COUNT

RBCs are produced in the bone marrow. After a maturation process, RBCs enter the blood circulation. For the first twenty-four hours in the circulation, they are still slightly immature and can be identified by the presence of **RNA** (ribonucleic acid) in the cell cytoplasm. When an immature RBC is exposed to certain stains, the RNA forms stained granular aggregates or filaments called a **reticulum** (Figure 2-68). For this reason, these immature RBCs are called **reticulocytes**.

The staining technique is called **supravital** staining, a procedure in which the cells are stained while still living. Two common dyes used for supravital stains are: New Methylene Blue and Brilliant Cresyl Blue. Reticulocytes appear as blue-tinged RBCs with dark bluish-purple granules or filaments. Mature RBCs appear uniformly bluish-green (see Color Plate 11).

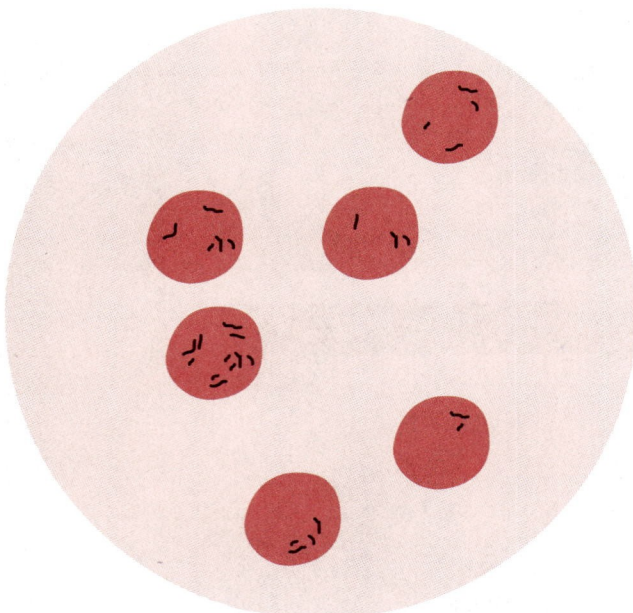

**FIGURE 2-68** Reticulocytes stained with New Methylene Blue and showing stained reticulum

## REFERENCE VALUES FOR RETICULOCYTE COUNTS

Normal reticulocyte count varies with age (Table 2-19). Newborn infants have high counts that decrease to adult levels by two weeks of age. In a healthy adult, approximately 1% of the RBCs will stain as reticulocytes when a supravital stain is applied to a blood sample. Reticulocyte counts above 3% in an adult indicate that RBCs are being produced at an increased rate. **Reticulocytosis**, an increased number of reticulocytes, may be a response to acute blood loss from hemorrhage, chronic blood loss such as from a bleeding ulcer, or anemia treatment.

Reticulocyte values below 0.5% indicate a decreased rate of RBC production. A decrease in reticulocytes, **reticulocytopenia**, may be seen in iron deficiency anemia, vitamin $B_{12}$ or folic acid deficiencies, or aplastic anemia.

| TABLE 2-19 Reference values for reticulocyte counts | | |
|---|---|---|
| | REFERENCE VALUE | UPPER LIMIT OF NORMAL |
| Adults | 0.5–1.5% | 3% |
| Newborns | 2.5–6.5% | 10% |

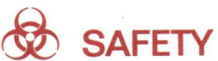 **SAFETY**

Standard and Universal Precautions must be observed to protect the worker from exposure to bloodborne pathogens when performing the reticulocyte count. Appropriate PPE must be worn while obtaining the blood sample, staining the cells, and making the smears.

### Quality Assurance

Recently collected blood must be used for the reticulocyte count, since the immature RBCs will continue to mature as the blood stands. If this occurs, the reticulocyte count may be falsely decreased.

When performing the reticulocyte count, the technician must be careful not to confuse artifacts and debris as reticulum. Filtering the stain frequently will keep debris and precipitate to a minimum. Fine reticulum that is faintly stained may be overlooked if the smears are not thoroughly examined. To avoid counting the same cells twice, a definite counting pattern must be used.

Reticulocyte control solutions are available for manual or automated counts. One control is Retic-Chex™ from Streck Laboratories, Inc., which is manufactured from human RBCs and serves as a positive control to meet federal and state regulations. Streck also markets Retic-Chex™ stain, a buffered and filtered New Methylene Blue stain that produces more even distribution of RBCs.

## PERFORMING THE RETICULOCYTE COUNT

The reticulocyte count may be performed manually using either capillary or venous blood. A few drops of blood are mixed with equal parts of New Methylene Blue stain in a small test tube and the mixture is allowed to stand for 15 minutes. The blood-stain mixture is then used to prepare blood smears.

After the blood smears air-dry, they are examined microscopically using the oil-immersion objective. A total of 1,000 RBCs are counted (500 per slide) and the number of reticulocytes seen per 1,000 RBCs is record-ed. (A reticulocyte is also counted as an RBC.) The percentage of reticulocytes is then calculated.

## Calculating the Reticulocyte Percentage

A reticulocyte count is reported as the percentage of RBCs that are reticulocytes. This count is only an estimate. The percentage of reticulocytes is calculated using the formula:

$$\frac{\text{\# Reticulocytes counted}}{\text{\# Erythrocytes counted}} \times 100 = \% \text{ Reticulocytes}$$

*or*

$$\frac{\text{\# Reticulocytes}}{1000} \times 100 = \% \text{ Reticulocytes}$$

*or*

$$\frac{\text{\# Reticulocytes}}{10} = \% \text{ Reticulocyte}$$

A sample calculation is shown in Figure 2-69.

## Correcting the Reticulocyte Count for Anemia

In order for the reticulocyte count to give valuable information about RBC production, it should be correlated with the RBC count or the hematocrit. For example, the normal reticulocyte count is approximately 1%. An individual with a RBC count of $5 \times 10^6$ RBC/µL and a reticu-locyte count of 1% would have approximately 50,000 reticulocytes/µL of blood. However, another individual with a 1% count and $3 \times 10^6$ RBC/µL would have only 30,000 reticulocytes per µL. Although the reticulocyte percentages are the same in the two individuals, the total numbers of reticulocytes are not. For this reason, reticulocyte counts are often corrected for anemia to give the physician a more accurate reflection of the status of RBC production in the patient.

### Absolute Reticulocyte Count

The absolute reticulocyte count is a calculation that corrects the observed reticulocyte count for anemia. It is obtained by multiplying the RBC count by the reticulocyte percentage. For example, if a patient has a reticulocyte count of 2% and an RBC count of $4 \times 10^6$ RBC/µL, the absolute reticulocyte count would be calculated as follows:

$$
\begin{aligned}
\text{Absolute} \\
\text{reticulocyte count} &= \text{RBC count} \times \% \text{ Reticulocytes} \\
&= 4 \times 10^6/\mu L \times 2\% \\
&= 8 \times 10^4/\mu L \text{ or} \\
&= 80,000 \text{ reticulocytes}/\mu L
\end{aligned}
$$

### Corrected Reticulocyte Count

Another way of correcting the reticulocyte percentage for anemia is to calculate the corrected reticulocyte count. This is done by multiplying the reticulocyte count (in %) times the hematocrit divided by 45 (the normal hematocrit). For example, a patient has a reticulocyte count of 3% and an hematocrit of 35%. The corrected reticulocyte count would be calculated as follows:

$$
\begin{aligned}
\text{Corrected retic count} &= \text{Retic count (\%)} \times \frac{\text{Hct}}{45} \\
&= 3\% \times \frac{35}{45} \\
&= 2.3\%
\end{aligned}
$$

## Automated Counts

Instrumentation makes it possible to count reticulocytes with more precision than provided by manual counts. Most instruments that perform reticulocyte counts use the principle of flow cytometry (see Lesson 2-13 for detailed discussion). These instruments make use of RNA-specific stains to identify reticulocytes in a blood sample as it flows through a special electronic counting chamber. In automated methods, large numbers of cells are counted, which should result in increased accuracy.

I. Count the reticulocytes using two smears:

|  | | Erythrocytes counted | Reticulocytes seen |
|---|---|---|---|
| Smear 1 | | 500 | 7 |
| Smear 2 | | 500 | 5 |
| | Total | 1000 | 12 |

II. Calculate the percentage of reticulocytes:

$$\% \text{ Retics} = \frac{\text{\# Reticulocytes counted}}{\text{\# RBC counted}} \times 100$$

$$\% \text{ Retics} = \frac{12}{1000} \times 100$$

$$\% \text{ Retics} = \frac{12}{10}$$

$$\% \text{ Retics} = 1.2$$

**FIGURE 2-69** Sample calculation of reticulocyte percentage

### Procedural Notes

- Examine cells carefully so reticulum is not overlooked.
- Do not confuse artifacts with reticulum.
- Use a definite counting pattern to ensure cells are not counted twice.
- Perform the reticulocyte count within four hours of blood collection.
- Filter stain to prevent precipitate from forming on smear.

### Safety Precautions

- Observe Universal and Standard Precautions when performing the reticulocyte count.
- Wear gloves, protective face wear, and a buttoned, fluid-resistant laboratory coat.

## LESSON REVIEW

1. What is a reticulocyte?
2. Why would a reticulocyte count be performed?
3. What is the normal reticulocyte count for adults; for newborns?
4. What are two dyes used to stain reticulocytes?
5. What conditions can cause a high reticulocyte count?
6. Why must Standard Precautions be observed during the reticulocyte count?
7. What conditions can cause a low reticulocyte count?
8. State the formula for calculating a reticulocyte count.
9. Calculate the absolute reticulocyte count and the corrected reticulocyte count from the following values: Hct = 32%; RBC = 3.8 x 10⁶/µL; Retic count = 3%
10. Define reticulocyte, reticulocytopenia, reticulocytosis, reticulum, RNA, and supravital stain.

## STUDENT ACTIVITIES

1. Reread the information on reticulocyte counts.
2. Review the glossary terms.
3. Practice performing reticulocyte counts and calculating reticulocyte percentages as outlined on the Student Performance Guide.

## *Student Performance Guide*

## **LESSON 2-11** Reticulocyte Count

Name _____  Date _____

  ### INSTRUCTIONS

1. Practice the procedure for performing a reticulocyte count following the step-by-step procedure.
2. Demonstrate your understanding of this lesson by:
   a. Completing a written examination successfully, and
   b. Performing the procedure for the reticulocyte count satisfactorily for the instructor. All steps must be completed as listed on the instructor's Performance Check Sheet.

## MATERIALS AND EQUIPMENT

- gloves
- hand disinfectant
- microscope
- microscope slides
- lens paper
- acrylic safety shield
- immersion oil
- Pasteur pipet with bulb
- New Methylene Blue stain, freshly filtered (or commercial kit such as Retic-Set® by Fisher Scientific)
- 70% alcohol or alcohol swabs
- sterile cotton or gauze
- sterile lancet
- capillary tubes, heparinized and plain
- test tube 10 x 75 mm
- tally counter
- surface disinfectant (10% chlorine bleach solution)
- biohazard container
- puncture-proof container for sharp objects
- commercially available stained reticulocyte slides (optional)
- reticulocyte count worksheet

***Optional:***
- freshly collected EDTA blood specimen
- materials for RBC count and microhematocrit
- reticulocyte controls

## PROCEDURE

Record in the comment section any problems encountered while practicing the procedure (or have a fellow student or the instructor evaluate your performance).

S = Satisfactory
U = Unsatisfactory

| You must: | S | U | Comments |
|---|---|---|---|
| 1. Wash hands and put on gloves | | | |
| 2. Assemble equipment and materials. Set up acrylic safety shield | | | |
| 3. Perform a capillary puncture and wipe away the first drop of blood with dry sterile cotton or gauze (or use freshly collected, well-mixed venous anticoagulated blood to perform the test) | | | |
| 4. Fill one or two heparinized capillary tubes with blood (use plain capillary tubes if using anticoagulated blood) | | | |

| You must: | S | U | Comments |
|---|---|---|---|
| 5. Dispense two to three drops of blood into the bottom of a small test tube | | | |
| 6. a. Add an equal amount of New Methylene Blue stain to the test tube and mix<br>b. Allow mixture to stand for 15 minutes at room temperature<br>c. Remix contents of test tube and fill a plain capillary tube with the blood-stain mixture<br>d. Follow manufacturer's guidelines if using a kit such as Retic-Set® | | | |
| 7. Prepare two blood smears from the blood-stain mixture and allow to air-dry | | | |
| 8. Place one slide on the microscope stage and secure it | | | |
| 9. Use the low-power (10X) objective to find a good area of the smear | | | |
| 10. Place one drop of immersion-oil on the slide and carefully rotate oil-immersion objective into position | | | |
| 11. Count all erythrocytes in one oil-immersion field and record the number of reticulocytes in the field. ***Note:*** A reticulocyte is also counted as a red blood cell | | | |
| 12. Move the slide to an adjacent microscopic field | | | |
| 13. Count all erythrocytes in the (adjacent) field and record the number of reticulocytes in the field | | | |
| 14. Continue steps 12–13 until 500 erythrocytes have been counted. Record count on worksheet | | | |
| 15. Repeat steps 8–14 using the second slide | | | |
| 16. Calculate the reticulocyte percentage using the worksheet:<br>$$\frac{\text{\# of retics counted}}{1000 \text{ RBCs}} \times 100 = \% \text{ reticulocytes}$$ | | | |
| 17. Record the results on the worksheet | | | |
| 18. Clean oil-immersion objective carefully and thoroughly with lens paper | | | |
| 19. Clean any oil from microscope stage with laboratory tissue | | | |
| 20. Optional: If specimen for reticulocyte count is from a tube of anticoagulated blood, perform an RBC count and microhematocrit from the same specimen. Record results on worksheet (if anticoagulated specimen is not available, go to step 21)<br>a. Calculate the absolute reticulocyte count using the worksheet | | | |

| You must: | S | U | Comments |
|---|---|---|---|
| b. Calculate the corrected reticulocyte count using the work sheet | | | |
| 21. Return equipment to proper storage | | | |
| 22. Store or discard slides as instructed | | | |
| 23. Clean work area with surface disinfectant | | | |
| 24. Remove and discard gloves in biohazard container | | | |
| 25. Wash hands with hand disinfectant | | | |

*Evaluator Comments:*

Evaluator _____ Date _____

## *Worksheet*

## **LESSON 2-11** Reticulocyte Count

Name _____ Date _____

Specimen I.D. _____

I. Perform the reticulocyte count and record the results

A.                  RBCs counted         Retics counted

     Slide 1          _____     _____

     Slide 2          _____     _____

     **Total**           _____     _____

B. Write the formula for the reticulocyte count:

C. Calculate the reticulocyte count:

_____ = % reticulocytes

II. Optional: If available, perform RBC count and hematocrit on the same blood specimen used for the reticulocyte count and record the results.

A. RBC/µL = _____ Hct (%) = _____

B. Calculate the absolute reticulocyte count:
     1. Write the formula for the absolute reticulocyte count:
     2. Calculate the absolute reticulocyte count:

       The absolute retic count is _____.

C. Calculate the corrected reticulocyte count:
     1. Write the formula for the corrected reticulocyte count:
     2. Calculate the corrected reticulocyte count:

       The corrected retic count is _____.

# Erythrocyte Sedimentation Rate

## LESSON OBJECTIVES

**After studying this lesson, you should be able to:**

■ *Explain the purpose of performing an erythrocyte sedimentation rate.*

■ *List four properties of blood that affect the erythrocyte sedimentation rate and explain how the rate is affected by each.*

■ *List five technical factors that may affect the erythrocyte sedimentation rate and explain how the rate is affected by each.*

■ *Discuss the relationship of the erythrocyte sedimentation rate to disease.*

■ *List five pathological conditions in which the erythrocyte sedimentation rate would be increased or decreased.*

■ *State the reference values for the erythrocyte sedimentation rate test.*

■ *Perform an erythrocyte sedimentation rate.*

■ *Define the glossary terms.*

## GLOSSARY

**acute phase proteins** / proteins that increase rapidly in serum during acute infection, inflammation, or following tissue injury

**aggregate** / the total substances making up a mass; a cluster or clump of particles

**inflammation** / tissue reaction to injury

**polycythemia** / an excess of RBCs in the peripheral blood

**rouleau(x)** / group(s) of RBCs arranged like a roll of coins

**sedimentation** / the process of solid particles settling to the bottom of a liquid

**Westergren tube** / a slender pipet marked from 0–200 mm, used in the Westergren erythrocyte sedimentation rate method

**Wintrobe tube** / a slender thick-walled tube marked from 0–100 mm, used in the Wintrobe method of macrohematocrit and Wintrobe erythrocyte sedimentation rate

# INTRODUCTION

The erythrocyte sedimentation rate (ESR) is a simple, frequently performed hematology test, often referred to as the "sed rate." The ESR test is not specific for a particular disease but is used as an indicator of **inflammation**, or tissue injury. The sedimentation rate results may also be used to evaluate treatment and follow the course of certain inflammatory diseases.

# PRINCIPLE OF THE ESR TEST

The ESR test is based on the principle of **sedimentation**, the process of solid particles settling to the bottom of a liquid. In a sample of anticoagulated blood that is left undisturbed, the erythrocytes will gradually separate from the plasma and settle to the bottom of the container. The rate at which the erythrocytes settle or fall under controlled laboratory conditions is known as the erythrocyte sedimentation rate.

To perform the manual ESR test, a sample of anticoagulated blood is placed in a calibrated tube of standard dimensions, and incubated in a vertical position for exactly one hour. At the end of the hour, the distance the erythrocytes have fallen from the plasma meniscus (at the zero mark) is measured in millimeters (mm) and reported (Figure 2-70). This is the erythrocyte sedimentation rate.

In blood samples from most healthy persons, erythrocyte sedimentation occurs slowly. In many diseases, particularly inflammatory diseases, the rate of sedimentation is rapid. In some cases, the rate is proportional to the severity of the disease.

# FACTORS AFFECTING THE ESR

Factors that affect the rate of erythrocyte sedimentation in a blood sample are: (1) properties of the plasma, (2) properties of the erythrocytes, and (3) technical factors.

## Properties of Blood Affecting the ESR

The rate of erythrocyte sedimentation is affected by the plasma proteins in the blood sample tested and by the size, shape, and number of erythrocytes.

### Plasma Proteins

The erythrocyte sedimentation rate is proportional to the RBC mass. In normal blood, erythrocytes suspended in the plasma form few, if any, **aggregates** or clusters. Therefore, the mass of the falling (settling) erythrocytes is small and the rate of sedimentation is slow. In abnormal blood, the erythrocytes sometimes form aggregates called **rouleaux**. This phenomenon is called rouleaux because the aggregates look like rolls or stacks of coins (Figure 2-71 and Color Plate 17). This causes an increase in effective mass and an increased rate of sedimentation. (Clumps or clusters of cells are heavier than single cells and will settle faster.)

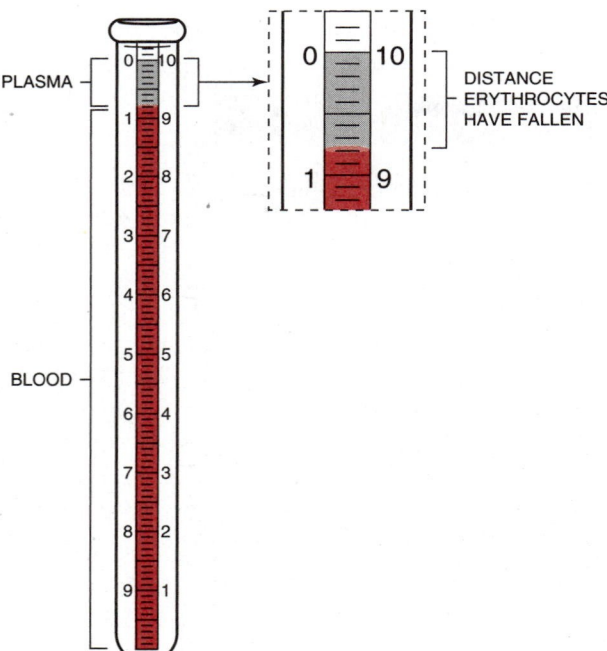

**FIGURE 2-70** Wintrobe tube showing sedimentation of cells. Example shown illustrates a sedimentation of 8 mm

PLASMA

BLOOD

0 10
1 9

DISTANCE ERYTHROCYTES HAVE FALLEN

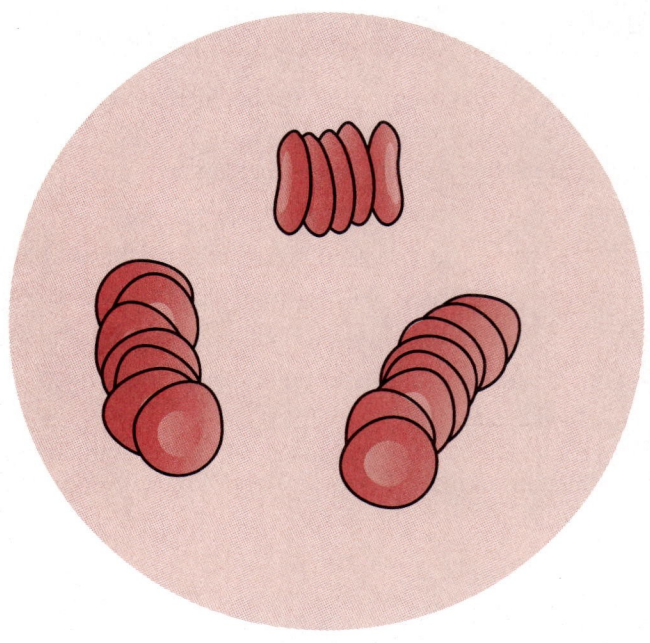

**FIGURE 2-71** Erythrocytes forming rouleaux

The amount and type of plasma proteins present in a blood sample affect the ESR by influencing rouleau formation. Increased levels of proteins such as fibrinogen, **acute phase proteins**, or other plasma globulins enhance the tendency of RBCs to form rouleaux and therefore increase the sedimentation rate.

### Size of Erythrocytes

Macrocytic cells sediment more rapidly than microcytic cells because of their large size (increased mass).

### Shape of Erythrocytes

Changes in the shape of the erythrocytes can also affect the ESR. For example, in sickle cell anemia the irregularly shaped erythrocytes cannot aggregate and the ESR may be low (or zero). Spherocytic cells also sediment at a slow rate.

### Number of Erythrocytes

The ESR is affected by the RBC count. The sedimentation rate may be rapid in some anemias because there are fewer erythrocytes in the sample. Therefore, the hematocrit or RBC count should be checked on samples that have elevated ESRs to determine if the elevated rate is due to inflammation or to anemia. When the erythrocyte number is increased, as in **polycythemia**, the erythrocytes settle slowly and the ESR is low.

## Technical Factors Affecting the ESR

Technical factors such as temperature, timing, tube size, pipetting technique, sample mixing, and tube tilting or vibration during incubation will affect the sedimentation rate and can be a source of error in the test (Table 2-20). The precautions listed below must be followed to perform the test correctly.

- The sedimentation tube must be kept exactly vertical during the test; even minor degrees of tilting may greatly increase the ESR.

- The test should be set up on a counter free from vibration. Vibrations, such as those occurring on a counter where a centrifuge is running, will cause a falsely increased ESR.

- The temperature in the testing area should be kept constant (20–25°C) while the test is being performed. Low temperatures cause erythrocytes to settle more slowly.

- The ESR test should be set up within two hours after the blood sample is collected. However, blood collected in EDTA may be stored at 4°C for up to six hours for most ESR methods, but must be brought to room temperature before the test is set up.

- The length and diameter of the sedimentation tube affect the rate of sedimentation. Therefore, standardized tubes must be used in the test.

- Anticoagulated blood samples must be mixed properly immediately before setting up the ESR test.

- Careful pipetting technique should be used when diluting blood samples and filling the sedimentation tube. Air bubbles in the tube will interfere with test accuracy.

- The test must be timed accurately. The ESR increases with time.

## REFERENCE VALUES FOR THE ESR

Each ESR method has its own set of reference values. It is necessary to follow specific instructions for the method used and to compare results with the appropriate reference values for the method.

Reference values for the Sediplast® ESR (Modified Westergren), Wintrobe ESR, and Zeta Sedimentation Ratio (ZSR) are given in Table 2-21. Sediplast® and Wintrobe results are reported in mm/hr. The reference values for the Wintrobe method are lower than for the Sediplast®, because blood is not diluted in the Wintrobe method.

The ZSR is calculated from the hematocrit and zetacrit, and is reported as a percentage. Since the ZSR value is corrected for RBC volume, the reference value is the same for males and females of all ages.

## RELATIONSHIP OF ESR TO DISEASE

The ESR is a nonspecific test. The ESR is elevated in several inflammatory conditions such as rheumatic fever, rheumatoid arthritis, and lupus erythematosus because these conditions are accompanied by changes in plasma proteins. Other conditions in which the ESR may be

**Table 2-20.** Technical errors that may cause a false increase or decrease in the ESR

| FALSE INCREASED RATE | FALSE DECREASED RATE |
| --- | --- |
| Tube tilted (not vertical) | Low temperature of blood |
| Vibration of tube during test | Air bubbles in tube |
| Test > one hour | Test < one hour |
| Improper blood dilution | Improper blood dilution |
| Improper mixing of blood | Improper mixing of blood |
| Room temp >25°C | Room temp <20°C |

**Table 2-21.** One-hour reference values for Sediplast® ESR (Modified Westergren) and Wintrobe ESR methods and reference ranges for ZSR

| | | SEDIPLAST® ESR (MM) | WINTROBE ESR (MM) | ZSR PERCENTAGE (ALL AGES) |
|---|---|---|---|---|
| Males: | < 50 years | 0–15 | 0–9 | 40–51 normal |
| | > 50 years | 0–20 | | 51–54 borderline |
| | | | | ≥ 55 elevated |
| Females: | < 50 years | 0–20 | 0–20 | |
| | > 50 years | 0–30 | | |
| Children: | | | 0–13 | |

increased include tuberculosis, acute and chronic infections, acute viral hepatitis, Hodgkin's disease, cancer, and multiple myeloma (Table 2-22). Pregnant females may have an increased ESR, usually due to increased plasma fibrinogen levels or a decreased erythrocyte count. Anemia may cause an increased ESR in the absence of inflammation. In polycythemia and sickle cell anemia, the ESR is low or sometimes zero.

Because the ESR test is nonspecific, it is not used as the basis for diagnosing disease, but is often used to follow the course of treatment of inflammatory diseases or to detect inflammation when WBC counts may not be elevated. For example, elderly patients may have normal WBC counts in the presence of acute infection.

Commercial control solutions for the ESR test are available from several suppliers. Polymedco markets two whole blood controls for ESR, SED-CHEX™ for manual methods and SED-CHEK2™ for automated systems and systems that use sodium citrate diluent. Streck Laboratories, Inc. manufactures ESR-Chex™, which can be used in either manual or automated methods. The regular use of controls ensures the ESR values reported by the laboratory are accurate.

 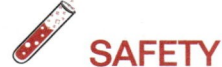 **SAFETY**

Performing the ESR involves working with a tube of whole blood; the technician may also perform the venipuncture to obtain the sample. Universal and Standard Precautions must always be observed to protect the worker from bloodborne pathogens. Appropriate personal protective equipment and engineering controls should be used. In addition, all sharps must be handled properly and disposed of in sharps containers.

*Quality Assurance*

The ESR is affected by environmental and technical factors and properties of the sample. Quality assurance procedures must include guidelines to check for these effects.

**Table 2-22.** Conditions in which the ESR may be increased or decreased

| INCREASED SEDIMENTATION RATE | DECREASED SEDIMENTATION RATE |
|---|---|
| Pregnancy | Presence of sickle cells |
| Anemia | Polycythemia |
| Macrocytosis | Spherocytosis |
| Inflammatory diseases | Increased plasma viscosity |
| Cancer | Microcytosis |
| Acute and chronic infections | |
| Multiple myeloma | |
| Increased plasma fibrinogen | |
| Increased plasma globulins | |

# METHODS OF PERFORMING THE ESR

There are several methods of measuring the ESR, each with advantages, disadvantages, and different levels of sensitivity. Each method has its own set of reference values because the methods differ in technique and the equipment used (see Table 2-21).

## Manual Methods

Two manual methods described in this lesson are the Wintrobe and the Westergren (Modified).

### Wintrobe Method

The Wintrobe ESR method is performed using a **Wintrobe tube** graduated from 0–100 mm (0–10 cm) and with a capacity of 1 mL of blood (Figure 2-70). The use of disposable Wintrobe tubes is recommended because of the biohazard involved in disinfecting and cleaning reusable tubes. A special rack, which holds the tube vertical, is also required (Figure 2-72).

The Wintrobe tube is placed in the sedimentation rack and is filled to the 0 mark with 1 mL of well-mixed anticoagulated blood using a long-stemmed pipet (Figure 2-72). At the end of one hour, the distance the erythrocytes have fallen in the blood sample is measured using the markings on the tube. The distance is recorded in mm (Figure 2-70).

The advantages of the Wintrobe method are its simplicity and the lack of expensive equipment. However, this method is not as sensitive as the Westergren ESR method.

### Westergren Method

The Westergren ESR method is performed using a **Westergren tube** (or pipet) graduated from 0–200 mm and a Westergren rack for holding the tubes. The Westergren test is more sensitive and complex than the Wintrobe method, requiring predilution of the blood with sodium citrate or saline before the pipet is filled. The test has been modified in recent years and most laboratories now perform the Modified Westergren method.

Modified Westergren kits are available that have closed systems with self-filling disposable tubes and premeasured diluent (Figure 2-73). These kits eliminate the biohazard risks present in the original Westergren method and also provide accurate filling of the tube. The use of one of these kits, the Sediplast® ESR System (Figure 2-73), is detailed in the Student Performance Guide at the end of this lesson and in Figure 2-74.

In the Sediplast® ESR System, anticoagulated blood is mixed with premeasured diluent in the sedivial. After mixing, the Westergren tube is inserted into the vial with a twisting motion until the tube reaches the bottom of the vial. The blood column will automatically zero itself and any extra blood will overflow into the sealed reservoir. The vial containing the tube is placed in the sedimentation rack for exactly one hour. At the end of the hour, the distance the erythrocytes have fallen is measured using the markings on the tube and is reported in millimeters per hour.

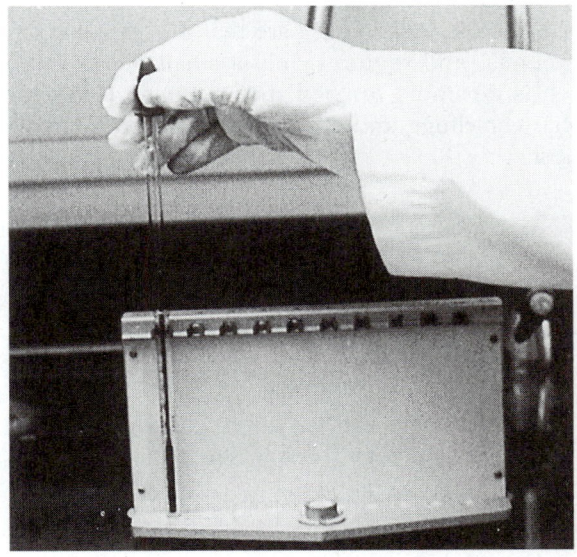

**FIGURE 2-72** Wintrobe ESR method (Photo courtesy of John Estridge)

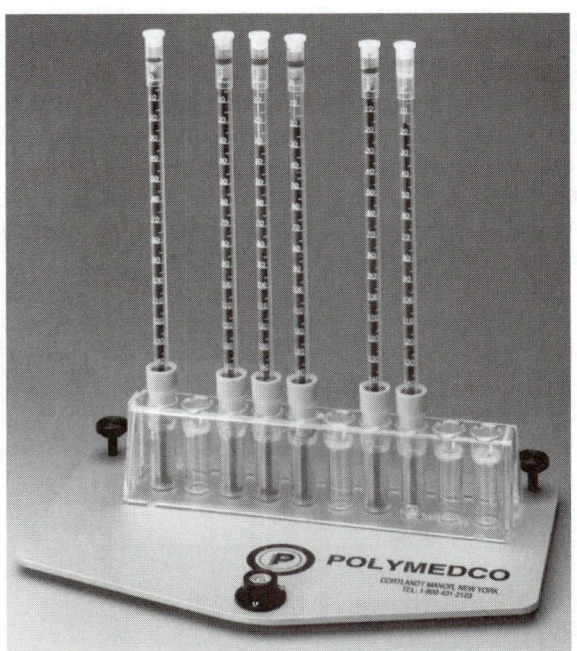

**FIGURE 2-73** Sediplast® ESR System (Photo courtesy of Polymedco, Inc.)

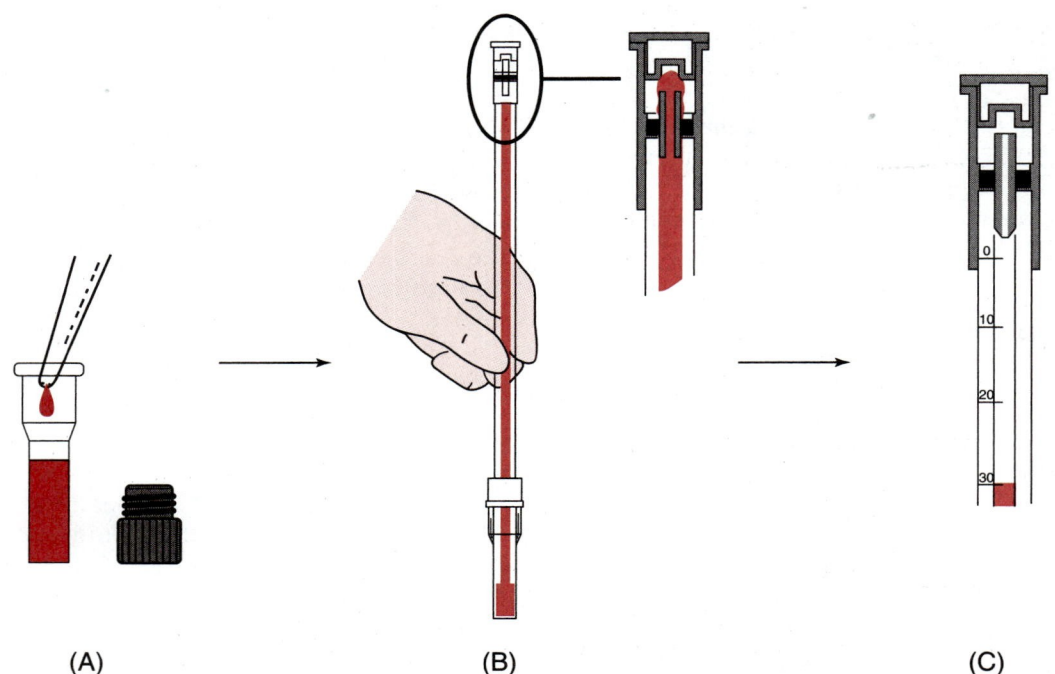

(A)  (B)  (C)

**FIGURE 2-74** Steps for Sediplast® ESR test. (A) pipet blood into vial containing diluent, (B) insert tube through vial stopper and tube will fill and autozero (inset), and (C) after one hour read sedimentation distance using markings on tube

## Automated Methods

### SEDIMAT™

The SEDIMAT™ system is manufactured by Polymedco and uses the principles, supplies, and procedures of the SEDIPLAST™ system. The filled SEDIPLAST™ Westergren tube is placed into the SEDIMAT™ automated ESR reader. The system is "walkaway;" the reader displays the reading of each sample on an LCD display. The results are also stored in memory and can be printed out using the attached thermal printer. The system eliminates technician bias and variability in technique among technicians.

### Ves-Matic™

The Ves-Matic™ ESR system is an automated walkaway analyzer. A venipuncture is performed using a special vacuum tube that draws one mL of blood into a solution of sodium citrate. The tube is placed directly into the analyzer; the ESR is determined by infrared light and the results are available in approximately 22 minutes.

### Zeta Sedimentation Ratio (ZSR)

The Zeta Sedimentation Ratio (ZSR) is performed using a special, small-bore capillary tube that is filled with blood and spun for three to four minutes in a centrifuge

called the Zetafuge® (Beckman Coulter). This centrifuge alternately compacts and disperses the RBCs under standardized centrifugal force. The tube is then read on a special reader to obtain a value called the zetacrit, which represents the percentage of sedimented erythrocytes. The zetacrit value is divided into the hematocrit value (also a percentage) and the result is the ZSR, expressed as a percentage.

The ZSR's advantages are that it is rapid, corrects for anemia, and requires only a small blood sample, which is desirable for pediatric patients. However, a special centrifuge and reader are required to perform the test.

*Procedural Notes*

- Follow the manufacturer's instructions for the test method being used.
- Be sure the blood has been properly mixed before setting up the ESR test.
- Read test results at the appropriate time interval after setup.
- Be sure to use reference values specific to the test method used.

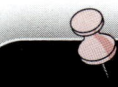

## *Safety Precautions*

- Follow Universal and Standard Precautions.
- Wear gloves, protective face wear, and buttoned, fluid-resistant laboratory coat.

## SUMMARY

The ESR is a nonspecific test. The results can be used to detect inflammation that may not be detected by other tests. The test can also be used to follow the progress of certain diseases. Since the test is affected by many factors, the worker must follow the instructions for the specific method and take care to eliminate environmental and technical factors that could cause erroneous test results.

## LESSON REVIEW

1. Why would an ESR be performed?
2. What four properties of blood affect the ESR? Explain how the ESR is affected by each of these factors.

3. Name five conditions or diseases in which the ESR would be increased.
4. What two conditions usually have a low ESR?
5. What are the reference values for the ESR using the Wintrobe method? Westergren method?
6. Name four technical factors that can affect the sed rate.
7. Name two automated methods for performing an ESR.
8. Define acute phase proteins, aggregate, inflammmation, polycythemia, rouleau(x), sedimentation, Westergren tube, and Wintrobe tube.

## STUDENT ACTIVITIES

1. Reread the information on ESR.
2. Review the glossary terms.
3. Practice performing the ESR as outlined on the Student Performance Guide.
4. Evaluate the effect of technical factors on the ESR: set up three ESR tests on the same blood sample. Treat one tube according to the test procedure, place one in the refrigerator, and place one at an angle at room temperature. At the end of one hour, compare the results from the three tests and explain them.

# Student Performance Guide

## LESSON 2-12 Erythrocyte Sedimentation Rate

Name _____    Date _____

### ☣ INSTRUCTIONS

1. Practice performing the ESR test following the step-by-step procedure.
2. Demonstrate your understanding of this lesson by:
   a. Completing a written examination successfully, and
   b. Performing the ESR procedure satisfactorily for the instructor. All steps must be completed as listed on the instructor's Performance Check Sheet.

*Note:* Consult the manufacturer's package insert for specific instructions for the ESR kit being used.

### MATERIALS AND EQUIPMENT

- gloves
- hand disinfectant
- sample of venous blood collected in EDTA
- Sediplast® Kit (or other ESR kit):
  sedivial and sedirack
  Sediplast® autozeroing pipet
  Pipet capable of delivering up to 1.0 mL
- Wintrobe method:
  Wintrobe sedimentation tube
  Wintrobe sedimentation rack
  long-stem Pasteur-type pipet with rubber bulb
- timer
- 10% chlorine bleach solution
- biohazard disposal container
- acrylic safety shield or protective facewear
- puncture-proof biohazard container for sharps

### PROCEDURE

Record in the comment section any problems encountered while practicing the procedure (or have a fellow student or the instructor evaluate your performance).

S = Satisfactory
U = Unsatisfactory

| You must: | S | U | Comments |
|---|---|---|---|
| 1. Wash hands and put on gloves | | | |
| 2. Assemble equipment and materials | | | |
| 3  Mix blood sample gently for two minutes | | | |
| 4. Perform either Sediplast® ESR (method a) or Wintrobe (method b):<br>a. Sediplast® ESR (Modified Westergren)<br>   (1) Remove stopper on sedivial and fill to the indicated mark with 0.8 mL blood. Replace stopper and invert vial several times to mix (or mix using pipet)<br>   (2) Place sedivial in Sediplast® rack on a level surface | | | |

| You must: | S | U | Comments |
|---|---|---|---|
| (3) Insert the disposable Sediplast® pipet gently through the piercable stopper with a twisting motion and push down until the pipet rests on the bottom of the vial.  The pipet will autozero the blood and any excess will flow into the sealed reservoir compartment<br>(4) Set timer for one hour<br>(5) Return blood sample to proper storage. (If no laboratory work will be performed during the incubation, remove gloves, discard appropriately, and wash hands. Reglove before handling test materials)<br>(6) Let the pipet stand undisturbed for exactly one hour and then read the results of the ESR: Use the scale on the tube to measure the distance from the top of the plasma to the top of the RBCs<br>(7) Record the sedimentation rate:<br>ESR (Mod. Westergren, 1 hr) = _____ mm<br>(8) Dispose of tube and vial in appropriate biohazard container | | | |
| b. Wintrobe method:<br>(1) Place tube in Wintrobe sedimentation rack<br>(2) Check the leveling bubble to ensure the Wintrobe rack is level<br>(3) Fill Wintrobe tube to the "0" mark with well-mixed blood using the Pasteur pipet, being careful not to overfill.<br>*Note:* Insert pipet tip to bottom of tube and fill from the bottom up to avoid air bubbles<br>(4) Set timer for one hour.  Be certain the tube is vertical<br>(5) Return blood sample to proper storage. (If no other laboratory work is scheduled, remove gloves, discard appropriately, and wash hands.  Reglove before handling test materials)<br>(6) Measure the distance the erythrocytes have fallen (in mm): after exactly one hour, use the scale on the tube to measure the distance from the top of the plasma to the top of the RBCs<br>(7) Record the sedimentation rate:<br>ESR (Wintrobe, 1 hr) = _____ mm<br>(8) Disinfect and clean equipment and return to storage<br>*Note:* Discard disposable equipment in bio-hazard container | | | |
| 5.  Clean work area with surface disinfectant. | | | |
| 6.  Remove gloves and discard in biohazard container | | | |
| 7.  Wash hands with hand disinfectant | | | |
| *Evaluator Comments:* | | | |

Evaluator _____ Date _____

# Principles of Automated Hematology

## LESSON OBJECTIVES

**After studying this lesson, you should be able to:**

- *Describe the history of the quantitation of blood cells.*
- *Compare the accuracy and precision of manual and automated blood cell-counting methods.*
- *Name two automated cell-counting technologies.*
- *Give an example of an instrument that uses each type of counting technology.*
- *Discuss quality control for these instruments.*
- *Discuss the principles of coagulation analyzers.*
- *List two examples of coagulation analyzers.*
- *Define the glossary terms.*

## GLOSSARY

**aperture** / an opening

**electrolyte** / a solution that conducts an electrical current

**fluorescent** / having the property of emitting light of one wavelength when exposed to light of another wavelength

**histogram** / a graph that illustrates the size and frequency of occurrence of articles being studied

**impedance** / resistance in an electrical circuit

**index of refraction** / the ratio of the velocity of light in one medium, such as air, to its velocity in another material

**laser** / a narrow and extremely intense beam of light of only one wavelength going in only one direction

## INTRODUCTION

Humans have long been fascinated with blood, associating it with life in themselves and animals. In the 1600s, William Harvey recorded his observations of RBCs as they passed through the capillaries. However, until the end of the 19th century, there was no way to quantitate the blood cells.

In 1855, researchers devised the first counting chambers (hemacytometers) for viewing and counting cells using a microscope. Hemacytometers were gradually improved by changing the background color of the glass, and adding some metal to the etched lines to make them brighter. By using special diluting pipets and these hemacytometers, blood cells in a specific volume of blood could be quantitated.

225

In laboratories today, manual cell counts continue to be performed for various reasons. Manual counts can be used to check hematological results from an instrument, although there are controls available for hematology instruments. In addition, cell counts on body fluids, such as spinal or joint fluid, are counted using a hemacytometer. If the laboratory does not have a backup instrument, manual counts must be performed if the main instrument is broken.

## THE BEGINNINGS OF AUTOMATED HEMATOLOGY

Blood cells were routinely counted by manual methods until the late 1950s. In 1956, W. H. Coulter patented a device that automatically counted blood cells using the method of *electrical impedance*, also known as *aperture impedance*. This invention has made performance of blood cell counts faster, easier, and more available. In addition, the instrument results are more accurate and precise. Manual counts have a coefficient of variation (CV) of approximately ±10%, whereas reliable instrument counts have a CV of about ± 1–2%.

The first automated hematology instruments performed only the RBC and WBC counts. The hemoglobin measurement was added later. Instruments now on the market provide direct or calculated values for 60 or more parameters. In these instruments, only the WBCs, RBCs, hemoglobin, platelets, and reticulocytes are directly counted or measured. The hematocrit and indices values are calculated from the RBC and hemoglobin results. Examples of the information available from various instruments is shown in Table 2-23.

| Table 2-23 Examples of results available on hematology analyzers | | |
|---|---|---|
| RBC | MCH | Left shift |
| WBC | MCHC | Atypical lymphs |
| HGB | RDW* | Hypochromia |
| HCT | immature granulocytes | RBC fragments |
| MCV | 3-part differential | Nucleated RBCs |
| PLT count | 5-part differential | Reticulocyte count |
| MPV** | | |

*RDW is red cell distribution width, a measure of RBC anisocytosis
**MPV is mean platelet volume, a measure of the volume of the average platelet
*Note:* Instruments are available that perform other measurements of blood components; many results are only performed for research purposes

## TWO BASIC CELL-COUNTING TECHNOLOGIES

Electrical impedance remained the only automated cell-counting method for about two decades. Then, in the 1970s, light-scatter cell-counting technology was developed and later, in the '80s, image processing was introduced.

### Electrical-Impedance Cell Counting

All electrical-impedance cell counters are based on Coulter's principles. The instruments have also been adapted for industrial use to count other types of particles in solutions.

#### Principle of Electrical-Impedance Counting

Blood cells to be counted by electrical impedance are diluted in an **electrolyte**, a solution that conducts electricity. An electrical current flows in the electrolyte from one electrode to another across the **aperture** (opening) (Figure 2-75).

The blood cells are poor conductors of electricity. As a cell suspended in the electrolyte (diluent) passes

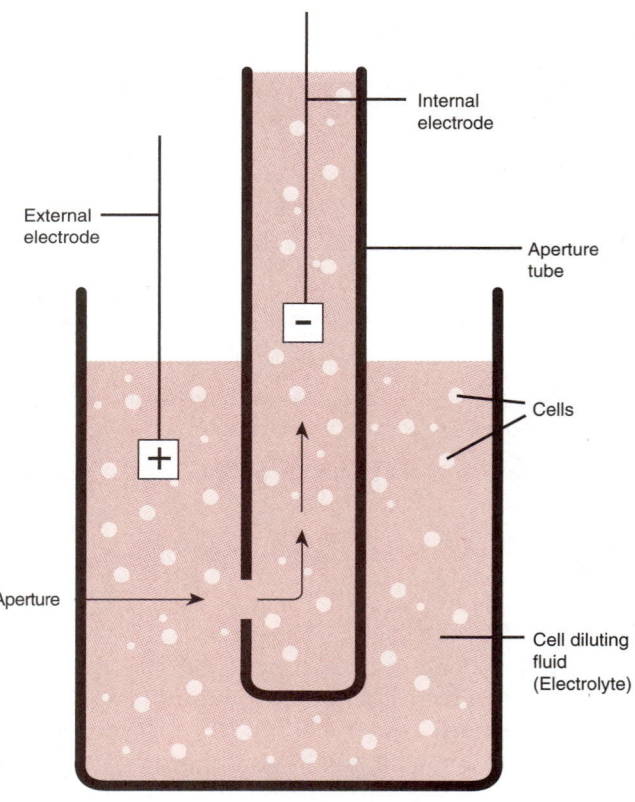

**FIGURE 2-75**   Illustration of electrical-impedance method of cell counting

through the aperture, the nonconducting cell causes an **impedance** or interruption of the electrical circuit. The impedance causes a pulse in the electrical circuit. These pulses are counted as cells. The size of the impedance is proportional to the size of the cell causing it. Therefore, the instrument not only records how many cells pass through the aperture, but also the size of each cell.

When cells pass through the aperture, they must be in the center of the aperture or they will register as being larger than their real size. Also, a cell that becomes stuck in the aperture is counted repeatedly.

### Improvements in Electrical-Impedance Counting

Accuracy and precision were improved by altering instruments to channel the flow to the center and also to electronically "edit" the pulses. The information gained is then more accurate for the purpose of sizing cells. Most cell counters display this information on a screen in a graph called a **histogram**. The relative numbers of cells are plotted on the "Y" axis and the sizes are plotted on the "X" axis (Figure 2-76).

### Examples of Electrical-Impedance Instruments

Hematology instruments manufactured by several companies use electrical-impedance technology (Figure 2-77). Beckman Coulter, Inc., markets a variety of such instruments, including the COULTER® ONYX™ for labs performing 10–100 CBCs per day and the COULTER® AᶜᐧT diff™ for labs performing 1–50 CBCs per day.

The Serono-Baker® 7000, 8000, and 9000 series are all suitable for the workload in a small laboratory or a hematology or oncology practice. The Sysmex® K series also uses electrical impedance. The ABBOTT Cell-Dyn® 3500 uses electrical impedance and an optical method; the combination is very useful for abnormal samples. Many of these automatic cell counters perform 50–110 tests per hour, require small quantities of blood for testing, and have closed-tube sampling capability to reduce risk of exposure to blood.

## Light-Scattering Cell Counting

### Principles of Light Scatter

In light-scatter cell counters, a **laser** beam or tungsten-halogen light beam is directed at a stream of blood cells passing through a narrow channel. The channel is narrow so the cells are forced to pass through in single file. When the light beam strikes a cell, the beam is scattered at an angle. Sensors detect how much light is scattered and how much of the beam was absorbed by the cell (Figure 2-78).

Each type of cell causes a different angle of scatter. This angle depends on the volume, shape, and **index of refraction** of the cell. However, the size of the cell has the most important effect on the scatter.

The laser light is monochromatic, which means it has only one wavelength, and travels in only one direction. These two characteristics allow it to be more finely tuned than the tungsten-halogen light and enable it to produce scatter patterns more useful in diagnostic hematology. One disadvantage is that laser-beam instruments cannot be calibrated with the same materials as other

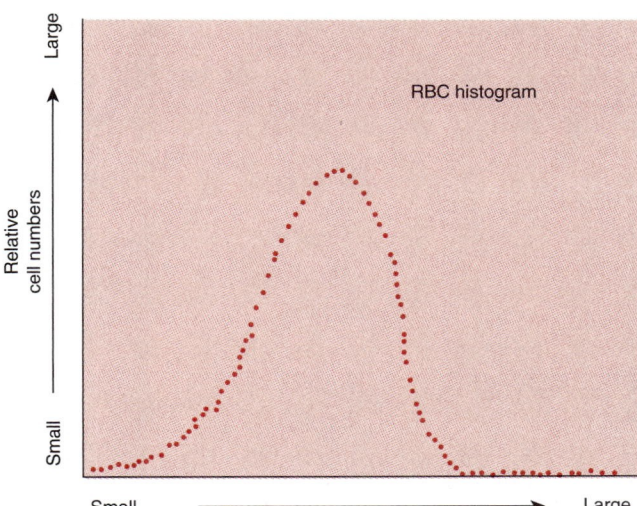

**FIGURE 2-76** Example of histogram showing relative RBC numbers plotted versus RBC size

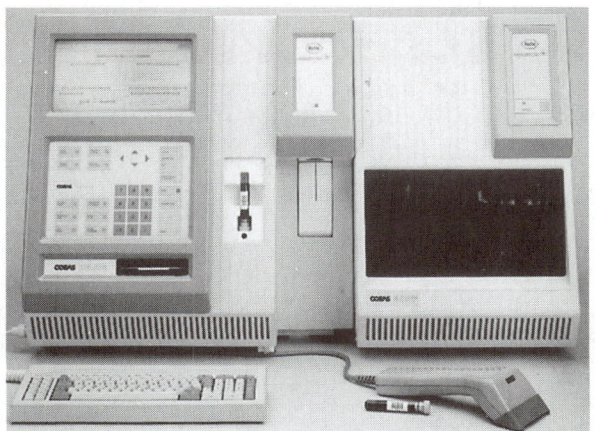

**FIGURE 2-77** COBAS HELIOS® cell counter (Photo courtesy of Roche Diagnostics Corporation, Branchburg, NJ)

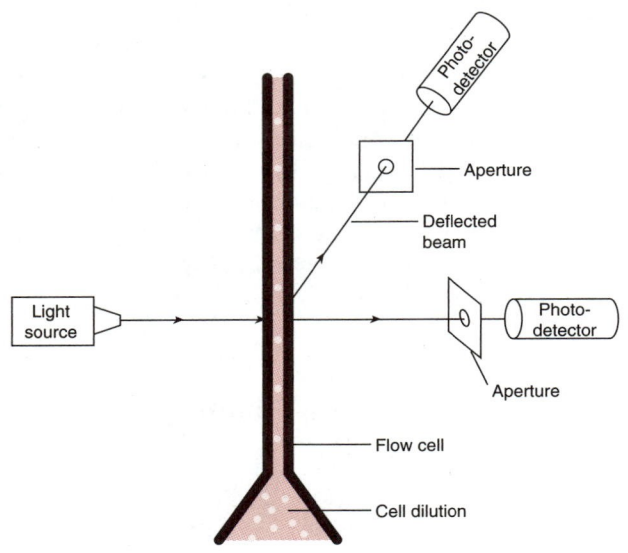

**FIGURE 2-78** Illustration of light-scatter method of cell counting

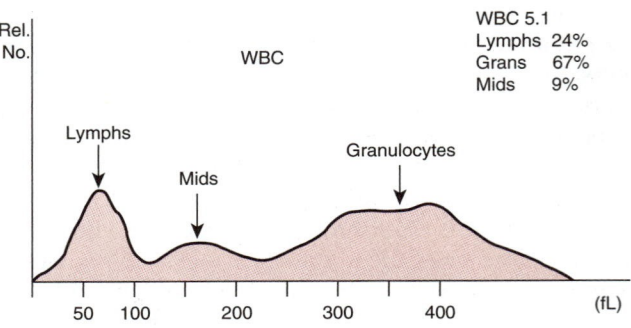

**FIGURE 2-79** Histogram of three-part differential illustrating normal WBC count and differential

cell counters. Only human blood cells may be used for calibrating the laser counters.

An important feature that manufacturers have added to light-scatter instruments is the sheath-flow, to focus the cells hydrodynamically. This improves performance and also avoids the maintenance and cleaning problems of the electrical-impedance models. Examples of instruments using light-scattering technology are the Technicon® models, the COULTER® GEN-S™, and the Bayer ADVIA® 120. The ABBOTT Cell-Dyn® 3500 combines aperture-impedance technology with light-scattering.

## AUTOMATED DIFFERENTIAL LEUKOCYTE COUNTING

### Three-Part Leukocyte Differential

Several instruments that incorporate a differential into the cell counter are now manufactured. As in the cell counters, two major technology types were developed: electrical-impedance and laser light scatter. Beckman Coulter produces the COULTER® AC•T diff™, a cell-impedance instrument that provides a three-part differential useful as a screening device. The Sysmex® CC-800 from TOA Medical Electronics produces a two-part differential; the "K" series offers a three-part differential. Serono-Baker's "Baker® 9000" series also performs a three-part differential count (Figure 2-79 and Table 2-24).

**Table 2-24.** Examples of hematology analyzers, the technology used, and the type of differential reported

| TECHNOLOGY USED | INSTRUMENT | TYPE OF DIFFERENTIAL REPORTED |
| --- | --- | --- |
| Electrical-impedance | COULTER® ONYX™ | 5 part |
| | COULTER® AC•T diff™ | 3 part |
| | Serono-Baker® | 3 part |
| Light-scattering | COULTER® VCS, STKS, GEN-S™ | 5 part |
| | Bayer ADVIA® 120 | 5 part |
| Combination of electrical-impedance and light-scattering | ABBOTT Cell-Dyn® 3500 | 5 part |

For these instruments to produce an automated differential, the cells must be subjected to a special reagent. This reagent shrinks the cytoplasm of each type of WBC to a different degree, with the lymphocytes shrinking the most. This sorts the cell sizes into three distinct classifications: lymphocytes, mononuclear cells, and granulocytes. Cells of 35–99 fL (femtoliters) are grouped as lymphocytes, cells of 100–200 fL are called mononuclear cells (mids), and cells greater than 200 fL are called granulocytes (Figure 2-79).

The three-part differential is a screening device. It does not separate the granulocytes into neutrophils, eosinophils, and basophils. The instrument "flags" abnormal results to alert the operator that an abnormal condition such as abnormalities in RBC or WBC count, atypical lymphocytes, or giant platelets, may be present.

## Five-Part Differential Counting

Several hematology analyzers are available that provide five-part differentials (Table 2-24). In the usual five-part differential, the WBCs are sorted into neutrophils, lymphs, monocytes, eosinophils, and basophils, creating a histogram (Figure 2-80, top). Any variant lymphs or other immature cells are included in an additional category called LUC (large unstained cells),

Beckman Coulter's VCS technology uses three cell parameters—volume (V), conductivity (C), and light scatter (S)—to count and classify WBCs. VCS modules can be incorporated into counters such as the COULTER® STKS, GEN-S™, and MAXM™ to produce a complete CBC with automated five-part differential. The instruments require as little as 100 μL of blood per sample, and can process up to seventy-five samples per hour. The GEN-S™ system, for the laboratory performing 100–1000 CBCs per day, provides thirty-three parameters, including five-part differential and reticulocyte analysis. A five-part differential and twenty-six parameters are available on the COULTER® MAXM™. The COULTER® ONYX™ provides eighteen parameters including a five-part differential and is suitable for labs performing 10–100 CBCs per day.

ABBOTT Diagnostics markets the Cell-Dyn® 3000 and 3500 instruments that provide a five-part differential by multi-angle polarized light-scatter separation (MAPSS). This method does not alter or shrink the cells. It characterizes each individual cell by the light-scatter pattern from four specific angles.

## Cytochemical Staining Differentials

The first instrument that used cytochemical staining to create a differential count was the Hemalog D™ from the Technicon Corporation in 1975. The instrument per-

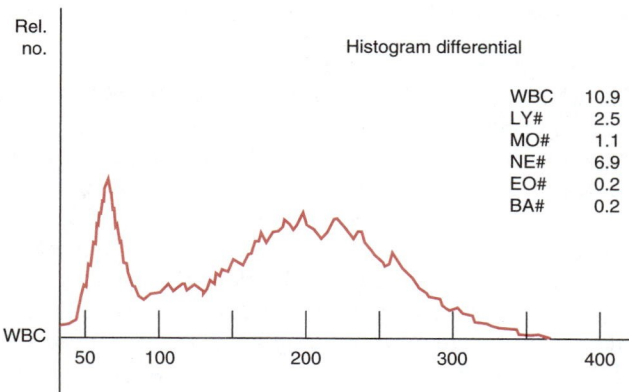

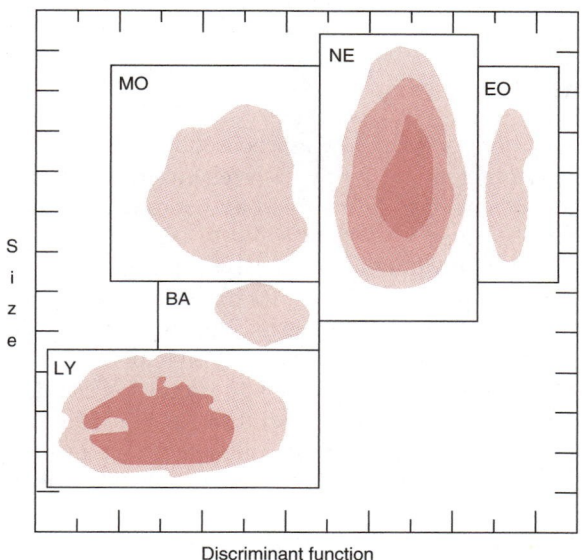

**FIGURE 2-80** Top, histogram and bottom, scattergram (cytogram) illustrating five-part differential formats

forms a CBC and five-part differential. Certain chemicals, such as peroxidase and alcian blue, which affect the various WBCs in specific ways, are added to the blood sample. The sample stream is then subjected to a light beam and the scatter is measured and recorded. From that information, the total WBC count and five-part differential are reported. The display of this information is called a "cytogram" (Figure 2-80, bottom). The Technicon H™ series multichannel analyzers incorporate this technology. Additional instruments of this type are available, such as the COBAS ARGOS® 5Diff by Roche Diagnostics Corp.

## Image-Processing Instruments

Another type of technology, popular in the 1980s, was image-processing of differentials. These instruments compared cells on a prepared blood smear with thousands of images of "normal" cells stored in computer memory. Although they could match the performance of a skilled technologist, the instruments had several disadvantages, such as the requirement that each abnormal cell be reviewed by a technologist. In addition, the results were limited by all the disadvantages of the visual counting system: reliance on a well-made smear, cell distribution, and staining technique. Two instruments produced using this technology were the LARC™ and the Hematrak™. Neither of these is currently produced or distributed in the United States.

## Flow Cytometry

Flow cytometry is the newest technique in hematology. Flow cytometers are particularly useful in situations in which cells need to be counted and sorted into subsets of populations. **Fluorescent stains** that attach to certain cell components, are combined with the blood sample. The sample is then processed by a light-scatter method. The scatter patterns from the fluorescent tagged cells are specific for certain cell types.

Flow cytometry is especially useful for classifying subsets of cells in leukemias and in AIDS. This method can also be used to count reticulocytes. Two examples of such instruments are the FACSCalibur™ (Becton Dickinson) and the EPICS® ALTRA™ (Beckman Coulter).

## Quality Assurance for Hematology Instruments

Instrument manufacturers have responded to laboratories' need for more quality control by designing instruments that can help the laboratory spot QC problems, correct failures, and store and retrieve QC data. Manufacturers provide calibrators, control specimens, and technical service hotlines.

Many instruments, especially larger ones, record the patient's I.D. from bar codes on the sample tube, helping to decrease transcription errors. Some instruments store up to 10,000 patient records at a time. A technologist can pull up a screen and compare a patient's results on one day with those from another day.

Instruments such as the BAKER® 9000 also prepare Levey-Jennings charts for each run of control samples. In addition, as each control sample is run, any value not within ±3 *sd* (standard deviation) is flagged. The Levey-Jennings screen can be accessed to see if a trend or shift might be developing. At the end of the month, the complete QC record can be printed out.

An inexpensive method of quality checks involves choosing 5–10 patient samples within reference ranges from a day's workload and reanalyzing them the next day on the same instrument. Statistical methods can then be used to calculate whether there is a significant change between the two sets of values.

# HEMOSTASIS TESTING

Coagulation analyzers range from relatively simple ones to more complex, fully automated ones. Two basic technologies are used. The one that has been used the longest is detecting a fibrin clot with a moving wire loop. Some newer instruments use photo-optical density to detect clot formation. Platelet aggregation function can be tested by an aggregometer. These instruments may use either plasma or whole blood.

## Plasma Tests

Tests for function of the plasma-coagulation factors have traditionally been performed on patient plasma samples. The FibroSystem™ by Becton Dickinson has been used for many years (Figure 2-81). It works on the principle of fibrin clot detection with a moving wire loop. This instrument can be used for prothrombin time (PT), activated partial thromboplastin time (APTT), and fibrin assays. The technologist must insert the samples into the fibrometer, add the reagents, and start the timer. The instrument stops when a clot is detected and displays the time elapsed.

Other more automated hemostasis instruments are now on the market. They range from semiautomated to fully automated (Figure 2-82). With the fully automated models, a tray or rack of plasma tubes can be placed into the machine with identification, such as bar coding. The technologist is then free to perform other duties in the laboratory. The CA-1000™ from Sigma Diagnostics can perform up to eight tests simultaneously. These include PT, APTT, fibrinogen, thrombin time, and tests of specific coagulation factors. Sigma markets the AccuStasis™ 1000 and 2000 for smaller laboratories (Figure 2-83).

Helena Laboratories markets the Cascade® 480, which automatically aspirates plasma samples directly from blood-collection tubes. The ELECTRA 1000C™, manufactured by Medical Laboratory Automation, Inc. (MLA), has an automated specimen-processing and identification system. The COAG-A-MATE® series of instruments, marketed by Organon Teknika, has been popular in both small and large laboratories.

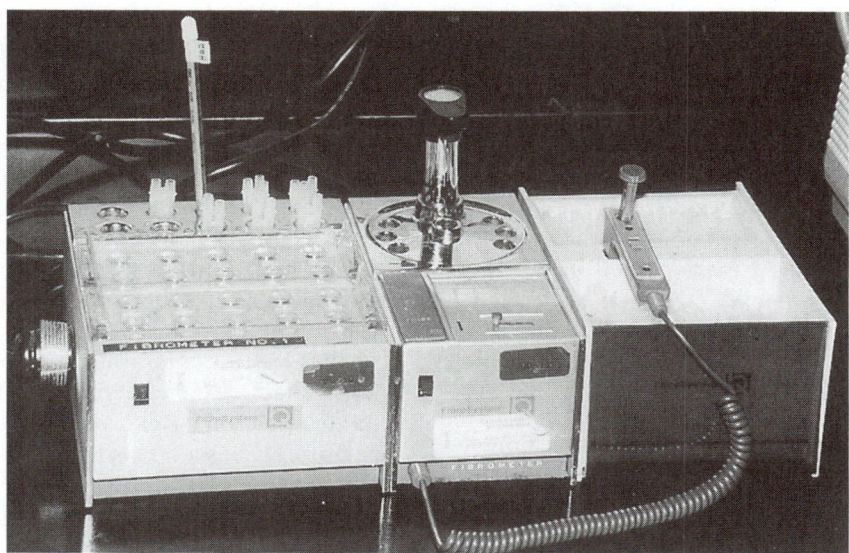

**FIGURE 2-81** Fibrometer

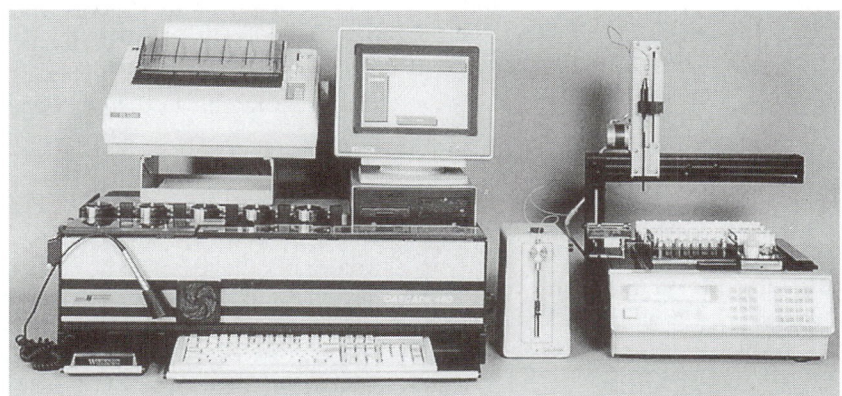

**FIGURE 2-82** Automated hemostasis analyzer (Photo courtesy of Helena Laboratories, Beaumont, TX)

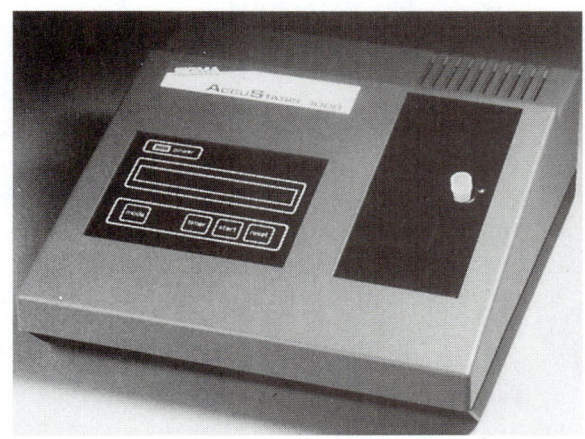

**FIGURE 2-83** AccuStasis™ hemostasis analyzer (Courtesy of Sigma Diagnostics)

An additional line of coagulation analyzers known as the ACL™ series is marketed by Beckman Coulter. The smallest and simplest of them is the ACL™. Its test menu includes PT fibrinogen, APTT, thrombin time, protein C, and protein S and clotting-factor assays. Other analyzers in the series, ACL™1000 through 7000, can sample directly from the blood-collecting tube, reducing technicians' exposure risk.

## Whole Blood Tests

Newer systems have been developed to meet the need for rapid testing. The Hemochron® Jr. Coagulation Analyzer from International Technidyne Corporation performs several rapid coagulation tests using whole blood. The results of some tests are available in less than two minutes.

Array Medical markets the Actalyke™ designed primarily for POCT. It performs the Activated Clotting Time test (ACT), which is used to monitor heparin anticoagulant therapy. Another POCT coagulation analyzer is the GEM™ PCL manufactured by Instrumentation Laboratory. The GEM™ PCL's test menu includes APTT, PT, and ACT. The sample size required is just 50 µL of whole blood available from capillary puncture. The APTT and the PT can also be performed on a blood sample drawn into a citrate tube.

## Platelet Aggregation Tests

Platelet aggregation can be tested using instruments specially made for the purpose. A tube containing a suspension of platelets is inserted into the instrument. Reagents that induce platelet aggregation, such as collagen, epinephrine, or ristocetin, are added to the suspension. The amount of light transmitted as the platelets aggregate into clumps is proportional to the degree of aggregation; as more platelets aggregate, the suspension clears. The instrument displays a graph illustrating the response. The PACKS™-4 is a platelet aggregometer made by Helena Laboratories (Figure 2-84).

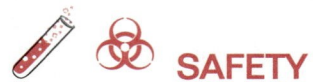 **SAFETY**

Instruments substantially increase accuracy and reduce the time required to complete hematology and coagulation testing. However, these instruments do pose physical, chemical, and biological hazards.

Routine maintenance or repair of an instrument can present several hazards. Some instruments automatically perform routine maintenance procedures, but if the technician must do them, the manufacturer's instructions must be closely followed. Repairs should be performed only by trained personnel. Removal of the outside case should be attempted only by authorized personnel because of the hazard of electrical shock.

Chemical hazards are present in the reagents used by the instruments when performing analyses. The MSDS sheets accompanying the chemicals must be read and understood by everyone using them. If differential slides must be stained, all chemical precautions must be observed to avoid injury.

Preparation of the blood sample for analysis and use of hematology controls and calibrators potentially exposes the worker to bloodborne pathogens (BBP). Instruments that have a through-the-cap sampler and produce an automated differential greatly reduce the risk. Standard and Universal Precautions must be followed and PPE worn when performing maintenance and repairs, since the internal parts of the instrument may be contaminated with blood.

## SUMMARY

Automated instruments for hematology and hemostasis have simplified and somewhat reduced the hematology workload. At the same time, they have increased the laboratory's capacity and capability to perform hematology testing.

Every laboratory professional should ensure that correct controls and calibration materials are used for all procedures. When a laboratory maintains a good QC program and participates in a certified proficiency program, the physician can have confidence in the results used to guide patient treatment.

## LESSON REVIEW

1. Describe the history of blood cell counting after Harvey's observations.
2. How does the coefficient of variation of manual blood cell counts compare to that of automated counts?
3. Name two types of technology used to count blood cells and give an example of each type.
4. Discuss the importance of QC for automated instruments.

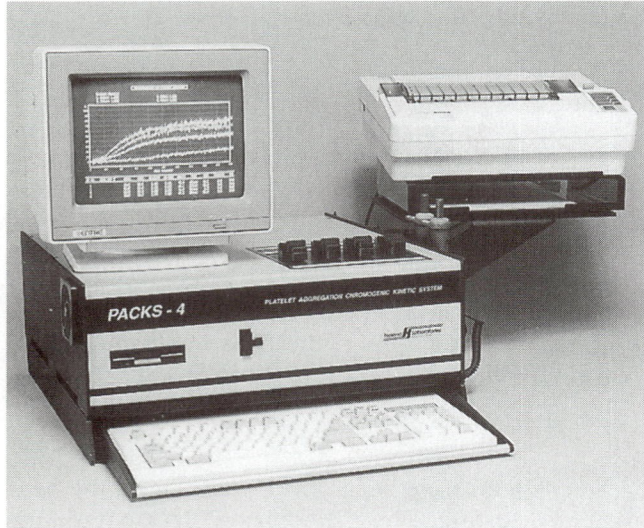

**FIGURE 2-84** Platelet aggregometer (Courtesy of Helena Laboratories, Beaumont, TX)

5. List two types of instruments used for plasma coagulation testing.

6. What is the difference between the technologies used for three-part differential counters and five-part differential counters?

7. Explain what information is illustrated by a histogram.

8. Explain how platelet aggregation can be tested.

9. Explain the advantages of the new whole blood coagulation tests.

10. Explain the uses of a flow cytometer.

11. Define aperture, electrolyte, fluorescent, histogram, impedance, index of refraction, and laser.

## STUDENT ACTIVITIES

1. Reread the information on principles of automated hematology.

2. Review the glossary terms.

3. Investigate the use of automation in large hematology laboratories and in small practices. How do their needs differ?

4. Interview someone who works in a hematology laboratory. Ask what type of hemostasis testing is performed there.

5. After consulting operating manuals for hematology instruments, calculate the amount of time required to manually perform fifty CBCs with differential counts; compare that with the time required if a hematology analyzer that performs a five-part differential is used.

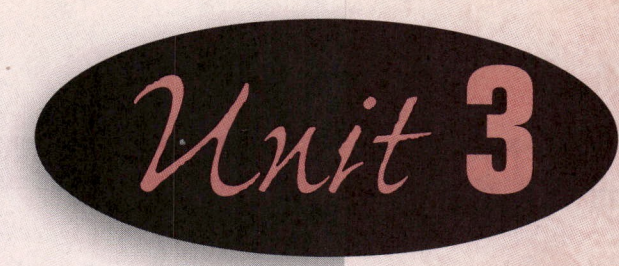

# Basic Hemostasis

## UNIT OBJECTIVES

**After studying this unit, you should be able to:**

- *Explain the mechanism of hemostasis.*
- *Discuss disorders of hemostasis.*
- *Perform a bleeding time test.*
- *Perform a prothrombin time (PT) test.*
- *Perform an activated partial thromboplastin time (APTT) test.*
- *Perform a rapid coagulation test.*

## UNIT OVERVIEW

Unit 3 is an introduction to the complex topic of hemostasis, the process of stopping bleeding. Lesson 3-1, Principles of Hemostasis, outlines the basic mechanisms of hemostasis and provides a foundation for understanding the principles of the routine coagulation screening procedures included in the unit.

Disorders of hemostasis, including inherited and acquired conditions of platelets and coagulation factors, are discussed in Lesson 3-2.

The bleeding time test, a screening procedure that can detect some blood-clotting disorders, is discussed in Lesson 3-3. The bleeding time test is not specific for a particular deficiency. It is presented in this unit as an introduction to the principles involved in hemostasis.

The prothrombin time and the activated partial thromboplastin time, frequently ordered coagulation screening tests, are covered in Lessons 3-4 and 3-5. These tests illustrate the ability of plasma proteins to form a fibrin clot. Lesson 3-6 includes the principles of some rapid tests for hemostatic function, such as the D-dimer and ACT tests. Both manual and automated methods are presented.

Units 2 and 3 cover several hematology and coagulation procedures performed in medical laboratories. However, these procedures actually represent only a few of the large number of tests performed in the hematology laboratory and are included to illustrate some basic principles of hematology and coagulation.

Addison, L. A. & Fischer, P. M. (1990). *The office laboratory.* East Norwalk, CT: Appleton and Lange.

Brown, B. A. (6th ed.). (1993). *Hematology: Principles and procedures.* Philadelphia: Lea & Febiger.

Harmening, Denise M. (Ed.). (3rd ed.). (1996). *Clinical hematology and fundamentals of hemostasis.* Philadelphia: F. A. Davis Company.

Henry, J. B. (Ed.). (19th ed.). (1996). *Clinical diagnosis & management by laboratory methods.* Philadelphia: W. B. Saunders Company.

Howanitz, J. H. & Howanitz, P. J. (Eds.). (1991). *Laboratory Medicine—test selection and interpretation.* New York: Churchill Livingstone, Inc.

Koepke, J. A. (Ed.). (1991). *Practical laboratory hematology.* New York: Churchill Livingstone, Inc.

Kovanda, Beverly M. (1998). *Point-of-care testing—capillary puncture.* Albany, NY: Delmar Publishers.

Lee, Richard G. et al. (10th ed.). (1998). *Wintrobe's clinical hematology.* Baltimore: Williams & Wilkins.

Miale, J. B. (6th ed.). (1982). *Laboratory medicine—hematology.* St. Louis: C. V. Mosby.

Ratnoff, O. D., & Forbes, C. D. (Eds.). (2nd ed.). (1991). *Disorders of hemostasis.* Philadelphia: W. B. Saunders.

Tilton, R. C., Balows, A., Hohnadel, D. C., & Reiss, R. R. (Eds.). (1992). *Clinical laboratory medicine.* St. Louis: Mosby Yearbook.

# Principles of Hemostasis

## GLOSSARY

**adhesion** / the act of two parts or surfaces sticking together

**aggregation** / the collecting of separate objects into one mass

**atherosclerosis** / a condition in which lipids, calcium, and other substances deposit on the inner surface of the arteries

**coagulation** / the process of forming a fibrin clot

**coagulation factors** / a group of plasma proteins involved in blood clotting

**collagen** / a protein connective tissue found in skin, bone, ligaments, and cartilage

**embolus (pl. emboli)** / a mass (clot) of blood or foreign matter carried in the circulation

**endothelium** / the layer of epithelial cells that lines blood vessels and the serous cavities of the body

**fibrin** / a protein formed from fibrinogen by the action of thrombin

**fibrinogen** / a plasma protein produced in the liver and converted to fibrin through the action of thrombin

**fibrinolysis** / enzymatic breakdown of a blood clot

**hemostasis** / the process of stopping bleeding

**intravascular** / inside the blood vessels

**plasmin** / an enzyme that binds to fibrin and initiates breakdown of the fibrin clot

**plasminogen** / the inactive precursor of plasmin

**prothrombin** / the precursor of thrombin; factor II

**thrombin** / a protein formed from prothrombin by the action of thromboplastin and other factors in the presence of calcium ions; factor $II_a$

**thromboplastin** / a lipoprotein found in endothelium and other tissue; coagulation factor III; also called tissue factor

**thrombus (pl. thrombi)** / a blood clot that obstructs a blood vessel

**vasoconstriction** / narrowing of the diameter of a blood vessel

## INTRODUCTION

Blood normally circulates through the body in a liquid form via the arteries, veins, and capillaries. Problems arise when blood is lost from the vessels by bleeding, or when an **intravascular** clot **(thrombus)** obstructs a blood vessel.

The process of stopping the loss of blood from blood vessels is **hemostasis**. This process involves four interrelated and interdependent systems, as shown below. These are the blood vessels, platelets, blood coagulation factors, and components of the clot degradation system (fibrinolysis).

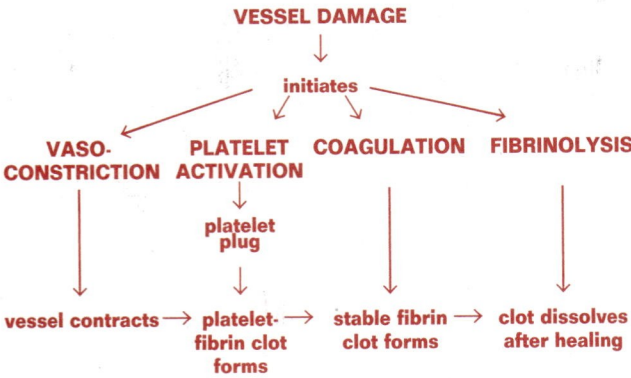

In the majority of patients, these systems function normally; bleeding is stopped by clot formation, and unwanted clot formation is prevented by the body's circulating inhibitors. However, congenital and acquired abnormalities can affect hemostasis. An abnormality may be minor and only result in inconvenience such as easy bruising, or it may cause a life-threatening incident, such as a hemorrhage.

## THE ROLE OF BLOOD VESSELS IN HEMOSTASIS

The "vascular phase" of hemostasis includes a variety of responses that may occur when a blood vessel is damaged. One reaction is **vasoconstriction**, the narrowing of the vessel to reduce blood flow to the damaged area. When a vessel is completely severed, the cut ends may retract and be compressed by the contraction of skeletal muscle. Small capillary vessels may seal themselves together if the damaged edges touch. **Collagen**, a protein connective tissue exposed when the **endothelium** lining the blood vessels is damaged, plays an important role in platelet activation.

## THE ROLE OF PLATELETS IN HEMOSTASIS

Platelets have a rounded disk-like shape while circulating in the bloodstream. However, platelets undergo a shape change when they come in contact with the exposed collagen in the wall of a damaged blood vessel. This contact with collagen initiates platelet **adhesion**, the act of the individual platelets sticking to the damaged edge of the vessel. Normal adhesion also requires a plasma protein, von Willebrand's factor (VIII:vWF).

As the platelets adhere to the vessel surface, they become activated, lose their normal disk-like shape, and become more spherical. At the same time, they form numerous spiny projections all around their edges and begin to stick to each other, a process called **aggregation**. Because of the large number of platelets present in circulating blood, a platelet plug forms in seconds to stop bleeding in the case of a small wound, such as a capillary puncture (Figure 3-1).

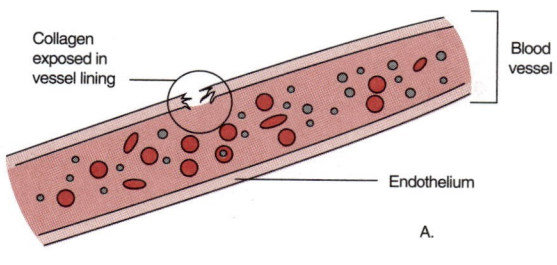

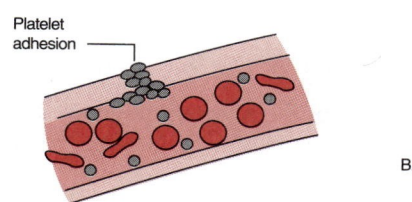

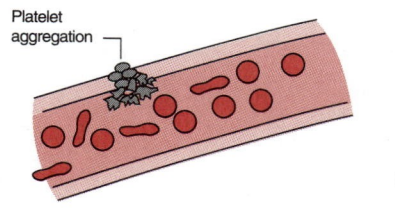

**FIGURE 3-1** Illustration of platelet action in a small wound: (A) collagen exposed in vessel lining, (B) platelet adhesion, and (C) platelet aggregation

Platelets are not complete cells, but are quite active chemically. Over forty substances are secreted from platelets during the "release" reaction that accompanies aggregation. Within one minute, fibrin strands begin to appear, trapping RBCs and WBCs into the clot, making it stronger.

## THE ROLE OF COAGULATION FACTORS IN HEMOSTASIS

The **coagulation factors** are plasma proteins, except for Factor IV, calcium, a mineral. The protein coagulation factors are produced in the liver and circulate in the blood in an inactive form. When a vessel becomes damaged, a series of complex reactions leads to the activation of coagulation factors, resulting in formation of a fibrin clot.

The coagulation factors are numbered I through XIII, in the order in which they were discovered, not in the order of their action. (The number VI is no longer used.) In addition, two of the factors are named, but

have no number. The active forms of the factors are designated by the subscript letter "a" after the number. For example, activated factor XII is $XII_a$. The coagulation factor numbers and names are listed in Table 3-1.

Coagulation factor interaction involves very complex reactions. However, the entire procedure can be expressed as follows:

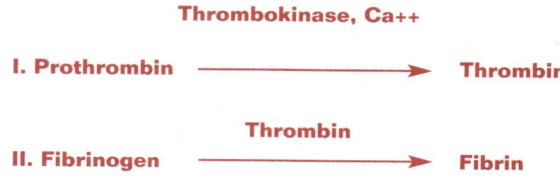

These two basic concepts developed in 1905 by Morowitz are still valid today. The only changes are the additions of the intermediate plasma-coagulation factors and calcium. The end results are the production of a stable fibrin clot to stop bleeding and then dissolution of the clot when it is no longer needed.

## THE COAGULATION PATHWAYS

The **coagulation** process involves activation of the common pathway by either the extrinsic or the intrinsic pathway. There also is some evidence of interaction between the extrinsic and the intrinsic pathways. Figure 3-2 illustrates the three pathways.

**Table 3-1.** The Coagulation Factors

| FACTOR NUMBER | NAME |
| --- | --- |
| Factor I | Fibrinogen |
| Factor II | Prothrombin |
| Factor III | Thromboplastin, tissue factor (TF) |
| Factor IV | Calcium ($Ca^{++}$) |
| Factor V | Prothrombin accelerator |
| Factor VII | Proconvertin |
| Factor VIII:C | Antihemophilic factor (AHF) |
| Factor IX | Christmas factor |
| Factor X | Stuart-Prower factor (PTC) |
| Factor XI | Plasma thromboplastin antecedent (PTA) |
| Factor XII | Hageman factor (contact factor) |
| Factor XIII | Fibrin-stabilizing factor |
| [no number assigned] | Fitzgerald factor (high molecular weight kininogen) |
| [no number assigned] | Fletcher factor (prekallikrein) |

Note: *Some references may use different names for the numbered factors.*

## The Extrinsic Pathway

The extrinsic system is so named because one of the coagulation factors involved is not present in circulating blood. This is factor III (called tissue factor or **thromboplastin**) that is released when blood vessel endothelium is damaged. Factor III, a lipoprotein composed of protein and phospholipid, acts as a co-factor in the activation of factor VII to $VII_a$. Calcium ($Ca^{++}$) is required for the reaction. Activated factor VII then participates in the reaction converting X to $X_a$ (Figure 3-2).

## The Intrinsic Pathway

All of the factors required in the intrinsic pathway are present in the circulating blood. This pathway is initiat-

ed when factor XII, called the contact factor, is activated by contact with certain surfaces to form $XII_a$. The final reaction in the intrinsic pathway is the conversion of factor VIII to $VIII_a$. Platelet factor 3 (PF3), a phospholipid released from the platelet membranes, is also required in the activation of factor VIII to factor $VIII_a$ by $IX_a$. Recent findings indicate that factor IX may also be activated by factor III (tissue factor). Factor $VIII_a$ converts factor X to $X_a$ (Figure 3-2). The intrinsic pathway is also activated when blood contacts a glass syringe or tube during blood collection.

## The Common Pathway

Whether the intrinsic or the extrinsic pathway is activated, the end result is activation of factor X to $X_a$. The

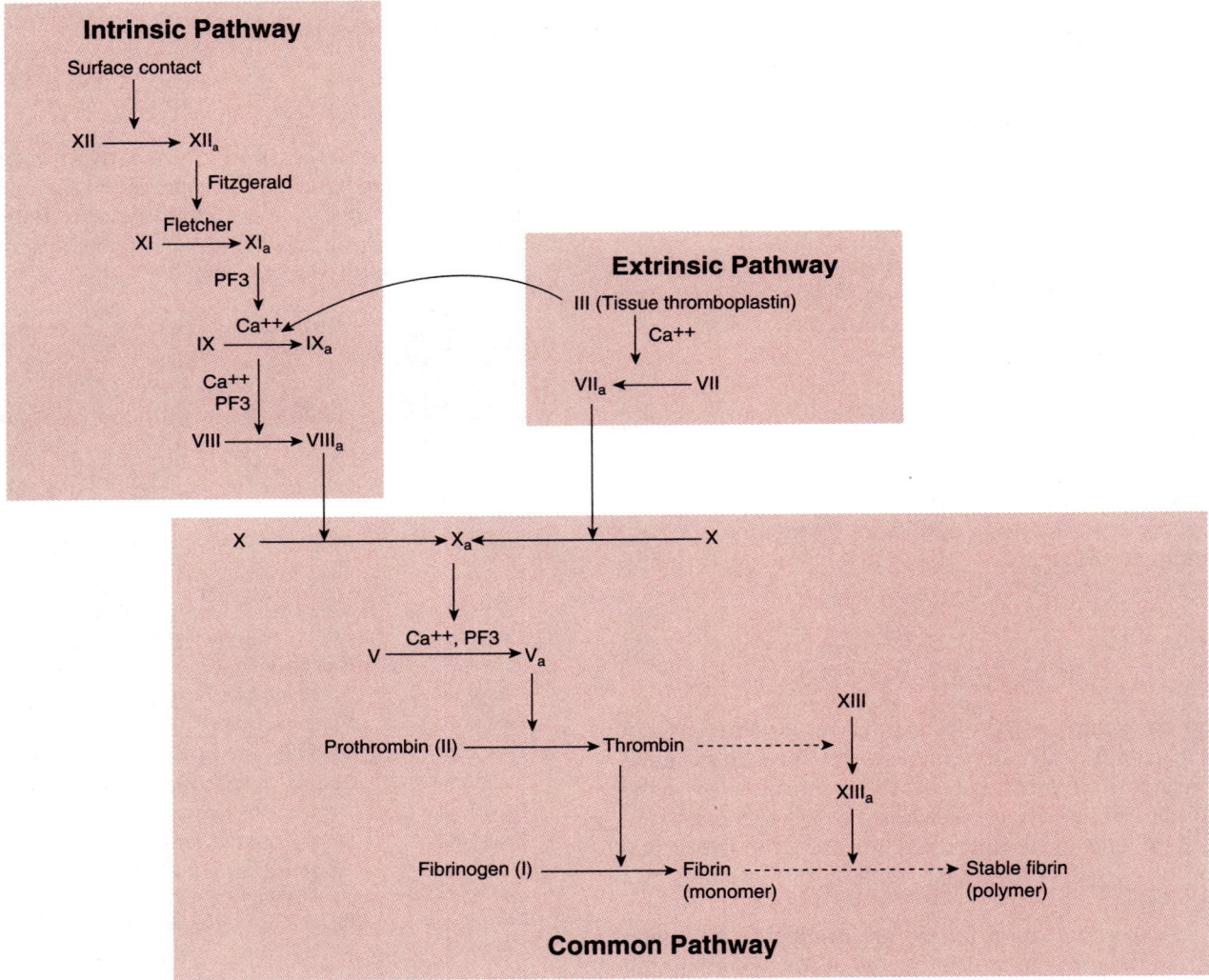

**FIGURE 3-2** A modification of the "cascade" or "waterfall" hypothesis of hemostasis of MacFarlane (1964) and Davie and Ratnoff (1964)

remainder of the activation sequences follow a "common pathway" (Figure 3-2). A complex reaction involving $X_a$, V, phospholipid, and calcium results in the activation of **prothrombin** to **thrombin**. Thrombin then acts as a catalyst in the conversion of **fibrinogen** to **fibrin**. The fibrin clot is stabilized by factor $XIII_a$.

# CONTROL MECHANISMS IN HEMOSTASIS

In normal patients, a clot forms only at the site of injury. Regulating systems prevent an isolated injury from initiating the clotting mechanism throughout the body. Normal endothelium lining the blood vessels can also act as a regulator, preventing platelets from adhering and aggregating. In addition, some plasma proteins act as circulating coagulation inhibitors to prevent the formation of unwanted clots.

## Intravascular Clotting

Sometimes the hemostasis mechanism goes amiss and intravascular blood clots become a problem. When blood vessel walls become rough and irregular, such as in **atherosclerosis**, platelets may become activated and initiate the formation of clots within the blood vessels (intravascular clotting). A blood clot attached to a vessel wall is called a **thrombus**, but when it breaks off and travels through the circulatory system it is called an **embolus**. Emboli are very dangerous because they become lodged in small vessels in the brain, lungs, and other organs. They can cause serious damage and sometimes death unless they are dissolved.

## Drug Therapy to Prevent Thrombosis

The two types of anticoagulants commonly used for preventing and treating thrombosis are heparin and coumarin (warfarin). Heparin administered intravenously is effective immediately, but is usually only used short term. The coumarin oral anticoagulants require up to a week to take effect and can be used long term. Heparin therapy can usually be discontinued after a patient has been taking an oral anticoagulant for a week. Patients with atherosclerosis or phlebitis may take an oral anticoagulant (sometimes called a "blood thinner") to prevent the formation of thrombi or clots.

## Fibrinolysis

After the blood clot has served its function of stopping bleeding, it must be dissolved. This complex process is called **fibrinolysis**. Two important components of the fibrinolytic system are **plasminogen** and **plasmin**.

Plasminogen is present in circulating blood and must be activated to become plasmin. On activation, plasmin binds to fibrin in the clot, initiating its breakdown. The complete mechanism of the fibrinolytic system is not yet completely understood.

# SUMMARY

Hemostasis involves the study of many factors and is very complex. The lessons in this unit present only the most basic theories and procedures. Tests for hemostatic function range from the more common tests, such as platelet count and prothrombin time, to assays for factor deficiencies and platelet aggregation tests. Family gene studies for inherited defects may also be performed. Lesson 3-2 discusses disorders of hemostasis and testing for hemostatic function.

The coagulation test procedures presented in this unit are intended as an introduction to some of the more common tests. These are tests that might be performed in a small laboratory, such as a physician office laboratory, in a small group practice laboratory, or in point-of-care testing.

# LESSON REVIEW

1. List the four interrelated systems that have a role in hemostasis.
2. Describe the blood vessels' role in hemostasis.
3. Outline the role of platelets in clot formation.
4. Describe the coagulation factors' role in hemostasis.
5. List the coagulation factors that are vitamin K dependent.
6. Explain how atherosclerosis can cause thrombus formation.
7. Name the two important components of the fibrinolytic system.
8. Name the three coagulation pathways.
9. Define adhesion, aggregation, atherosclerosis, coagulation, coagulation factors, collagen, embolus, endothelium, fibrin, fibrinogen, fibrinolysis, hemostasis, intravascular, plasmin, plasminogen, prothrombin, thrombin, thromboplastin, thrombus, and vasoconstriction.

# STUDENT ACTIVITIES

1. Reread the information on principles of hemostasis.
2. Review the glossary terms.
3. Research and report on a test that may be used to evaluate the intrinsic, extrinsic, or common coagulation pathway.

# Disorders of Hemostasis

## LESSON OBJECTIVES

**After studying this lesson, you should be able to:**

- *Name two acquired and two inherited disorders of platelets.*
- *Name two acquired and two inherited disorders of coagulation factors.*
- *List the coagulation factors that are vitamin K dependent.*
- *Name three tests for evaluating hemostatic function.*
- *Discuss disseminated intravascular coagulation (DIC).*
- *Define the glossary terms.*

## GLOSSARY

**disseminated intravascular coagulation (DIC)** / a bleeding disorder characterized by widespread thrombotic and secondary fibrinolytic reactions

**hemophilia** / a bleeding disorder resulting from a hereditary coagulation factor deficiency or dysfunction

**petechiae** / small, purplish hemorrhagic spots on the skin

## INTRODUCTION

Hemostasis disorders have a variety of causes. A disorder may be inherited, such as classic hemophilia, or acquired, such as abnormalities resulting from a vitamin K deficiency. Acquired abnormalities may also arise because of medications, such as the effect of aspirin on platelet aggregation. Other drugs or treatments may accelerate clot formation. These inherited and acquired disorders of hemostasis affect patients' lives and require clinical examination, laboratory tests, and investigation into family medical history for diagnosis.

## HEREDITARY HEMOSTASIS DISORDERS

### Hemophilia

The **hemophilias** are inherited diseases in which there is a deficiency or functional disorder in one or more of the coagulation factors. Classic hemophilia, called *hemophilia A*, is caused by a functional deficiency of coagulation factor VIII, the VIII:C protein.

*Hemophilia B*, also called Christmas disease, is named after the first patient in which it was studied. The defect in Christmas disease is a functional deficiency of coagulation factor IX.

Hemophilias A and B are inherited as sex-linked recessive genes carried on the X chromosome. Since males inherit one X and one Y, if the inherited X chromosome carries the recessive hemophilia gene, the disease will be expressed. Since females have two X chromosomes, those who carry the recessive hemophilia gene on one X chromosome will not manifest the disease because the normal X chromosome will be dominant. These females are called "carriers" and may pass the recessive gene to their offspring. Therefore, the diseases are limited almost exclusively to males, although there have been rare cases documented in females.

The clinical symptoms of hemophilias A and B are identical. Affected infants do not have symptoms unless they undergo circumcision or other surgery. However, as the child grows and is subject to bumps and falls, large bruises appear. Abnormal bleeding occurs into the joints, causing swelling and pain. In addition, bleeding occurs in the mouth, muscles, renal tract, gut, and after dental extractions.

## Inherited Platelet Disorders

Several inherited disorders of platelets cause prolonged bleeding in the patient. *Bernard-Soulier syndrome* is a disorder in which the platelets are larger than normal and are present in normal or decreased numbers. The platelets' ability to adhere is decreased because of a defect in the surface membrane. Affected patients develop small, purplish spots on the skin called **petechiae**. They also suffer gastrointestinal bleeding, nosebleeds, abnormal menstrual bleeding, or intracranial bleeding. The disease may be severe and even fatal.

The defect in *von Willebrand's disease* is due to deficiency or functional abnormality in a portion of the coagulation factor VIII molecule, the VIII:vWF segment. This defect alters the platelets' ability to aggregate.

In *Glanzmann's thrombasthenia*, the platelet count and platelet morphology are usually normal. The platelets have the ability to adhere to collagen but do not have normal aggregation. If a smear is made from the patient's capillary blood or venous blood without an anticoagulant, the platelets do not form the characteristic clumps. The defect has been found to be in the surface membrane of the platelets. The patient's bleeding problems are similar to those of the Bernard-Soulier patient.

# ACQUIRED DISORDERS OF HEMOSTASIS

Acquired disorders of hemostasis may cause either abnormal bleeding or thrombus formation. The disorders may affect one or more of the coagulation factors or the platelets (Table 3-2).

## Acquired Coagulation Factor Disorders

Included among the causes of acquired bleeding problems are certain conditions in which the patient develops circulating inhibitors to coagulation factors. Severe deficiency of vitamin K causes decreased production of the vitamin K dependent coagulation factors. The vitamin K dependent factors are II, VII, IX, and X.

**Disseminated intravascular coagulation (DIC)** is a serious condition in which a pathological process initiates coagulation and secondary fibrinolysis.

Depending on the balance between the two systems, there may be thrombosis or bleeding, or a combination of the two. Some conditions that may contribute to DIC are crushing injuries, certain bacterial, viral, or rickettsial infections, and drug reactions.

DIC occurs when intravascular coagulation is triggered. This causes fibrin deposition in blood vessels, which in turn uses up the available supply of coagulation factors. Microthrombi form in vital organs, including the kidneys, lungs, heart, and brain. The fibrinolytic system is then activated, releasing fibrin fragments that can act as coagulation inhibitors.

## Acquired Platelet Disorders

Acquired platelet disorders can arise from several sources. *Idiopathic thrombocytopenic purpura (ITP)* occurs when the immune system makes antibodies against the patient's own platelets. Acquired thrombocytopenia can occur when the spleen enlarges from disease. The enlarged spleen traps many platelets inside the spleen (sequestration), reducing the number of circulating platelets. Infection by certain viruses can decrease the bone marrow production of megakaryocytes. Ingestion of aspirin affects the aggregation of platelets for up to eight days by inhibiting the platelet-release reaction (Table 3-2).

**Table 3-2.** Acquired and Inherited Disorders of Hemostasis

### COAGULATION FACTOR DISORDERS

| ACQUIRED | INHERITED |
|---|---|
| Vitamin K deficiency | Hemophilia A |
| Disseminated intravascular coagulation (DIC) | Hemophilia B |
| Anticoagulant therapy | Deficiencies or dysfunction of coagulation factors |

### PLATELET DISORDERS

| ACQUIRED | INHERITED |
|---|---|
| Aspirin ingestion | Bernard-Soulier syndrome |
| Decreased megakaryocyte production | von Willebrand's disease |
| Idiopathic thrombocytopenic purpura (ITP) | Glanzmann's thrombasthenia |

This table lists only a few disorders and is not meant to be a comprehensive list.

**Table 3-3.** Expected coagulation test results for some disorders of hemostasis

| CONDITION | TEST RESULTS | | |
|---|---|---|---|
| | Bleeding Time | PT | APTT |
| Hemophilia A | Normal | Normal | Abnormal |
| Hemophilia B | Normal | Normal | Abnormal |
| von Willebrand's disease | Prolonged | Abnormal | Abnormal |
| Anticoagulant therapy | Normal | Abnormal | Abnormal |
| Glanzmann's thrombasthenia | Prolonged | Normal | Normal |

# TESTS OF HEMOSTATIC FUNCTION

Examination of hemostatic function may involve testing the platelets, the blood vessels, or the coagulation factors. The tests most often performed are prothrombin time (PT), activated partial thromboplastin time (APTT), bleeding time, and platelet count. Expected laboratory results for some disorders of hemostasis are shown in Table 3-3.

The platelet count, discussed and performed in Lesson 2-6, is a quantitative test for platelets. However, even if the platelet count is in the normal reference range, a bleeding problem can still exist if the platelets do not function normally.

Bleeding time is a screening test for quantitative or qualitative abnormalities in the platelets, and also for vascular integrity of the capillaries (Lesson 3-3). Whenever bleeding time is prolonged, more definitive tests, such as platelet adhesion, platelet aggregation, and clot retraction, must be performed.

Prothrombin time is a measure of the extrinsic pathway and is discussed at length in Lesson 3-4. The APTT, discussed in Lesson 3-5, is a test of intrinsic pathway function. Instruments used in coagulation testing are discussed in Lesson 2-13, Principles of Automated Hematology, and Lesson 3-6, Rapid Tests for Hemostasis Disorders.

## Quality Assurance for Hemostasis Tests

Specimen collection for hemostasis tests must be done carefully. Venipuncture must be performed with minimum trauma to the vein and surrounding tissues. Tests of the coagulation pathways, such as prothrombin time, are designed to artificially activate the coagulation factors in a plasma sample to measure the clotting time. Tissue or vessel damage during venipuncture releases thromboplastin into the sample, activating the extrinsic pathway prematurely, causing erroneous test results. In addition, the blood-collecting tube must contain the correct type and amount of anticoagulant.

## SUMMARY

The study of the causes, test methods, and treatment of hemostasis disorders is complex, but exciting. Many advances have been made since the two basic concepts were outlined by Morowitz in 1905. Advances in technology have allowed scientists to understand the structures and functions of an increasing number of the protein molecules involved in coagulation and fibrinolysis. This has led to new understandings of the causes and treatments of hemostasis disorders.

## LESSON REVIEW

1. Name two acquired disorders of platelets.
2. What is the effect of aspirin on platelets?
3. List the vitamin K dependent coagulation factors.
4. Name two hereditary disorders of coagulation factors.
5. Explain the differences between hemophilia A and hemophilia B.
6. Explain why hemophilia A and hemophilia B are almost exclusively limited to males.
7. Name two inherited platelet disorders.
8. Discuss conditions that contribute to disseminated intravascular coagulation (DIC).
9. How does the defect in von Willebrand's disease affect platelets?
10. Define disseminated intravascular coagulation, hemophilia, and petechiae.

## STUDENT ACTIVITIES

1. Re-read the information on hemostasis disorders.
2. Review the glossary terms.
3. Research and report on a hemostasis disorder.

# Bleeding Time

## LESSON OBJECTIVES

**After studying this lesson, you should be able to:**

- *State the purpose of the bleeding-time test.*
- *Name and describe two methods used to determine bleeding time and list the reference values of each.*
- *List three conditions in which bleeding time will be prolonged.*
- *Report the results of a bleeding time.*
- *List the precautions to be observed in performing a bleeding time.*
- *Define the glossary terms.*

## GLOSSARY

**dysfunction** / impaired or abnormal function

**hemorrhage** / excessive or uncontrolled bleeding

## INTRODUCTION

The bleeding-time test is a screening procedure used to evaluate the function of platelets and small blood vessels. The test is performed by making a small standardized incision of the capillaries. The length of time required for the bleeding to stop is noted and recorded.

## PRINCIPLE OF THE BLEEDING TIME TEST

Hemostasis, the cessation of bleeding, involves a series of complex interactions. The components that must interact are (1) blood vessels, (2) blood platelets, and (3) plasma proteins known as coagulation factors. The blood vessels must be able to constrict and slow blood flow after an injury. This property is known as vasoconstriction. The platelets react within seconds after an injury to form a plug and release certain chemical acti-

vators. The coagulation factors, proteins in the plasma in inactive form, are activated by the platelets and the tissue factor released from the injured tissue.

When all the hemostasis components interact and function properly, a clot is formed and bleeding stops. Failure of the clotting mechanism can be due to the absence, deficiency, or improper function of any of the components. Failure of the hemostatic or clotting mechanism may result in **hemorrhage**, uncontrolled bleeding.

Several laboratory tests can be performed to detect deficiencies of the hemostatic system. Bleeding time is one of these tests. It is influenced by the number and function of platelets and the condition of the vessels.

Decreased numbers of platelets (thrombocytopenia), platelet **dysfunction**, and ingestion of aspirin or other drugs may prolong bleeding time. Aspirin can affect platelet function for up to eight days. Except for von Willebrand's disease, abnormality or deficiency of one of the coagulation factors does not usually affect the bleeding time.

## METHODS OF MEASURING BLEEDING TIME

Two ways of measuring bleeding time are the Ivy method and the Duke method. The Ivy method, although the more difficult to perform correctly, is preferred because it can be somewhat standardized. The Duke method is rarely performed. Both methods present difficulties in obtaining reproducible results. All coagulation tests must be performed carefully and accurately by well-trained technicians.

 ### Safety

Universal and Standard Precautions must be observed while performing the bleeding-time test. Appropriate personal protective equipment, including gloves and a fluid-resistant laboratory coat, must be worn by the technician. In addition, the blades of the bleeding-time device or lancet are potentially dangerous. All sharps must be handled carefully and discarded in a puncture-proof sharps container. The filter paper should be disposed of in the biohazard waste container.

> ### Quality Assurance
>
> Quality assurance is involved in several aspects of the bleeding-time test. The proper area of the arm must be used, and the alcohol-cleansed site must be allowed to dry completely before the test is performed. Pediatric-sized bleeding-time devices should be used when performing the test on infants and children. In addition, the filter paper should touch only the drop of blood, not the wound itself. Stopwatches must be checked for accuracy on a regular basis.

### Ivy Bleeding Time

The Ivy bleeding-time test is performed by making an incision in the forearm and measuring the time required for bleeding to stop.

This method is usually performed using devices such as Simplate® or Surgicutt®, which make a more standardized incision than a lancet or blade (Figures 3-3 and 3-4). Proper incision depth and length differs for infants and children and for adults. Bleeding-time devices are available in sizes appropriate for these groups. Patients must be informed that this procedure may cause scarring.

A blood-pressure cuff is placed around the patient's arm above the elbow, and the pressure is increased to 40 mm of mercury to standardize the pres-

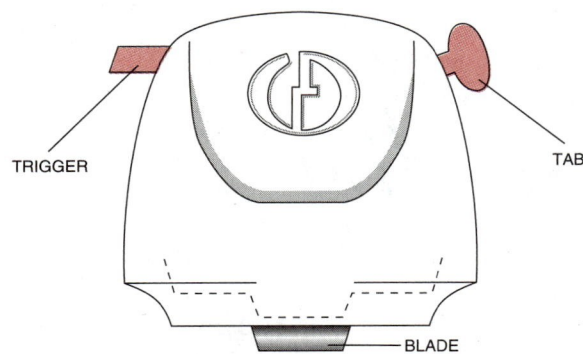

**FIGURE 3-3** Illustration of Simplate® device used in bleeding-time test

sure in the capillaries. This pressure is held constant for the entire procedure.

The forearm is cleansed with 70% alcohol. A standardized incision is made in an area free of large superficial blood vessels (Figure 3-4). A stopwatch is started when the first drop of blood appears. At thirty-second intervals, the blood is blotted with filter paper without touching the puncture site. When bleeding ceases, the time is noted and the pressure cuff removed. The time between the first appearance of blood and the stopping of blood flow is the bleeding time.

Normal bleeding time by the Ivy method is two to nine minutes (Table 3-4).

### Duke Bleeding Time

The Duke bleeding-time test was used for many years but is rarely performed today. The Duke bleeding time test is performed by making an incision in the earlobe and measuring the time required for bleeding to cease.

To perform the test, the earlobe is cleansed with alcohol and allowed to dry. A puncture is made with a sterile lancet and timing is begun when the first drop of blood appears. The blood is blotted every thirty seconds with filter paper without touching the actual puncture site. The watch is stopped when bleeding ceases. The time elapsed is reported as the bleeding time. Normal bleeding time by the Duke method is one to three minutes (Table 3-4).

**Table 3-4.** Reference ranges for bleeding time tests*

| METHOD | REFERENCE RANGE |
| --- | --- |
| Ivy | 2–9 minutes |
| Duke | 1–3 minutes |

*Each laboratory should establish its own reference ranges for bleeding time.

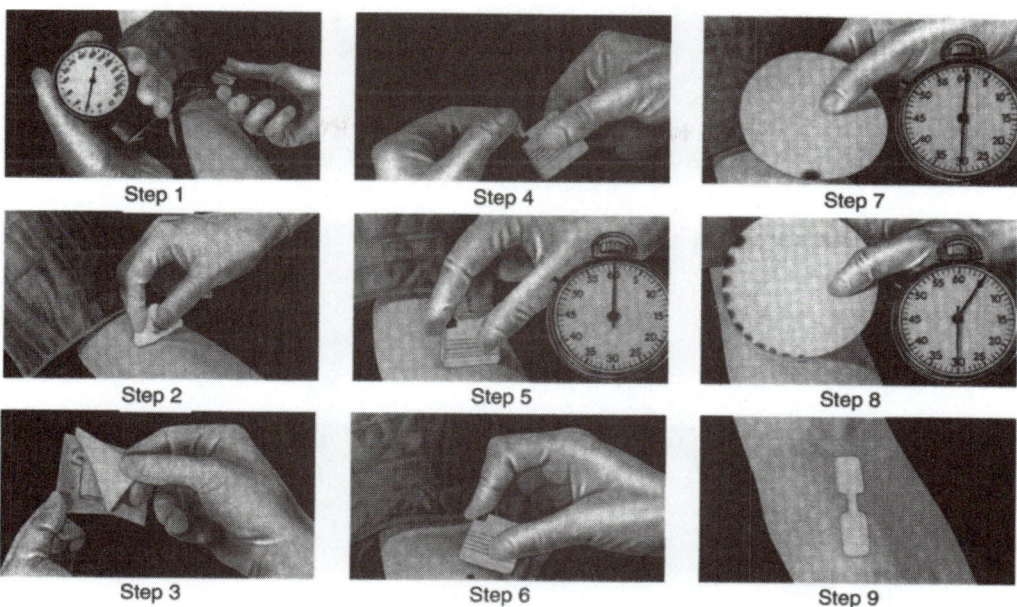

Step 1 · Step 4 · Step 7
Step 2 · Step 5 · Step 8
Step 3 · Step 6 · Step 9

**FIGURE 3-4** Surgicutt® bleeding time procedure

## Procedural Notes

- Do not perform the bleeding-time test if the patient has taken aspirin products within the last seven days.
- Ensure that the incision site is warm before performing the test.
- Choose an incision site free of superficial veins.
- Allow the alcohol-cleansed puncture site to dry completely before making the incision.
- Do not wipe away the first drop of blood that appears after the incision is made.
- Touch only the drop of blood, not the incision, with the filter paper.
- Stop the test if bleeding continues more than fifteen minutes in the Ivy test.

## Safety Precautions

- Observe Universal and Standard Precautions.
- Discard the used puncture device in the biohazard sharps container.
- Discard the used filter paper in the appropriate biohazard waste container.

## LESSON REVIEW

1. What functions are measured by the bleeding-time test?
2. What three components interact to produce hemostasis?
3. How do the number and function of platelets affect the bleeding time?
4. Explain the procedure for the Ivy bleeding-time test.
5. Describe the quality assurance procedures that must be observed when performing the bleeding-time test.
6. State the reference range for bleeding time by the Ivy method.
7. List safety precautions that should be observed when performing a bleeding-time test.
8. What incision site is used for the Ivy method? For the Duke method?
9. Define dysfunction and hemorrhage.

## STUDENT ACTIVITIES

1. Reread the information on bleeding time.
2. Review the glossary terms.
3. Practice explaining the bleeding-time procedure to a patient.
4. Practice performing a bleeding-time test as outlined on the Student Performance Guide.

## Student Performance Guide

### LESSON 3-3 Bleeding Time

Name _____ Date _____

### ☣ INSTRUCTIONS

1. Practice performing a bleeding-time test (Ivy method) following the step-by-step procedure.
2. Demonstrate your understanding of this lesson by:
   a. Completing a written examination successfully, and
   b. Performing the bleeding-time procedure satisfactorily for the instructor. All steps must be completed as listed on the instructor's Performance Check Sheet.

*Note: Always follow manufacturer's directions.*

### MATERIALS AND EQUIPMENT

- gloves
- hand disinfectant
- sterile cotton balls or gauze
- 70% alcohol or alcohol swabs
- blood-pressure cuff
- filter paper
- stopwatch
- surface disinfectant (10% chlorine bleach solution)
- biohazard container
- puncture-proof container for sharps
- butterfly bandage
- commercial bleeding-time device such as Simplate® or Surgicutt®

### PROCEDURE

Record in the comment section any problems encountered while practicing the procedure (or have a fellow student or the instructor evaluate your performance).

S = Satisfactory
U = Unsatisfactory

| You must: | S | U | Comments |
|---|---|---|---|
| 1. Wash hands and put on gloves | | | |
| 2. Assemble equipment and materials | | | |
| 3. Explain the procedure to the patient | | | |
| 4. Seat the patient and explain that the test can cause a small scar; have the patient rest the arm palm side up | | | |
| 5. Choose a site containing no visible blood vessels on the volar surface approximately 5 cm below the cubital crease | | | |
| 6. Cleanse the site with 70% alcohol. Wait for the alcohol to dry completely | | | |
| 7. Place the blood-pressure cuff on the arm above the elbow and inflate to 40mm Hg pressure (for adults). Maintain that pressure during the test | | | |

| You must: | S | U | Comments |
|---|---|---|---|
| 8. Set a sharps-disposal container within reach | | | |
| 9. Prepare the incision device following manufacturer's instructions; place the device on the surface of the clean site within 30 seconds of inflating the cuff. The incision should be either parallel or perpendicular to the bend of the elbow | | | |
| 10. Push the trigger to release the blade(s); start the stopwatch | | | |
| 11. Discard the device into the sharps container | | | |
| 12. Touch the filter paper to the drop of blood after 30 seconds; do not touch the wound | | | |
| 13. Repeat step 12 every 30 seconds until no blood appears on the filter paper | | | |
| 14. Stop the watch | | | |
| 15. *Remove the blood pressure cuff.* | | | |
| 16. Wash the site gently with a non-alcohol wipe; when dry, apply a butterfly bandage to minimize the chance of scarring. Advise the patient to leave the bandage in place for twenty-four hours | | | |
| 17. Discard filter paper in biohazard container | | | |
| 18. Wipe the work area with surface disinfectant | | | |
| 19. Remove and discard gloves in biohazard container. Wash hands with hand disinfectant | | | |
| 20. Report results as the time on the stopwatch | | | |

*Evaluator Comments:*

Evaluator _____  Date _____

# Prothrombin Time

## LESSON OBJECTIVES

**After studying this lesson, you should be able to:**

■ *Discuss the role of prothrombin in blood coagulation.*
■ *Explain the major use of the prothrombin time test.*
■ *Perform a prothrombin time test.*
■ *State the reference values for the prothrombin time test.*
■ *Name three POCT instruments for prothrombin time.*
■ *Define the glossary terms.*

## GLOSSARY

**coumarin** / an anticoagulant administered orally to prevent or slow clotting

**enzyme** / a protein that causes or accelerates changes in other substances without being changed itself

**prothrombin time (PT)** / a coagulation-screening test used to monitor oral anticoagulant therapy

## INTRODUCTION

The **prothrombin time (PT)** or "pro time," one of the most frequently performed coagulation tests, evaluates the function of the extrinsic and common pathways of hemostasis. It is used not only as a coagulation screening test, but also to monitor oral anticoagulant therapy. The PT is especially effective for monitoring patients receiving **coumarin**. Patients may have the PT performed in a physician office laboratory (POL), a hospital outpatient laboratory, or a reference laboratory. PT results can be used to guide the physician in regulating the patient's anticoagulant dosage.

## PRINCIPLE OF THE PROTHROMBIN TIME

The hemostasis pathway is normally activated when damage occurs to blood vessel endothelium or to body tissue. The extrinsic pathway converts Factor X, a proenzyme, to the enzyme $X_a$ which in turn converts prothrombin to the enzyme thrombin. An **enzyme** is a

protein that is able to cause or accelerate changes in other substances without being changed. Thrombin acts on fibrinogen to form fibrin monomers that make up the initial unstable clot. The simplified reactions are:

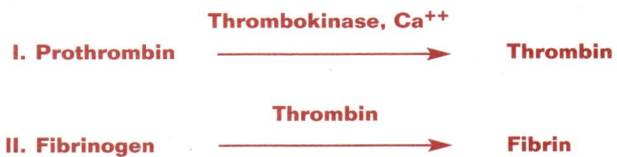

**I. Prothrombin** $\xrightarrow{\text{Thrombokinase, Ca}^{++}}$ **Thrombin**

**II. Fibrinogen** $\xrightarrow{\text{Thrombin}}$ **Fibrin**

## PROTHROMBIN TIME TEST

Prothrombin (Factor II) is produced in the liver and is vitamin K dependent. A deficiency of vitamin K causes reduced amounts of the factor to be produced and can result in bleeding. The prothrombin time is used as a coagulation-screening test to measure the extrinsic pathway. Its major use is to monitor oral anticoagulant therapy since these anticoagulants decrease the production of prothrombin and factors VII, IX, and X in the liver. The test was developed by Dr. A. J. Quick, who named it "prothrombin time" because he thought it measured only prothrombin. Even though it was later discovered that the test actually measures prothrombin plus additional factors, it is still called the prothrombin time.

## Reference Values for Prothrombin Time

The reference values for prothrombin time vary slightly from one laboratory to another because of different techniques used. When the manual-tilt method or a fibrometer method is used, the expected value on citrated samples from healthy individuals is commonly accepted to be 11 to 13 seconds. When other techniques are used, the laboratory must determine its own reference values. Table 3-5 gives examples of the effects of certain conditions on the prothrombin time.

## Use of Prothrombin Time Results

When a patient is receiving oral anticoagulants, a prothrombin time is performed at regular intervals, sometimes weekly. The physician can use the results to regulate the anticoagulant dose. The usual goal is to keep the patient's prothrombin time at about 16 to 18 seconds, or 1.3 to 1.5 times the normal control value. This degree of prolongation is usually sufficient to prevent unwanted clotting, but not so long that the patient suffers abnormal bleeding.

Prothrombin times may be reported in three ways: (1) in seconds, (2) as the prothrombin time ratio (PT ratio), or (3) as the International Normalized Ratio (INR). The PT ratio is obtained by dividing the patient's prothrombin time by the prothrombin time of the normal control. The INR is calculated by using the patient's prothrombin time, the prothrombin time of the normal control plasma, and an index supplied by the manufacturer for each lot of thromboplastin.

## PERFORMING THE PROTHROMBIN TIME

To perform the PT, a commercial reagent, thromboplastin-CaCl$_2$, is added to patient plasma and the time required for a fibrin clot to form is measured. The prothrombin time has been automated for several years; however, some laboratories still perform the test manually. Most commercial reagents can be used for either method, but the instructions for each must be followed carefully.

Many coagulation analyzers are on the market. A fibrometer such as the Fibrosystem® from Becton Dickinson is a popular choice if the prothrombin time is the only coagulation assay desired.

 **Safety**

Performing the prothrombin time involves handling patient blood and control plasmas. In addition, the technician may also perform the venipuncture and process the specimen before testing it. Universal and Standard Precautions must be observed to protect the worker from bloodborne pathogens.

| **Table 3-5.** Prothrombin time results in various conditions | |
| --- | --- |
| **CONDITION** | **PROTHROMBIN TIME RESULTS** |
| **Factor Deficiencies** | |
| VIII | Normal |
| XI | Normal |
| XII | Normal |
| II | Prolonged |
| V | Prolonged |
| VII | Prolonged |
| X | Prolonged |
| **Other Conditions** | |
| Coumarin therapy | Prolonged |
| Heparin therapy | Prolonged |
| Liver disease | Prolonged |
| Vitamin K deficiency | Prolonged |

### *Quality Assurance*

Quality assurance for the prothrombin-time test includes collecting and processing the specimen, analyzing control plasmas, and performing the test procedure. The venipuncture must be clean, since trauma to the vein or surrounding tissues releases tissue factor into the specimen. The ratio of anticoagulant to blood is critical: one part anticoagulant to nine parts blood. The filled tube should be immediately inverted *gently* to mix the blood and anticoagulant. In the process of separating the plasma from the blood cells by centrifugation, the tube of blood must be stoppered to prevent exposure to the air. All specimens, controls, and instruments must be at the proper temperature before the test is performed.

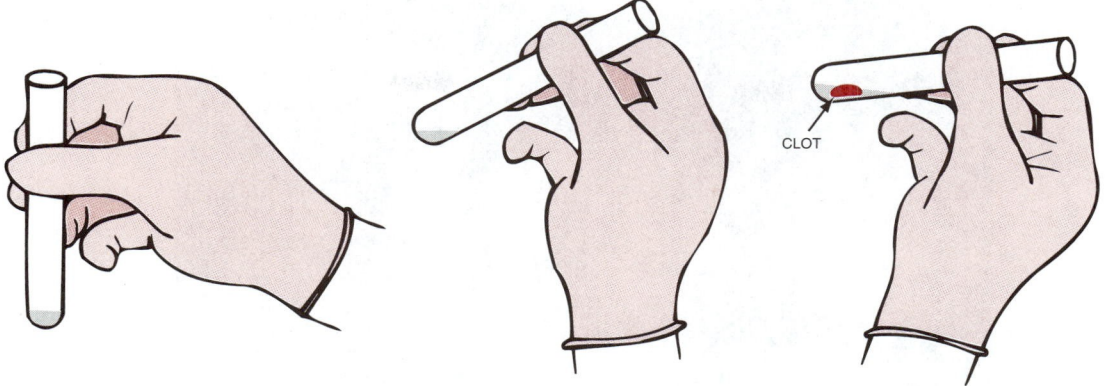

**FIGURE 3-5** Illustration of the manual tilt-tube prothrombin time method: (Left) lift tube out of waterbath; (center) tilt tube horizontally; and (right) observe formation of fibrin clot

## Collecting the Specimen

The prothrombin time specimen must be drawn with minimal trauma to the vein and surrounding tissue to prevent the release of tissue thromboplastin into the sample. The blood is drawn into a tube or syringe containing an anticoagulant compatible with the commercial reagent system being used. Most systems for prothrombin time are compatible with a 3.8% solution of sodium citrate, but the instructions for each method must be consulted. Vacuum tubes that contain the proper quantity and concentration of citrate are available (Table 2-1 page 114). The blood must be centrifuged as soon as possible and the plasma transferred to a clean tube for use in the assay. The plasma should be assayed within four hours of blood collection and should not stand at 37°C for more than five minutes before being tested.

## Manual Method

To perform a manual prothrombin time, the patient's plasma and the thromboplastin reagents are pipetted into separate labeled test tubes that are warmed by being placed in a 37°C waterbath for a prescribed amount of time. When the warming time has elapsed, 0.1 mL of the patient's plasma is forcibly added to 0.2 mL of reagent. A stopwatch is started at the same time. The tube is allowed to remain in the waterbath about 10 seconds. It is then removed and the outside is quickly wiped to remove water droplets. The tube is held horizontally at eye level in front of a good light source. The tube is immediately tilted back and forth until a thickening appears (Figure 3-5). This is the fibrin clot. At the first appearance of the clot, the stopwatch is stopped and the time recorded in seconds. It is generally recom-

mended that manual determinations be performed in triplicate. Timing of the first one will be approximate and the other two should agree with each other.

## Automated Method–Fibrometer

The use of an instrument to determine prothrombin time eliminates the need for a waterbath. Fibrometers have built-in heat blocks to warm the samples, controls, and reagents (Figure 3-6). The samples and reagents are pipetted into special cups that fit into the heat wells of the instrument. After the specified warming time has elapsed, the cup containing the reagent is placed in the center well of the instrument. The automatic pipetter on the instrument is used to draw up and then expel the patient sample into the reagent. The timer automatically starts when the sample is expelled. Two wire probes detect the formation of the clot and stop the timer. The elapsed time is read directly off the instrument. Automated determinations should be performed in duplicate and the results averaged. Abnormal and normal plasma controls are analyzed in the same manner.

## Other Prothrombin Analyzers

Many coagulation analyzers are available with large test menus for patient specimens. The majority of these are designed for high-volume laboratories and are discussed in Lesson 2-13, Principles of Automated Hematology. However, the prothrombin time is available on several of the smaller handheld devices used in home and POCT. Examples of these are the CoaguChek™ (distributed by Roche Diagnostics Corporation), the Hemochron® Jr. (International Technidyne Corp), and GEM™ PCL (Instrumentation Laboratory). These instruments are discussed in more detail in Lesson 3-6.

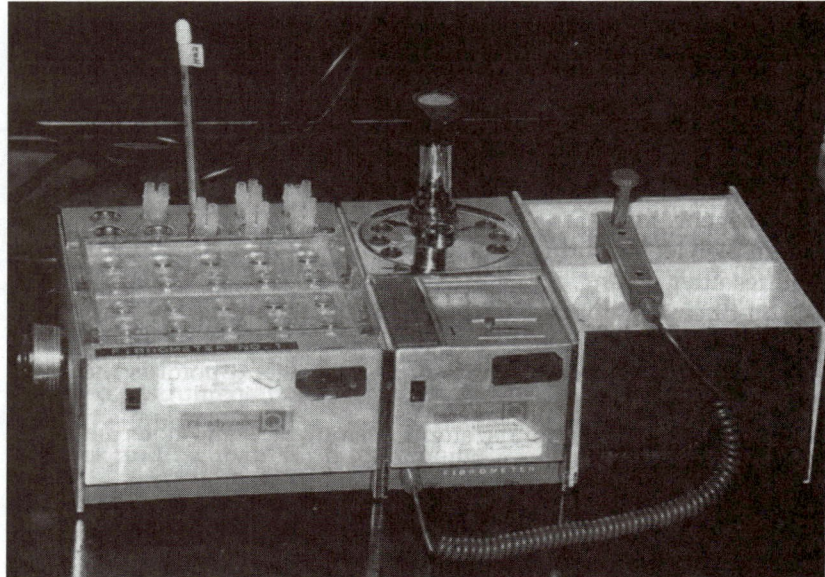

**FIGURE 3-6** Fibrometer

## Procedural Notes

- Keep waterbath or heat block temperature at 37°C.

- Warm test sample and reagents for the times specified in the package inserts and manufacturer's instructions.

- Follow an established quality-control program, testing both normal and abnormal plasmas.

- Avoid trauma to vein and surrounding tissues when performing a venipuncture for prothrombin time.

## Safety Precautions

- Observe Universal and Standard Precautions.

- Treat all control solutions as if potentially infectious.

## LESSON REVIEW

1. What is the role of prothrombin in blood coagulation?

2. How does the physician use results from the prothrombin time?

3. Explain how a manual prothrombin time is performed.

4. Explain how to perform a prothrombin time using a fibrometer.

5. What is the reference value for the prothrombin time test?

6. List three ways of reporting prothrombin times.

7. What is the desired range for the prothrombin time of a patient receiving oral anticoagulant therapy?

8. What anticoagulant is used to collect blood for a prothrombin time?

9. List four conditions in which the prothrombin time is prolonged.

10. Define coumarin drugs, enzyme, and prothrombin time.

## STUDENT ACTIVITIES

1. Reread the information on prothrombin time.

2. Review the glossary terms.

3. Practice performing the prothrombin time as outlined on the Student Performance Guide.

# Student Performance Guide

## LESSON 3-4 Prothrombin Time

Name _____    Date _____

  ### INSTRUCTIONS

1. Practice performing the prothrombin time test following the step-by-step procedure.
2. Demonstrate your understanding of this lesson by:
   a. Completing a written examination successfully, and
   b. Performing the prothrombin time test satisfactorily for the instructor. All steps must be completed as listed on the instructor's Performance Check Sheet.

*Note:* Follow manufacturer's directions for instrument and reagents used

## MATERIALS AND EQUIPMENT

- gloves
- centrifuge
- commercial source of thromboplastin-$CaCl_2$
- fresh citrated human plasma
- normal controls
- abnormal controls
- distilled water for reconstituting controls
- biohazard container
- surface disinfectant (10% chlorine bleach solution)
- laboratory tissue
- hand disinfectant
- test tube rack

### For Manual Method
- test tubes (13 x 75 mm)
- waterbath at 37°C
- pipets to transfer 0.1 and 0.2 mL
- stopwatch

### For Automated Method
- coagulation instrument, such as fibrometer
- supplies for instrument

## PROCEDURE

Record in the comment section any problems encountered while practicing the procedure (or have a fellow student or the instructor evaluate your performance).

S = Satisfactory
U = Unsatisfactory

| You must: | S | U | Comments |
|---|---|---|---|
| 1. Wash hands and put on gloves | | | |
| 2. Obtain citrated blood sample (if not provided) | | | |
| 3. Centrifuge the specimen as specified in reagent package insert | | | |
| 4. Remove the plasma and transfer to a clean test tube. Label with patient identification | | | |
| 5. Perform a manual prothrombin time:<br>a. Check that waterbath temperature is 37°C | | | |

| You must: | S | U | Comments |
|---|---|---|---|
| b. Pipet 0.2 mL of thromboplastin-CaCl$_2$ reagent into seven labeled tubes (three for the patient, two for each normal and abnormal control) <br><br> c. Place tubes in rack in waterbath <br><br> d. Pipet sufficient patient plasma and control plasmas (0.4-0.5 mL each) to perform the test in triplicate in another set of appropriately labeled tubes <br><br> e. Place tubes in rack in waterbath <br><br> f. Allow patient sample, controls, and reagent to warm for the prescribed amount of time <br><br> g. Draw up 0.1 mL patient plasma and forcibly expel into tube containing reagent, starting stopwatch simultaneously <br><br> h. Allow tube to remain in waterbath about ten seconds before picking it up and rapidly wiping water from outside of tube <br><br> i. *Work quickly*—pick up the tube, wipe the outside with tissue, start tilting tube slowly back and forth in front of good light source <br><br> j. Stop the watch at the first sign of thickening (clot) in the moving liquid and record the time <br><br> k. Repeat steps g–j using another tube of warmed reagent. Remember that the first time is approximate, and the second and third should agree with each other <br><br> l. Perform steps g–j in duplicate for each control sample <br><br> m. Report results: Report average of patient's second and third times; record the times for the controls | | | |
| 6. Perform an automated prothrombin time: <br> (If instrument is not available, proceed to step 7) <br><br> a. Turn on instrument. If using the instrument's pipetter, be certain it is turned "OFF" <br><br> b. Label desired number of sample cups and place in heat block (patient samples should be run in duplicate) <br><br> c. Pipet 0.2 mL of thromboplastin-CaCl$_2$ into cups, following manufacturer's instructions <br><br> d. Pipet sufficient patient plasma and controls (0.4–0.5 mL) into separate cups to allow for duplicate testing of patient and controls <br><br> e. Allow all components to warm the prescribed amount of time. Place one sample cup with measured thromboplastin-CaCl$_2$ into center well of fibrometer <br><br> f. Draw up 0.1 mL of patient plasma <br><br> g. Turn pipetter "ON" <br><br> h. Expel plasma into center cup containing 0.2 mL thromboplastin-CaCl$_2$. The timer will start automatically when the plunger is depressed, if using instrument's pipet | | | |

| You must: | S | U | Comments |
|---|---|---|---|
| i.  Wait for timer to stop, signaling the formation of a clot<br>j.  Record the time in seconds<br>k.  Gently wipe probe wires with laboratory tissue between determinations<br>l.  Repeat steps e–k using patient plasma<br>m. Average the two times and report the results<br>n.  Repeat steps e–k for each control<br>o.  Record the times for the controls<br>p.  Turn off instrument | | | |
| 7.  Return all equipment to proper storage | | | |
| 8.  Dispose of all contaminated articles in biohazard container and contaminated sharps in sharps container | | | |
| 9.  Wipe counter with surface disinfectant | | | |
| 10. Remove and discard gloves in biohazard container | | | |
| 11. Wash hands with hand disinfectant | | | |

*Evaluator Comments:*

Evaluator _____ Date _____

# Activated Partial Thromboplastin Time

## LESSON OBJECTIVES

After studying this lesson, you should be able to:

- *Explain the principle of the activated partial thromboplastin time (APTT).*
- *Explain the reasons for performing an APTT.*
- *Explain which parts of the coagulation pathway are checked in the APTT.*
- *List the coagulation factor deficiencies detected by the APTT.*
- *Give the reference values for the APTT.*
- *List precautions to be observed when performing the APTT.*
- *Define the glossary terms.*

## GLOSSARY

**cephaloplastin** / a commercial preparation of partial thromboplastin

**partial thromboplastin** / the lipid portion of thromboplastin, available as a commercial preparation

## INTRODUCTION

The activated partial thromboplastin time (APTT) is used to monitor heparin therapy and screen for function of the intrinsic and common pathways of hemostasis. The APTT is named because the test reagent contains activators such as kaolin or silica to activate the contact factors in the intrinsic pathway. The test is sensitive to mild deficiencies of factors XII, XI, IX, and VIII and Fletcher and Fitzgerald factors. It is also useful for detecting deficiencies of factors X, V, II, and fibrinogen (I), although these factor deficiencies must be slightly more severe to cause a prolonged APTT. Factors VII, XIII, and platelet factor 3 (PF3) are not assayed in the APTT.

**Partial thromboplastin (cephaloplastin)** is the reagent used in performing the APTT. Partial thrombo-plastin, the lipid portion of tissue thromboplastin, is manufactured from human or bovine brain tissue or derived from soybeans. Since partial thromboplastin performs the function of PF3 in the APTT test, platelet abnormalities will have no effect on the APTT.

The formation of a fibrin clot in the APTT can occur only if factors in the intrinsic pathway—XII, XI, IX, and VIII—and those in the common pathway—I, II, V, and X—are present in sufficient amounts and are functional (Table 3-6).

## PERFORMING THE ACTIVATED PARTIAL THROMBOPLASTIN TIME

The APTT can be performed manually or by instrumentation. In a laboratory where only a few of the tests are

**Table 3-6.** Hemostasis pathways and coagulation factors tested by the APTT

| FACTORS OF INTRINSIC PATHWAY | FACTORS OF COMMON PATHWAY |
|---|---|
| XII | I |
| XI | II |
| IX | V |
| VIII | X |
| Fitzgerald | |
| Fletcher | |

performed, the manual method may be used. However, most laboratories use a fibrometer or other instrument to perform the APTT. When instrumentation is not available, the specimen may be sent to a reference laboratory.

In larger laboratories, automated instruments are available that perform the PT, APTT, and other tests on the same instrument. The patient and control plasma samples and reagents are usually pipetted into small plastic cups and preheated in a heat block provided with the instrument. However, some instruments automatically sample directly from the tube of plasma.

 ## Safety

Universal and Standard Precautions must be observed to protect the worker from exposure to bloodborne pathogens. Performing the APTT (aPTT) may expose the worker to the patient's blood specimen unless the coagulation instrument can sample through the stopper. Appropriate personal protective equipment must be used.

### Quality Assurance

The specimen used for coagulation testing must be collected with care. The venipuncture must be performed with as little trauma as possible to avoid contaminating the sample with tissue factor released when the vein is punctured. When possible, the blood should be collected without using a blood pressure cuff or tourniquet. If a tourniquet is used, it should be left on less than a minute to prevent blood concentrating in that area. Hemoconcentration can activate some clotting factors and cause platelet release reactions, interfering with test results. Control plasmas must be run and be within assay limits before results are reported.

## Collecting the Specimen

Blood is collected using sodium citrate anticoagulant. The proportions are one part sodium citrate (0.5 ml) to nine parts (4.5 ml) blood. Vacuum tubes are available containing this volume and also in a smaller size for pediatric use. After collection, the whole blood sample is centrifuged, and the plasma is removed and placed in another tube. The plasma should be stored covered at 4°C until used for the test. The test should be run within four hours of collection.

## Using the Fibrometer to Perform the APTT

The APTT is performed using the patient's plasma, the activated partial thromboplastin (cephaloplastin), and $CaCl_2$. The $CaCl_2$ is added to replace the $Ca^{++}$ removed from the plasma by the anticoagulant. Normal and abnormal control plasmas are also run. The cephaloplastin, $CaCl_2$, and plasmas are pipetted into the fibrometer cups, which are placed in the heat block to prewarm to 37°C for three to five minutes, but no longer than ten minutes.

When all reagents have been prewarmed, 0.1 mL cephaloplastin is pipetted into enough cups for each sample to be run in duplicate. To perform a control APTT assay, 0.1 mL of normal control plasma is added to one of the cups of cephaloplastin. The mixture of plasma-cephaloplastin is allowed to warm and activate for three minutes. To initiate the clotting reaction, 0.1 mL of the prewarmed $CaCl_2$ is added to the plasma-cephaloplastin mixture using the automatic pipet of the fibrometer. The probe is lowered into the sample, and the timer on the instrument will start and continue running until the probe detects a fibrin clot. The time in seconds is displayed on the instrument.

When the control plasmas have been run (in duplicate) and have been determined to be within control limits, the patient samples are run in duplicate using the same procedure. The times from the duplicate patient assays are averaged and the average time in seconds is reported.

## REFERENCE VALUES FOR THE APTT

The mean reference value for the normal APTT is usually about thirty-five seconds. Some laboratories use a range of 31–39 seconds. It is best if each laboratory establishes its own normal range by periodically running a batch of "normal" plasmas. When these normals are performed using the exact procedure used for patient samples, the test results are more reliable. Table

3-7 gives examples of conditions that affect the APTT. When the APTT is used to monitor heparin therapy, the usual goal is to keep the patient's APTT 1.5–2.0 times the APTT of the normal plasma control.

**Table 3-7.** Various conditions that affect the APTT

| CONDITIONS | EFFECTS ON APTT |
|---|---|
| **Factor Deficiencies** | |
| I, II, V, VIII, IX, X, XI, XII | Prolonged |
| VII, XIII | No effect |
| **Other Conditions** | |
| Heparin therapy | Prolonged |
| Vitamin K deficiency | Prolonged |

### Procedural Notes

- Read and follow the manufacturer's instructions for the reagents and instruments used.
- Perform venipuncture with care.
- Use the proper ratio of blood to anticoagulant.
- Remove plasma from RBCs promptly and perform test within four hours of collection.

### Safety Precautions

- Observe Universal and Standard Precautions.
- Handle control plasma as if potentially infectious.
- Discard used needles in biohazard sharps container.

## LESSON REVIEW

1. Which hemostasis pathway is measured by the APTT?
2. What conditions could cause a prolonged APTT?
3. What is one use of the APTT?
4. List two coagulation factors not measured by the APTT.
5. Why does the APTT not measure the extrinsic pathway of hemostasis?
6. Why is $CaCl_2$ added in the APTT?
7. Why is the activating agent added to the plasma during the APTT?
8. Define cephaloplastin and partial thromboplastin.

## STUDENT ACTIVITIES

1. Reread the information on the APTT.
2. Review the glossary terms.
3. Practice performing the APTT as outlined on the Student Performance Guide.

## *Student Performance Guide*

## **LESSON 3-5** Activated Partial Thromboplastin Time

Name _____   Date _____

### ☣ INSTRUCTIONS

1. Practice performing the APTT following the step-by-step procedure.
2. Demonstrate your understanding of this lesson by:
   a. Completing a written examination successfully, and
   b. Performing the APTT satisfactorily for the instructor. All steps must be completed as listed on the instructor's Performance Check Sheet.

*Note:* Follow manufacturers' instructions for instrument and reagents used.

### MATERIALS AND EQUIPMENT

- gloves
- venipuncture materials required for obtaining citrated blood, or citrated blood sample
- clinical centrifuge
- commercial control plasma
- biohazard container
- puncture-proof container for sharps
- hand disinfectant
- surface disinfectant (10% chlorine bleach solution)
- fibrometer and pipetter (or other coagulation analyzer)
- fibrometer tips and cups
- 37°C heat block
- commercial activated cephaloplastin (partial thromboplastin)
- $CaCl_2$, 0.02 M

### PROCEDURE

Record in the comment section any problems encountered while practicing the procedure (or have a fellow student or the instructor evaluate your performance).

S = Satisfactory
U = Unsatisfactory

| You must: | S | U | Comments |
|---|---|---|---|
| 1. Wash hands and put on gloves | | | |
| 2. Assemble materials and equipment and turn on instrument to warm up | | | |
| 3. Obtain citrated blood sample by venipuncture and label with patient's name (or use commercial plasma controls) | | | |
| 4. Centrifuge the blood sample for five minutes at 1,500 rpm to obtain the plasma | | | |
| 5. Follow instructions for the instrument being used. Check to see that heat block is at 37°C | | | |
| 6. Reconstitute the activated cephaloplastin according to manufacturer's instructions | | | |

| You must: | S | U | Comments |
|---|---|---|---|
| 7. Label instrument cups: normal control, abnormal control, patient name, cephaloplastin, and $CaCl_2$ | | | |
| 8. Pipet enough cephaloplastin into reagent cup(s) to have 0.1 mL for each test (which should be run in duplicate) | | | |
| 9. Pipet enough control plasma into labeled cups to have 0.1 mL for each test | | | |
| 10. Pipet into the reagent cups enough $CaCl_2$ to have 0.1 mL for each test | | | |
| 11. Allow reagents and plasmas to prewarm for at least three minutes and not more than ten minutes | | | |
| 12. Place a clean cup in the reaction well of the instrument and pipet 0.1 mL cephaloplastin into it | | | |
| 13. Perform the APTT on a normal control plasma by pipetting 0.1 mL of normal control into the cup containing the 0.1 mL of prewarmed cephaloplastin (in the reaction well) | | | |
| 14. Let the mixture warm and activate for three minutes | | | |
| 15. Draw up 0.1 mL prewarmed $CaCl_2$, turn on pipetter, and dispense $CaCl_2$ into the cup in the reaction well. The probe will lower into the cup and the timer will start automatically and stop when a fibrin clot is detected | | | |
| 16. Record the time from the instrument's timer | | | |
| 17. Repeat the test (steps 13–16) on the normal control plasma | | | |
| 18. Average the results and report the APTT in seconds | | | |
| 19. Perform the APTT in duplicate using the abnormal control plasma, following steps 13–18 | | | |
| 20. If all control values are within acceptable limits, repeat steps 13–18, using patient plasma | | | |
| 21. Dispose of all biohazard waste in biohazard container | | | |
| 22. Dispose of contaminated sharps in sharps container | | | |
| 23. Turn instrument off and return all equipment to proper storage | | | |
| 24. Wipe counter with surface disinfectant | | | |
| 25. Remove and discard gloves in biohazard container; wash hands with hand disinfectant | | | |

*Evaluator Comments:*

Evaluator _____ Date _____

# *Rapid Tests for Hemostasis Disorders*

**After studying this lesson, you should be able to:**

- *List two conditions that could require rapid hemostasis testing.*
- *Discuss the role of heparin in heart diagnostic procedures.*
- *Discuss the reasons for close monitoring of heparin levels.*
- *Explain the breakdown of fibrinogen and fibrin into smaller molecules.*
- *Perform a test for the degradation products of cross-linked fibrin.*
- *Perform a test for activated clotting time.*
- *Define the glossary terms.*

## GLOSSARY

**angioplasty** / surgical repair of a vessel

**D-dimer** / a small molecule cleaved from cross-linked fibrin in a clot by plasmin during fibrinolysis

**disseminated intravascular coagulation** / a bleeding disorder characterized by widespread thrombotic and secondary fibrinolytic reactions

**FDP** / fibrinogen-degradation products formed when plasmin cleaves fibrinogen

**XDP** / fibrin-degradation products that contain the D-dimer cross-linked region

## INTRODUCTION

Many situations may arise that require quick and easily obtainable hemostasis test results. For example, patients undergoing cardiac **angioplasty** are given the anticoagulant heparin to prevent thrombosis. Heparin is also administered to patients for other conditions. Heparin inhibits the activated forms of Factors IX, X, XI, and XII, as well as platelet release factor.

Not only do patients vary in their sensitivity to heparin, but heparin from different sources has varying activity. Because of this, heparin levels must be closely monitored to maintain the proper balance between bleeding and thrombosis. Two hemostasis tests used to monitor heparin therapy are the activated clotting time (ACT) and the activated partial thromboplastin time (APTT). New technologies allow the specimen to be analyzed at or near the patient's bedside, decreasing the time required to obtain results. These POCT are performed on small, portable instruments. Less than 50 µL of blood is required for many of the tests, an important consideration if the patient's condition demands frequent testing.

Mechanisms that normally keep clotting and dissolution of the clot in balance sometimes malfunction. Pathological clotting or excessive dissolution (lysis) of clots may occur. Degradation of the fibrin clot releases products that can be measured using rapid slide tests. These tests are useful in conditions such as disseminated intravascular coagulation, deep vein thrombosis, and pulmonary embolism.

**Disseminated intravascular coagulation (DIC)** is a serious situation in which widespread thromboses and a secondary hemorrhagic condition occur. Bleeding develops as a result of fibrinolysis combined with depletion of platelets and coagulation factors used up in the formation of the many clots. Patients can develop DIC from injuries that cause widespread damage to the vascular system, such as those received in construction mishaps, auto accidents, explosions, and earthquakes. Certain bacterial and viral infections can also cause DIC. As clotting progresses, fibrinolysis occurs, releasing fibrin- and fibrinogen-degradation products that have a further anticoagulant effect.

Deep vein thrombosis and pulmonary embolism are sometimes difficult to diagnose by clinical symptoms alone. If thrombi do exist, a slide test can detect an elevated level of fibrin- and fibrinogen-degradation products caused by increased fibrinolysis.

# RAPID HEMOSTASIS TESTS

## Manual Tests for Fibrinogen and Fibrin Degradation Products

In the common pathway of the coagulation "cascade," the enzyme thrombin acts as a catalyst for transforming fibrinogen to fibrin, forming an unstable clot. The fibrin strands in the unstable clot then begin to gel and are acted upon by Factor XIII$_a$. This forms a stable insoluble clot, in which the fibrin strands become cross-linked to each other in their D-Domain (D-dimer) region.

The balance between formation of clots and fibrinolysis is regulated by limiting factors such as plasmin. Both fibrin and fibrinogen are cleaved by plasmin to yield various degradation products. There are tests for fibrinogen-degradation products (**FDP**) and for fibrin-degradation products (**XDP**, for *cross*-linked). The FDP are formed from the action of plasma on circulating fibrinogen. XDP, derivatives of cross-linked fibrin containing D-dimers, are formed by the lysis of the stable fibrin clot (Figure 3-7). It is important to distinguish between FDP and XDP, since the presence of elevated XDP indicates a more serious condition.

### DADE® Dimertest® Latex Assay

The DADE® Dimertest® Latex Assay is specific for the D-dimers (XDP) formed from the degradation of stable fibrin. A highly specific monoclonal antibody (anti-D dimer) binds to any D-dimer present in the specimen. The quantity of D-dimer in the patient's plasma is proportional to the quantity of fibrin being cleaved.

The test can be used when conditions such as DIC, pulmonary embolism, and deep venous thrombosis are suspected, but cannot be diagnosed by clinical examination alone. The reference values for fibrin-degradation products are: any value less than 0.20 µg/mL is considered negative; any value greater than 0.20 µg/mL is considered positive.

## Portable Instruments

Many small handheld analyzers are available for performing hemostasis testing. Some of these test whole blood, while others require a plasma specimen. These instruments include International Technidyne Corporation's HEMOCHRON® Jr., Instrumentation Laboratory's GEM™ PCL and Array Medical's Actalyke™. All of these perform tests on small quantities of whole blood or plasma.

### HEMOCHRON® Jr. Whole Blood Microcoagulation System

The HEMOCHRON® Jr. Whole Blood Microcoagulation System performs the PT, the APTT, and the ACT (Figure 3-8). For each test, approximately 200 µL of whole blood is collected. This is added to a cuvette that has been prewarmed in the instrument. A 15 µL aliquot (of the 200 µl) is analyzed by the instrument.

To perform the PT, 15 µL of whole blood is automatically mixed with reagents contained in the cuvette

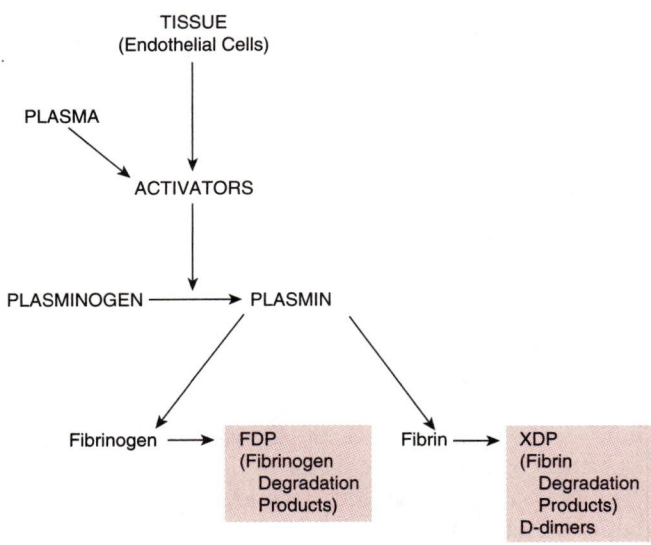

**FIGURE 3-7** Illustration of the fibrinolytic pathway showing formation of D-dimers

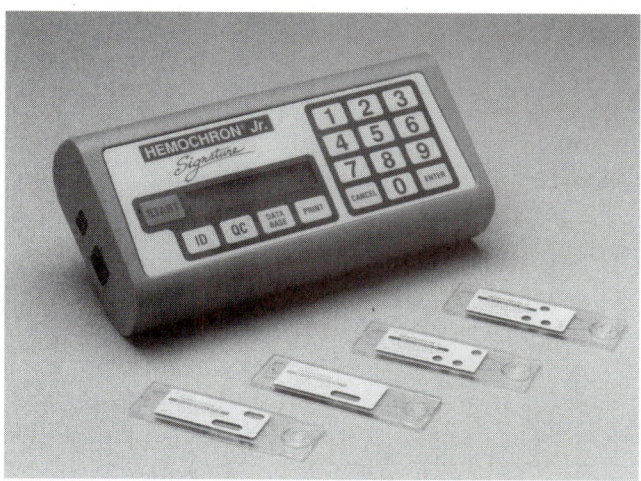

**FIGURE 3-8** HEMOCHRON® Jr. coagulation analyzer (Courtesy International Technidyne, Edison, NJ)

after it is inserted into the instrument. Inside the instrument, the sample is moved back and forth in test channels and monitored for clot formation. As the clot begins to form, a photometer with two optical detectors registers the endpoint when movement of the blood has slowed. The PT time is displayed as converted plasma value and as the International Normalized Ratio (INR).

The APTT is performed in a similar manner with a whole blood sample. The APTT result is displayed as a mathematically converted plasma equivalent value and as the whole blood APTT in seconds.

The ACT is a diagnostic test in which whole blood is added to a test tube containing a clotting activator such as kaolin, celite, silica, or glass particles. The ACT+ performed by the HEMOCHRON® Jr. uses a mixture of silica, kaolin, and phospholipid as the activator. The reaction takes place in the cuvette within the instrument. Detection of a clot by the photometer determines the test endpoint. The ACT+ test result is automatically converted to a reference celite-ACT value reported in seconds.

### Actalyke™ ACT System

The Actalyke™ Activated Clotting Time (ACT) Test System (Array Medical) is a portable battery-powered analyzer used to monitor heparin therapy. The protocol is similar to that for standard ACT test methods. The instrument is available in single- or dual-test well models. Whole blood is tested and the results are available in minutes.

### GEM™ PCL

The GEM™ PCL (Instrumentation Laboratory) requires 50 μL of whole blood each for the ACT, PT, and APTT.

Plasma samples from citrated blood can also be used for the PT and the APTT. Results are available in less than five minutes.

## PERFORMING THE TESTS

 **Safety**

Universal and Standard Precautions must be observed when handling patient specimens and the control blood or plasmas. Appropriate personal protective equipment should be used when collecting the blood specimen and performing the test. The fresh whole blood is obtained by venipuncture, presenting the danger of needlesticks. The positive controls for D-dimer tests are made from human D-dimer, and should be considered potentially infectious.

### *Quality Assurance*

Specimen collection must be performed following the manufacturer's instructions. Plasma from blood collected in citrate anticoagulant should be used for the D-dimer test and for PT and APTT plasma tests. Heparin or EDTA anticoagulants must not be used; they can cause a false positive reaction in the D-dimer test. The venipuncture must be clean to avoid the release of tissue thromboplastin into the specimen.

All reagents must be brought to room temperature before the tests are performed. Controls must be run with each batch of patient tests that are performed.

The pipetting for the D-dimer test must be very precise. Also, the test must be read immediately at the end of three minutes or the latex will dry out and cause a false positive reaction. Manufacturers' instructions for all test systems must be carefully followed.

### Performing the DADE® Dimertest® Latex Assay

The reagents are mixed with the patient's plasma on the slide provided in the test kit. The slide is rotated manually or on a rotator for three minutes. Under a strong light source, the reaction is checked for white agglutination (clumping) against the black background of the slide. Agglutination demonstrates the binding of the antibody on the latex beads to D-dimers in the specimen (Figure

3-9). If the result is positive, the results may be quantified by making serial dilutions of the plasma, using a buffer included in the kit.

## Performing the Activated Clotting Time Plus (ACT+) Using the HEMOCHRON® Jr.

The HEMOCHRON® Jr. test system requires a warmup period of approximately 90 seconds before the test is performed. One of the cuvettes provided is inserted into the instrument to initiate the pre-warm/self-check mode. If the specimen is from a capillary puncture, the second drop of blood is used to fill the fingerstick collection cup of the test cuvette. Venous blood can be drawn into a syringe and then dispensed into the center well of the cuvette.

After the sample has been added to the cuvette, the "start" key is pressed. A single beep signals completion of the test. The result is reported in seconds and is displayed on the screen; the instrument automatically

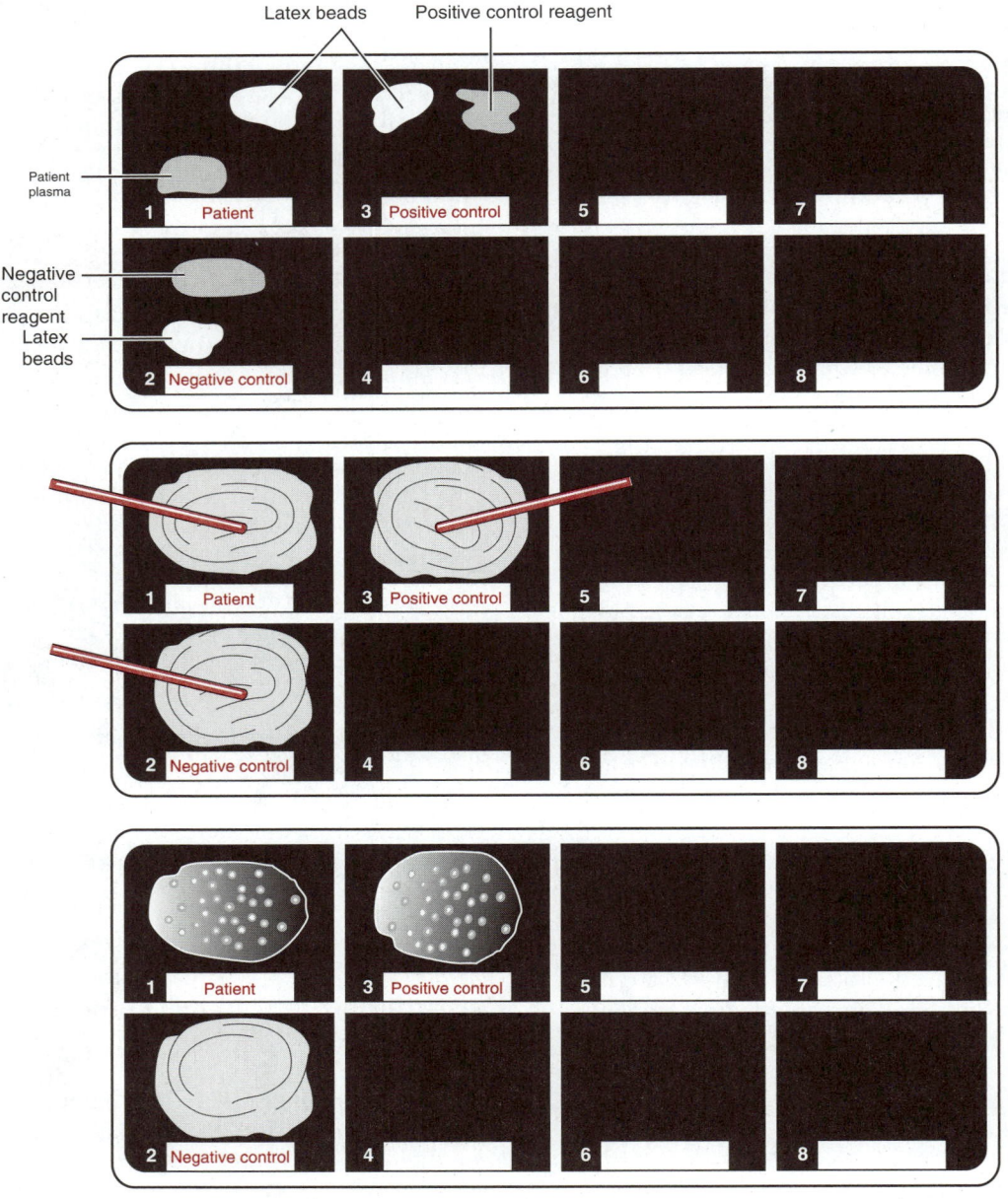

**FIGURE 3-9** Rapid slide test for D-dimers. Top, add one drop of latex reagent next to patient plasma, positive control and negative control; center, mix the test plasmas and latex reagent; bottom, illustration of positive patient reaction and negative and positive control reactions.

**Table 3-8.** Reference values for PT, APTT, and ACT using the HEMOCHRON® Jr.

| TEST | WHOLE BLOOD | | PLASMA EQUIVALENT | |
| --- | --- | --- | --- | --- |
| | Mean | Range | Mean | Range |
| PT | 19 sec | 17-22 sec | 12.5 sec | 11.3-13.6 sec |
| APTT | 110 sec | 93-127 sec | 24 sec | 24-30 sec |
| ACT+ | 121 sec | 89-153 sec | None | None |

converts the result to a reference celite-ACT value (Table 3-8).

### Procedural Notes

■ Follow manufacturer's directions for specimen collection.

■ Collect specimens for the D-dimer rapid slide test and HEMOCHRON® Jr. plasma tests in citrate anticoagulant only.

■ Equilibrate all specimens and reagents to room temperature before using.

■ Run two levels of controls with each batch of patient samples.

### Safety Precautions

■ Observe Universal and Standard Precautions when handling patient and control samples.

■ Discard all used materials in appropriate biohazard containers.

## SUMMARY

Several tests and POCT instruments are available to quickly and conveniently obtain test results for patients with hemostasis disorders. This ensures improved monitoring of patient status during procedures, such as open-heart surgery.

## LESSON REVIEW

1. List two conditions that could require rapid hemostasis testing.
2. What anticoagulant is administered to patients undergoing cardiac angioplasty?
3. How does heparin inhibit clotting?
4. Why is it important to monitor heparin levels?
5. List two tests used to monitor heparin therapy.
6. What is DIC?
7. The D-dimer test detects degradation products from the breakdown of which clotting proteins?
8. Name three conditions the D-dimer test can help to diagnose.
9. Name three small handheld analyzers that perform the ACT.
10. Define angioplasty, D-dimer, disseminated intravascular coagulation, FDP, and XDP.

## STUDENT ACTIVITIES

1. Reread the information on rapid tests for disorders of hemostasis.
2. Review the glossary terms.
3. Practice performing a rapid test for fibrin-degradation products or ACT as outlined on the Student Performance Guide.

## *Student Performance Guide*

## **LESSON 3-6** Rapid Tests for Disorders of Hemostasis

Name _____    Date _____

 ### INSTRUCTIONS

1. Practice performing a rapid test for fibrin-degradation products or ACT following the step-by-step procedure.

2. Demonstrate your understanding of this lesson by:
   a. Completing a written examination successfully, and
   b. Performing the procedure for either fibrin-degradation products or the ACT as directed by the instructor. All steps must be completed as listed on the instructor's Performance Check Sheet.

***Note:*** The following is a general procedure for detecting D-dimer fragments using the DADE® Dimertest® and a general procedure for the performance of an ACT using the HEMOCHRON® Jr. system. The manufacturers' instructions for the specific methods or instruments being used must be followed.

### MATERIALS AND EQUIPMENT

- gloves
- marking pencil
- blood-collection equipment:
  syringe venipuncture (ACT test)
  vacuum tube blood collection equipment (D-dimer test), including citrate collection tube
- capillary puncture materials
- commercial kit for detecting D-dimer fragments
- pipets and tips to deliver 20 and 100 μL
- disposable plastic test tubes and test tube rack (optional, for semi-quantitative D-dimer test)
- mechanical slide rotator (optional)
- HEMOCHRON® Jr. or other handheld instrument for determining ACT, including cuvettes and whole blood controls
- surface disinfectant
- biohazard container
- biohazard sharps container

### PROCEDURE

Record in the comment section any problems encountered while practicing the procedure (or have a fellow student or the instructor evaluate your performance).

S = Satisfactory
U = Unsatisfactory

| You must: | S | U | Comments |
|---|---|---|---|
| 1. Assemble equipment and materials | | | |
| 2. Wash hands and put on gloves | | | |
| 3. Perform the manual test for D-dimers (DADE® Dimertest® Latex Assay). If manual test is not available skip to step 4<br>a. Obtain plasma from a citrated specimen<br>b. Allow the reagents and specimen to equilibrate to room temperature<br>c. Mark patient identifications and control in white areas of the slide<br>d. Hold the latex beads bottle vertically and add one drop of latex beads to each test area | | | |

| You must: | S | U | Comments |
|---|---|---|---|
| e. Dispense 20 µL of undiluted patient plasma or control solution adjacent to the latex beads in each test area <br> f. Promptly mix the suspensions together until the test area is covered; *use a new stirrer for each test area and discard after use* <br> g. Rotate the slide gently for three minutes, manually or using a rotator <br> h. Exactly three minutes after mixing, check for agglutination (clumping); make observations before the suspension begins to dry out to avoid a false positive reaction. (A positive result is white agglutination on a black background; a negative result is a homogeneous white mixture on a black background) <br> i. Record the results for the patient and the positive and negative controls <br> j. Optional: if test is positive, perform the semi-quantitative test following the manufacturer's instructions <br> k. If controls are within acceptable limits, report the patient results | | | |
| 4. Perform activated clotting time (ACT+) using HEMOCHRON® Jr. (The whole blood controls must be prepared 15 minutes before use; follow the manufacturer's instructions for rehydration and use) <br> a. Insert the cuvette into the slot to start the instrument <br> b. Obtain a fresh whole blood specimen (1-2 mL) <br> c. Wait for message "ADD SAMPLE" to appear and add the sample to the center well of the cuvette using a syringe, with or without the needle attached <br> d. Fill the well to the top; avoid bubble formation. Allow excess sample to spill over into the outer well <br> e. Depress the START button <br> f. Wait for the result to be displayed <br> g. Repeat steps 4a through 4f for both levels of controls or as directed by the instructor. Refer to acceptable range provided with each quality control kit <br> h. If the controls are within the acceptable range, report the patient results | | | |
| 5. Use safety disposal device to discard syringe needle | | | |
| 6. Discard used slides, stirrers, cuvettes, and syringes in biohazard container | | | |
| 7. Discard used sharps in biohazard sharps container | | | |
| 8. Disinfect the work area with surface disinfectant | | | |
| 9. Remove and discard gloves in biohazard container and wash hands with hand disinfectant | | | |
| 10. Return other equipment to storage | | | |

*Evaluator Comments:*

Evaluator _____    Date _____

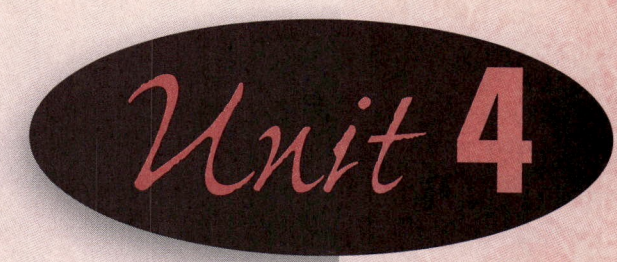

# Unit 4

# Basic Immunology and Serology

## UNIT OBJECTIVES

**After studying this unit, you should be able to:**

- *Discuss the use of immunological tests in the medical laboratory.*
- *Explain the mechanisms of humoral and cell-mediated immunity.*
- *Explain the principles of three types of immunological tests.*
- *Perform ABO grouping.*
- *Perform Rh typing.*
- *Perform a slide test for infectious mononucleosis.*
- *Perform a test for rheumatoid factors.*

## UNIT OVERVIEW

Immunology, the study of the body's protective responses, is a young, rapidly growing discipline. Even though most laboratories have a separate immunology or serology department, every section of the laboratory uses immunological principles and procedures in some way. Therefore, a basic knowledge of immunology is necessary to understand the principles of many of the new generation of laboratory tests. This unit provides a brief introduction to principles of immunology and to basic techniques commonly used in immunology, immunohematology, and serology.

Serology was the term first used for the laboratory branch of immunology because early laboratories used serum for testing. Today, serological procedures use serum, whole blood, urine, or other body fluids in tests designed around the antigen-antibody reaction. These tests are often called immunoassays. Principles of immunology and immunoassays are described in Lesson 4-1.

Modern serology laboratories detect, identify, and measure serum antibodies to aid in diagnosing of diseases such as hepatitis, AIDS, influenza, infectious mononucleosis (Lesson 4-4), and rheumatoid arthritis (Lesson 4-5). Other procedures use antibodies to measure hormones, identify subsets of blood cells, identify microbial pathogens, or monitor drug levels. These types of tests would be performed in the chemistry, hematology, microbiology, and toxicology departments, respectively.

Immunohematology, or blood banking, is the branch of immunology that uses immunological principles to identify and study the blood groups. While some blood banking procedures are relatively simple, such as routine ABO grouping and Rh typing (described in Lessons 4-2 and 4-3), blood banking also involves more complex procedures such as compatibility testing for blood transfusion, antibody identification, and tissue typing of organ donors.

Immunological principles are used throughout the clinical laboratory, so a good foundation and understanding of immunology is necessary for laboratory workers in all departments.

# SUGGESTED READINGS AND REFERENCES

American Association of Blood Banks. (1996). *Technical manual of the American Association of Blood Banks*. Bethesda, MD.

Bryant, Neville J. (3rd ed.).(1994). *An introduction to immunohematology*. Philadelphia: W. B. Saunders.

Diamandis, E. P. & Christopoulos, T. K. (1994). *Textbook of immunological assays*. Washington, D.C.: AACC Press.

Flynn, J. C., Jr. & Kaszczuk, S. (Eds.). (1997). *Essentials of immunohematology*. Philadelphia: W. B. Saunders Co.

Forbes, B. A., Sahm, D. F., Trevino, E. & Weissfeld, A. (10th ed.). (1998). *Bailey & Scott's diagnostic microbiology*. St. Louis: Mosby Year Book.

Harmening, D. (Ed.) (4th ed.). (1999). *Modern blood banking and transfusion practices*. Philadelphia: F. A. Davis Company.

Henry, J. B. (Ed.). (19th ed.). (1997). *Clinical diagnosis & management by laboratory methods*. Philadelphia: W. B. Saunders Company.

Keren, D. F. & Warren, J. S. (2nd ed.). (1994). *Diagnostic immunology*. Baltimore: Williams & Wilkins.

Lefkovits, I. (Ed.) (1999). *Immunology methods manual: The comprehensive sourcebook of techniques*. San Diego: Academic Press.

Marshall, J. (1993). *Fundamental skills for the clinical laboratory professional*. Albany, NY: Delmar Publishers Inc.

Miller, L. E., Ludke, H. R., Peacock, J. E., & Tomar, R. H. (2nd ed.). (1991). *Manual of laboratory immunology*. Philadelphia: Lea & Febiger.

Monospot™ package insert, Meridian Diagnostics, Inc., Cincinnati, OH.

Peakman, M. & Vergani, D. (1997). *Basic and clinical immunology*. London: Churchill Livingstone.

Ravel, R. (6th ed.). (1995). *Clinical laboratory medicine: Clinical application of laboratory data*. Chicago: Mosby Year Book.

Rose, N. R., deMacario, E. C., Folds, J. D., Lane, H. C., & Nakamura, R. M. (Eds.). (5th ed.). (1997). *Manual of clinical laboratory immunology*. Washington, D.C.: American Society for Microbiology.

Sacher, R. A. & McPherson, R. A. (11th ed.). (1999). *Widmann's clinical interpretation of laboratory tests*. Philadelphia: F. A. Davis Company.

Sheehan, C. (2nd ed.). (1997). *Clinical immunology: Principles and laboratory diagnosis*. Philadelphia: Lippincott-Raven.

Stites, D. P., Terr, A. I., & Parslow, T. G. (Eds.). (8th ed.). (1994). *Basic and clinical immunology*. Norwalk, CT: Appleton & Lange.

Turgeon, M. L. (2nd ed.). (1995). *Fundamentals of immunohematology: Theory and technique*. Baltimore: Williams & Wilkins.

Whitlock, S. A. (1997). *Immunohematology: Delmar's clinical laboratory manual series*. Albany, NY: Delmar Publishers.

Widmann, F. K. & Itatani, C. A. (1998). *An introduction to clinical immunology and serology*. Philadelphia: F. A. Davis Company.

Widmann, F. K. (16th ed.). (1995). *Standards for blood banks and transfusion services*. Washington, D.C.: American Association of Blood Banks.

# Introduction to Immunology and Serology

## LESSON OBJECTIVES

**After studying this lesson, you should be able to:**

- *Explain the difference between natural resistance and acquired immunity.*
- *State the three characteristics of specific immunity.*
- *Name the major cells that bring about specific immunity.*
- *Name the sites in the body where lymphoid tissue is found.*
- *Describe the structure of an immunoglobulin molecule.*
- *Name the five immunoglobulin classes and give characteristics of each.*
- *Explain the principle of agglutination.*
- *Explain the principle of precipitation.*
- *Explain the principles of enzyme immunoassays and radioimmunoassays.*
- *Define the glossary terms.*

## GLOSSARY

**agglutination** / the clumping or aggregation of particulate antigens due to reaction with a specific antibody

**allergy** / a condition resulting from an exaggerated immune response; hypersensitivity

**anamnestic response** / rapid increase in blood immunoglobulins following a second exposure to an antigen; booster response or secondary response

**antibody (Ab)** / serum protein that is induced by and reacts specifically with a foreign substance (antigen); immunoglobulin

**antigen (Ag)** / "foreign" substance that induces an immune response by causing production of antibodies or sensitized lymphocytes that react specifically with that substance; immunogen

**autoimmune disease** / disease resulting when the immune response is directed at one's own tissues (self-antigens)

**B lymphocyte, B cell** / a type of lymphocyte primarily responsible for the humoral immune response

**complement** / a group of plasma proteins that participates in immune reactions to cause cell lysis and the inflammatory response

**enzyme immunoassay (EIA)** / a serological test that uses an enzyme-labeled antibody as a reactant

**epitope** / the portion of an antigen that reacts specifically with an antibody; antigenic determinant

**immunocompetent** / capable of producing a normal immune response

**immunocompromised** / having reduced ability or inability to produce a normal immune response

**immunoglobulins (Ig)** / antibodies; serum proteins that are induced by and react specifically with antigens (immunogens)

**immunohematology** / the study of the blood group antigens and antibodies; blood banking

**immunology** / the branch of medicine involved in the study of the immune processes and immunity

**immunosuppression** / suppression of the immune response by physical, chemical, or biological means

**lymphokine** / any of several small molecules that are produced by lymphocytes and help regulate the immune response

**monoclonal antibody** / antibody derived from a single cell line or clone

**plasma cell** / a cell that produces antibodies and is derived from a B lymphocyte

**polyclonal antibodies** / antibodies derived from more than one cell line

**precipitation** / formation of an insoluble antigen-antibody complex

**primary lymphoid organs** / organs in which B and T lymphocytes acquire their special characteristics; in humans, the bone marrow and thymus

**radioimmunoassay (RIA)** / a serological test using a test component labeled with a radioisotope

**secondary lymphoid tissue** / tissues in which lymphocytes are concentrated, such as the spleen, lymph nodes, and tonsils

**seroconversion** / the appearance of antibody in the serum of an individual following exposure to an antigen

**serology** / the study of antibodies and antigens in serum using immunological methods

**T lymphocyte, T cell** / a type of lymphocyte responsible for the cell-mediated immune response

**thymus** / a gland located near the thyroid and considered a primary lymphoid tissue

**titer** / in serology, the reciprocal of the highest dilution that gives the desired reaction; concentration of a substance determined by titration

## INTRODUCTION

**Immunology**, the study of the immune system, is a relatively new branch of medicine that developed from the study of immunity. Early immunologists were physicians who worked to develop ways of providing immunity to infectious disease. They produced vaccines for bacterial and viral diseases such as smallpox, diphtheria, and tetanus.

As knowledge has advanced, it has become evident that the immune system has much broader functions than just providing protection from invading microorganisms. A healthy immune system is fundamental to overall good health. The immune system is involved not only in preventing or fighting infectious disease but also in providing protection from toxins and tumors (cancers).

The immune system may also be involved in the initiation of disease. For example, **allergies** such as hay fever or a poison ivy rash are brought on by an exaggerated immune response. **Autoimmune diseases** such as rheumatoid arthritis and lupus erythematosus result when components of the immune system react against one's own tissues.

Deficiencies or malfunctions of the immune system may permit the growth of cancer cells or allow the development of life-threatening infections by normally non-pathogenic (opportunistic) organisms.

This lesson presents an overview of immunology and serology and an introduction to principles of common immunological or serological tests. A basic understanding of immunology is required to be able to generate or use much of the data in today's clinical laboratory.

# IMMUNOLOGY IN THE MEDICAL LABORATORY

Immunology in the medical laboratory has many facets. Assays based on immunological principles are common in all departments of the laboratory. Tests that evaluate immune function are performed when patients have recurring infections, have problems healing, or have other symptoms indicating a possible problem with their immune response. Diagnosis of infectious diseases is aided by the use of serological tests that measure antibody levels to bacteria, viruses, and parasites. Many assays use the antigen-antibody reaction to test substances unrelated to the immune system. For example, in the clinical chemistry department, drug and hormone levels may be measured using immunoassays.

# THE IMMUNE SYSTEM

The immune system is a remarkably complex organization of tissues, cells, cell products, and biologically active chemicals, all of which interact to produce the *immune response*. The immune system provides specific defense mechanisms against a variety of foreign substances called **antigens**. These antigens may be molecules, viruses, blood cells, bacteria, or fungi.

## Natural Resistance vs. Specific Immunity

*Natural resistance* to various harmful agents is provided by physical barriers such as the skin and mucous membranes, the phagocytic action of cells such as neutrophils, and natural biochemicals and **complement** proteins that produce reactions such as inflammation. These types of responses are nonspecific. Previous exposure to an antigen is not required for the body to respond, and the body responds in the same way to many substances and organisms.

The *specific immune response* (specific immunity) is the type of immune response that recognizes and remembers different antigens. Specific immunity is characterized by three properties:

- recognition
- specificity
- memory

*Recognition* refers to the immune system's ability to recognize differences in vast numbers of antigens in the environment and to distinguish them from self (one's own tissues).

*Specificity* refers to the ability to direct a response toward a specific antigen without reacting with other similar antigens.

*Memory* refers to the immune system's ability to remember an antigen long after initial exposure. This ability, also called the **anamnestic response**, is the basis for immunizations. For example, a childhood immunization against the mumps virus will provide years of protection because the body's immune cells remember the viral antigens and will respond if they contact the virus again, even years after the immunization. After a child has a disease such as chickenpox, he or she usually develops lifelong immunity to the disease because of the memory response.

## Cells, Tissues, and Organs of the Immune System

Lymphocytes are the major cells that bring about the specific immune response. The two major types of lymphocytes are T lymphocytes (T cells) and B lymphocytes (B cells), each of which has different functions in immunity. Lymphocytes circulate in the blood and in the lymph fluid and are also concentrated in lymphoid tissues throughout the body.

The **primary lymphoid organs** are the bone marrow and the **thymus**. The spleen, lymph nodes, and tonsils are examples of **secondary lymphoid tissues** where lymphocytes can be found (Table 4-1).

## Humoral Immunity and Cell-Mediated Immunity

There are two types of specific immune response, the *humoral response* and the *cell-mediated* (cellular) *response* (Table 4-2). Both of these responses display recognition, specificity, and memory. The type of response that predominates is determined by which type of lymphocyte gives the major response to an

**Table 4-1.** Primary and secondary lymphoid organs and tissues

**PRIMARY LYMPHOID ORGANS**
Thymus
Bone marrow (bursa equivalent)

**SECONDARY LYMPHOID ORGANS AND TISSUES**
Lymph nodes
Spleen
Gut-associated lymphoid tissue (GALT)
   Peyer's patches
   Appendix
   Tonsils
Bronchus-associated lymphoid tissue (BALT)

**Table 4-2**. Comparison of humoral and cell-mediated immunity

| IMMUNITY | CELLS RESPONSIBLE | MEDIATED BY | PROTECTION PROVIDED |
|---|---|---|---|
| Humoral | B cells | Antibodies | Bacteria, toxins |
| Cellular | T cells | Cells and lymphokines | Viruses, fungi, tumors |

antigen. Other cells that contribute to and participate in immune responses and overall immunity are blood granulocytes, monocytes, and tissue macrophages. The interactions among lymphocytes, macrophages, and granulocytes and cell-mediated and humoral immunity are complex. For good immunity, all components of the immune response must function properly and be in proper balance.

**B lymphocytes** are responsible for humoral immunity and provide good protection against bacteria, toxins, and circulating antigens. B cells produce **antibodies (Ab)**, serum proteins that react specifically with antigens. **Plasma cells** are specialized B lymphocytes and are the most efficient antibody-producing cells.

**T lymphocytes** help bring about cell-mediated immunity, providing protection against viruses, fungi, tumor cells, and intracellular organisms. Cell-mediated immunity is initiated by the interaction of T cells with antigens and "foreign" cells. T lymphocytes secrete **lymphokines**, small molecules that help regulate the immune response (Table 4-2).

The designation "T lymphocyte" actually refers to several subsets of lymphocytic cells, each with different functions. These cells are identified by surface markers (CD markers). Human immunodeficiency virus (HIV), the virus that causes AIDS, infects and kills the subset of T lymphocytes called helper (CD4) cells, which causes an immune deficiency in infected persons.

## IMMUNOGLOBULINS

**Immunoglobulins (Ig)**, or antibodies, are proteins produced by plasma cells and secreted into body fluids in response to antigen exposure. Immunoglobulins circulate in the blood and make up approximately 10-15% of serum protein.

Antibodies are named by placing the prefix *anti* before the antigen with which the antibody reacts. For example, one type of test for AIDS detects the presence of antibodies to HIV (anti-HIV). The antibody specific for the A blood group antigen on group A red blood cells is called "anti-A."

### Structure and Function of Immunoglobulins

A typical antibody molecule consists of four protein chains, bound together so they form a shape similar to the letter "Y" (Figure 4-1). Each arm of the Y contains a binding site, that reacts with the **epitope**, or specific antigenic determinant, on an antigen.

An antigen entering the body triggers the production of immunoglobulins that react specifically with that antigen. This specific antigen-antibody reaction is a physical binding. It can be compared to a lock-and-key fit, with the antibody being the lock and the antigen the key (Figure 4-2). In this way, antibodies destroy or inactivate antigens, an important defense mechanism.

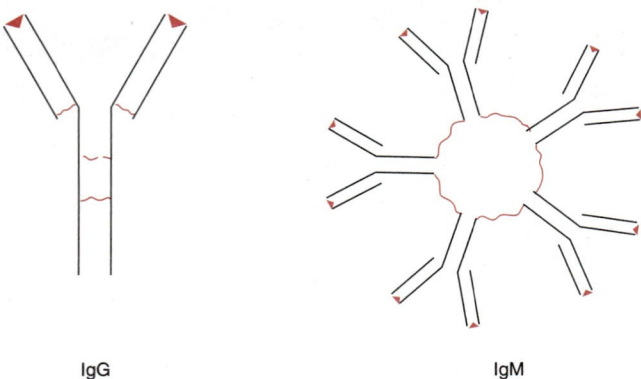

**FIGURE 4-1** Structure of IgG monomer (left) and IgM pentamer (right). Arrowheads point to antigen-binding sites

IgG

IgM

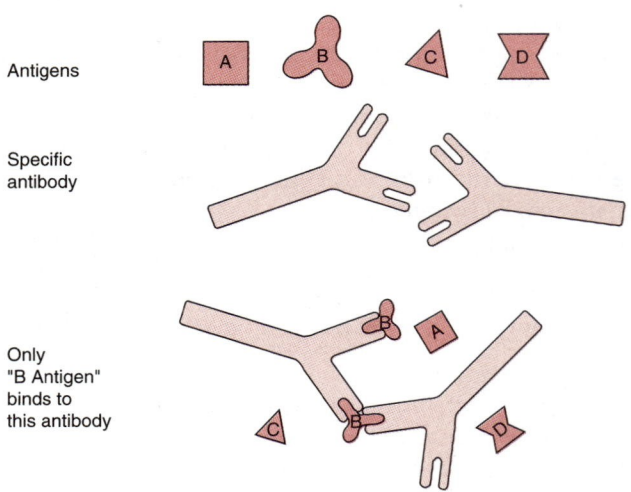

Antigens

Specific antibody

Only "B Antigen" binds to this antibody

**FIGURE 4-2** Illustration of the lock-and-key specificity of the antigen-antibody reaction

## Classes of Immunoglobulins

Five classes of immunoglobulins (Ig) in humans are immunoglobulin G (IgG), immunoglobulin M (IgM), immunoglobulin A (IgA), immunoglobulin D (IgD), and immunoglobulin E (IgE). Although the antibody classes are structurally similar, each has particular characteristics and functions (Table 4-3).

### IgG

IgG is the antibody class in highest concentration in serum. It is also called gamma globulin or immune globulin. IgG remains in serum for a long time and provides long-lasting immunity. It is also the only immunoglobulin class that crosses the placenta and provides the newborn with immunity that lasts several months.

### IgM

IgM is the second most abundant antibody. The IgM molecule is approximately five times as large as IgG. IgM is a pentamer, five Ig molecules bound together (Figure 4-1). IgM is the first antibody produced in response to an antigen, but does not provide long-lasting immunity. IgM is also the first class of antibody to be produced in newborns after birth. Because of its large size, IgM is useful in agglutination reactions. Serological tests that measure antibody levels in serum are usually measuring IgG or IgM.

### IgA

IgA is called the secretory antibody because it is the predominant immunoglobulin in tears, saliva, breast milk, and secretions of the respiratory and intestinal tract. IgA provides protection against organisms that invade through these sites.

**Table 4-3.** Characteristics and Functions of Ig classes

| CLASS | CHARACTERISTICS/ FUNCTIONS |
|-------|----------------------------|
| IgG | Long-lasting immunity, crosses placenta |
| IgM | First response antibody |
| IgA | Present in secretions |
| IgD | Function unknown |
| IgE | Allergic reactions |

### IgD

IgD is present in very small amounts in serum. Little is known of the biological function of IgD.

### IgE

IgE is present in very small amounts in serum. IgE is involved in some allergic reactions. Certain allergy tests measure the IgE levels or specificity in serum. IgE production may increase in parasitic infections.

## Primary vs. Secondary Antibody Response: Anamnestic Response

The *primary antibody response* is the response occurring after the first exposure to an antigen. The first antibody detectable in plasma after initial exposure to an antigen is IgM, which usually appears in serum three to four days after exposure. The IgM titer (concentration) quickly peaks and then drops rapidly over a few weeks.

IgG is detectable one to two weeks after antigen exposure. The IgG level peaks within a few weeks and decreases over a period of months (Figure 4-3).

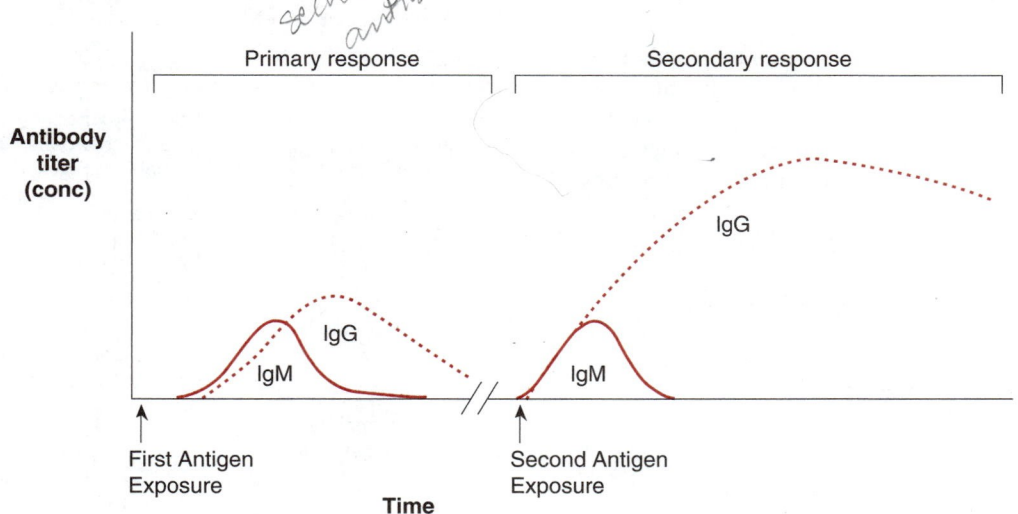

**FIGURE 4-3** Comparison of IgM and IgG levels in the primary and secondary antibody responses

Measurement or detection of IgM can provide information about when an individual was exposed to an organism or antigen. Since IgM is produced early and declines quickly, detection of IgM indicates acute disease (recent exposure). A rising IgG titer in serum samples collected two to three weeks apart also indicates recent exposure. **Seroconversion** is the term used when an antibody becomes detectable in the serum of a patient who has previously tested negative.

The *secondary antibody response* or **anamnestic response** is seen after reexposure to an antigen. Because immune cells remember the antigen, antibody production increases rapidly and IgM and IgG levels rise quickly (within two to three days) following antigen reexposure. In the secondary response, IgG reaches higher levels than in the primary response, and remains detectable in the serum for months to years (Figure 4-3).

## DISEASES INVOLVING THE IMMUNE SYSTEM

The immune system provides important protection from disease in **immunocompetent** individuals. Any deficiency or damage to the immune system makes an individual susceptible to disease, or **immunocompromised**.

Most abnormalities of the immune system are acquired. Many drugs, especially cancer chemotherapies, cause **immunosuppression** as an unwanted side effect. The HIV virus causes disease by interfering with immune function, causing infected persons to become susceptible to opportunistic organisms such as *Pneumocystis* that cause no problems for healthy individuals.

Malignancies of the immune system such as leukemias and lymphomas may occur. Disease or abnormalities can also occur when the immune system is overactive, as in allergies (hypersensitivities), or is misdirected, as in autoimmune diseases.

Immune deficiencies can be a result of inherited genes or of a developmental abnormality in the fetus. While these conditions are not common, the effect is usually severe, causing a shortened life expectancy. Table 4-4 lists some diseases and conditions involving the immune system.

## TYPES OF IMMUNOLOGICAL TESTS

### Tests of Immune Function

In the medical laboratory, tests based on principles of immunology are diverse and in wide use. Some of these tests are designed to measure immune function and to detect immune deficiencies or irregularities. These would include quantitation of CD4 and CD8 cells, quantitation of immunoglobulin subgroups, tests of leukocyte function, allergy tests, and tests for complement components. Most tests of immune function are performed in special immunology laboratories, usually located only in larger hospitals or reference laboratories.

### Tests Based on Antigen-Antibody Reactions

Because of their unique property of recognizing and distinguishing among closely related antigens, antibodies are widely used in designing clinical laboratory tests. Immunological tests may be used to detect an antigen or antibody in a patient, as in tests for hepatitis, HIV, influenza, or infectious mononucleosis. Tests may also use the antigen-antibody reaction to measure or detect a substance that is not part of the immune system; for example, using antibodies to measure drug or hormone levels.

#### Monoclonal and Polyclonal Antibodies

Antibodies used in immunological tests may be monoclonal or polyclonal. **Monoclonal antibodies** are antibodies of one specificity and class and are derived from one (mono) clone, or cell line. Monoclonal antibodies are produced in laboratories and used as reagents in many immunodiagnostic kits. **Polyclonal antibodies** are antibodies of more than one epitope specificity or from more than one (poly) cell line. Serum antibodies are polyclonal.

**Table 4-4.** Categories of diseases or conditions associated with immune system abnormalities

| CATEGORY | EXAMPLES |
| --- | --- |
| Autoimmune diseases | Rheumatoid arthritis, lupus erythematosus, juvenile diabetes, myasthenia gravis |
| Hypersensitivities | Rhinitis, asthma, dermatitis |
| Malignancies | Lymphomas, leukemias, multiple myeloma |
| Acquired immuno-deficiencies | Infections, systemic disease, malignancies, reactions to drugs, irradiation |
| Congenital immuno-deficiencies | DiGeorge syndrome, agammaglobulinemia, SCID (severe combined immune deficiency) |

## Test Sensitivity and Specificity

Laboratories should choose test methods based on the sensitivity and specificity of the method. *Specificity* refers to the ability to detect only the antibody or antigen for which the test is designed. Detection of other substances (cross-reactivity) decreases the specificity of the test and causes false positive reactions.

*Sensitivity* refers to the lower limit of detection, or the lowest concentration capable of being detected by the method (Table 4-5). Failure to detect small amounts of a substance in a test will result in false negative reactions.

## Quantitative Tests

Immunological procedures may be reported as negative or positive, or the tests may be quantitative. Quantitative procedures usually require serial dilutions of serum to estimate the immunoglobulin concentration to a specific antigen. The immunoglobulin concentration is expressed as the **titer**, or the reciprocal of the highest dilution showing a reaction. The procedure for serial dilutions is given in Lesson 6-3.

# PRINCIPLES OF IMMUNOLOGICAL TESTS

Examples of tests that use immunological principles include agglutination and agglutination inhibition tests, precipitation tests, fluorescent antibody techniques, enzyme immunoassays, and radioimmunoassays.

## Agglutination and Agglutination Inhibition

**Agglutination** is the visible clumping or aggregation of cells or particles due to their reaction with an antibody. When cells or particles, such as latex beads, have antigen molecules on their surface, they will agglutinate when reacted with a specific antibody. The presence of agglutination indicates a positive test. Blood typing is

based on this principle. Other tests that use the principle of agglutination include slide tests for rheumatoid factor, infectious mononucleosis, and bacterial identification in the microbiology laboratory.

A variation of the agglutination test is agglutination inhibition. In inhibition tests, a positive reaction is indicated by *absence* of agglutination. Some pregnancy tests are based on this principle.

## Precipitation

**Precipitation** is the formation of an insoluble complex when a specific antibody is reacted with a soluble antigen. These reactions are usually carried out in a gelatin-like substance called agarose. The formation of a visible white precipitate is a positive reaction. IgG is the antibody class that reacts best in precipitation reactions.

The precipitation reaction may be used in simple or complex tests. Techniques such as radial immunodiffusion and immunoelectrophoresis are based on the precipitation reaction (Figure 4-4). Tests for C-reactive protein, haptoglobin, and α-1 antitrypsin can be performed using precipitation methods. Many precipitation tests have been replaced by enzyme immunoassay methods.

## Complement Fixation

Complement fixation (CF) is a sensitive method for detecting an antigen-antibody reaction. In the clinical laboratory it is usually used to detect an antibody (IgG or IgM) in patient serum. CF assays are more sensitive than precipitation and agglutination methods but less sensitive than labeled antibody techniques.

---

**Table 4-5.** Immunological-based diagnostic methods in order of decreasing sensitivity

Radio immunoassay (RIA)/Enzyme immunoassay (EIA)

Fluorescent antibody (FA) techniques

Complement fixation (CF)

Agglutination

Precipitation

---

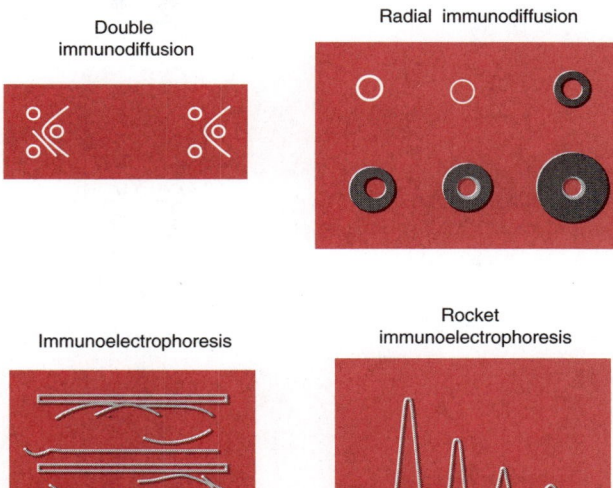

Double immunodiffusion

Radial immunodiffusion

Immunoelectrophoresis

Rocket immunoelectrophoresis

**FIGURE 4-4** Examples of precipitation techniques

The procedure for complement fixation is lengthy, complicated to perform, and requires many controls. Therefore, most laboratories do not routinely perform CF tests; the method is only used to detect unusual viral or fungal infections for which simpler tests are not available.

The CF test is a type of inhibition test. The CF test is based on the ability of complement proteins to interact with antibody and specific antigen to cause cell lysis.

The test is performed in two parts, the test system and the indicator system. In the test system, patient serum and an antigen (for example, a viral or fungal antigen) are reacted in the presence of a complement. If antibody specific for the antigen is present, the complement will be "fixed," or depleted, in the antigen-antibody reaction and will be unable to react in the second part of the test, the indicator system. The indicator system is added to the tubes after the serum, complement, and antigen have reacted. The indicator system is sheep red blood cells (SRBC) and an antibody against SRBC. The anti-SRBC will lyse the SRBC if active complement is present. *A negative test is indicated by hemolysis*, which can only occur if the antibody in the test serum is absent.

*Absence of hemolysis is a positive result*, indicating presence of the antibody in the test serum.

## Labeled Antibody Techniques

Several types of immunological tests use "labeled" antibodies. Molecules (labels) are conjugated (attached) to the antibodies, producing a visible reaction. The labels may be dyes, enzymes, or radioisotopes (Figure 4-5). Attaching labels to the immunoglobulins does not interfere with the immunoglobulins' ability to bind to antigens. Labeled antibody techniques are among the most sensitive immunoassays available.

### Enzyme Immunoassay

The **enzyme immunoassay (EIA)** is a more complex procedure than precipitation or agglutination. The test can be designed in several different ways, but it always involves an antigen, an antibody specific for the antigen, and a second antibody conjugated to an enzyme (Figure 4-5). The test may be designed to detect a particular antibody in a patient's serum or to detect an antigen in a patient specimen.

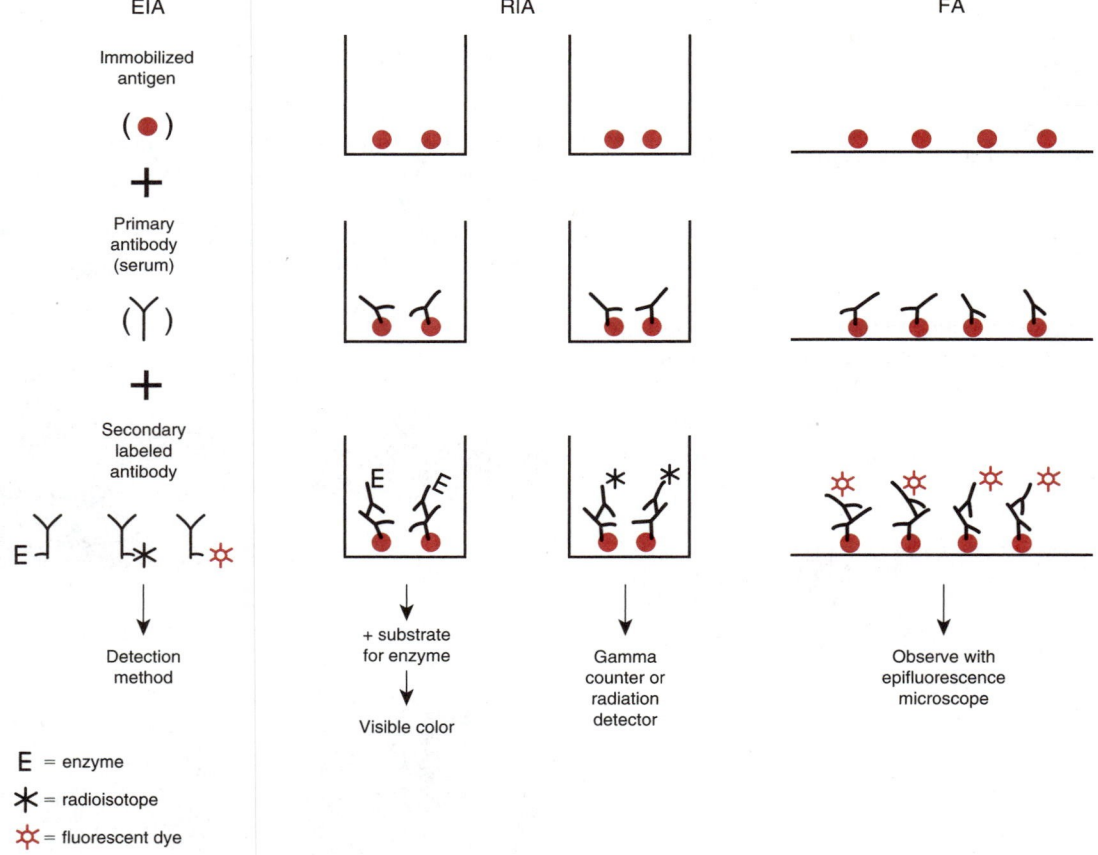

**FIGURE 4-5** Comparison of antibody labeling techniques. Left, enzyme immunoassay; center, radioimmunoassay; right, fluorescent antibody assay

## Example of EIA Test

An example of an EIA is a test for antibodies to rubella (German measles). Serum is added to a plastic incubation well that has been coated with inactivated rubella virus. If rubella antibodies are present in the serum, they will bind to the virus particles. After incubation, the well is rinsed to remove any unbound antibody, and a second antibody directed against (specific for) human antibody is placed in the well. This second antibody has an enzyme attached to it. If anti-rubella was present in the patient serum and became bound to the virus particles, the second labeled antibody will bind to the first layer of antibody (anti-rubella). If no antibody was present in the serum, the anti-human globulin will not bind. After this incubation, the well is again washed and a substrate specific for the enzyme is added. The substrate will form a color in the presence of the enzyme. Therefore, any color formed in the well indicates a positive test.

## Rapid Immunoassays

Numerous tests are based on variations of the EIA. In membrane EIAs, most or all of the reagents are incorporated in an absorbent membrane enclosed in a plastic cassette. When a sample (serum or urine) is added, it migrates through the membrane reacting with the reagents and forming a color (Figure 4-6). Most of these tests are simple to perform and interpret, even though the technology is complex. Examples of membrane EIAs include over-the-counter pregnancy test kits, tests for Group A *Streptococcus*, influenza, *Helicobacter pylori*, and HIV. Many EIAs are CLIA-waived..

## Radioimmunoassay

The **radioimmunoassay (RIA)** is similar in principle to the EIA. However, instead of an enzyme-labeled antibody, a radioisotope is used as the label (Figure 4-5). RIAs were developed before immunoassays and in the past were commonly used to test for hepatitis or to measure drug or hormone levels. However, EIAs have replaced many RIAs because the EIA reagents are more stable and the hazards of using radioactive materials are eliminated.

## Fluorescent Antibody Techniques

In fluorescent antibody (FA) tests, the label conjugated to the antibody is a fluorescent dye. This dye may be seen with the use of epifluorescence microscopes (Figure 4-5). Many serological tests rely on the use of fluorescent dyes to visualize the reaction. Microorganisms such as *Treponema* (which causes syphilis), mycobacteria (cause of tuberculosis), and *Cryptosporidium* are usually detected using fluorescent antibodies. Autoimmune diseases such as lupus erythematosus are diagnosed with the aid of immunofluorescence techniques. FA techniques, in general, require more expertise to perform and interpret than EIAs.

## SUMMARY

This lesson is a brief introduction to the basic principles of immunology and serology needed to understand procedures in the remaining lessons in this unit. It is impossible to cover all aspects of immunology and serology in a single lesson. The tests described in this unit are some of the simpler immunological tests. Numerous immunological tests are in wide use, from lymphocyte function assays to tests for tumor markers. A textbook of clinical immunology should be consulted for more comprehensive information.

## LESSON REVIEW

1. What is natural resistance?
2. What is specific immunity?
3. What are the three characteristics of specific immunity?
4. What is the type of immunity that develops from vaccinations?
5. Draw an antibody molecule. Show where the antigen binding sites are.
6. Name the five classes of immunoglobulins. Which is the most abundant?
7. Which immunoglobulin class gives long-lasting immunity?
8. Which immunoglobulin class participates in allergic reactions?
9. Explain the principle of agglutination. What is a positive reaction in an agglutination inhibition test?
10. What is precipitation?
11. What is a labeled antibody? What types of labeled antibodies are used in immunological tests?
12. Define agglutination, allergy, anamnestic response, antibody, antigen, autoimmune disease, B lympho-

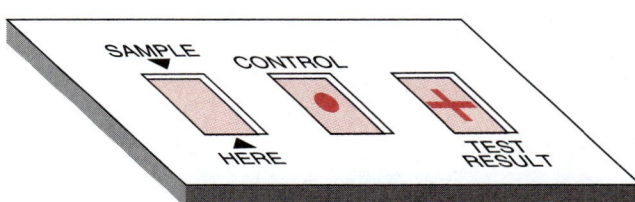

**FIGURE 4-6** Example of a membrane EIA test cartridge

cyte, complement, enzyme immunoassay, epitope, immunocompetent, immunocompromised, immunoglobulins, immunohematology, immunology, immunosuppression, lymphokine, monoclonal antibody, plasma cell, polyclonal antibodies, precipitation, primary lymphoid organs, radioimmunoassay, secondary lymphoid tissue, seroconversion, serology, T lymphocyte, thymus, and titer.

## STUDENT ACTIVITIES

1. Reread the introduction to immunology and serology.
2. Review the glossary terms.
3. Research an autoimmune disease, immune deficiency disease, or infectious disease diagnosed by immunological methods. Report on the cause of the disease, symptoms, methods of diagnosis, and appropriate clinical laboratory tests.

# Immunohematology— ABO Grouping

**After studying this lesson, you should be able to:**

■ *Name the four blood groups in the ABO system.*
■ *State the frequencies of the four ABO blood groups in the United States.*
■ *Name the blood group antigens and antibodies present in each of the four groups.*
■ *Explain forward grouping and reverse grouping*
■ *Perform ABO slide grouping and interpret the results.*
■ *Perform ABO tube grouping and interpret the results.*
■ *Explain grading of agglutination in tube grouping.*
■ *Define the glossary terms.*

## GLOSSARY

**antiserum** / serum that contains antibodies

**blood bank** / department in the medical laboratory where blood components are tested and stored until needed for transfusion; refrigerated unit used for storing blood components

**blood group antibody** / a serum protein (immunoglobulin) that reacts specifically with a blood group antigen

**blood group antigen** / a substance or structure on the red blood cell membrane that causes antibody formation and reacts with that antibody

**serofuge** / a centrifuge that spins small tubes such as those used in blood banking

## INTRODUCTION

Immunohematology, or blood banking, is the study of the human blood groups. A patient's blood group must be determined before a blood transfusion can be given. Blood groups must also be considered in organ transplantation, questions of paternity, forensic investigations, and genetic studies.

ABO grouping may be performed using slide tests or tube tests based on the principle of agglutination. The slide grouping method is quick and easy, and requires no special equipment. However, the tube test is the preferred method and is used most commonly in medical laboratories.

# BLOOD BANKING

The medical laboratory department that performs blood grouping and typing is called the **blood bank**, immunohematology department, or transfusion services. The name blood bank comes from the fact that donated blood to be used for transfusion is stored (or banked) in that department in a special refrigerated unit with a temperature control and alarm system (Figure 4-7).

## Obtaining Donor Blood

Most hospital blood banks obtain donor blood from blood donor processing centers, such as those operated by the American Red Cross or other independent blood-donation agencies. These processing centers draw blood from donors into sterile closed bags (Figure 4-8). A portion of the blood remains in "pigtails," sealed, segmented tubing that is external to the blood unit (Figure 4-8). Each tubing segment is coded to match the code on the unit. The blood in these segments of tubing is used for testing so the unit's sterility is maintained until it is transfused. By using these tubing segments, several tests can be performed on blood before it is transfused.

Technologists at the donor processing centers type and perform several other tests on the blood before releasing it to hospitals. Most of these tests are designed to eliminate potentially infectious units from being transfused. Blood is tested for syphilis and for antibodies against hepatitis B and C viruses, HIV, and human T-cell lymphotropic virus types I and II (HTLV-I, HTLV-II). Units are also tested for HIV and hepatitis viral antigens. Processing centers are not permitted to release units to blood banks if they have a positive reaction for any of these tests.

## Blood Components

Donated blood can be separated into several components, depending on the needs of the medical community in the region. Blood units may be left as whole blood but more commonly are separated into red cells, platelets, and plasma. In this way, several patients can benefit from the donation of one "unit" of blood.

After testing and processing, the blood components are distributed to hospitals for use in transfusion. Hospital blood banks retype the donor components and test them for compatibility with the patient before they are used.

## Procedures Performed in the Hospital Blood Bank Department

Blood banking is the term commonly used to refer to the techniques performed in this department. These procedures include ABO grouping and Rh typing, compatibility testing for blood transfusion, typing of donor blood, screening for and identification of unusual blood group antibodies, and tests for hemolytic disease of the newborn (HDN).

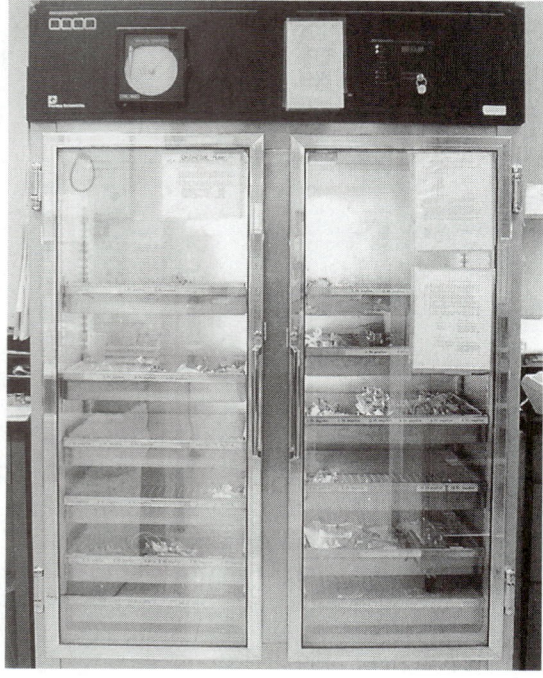

**FIGURE 4-7** Refrigerated unit for storing blood

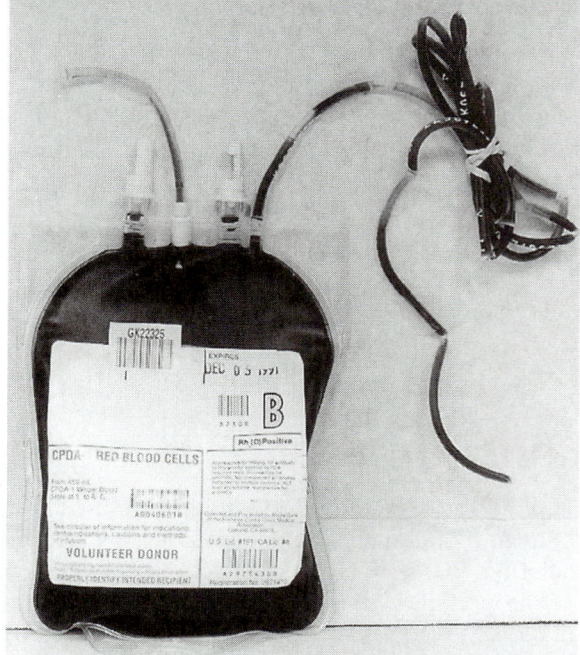

**FIGURE 4-8** Donor blood bag with segmented tubing (pigtails)

 **Safety**

Universal and Standard Precautions must be followed when performing all procedures in the blood bank. Gloves and protective clothing must be worn to protect against exposure to blood and blood products. Since blood grouping reagents originate from human blood products, all reagents must be handled as if potentially infectious. All contaminated supplies must either be decontaminated before washing or discarded in appropriate biohazard containers. Counter surfaces should be disinfected frequently with surface disinfectant. Safety rules must be followed when using electrical equipment and instruments with moving parts, such as serofuges.

### Quality Assurance

Strict quality control procedures must be followed in the blood bank department. Because the department is responsible for testing components that will be administered intravenously to patients, the department is regulated by the Food and Drug Administration (FDA). Care must be taken to ensure that patients receive transfusions of the highest quality and that all testing is conducted according to standard practices.

Quality control guidelines must ensure the proper working condition of refrigerators, freezers, water baths, centrifuges, and any other equipment used in preparing and testing blood components. Temperature monitors must be in place at all times to ensure that components are constantly stored within acceptable temperature ranges. Reagents must be inspected visually and tested at designated intervals and the results recorded. Reagent expiration dates must be observed and appropriate controls must be run. Standards for good blood-banking practice are issued by the American Association of Blood Banks (AABB), an agency that also accredits blood banks.

Special attention must be paid to patient and specimen identification. Observations and interpretations of results must be carefully recorded. Manufacturers' instructions must be followed for the particular reagents used.

In immunohematology, the quality of laboratory testing can have a direct, immediate impact on the patient. A blood transfusion, a potentially lifesaving event, is, in effect, a tissue transplant. Errors or

mistakes in matching blood for transfusion can lead to serious damage to the patient and sometimes may be fatal. For this reason, the technologists who work in the blood bank must be highly trained, conscientious, and vigilant.

## THE ABO SYSTEM

The ABO blood group system, the major human blood group system, was discovered around 1900. All individuals can be placed into one of four major groups: A, B, AB, or O. In the United States, approximately 45% of the population is group O and 41% is group A. Only 10% of the population is B, and 4% is AB (Table 4-6).

### Blood Group Antigens

ABO grouping is based on the presence or absence of two **blood group antigens**, substances found on the surface of the red blood cells. These blood group antigens are designated A and B and are products of inherited genes.

Individuals are grouped according to the antigens present on their blood cells: a person who is group A has A antigen; a person who is group B has B antigen; a person who is group AB has A and B antigens; and a person who is group O has neither A nor B antigen (Table 4-7). The slide and tube tests detect A or B antigen on red blood cells, a procedure called *forward* or *direct grouping* (or testing).

### Blood Group Antibodies

The discovery of the A and B antigens was accompanied by the discovery of the corresponding **blood group antibodies** in human blood. Antibodies (immunoglobulins) are serum proteins that react with

**Table 4-6.** ABO blood group frequencies in the United States

| GROUP | PERCENTAGE OF POPULATION |
|-------|--------------------------|
| A | 41% |
| B | 10% |
| O | 45% |
| AB | 4% |

**Table 4-7.** Table of ABO antigens and antibodies

| ABO GROUP | ANTIGEN ON RED BLOOD CELLS | ANTIBODY IN SERUM |
|---|---|---|
| A | A | Anti-B |
| B | B | Anti-A |
| AB | A and B | Neither anti-A nor anti-B |
| O | Neither A nor B | Both anti-A and anti-B |

an antigen. Antibodies of the ABO system are of the IgM class.

Antibodies are named according to the antigen with which they react: an antibody that reacts with A antigen (A red blood cells) is called anti-A; an antibody that reacts with B antigen (B red blood cells) is called anti-B. O cells are named because they have no A or B antigen; therefore, there is no anti-O antibody.

Blood group antibodies of the ABO system occur naturally in serum. If an antigen is missing from an individual's cells, the antibody specific for the missing antigen will be present. For example, group A individuals have anti-B antibody in their serum. An individual who is group O has both anti-A and anti-B since O cells have neither A nor B antigen (Table 4-7). Testing serum for the presence of the blood group antibodies is called *reverse, confirmatory* or *indirect grouping,* and is performed by tube test.

Although the blood group *antigens* of newborns are already developed, this is not the case with the blood group antibodies. The blood group antibodies of the ABO system may not be easily detectable until the age of about six months. For this reason, only forward grouping is reliable in newborns and young infants.

## Importance of ABO Grouping

ABO grouping is performed before procedures such as blood transfusion or organ transplantation. An individual should be transfused with blood of the same ABO group. The rule to follow in transfusing blood is to *avoid giving the patient an antigen he does not already have.* In an emergency, O blood may be used because it contains neither A nor B antigen. For this reason, people of blood group O are called *universal donors.*

## PRINCIPLE OF ABO SLIDE GROUPING

The slide test detects the A or B antigens on red cells using the principle of agglutination. This procedure is called direct or forward grouping and is accomplished

by combining the patient's blood cells with a known **antiserum** and observing for agglutination. If the antigen present on the cells corresponds to the antibody in the antiserum, the antibody will bind to the antigen and cause clumping of the cells, or agglutination. If the antigen is not present on the cells, no agglutination will be observed.

## Performing ABO Slide Grouping

ABO slide grouping is performed using a commercial typing slide or a clean microscope slide that has been marked into two halves using a wax pencil. One drop of commercial anti-A serum is added to the left side and one drop of anti-B serum to the right side. A small drop of well-mixed blood, capillary or venous, is placed on each side of the slide (Figure 4-9). The anti-A is mixed

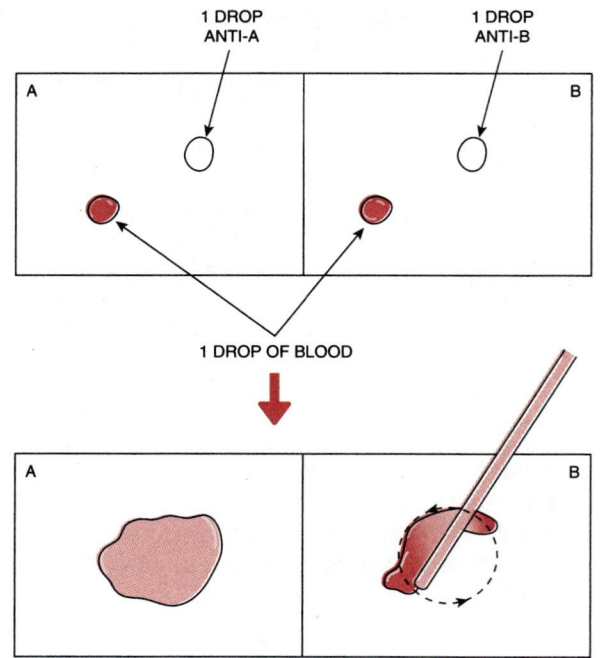

**FIGURE 4-9** ABO slide grouping procedure: (top) microscope slide with antisera and blood added; (bottom) mixing antisera and blood

with one drop of the blood using an applicator stick. The procedure is repeated for anti-B and the other drop of blood (Figure 4-9) using a clean applicator.

The slide is then rocked gently for two minutes and observed under good light for agglutination. Agglutination, a positive reaction, will appear as a clumping together of the red blood cells (Figure 4-10). The results should be recorded as positive (+) or negative (0).

## Interpretation of Slide Grouping Results

If only the A antigen is present on the red blood cells, the cells will agglutinate with anti-A but not with anti-B. If only B antigen is present, the cells will agglutinate with anti-B but not with anti-A. Group O blood will show no agglutination with either anti-A or anti-B. Group AB blood will agglutinate with both anti-A and anti-B (Table 4-8).

## PRINCIPLE OF ABO TUBE GROUPING

Tube testing is a more sensitive and reliable method of determining a patient's blood group than slide testing. Tube testing is used in blood banks and in clinical laboratories; slide testing is more likely to be used in physician office laboratories (POLs). Slide grouping uses whole blood from capillary puncture or venipuncture; tube grouping requires dilution of the blood with saline to make a 2-5% suspension of cells.

ABO tube grouping consists of (1) direct or forward grouping, which identifies the antigens on the cells, and (2) confirmatory or reverse grouping, which identifies the blood group antibodies in the serum. A centrifuge or serofuge may be used to speed up the reaction (Figure 4-11). A **serofuge** is a specialized centrifuge that spins small test tubes.

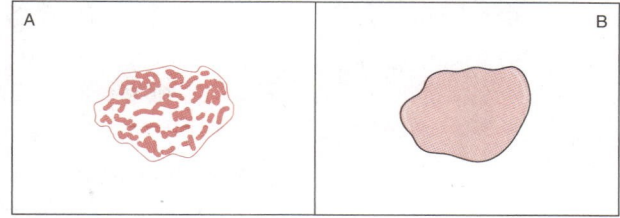

**FIGURE 4-10** Illustration of agglutination of blood cells by anti-A in ABO slide grouping. Reaction shown indicates the patient is group A.

## Direct or Forward Grouping

Forward or direct grouping identifies the antigens present on red blood cells by reacting a suspension of cells with anti-A and anti-B sera and observing for agglutination after centrifugation. If a centrifuge is not available, the reactions may be observed after allowing the tubes to sit at room temperature for fifteen to thirty minutes.

A 2–5% red blood cell suspension is made by adding eighteen to nineteen drops of saline to one drop of the patient's blood. Two tubes labeled "A" and "B" are set up: one drop of anti-A serum is placed in the "A" tube and one drop of anti-B serum is placed in the "B" tube. One drop of the patient's 2–5% cell suspension is added to each tube and the contents are mixed. The tubes are

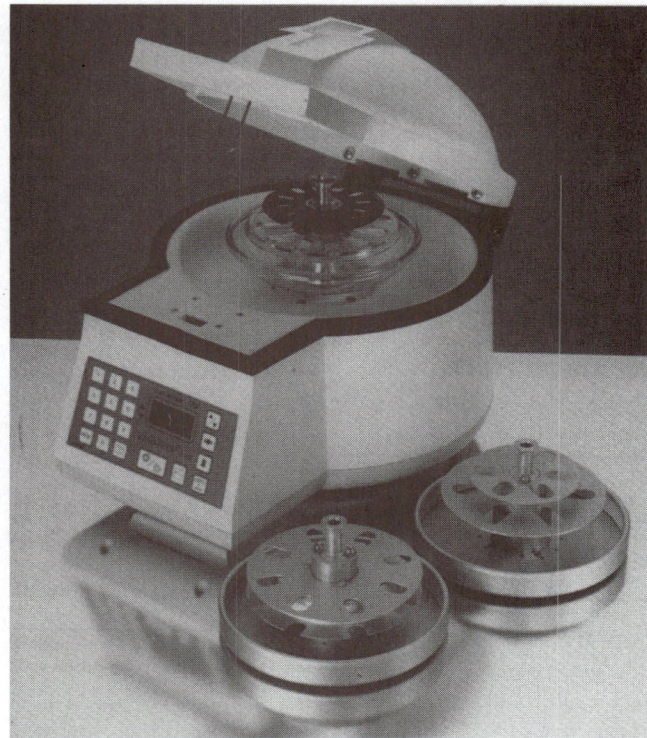

**FIGURE 4-11** Serological centrifuge. (Courtesy of Becton Dickinson Primary Care Diagnostic: Clay Adams and SEROFUGE are trademarks of Becton.

**Table 4-8.** Reactions of ABO groups with Anti-A and Anti-B sera

| BLOOD GROUP | REACTIONS OF CELLS WITH: | |
|---|---|---|
| | ANTI-A | ANTI-B |
| A | + | 0 |
| B | 0 | + |
| AB | + | + |
| O | 0 | 0 |

+ = agglutination
0 = no agglutination

**Table 4-9.** ABO forward and reverse grouping results

| ABO GROUP | FORWARD GROUPING | | REVERSE GROUPING | | |
|---|---|---|---|---|---|
| | Reactions of Cells with: | | Reactions of Plasma with: | | |
| | Anti-A | Anti-B | A Cells | B Cells | 0 Cells |
| O | 0 | 0 | + | + | 0 |
| A | + | 0 | 0 | + | 0 |
| B | 0 | + | + | 0 | 0 |
| AB | + | + | 0 | 0 | 0 |

0 = no agglutination
+ = agglutination

centrifuged for thirty seconds to enhance the reaction. The tubes are then removed from the centrifuge.

## Interpretation of Results

The tubes are tapped gently to loosen the cells from the bottom of the tube and the cells are observed for agglutination. Clumping of the cells is a positive reaction indicating the antigen present on the cells corresponds to the antibody placed in the test tube (Table 4-9). Reactions should be graded using a plus system: neg (no agglutination), w+, 1+, 2+, 3+, and 4+ (strongest agglutination). Figure 4-12 gives an illustration and description of each grade of reaction.

## Reverse or Indirect Grouping

Reverse (indirect or confirmatory) grouping identifies the antibodies present in a patient's serum or plasma by reacting the plasma with a commercial 2–5% suspension of group A cells and a commercial 2–5% suspension of group B cells and observing for agglutination.

Two drops of the patient's plasma are added to each of three tubes marked "a," "b," and "control." One drop of the group A cell suspension is added to tube "a," one drop of group B cell suspension is added to tube "b," and one drop of a 2–5% suspension of patient cells is added to the "control" tube. The contents of the tubes are mixed and the tubes are centrifuged for thirty seconds.

## Interpretation of Results

The tubes are tapped gently and the cells are observed for agglutination and the reactions graded (Figure 4-12). A positive test, agglutination, indicates that the antibody present in the patient's plasma corresponds to the antigen on cells added to the tube. The control tube should always be negative for agglutination since it contains

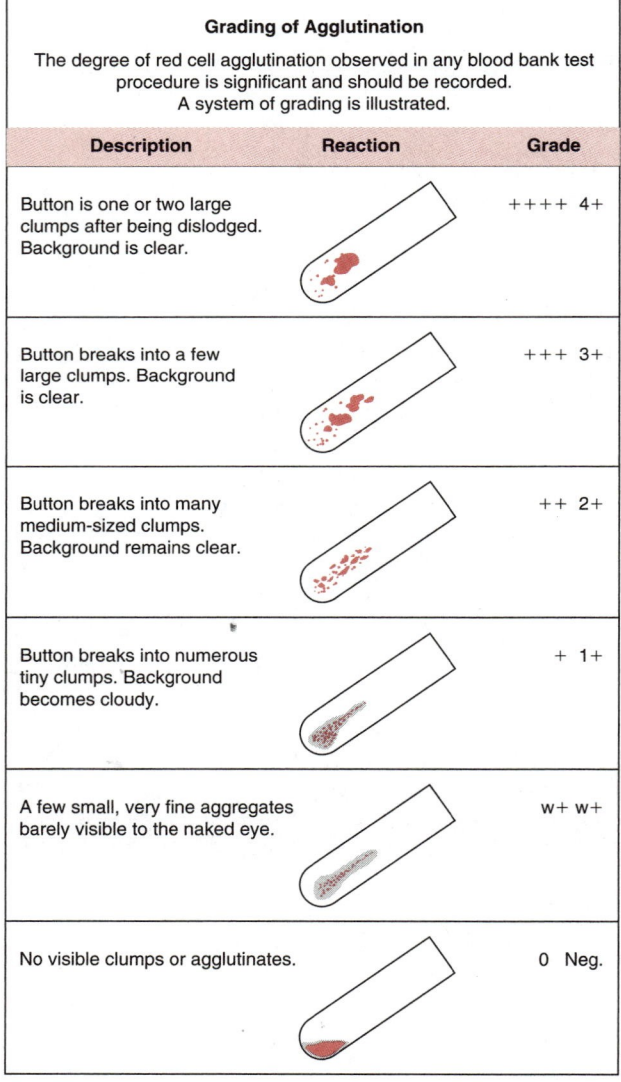

**Grading of Agglutination**

The degree of red cell agglutination observed in any blood bank test procedure is significant and should be recorded. A system of grading is illustrated.

| Description | Reaction | Grade |
|---|---|---|
| Button is one or two large clumps after being dislodged. Background is clear. | | ++++ 4+ |
| Button breaks into a few large clumps. Background is clear. | | +++ 3+ |
| Button breaks into many medium-sized clumps. Background remains clear. | | ++ 2+ |
| Button breaks into numerous tiny clumps. Background becomes cloudy. | | + 1+ |
| A few small, very fine aggregates barely visible to the naked eye. | | w+ w+ |
| No visible clumps or agglutinates. | | 0 Neg. |

**FIGURE 4-12** Illustration of grading of agglutination reactions

only the patient's plasma and cells. Reverse grouping results should confirm the results of forward grouping (Table 4-9).

## ADVANCES IN BLOOD BANK TECHNOLOGY

As in other departments of laboratory medicine, improvements are constantly being made in the technology of blood bank testing. Semi-automated systems are available for blood grouping and crossmatching. New gel methods allow some walk-away testing and are particularly helpful when staffing is low and technologists must work in more than one department on their shift. Since some of these reactions are stable for several hours, tests can be retained and reread if necessary. Although cost containment is an important issue in health care today, the blood bank must continue to maintain strict standards and use the best available methods, even if it means the cost of services must rise.

### Procedural Notes

- Follow manufacturer's directions regarding the storage and use of all commercial reagents.
- Do not use reagents beyond expiration dates.
- Perform quality control procedures at specified intervals and record.
- Observe timing carefully when performing slide tests.
- Use a 2–5% cell suspension for tube grouping.
- Use good lighting to observe reactions.
- Do not shake tubes too vigorously; weak agglutination reactions can be dispersed and misinterpreted.
- Record results as soon as they are observed.

### Safety Precautions

- Observe Universal and Standard Precautions when performing blood-grouping procedures.
- Wear buttoned fluid-resistant laboratory coat and other appropriate PPE.
- Discard all used glassware in biohazard sharps container.
- Observe safety rules when operating the serofuge.

## LESSON REVIEW

1. What department in the hospital laboratory performs blood grouping?
2. Name two other tests performed in this department.
3. What are four viral tests performed on donated blood before it can be released for transfusion?
4. Name three components that can be obtained from a unit of blood.
5. What antigens present on red blood cells determine the ABO groups?
6. Name the four groups in the ABO system and give the frequency of each.
7. What antibody is present in the serum of a person who is group B? Group 0?
8. What agglutination results would be observed when testing group A blood with anti-A and anti-B? When testing group AB blood?
9. How does ABO tube testing differ from ABO slide testing?
10. What is forward grouping?
11. What is reverse grouping?
12. How are the results of tube grouping tests interpreted? Explain the system of grading agglutination.
13. What safety precautions should be observed in ABO grouping?
14. Define antiserum, blood bank, blood group antibody, blood group antigen, and serofuge.

## STUDENT ACTIVITIES

1. Reread the information on ABO grouping.
2. Review the glossary terms.
3. Practice performing ABO groupings as outlined on the Student Performance Guide, using the worksheets for slide and tube grouping.

## Student Performance Guide

## LESSON 4-2 Immunohematology—ABO Grouping

Name _____   Date _____

### INSTRUCTIONS

1. Practice performing ABO grouping following the step-by-step procedure.
2. Demonstrate your understanding of this lesson by:
   a. Completing a written examination successfully, and
   b. Performing ABO grouping satisfactorily for the instructor. All steps must be completed as listed on the instructor's Performance Check Sheet.

*Note:* Package inserts should be consulted for specific instructions before test is performed.

### MATERIALS AND EQUIPMENT

- gloves
- hand disinfectant
- EDTA anticoagulated specimens
- stopwatch or timer
- wax pencil
- applicator sticks or stirrers
- physiological saline (0.85% or .15M NaCl)
- Pasteur pipets and rubber bulb or disposable plastic pipets
- anti-A (commercially available)
- anti-B (commercially available)
- A cells (2–5% suspension, commercially available)
- B cells (2–5% suspension, commercially available)
- serofuge or centrifuge capable of spinning 13 x 75 mm tubes at 2000–2500 rpm (optional)
- test tubes, 13 x 75 mm (disposable)
- test tube racks
- blood-grouping worksheets
- surface disinfectant (10% chlorine bleach solution)
- biohazard container
- puncture-proof container for sharps
- clean microscope slides or grouping slides

### PROCEDURE

| Record in the comment section any problems encountered while practicing the procedure (or have a fellow student or the instructor evaluate your performance). | | | S = Satisfactory<br>U = Unsatisfactory |
|---|---|---|---|
| **You must:** | **S** | **U** | **Comments** |
| 1. Wash hands and put on gloves. | | | |
| 2. Assemble equipment and materials | | | |
| 3. Perform slide grouping following steps 4–14 | | | |
| 4. Obtain a clean slide, mark the slide into two halves using a wax pencil. | | | |
| 5. Label the left side "A" and the right side "B" | | | |
| 6. Place one drop of anti-A serum on the "A" side (do not allow dropper to touch slide) | | | |

| You must: | S | U | Comments |
|---|---|---|---|
| 7. Place one drop of anti-B serum on the "B" side (do not allow dropper to touch slide) | | | |
| 8. Add one drop of well-mixed blood to each side of the slide using the Pasteur pipet (the drop of blood should be no larger than the drop of antibody) | | | |
| 9. Mix the blood and antiserum on side A and spread into a smooth round circle about the size of a nickel using a clean applicator stick. | | | |
| 10. Repeat the same procedure on side B using a clean applicator stick | | | |
| 11. Rock the slide gently for two minutes and look for agglutination using strong light | | | |
| 12. Record agglutination results on worksheet: agglutination = +; no agglutination = 0 | | | |
| 13. Determine the blood group and record | | | |
| 14. Repeat steps 4–13 on additional blood samples | | | |
| 15. Perform ABO forward tube grouping following steps 16–25 | | | |
| 16. Place one drop of a well-mixed blood specimen into a test tube; add eighteen to nineteen drops of saline, and label the tube "patient cells" (2–5%) | | | |
| 17. Label two test tubes "A" and "B" | | | |
| 18. Place one drop of anti-A in tube "A" | | | |
| 19. Place one drop of anti-B in tube "B" | | | |
| 20. Place one drop of the 2–5% patient cell suspension in each tube and mix | | | |
| 21. Place tubes in serofuge and spin thirty seconds. **Note:** balance the serofuge by placing tubes opposite each other. (If no serofuge is available, allow tubes to stand at room temperature for fifteen to thirty minutes and go to step 23) | | | |
| 22. Allow the serofuge to come to a complete stop and remove the tubes | | | |
| 23. Tap each tube gently to loosen cells from the bottom and observe cells for agglutination using good light. Grade agglutination (See Figure 4-12) | | | |
| 24. Record results from each tube on worksheet | | | |
| 25. Determine the blood group of the sample and record | | | |
| 26. Perform ABO reverse grouping on the blood sample following steps 27–38 | | | |
| 27. Centrifuge the blood sample, remove plasma from the sample, and place it in a clean test tube | | | |

| You must: | S | U | Comments |
|---|---|---|---|
| 28. Label three test tubes "a," "b," and "control" | | | |
| 29. Place two drops of plasma into each of these tubes | | | |
| 30. Place one drop of a 2–5% suspension of A cells into tube "a" and mix | | | |
| 31. Place one drop of a 2–5% suspension of B cells into tube "b" and mix | | | |
| 32. Place one drop of the patient's 2–5% cell suspension into "control" tube and mix | | | |
| 33. Place tubes in serofuge (be sure tubes are balanced) and spin thirty seconds (or allow tubes to sit at room temperature 15–30 minutes) | | | |
| 34. Remove the tubes from the serofuge after it stops completely | | | |
| 35. Tap each tube gently and observe cells for agglutination. Grade agglutination (See Figure 4-12) | | | |
| 36. Record the results from each tube on worksheet | | | |
| 37. Determine the blood group of the sample and record | | | |
| 38. Compare results of forward grouping with results of reverse grouping of the same sample. Reverse grouping should agree with results of forward grouping. | | | |
| 39. Repeat forward and reverse grouping on additional blood specimens if available | | | |
| 40. Discard all specimens appropriately | | | |
| 41. Soak reusable glassware in 10% chlorine bleach solution in a minimum of ten minutes and wash. Discard disposable tubes into biohazard sharps container | | | |
| 42. Clean equipment and return to proper storage. Return all reagents to proper storage | | | |
| 43. Clean work area with surface disinfectant | | | |
| 44. Remove gloves and discard in biohazard container | | | |
| 45. Wash hands with hand disinfectant | | | |

*Evaluator Comments:*

Evaluator _____ Date _____

## *Worksheet*

## **LESSON 4-2** ABO Grouping—Slide Method

Name _____   Date _____

| | AGGLUTINATION RESULTS* | | INTERPRETATION |
|---|---|---|---|
| Specimen I.D. | Anti-A | Anti-B | ABO group |
| _____ | _____ | _____ | _____ |
| _____ | _____ | _____ | _____ |
| _____ | _____ | _____ | _____ |
| _____ | _____ | _____ | _____ |
| _____ | _____ | _____ | _____ |

*Record results as:
0 = no agglutination
+ = agglutination

# Worksheet

## LESSON 4-2 ABO Grouping—Tube Method

Name _____   Date _____

| Specimen I.D. | DIRECT (FORWARD) GROUPING* | | INTERPRETATION | INDIRECT (REVERSE) GROUPING* | | | INTERPRETATION |
|---|---|---|---|---|---|---|---|
| | Anti-A | Anti-B | ABO Group | A Cells | B Cells | Control | ABO Group |
| _____ | _____ | _____ | _____ | _____ | _____ | _____ | _____ |
| _____ | _____ | _____ | _____ | _____ | _____ | _____ | _____ |
| _____ | _____ | _____ | _____ | _____ | _____ | _____ | _____ |
| _____ | _____ | _____ | _____ | _____ | _____ | _____ | _____ |
| _____ | _____ | _____ | _____ | _____ | _____ | _____ | _____ |

*Record results as:

0 = no agglutination
w+ = fine agglutinates, most cells not agglutinated
1+ = tiny clumps, cloudy background
2+ = several small clumps, clear background
3+ = several large clumps, clear background
4+ = 2-3 large clumps, clear background

# Immunohematology— Rh Typing

## GLOSSARY

**hemolytic disease of the newborn (HDN)** / a condition in which antibody from the mother destroys the red blood cells of the fetus

**immunization** / the process of producing immunity to an antigen

**Rh (D) immune globulin (RhIG)** / a concentrated, purified solution of human anti-D antibody used for injection

## INTRODUCTION

The Rh blood group, discovered in the 1940s, is the second most important human blood group system. The system is named Rh because the rhesus monkey was being used in the experiments when the system was discovered. Testing for antigens of the Rh system is a routine procedure in blood banks and clinical laboratories. A patient's Rh type must be determined before a blood transfusion is performed.

The Rh antigens may be detected by the slide method or the tube method. The tube method is the preferred method used in blood banks.

## THE Rh BLOOD GROUP SYSTEM

### Rh Antigens

The antigens of the Rh system are products of inherited genes and are present on the surface of red blood cells.

The major antigen in the Rh system is the D antigen. Red blood cells that possess the D antigen are called Rh (D) positive. Cells that lack the D antigen are called Rh (D) negative.

Eighty-five percent of the U.S. population are Rh (D) positive (D+) and 15% are Rh (D) negative (D-). Several other antigens are part of the Rh system but routine typing only tests for the D antigen.

### Weak D Antigen (D^U)

Some individuals have a form of the D antigen that reacts weakly in the typing procedure. Blood giving a weak reaction with anti-D is called weak D, or $D^U$, and is considered D positive.

Blood cells carrying the weak form of the D antigen may sometimes give a negative reaction in routine slide or tube typing even though the cells have a small amount of the antigen present. The typing test must be enhanced to detect these forms of weak D. The test to detect weak D is performed using the principles of the antiglobulin test and is not covered in this lesson. Laboratories allow only specially qualified workers to perform the weak D ($D^U$) test.

## Nomenclature of the Rh System

Two methods of naming the antigens in the Rh system are the Fisher-Race method and the Wiener method. The names of the antigen and antibody in each system are given in Table 4-10. Manufacturers of blood bank reagents may use one or both systems in labeling reagents.

## Rh Antibodies

Unlike the ABO system, the Rh system does not have antibodies that occur naturally. However, antibody to the D antigen (anti-D) may be produced by an Rh (D) negative person who becomes immunized or sensitized to the D antigen. This may occur during pregnancy or following blood transfusion.

### Hemolytic Disease of the Newborn (HDN)

Immunization to the D antigen during pregnancy may cause a condition called **hemolytic disease of the newborn (HDN)**. When an Rh (D) negative mother is pregnant with an Rh (D) positive baby, some of the baby's D positive blood cells may enter the mother's circulation during pregnancy or the birth process. This exposure to the D-positive cells may stimulate production of anti-D antibody by the mother.

The first Rh (D) positive child born to the Rh (D) negative mother is usually not affected because the mother's exposure to the D antigen does not usually occur until she gives birth. However, the effect may be seen in subsequent pregnancies in which the RBCs of the fetus carry the D antigen. In these cases, the mother's anti-D antibodies (stimulated by the earlier pregnancy) may enter the fetus' bloodstream and damage the unborn baby's red blood cells. This causes hemolysis of the baby's blood cells, thus the name hemolytic disease of the newborn (HDN). The effect on the fetus may be mild or severe, ranging from mild jaundice to anemia or brain damage. In severe cases, stillbirth or miscarriage may occur.

### Prevention of HDN

It is possible to prevent most cases of Rh HDN by administering **Rh (D) immune globulin (RhIG)** to the mother. RhIG is a concentrated solution of anti-D antibody that, when injected into the (D-) mother, will prevent anti-D antibody from forming. This injection must be given within seventy-two hours after delivery of a D positive baby or after termination of a pregnancy.

Women who have the weak D antigen are considered D positive and do not receive RhIG. Expectant mothers should have their Rh type determined during the first trimester of pregnancy. This helps to identify mothers who are at risk of having a baby with HDN so that the fetus may be monitored during the pregnancy for signs of stress.

## IMPORTANCE OF Rh TYPING

It is important to test all patients who are to receive transfusions for the D antigen so the proper type of blood will be given. Rh (D) negative patients should only be transfused with Rh (D) negative blood. Testing for the D antigen is also used to identify females at risk of giving birth to an infant with HDN, in family genetic studies, and in establishing parentage in legal cases.

## Rh TYPING PROCEDURES

The Rh (D) antigen may be identified using slide typing or tube typing techniques. Venous anticoagulated blood is the preferred specimen, but capillary blood may also be used.

**TABLE 4-10.** Fisher-Race and Wiener nomenclature for the Rh system

| NOMENCLATURE | ANTIGEN | ANTIBODY |
|---|---|---|
| Fisher-Race | D | Anti-D |
| Wiener | $Rh_O$ | Anti-$Rh_O$ |

**Safety**

Universal and Standard Precautions must be adhered to when collecting blood specimens and when performing typing. Gloves and other appropriate personal protective equipment must be worn when performing the procedures. Used slides or tubes must be discarded in a biohazard container for sharps.

---

### *Quality Assurance*

Patient identification, blood specimen identification, and slide or tube labeling must be done with accuracy. Typing antisera must be visually inspected and tested at designated intervals using appropriate control cells. Reagents must be used and stored according to manufacturers' directions and should not be used beyond their expiration dates. Timing limits for slide typing tests must be observed so that cell drying will not be mistaken for cell agglutination. Results and interpretation of results must be carefully recorded. When using high protein anti-D, a protein control should be included as part of the Rh typing test.

---

## Performing Rh Slide Typing

To perform Rh (D) typing, a drop of anti-D antiserum is added to a labeled microscope slide. A large drop of blood is added to the slide and the blood and antiserum are mixed with an applicator stick and spread over at least one-half of the slide. The slide is placed on a heated, lighted viewbox to heat it to 37°C and is rocked back and forth for two minutes while observing for agglutination (Figure 4-13). The presence or absence of agglutination is recorded. If agglutination is present, the reaction should be graded.

Several types of commercial anti-D are available for Rh typing, including high protein anti-D, chemically modified anti-D, monoclonal anti-D, and saline anti-D. Quality control procedures and instructions for use may differ for each type of antiserum. Recommendations in package insert(s) for the reagents being used must be followed.

A control slide is usually prepared and tested along with the patient sample when using high protein anti-D. This slide is prepared similarly to the test sample except that a control (protein) diluent is mixed with the blood instead of the antiserum.

## Performing Rh Tube Typing

Rh D tube typing is performed as for ABO grouping. A 2–5% suspension is made from the patient's cells. A drop of this suspension is mixed with a drop of anti-D

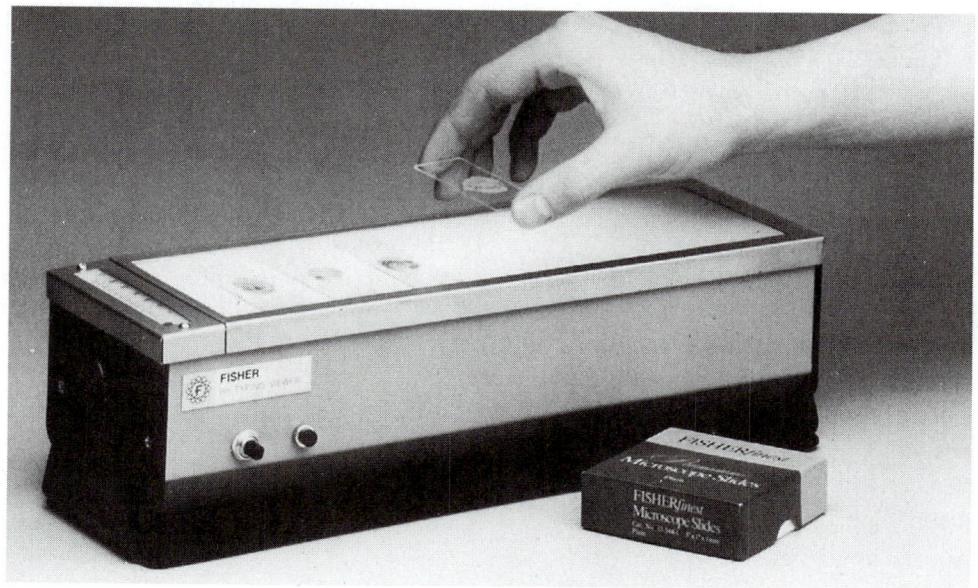

**FIGURE 4-13** A slide is placed on a heated, lighted box to check for the presence of agglutination

and the tube is centrifuged. The cell pellet is gently dispersed and observed for agglutination, and the reaction is graded. (Since the patient serum contains no natural anti-D antibody, reverse or confirmatory typing is not performed.)

## Interpreting Results of Rh Typing

If the patient is Rh (D) positive, the patient's cells will agglutinate when reacted with anti-D. If the patient is Rh (D) negative, no agglutination will be present (Table 4-11). Negative Rh (D) slide typing results must be confirmed with a tube test or weak D (D^u) test before being reported.

The control slide or tube should always be negative for agglutination. If the control is positive, the test is invalid and must be repeated using a different method or different reagents. Positive control results may be due to contaminated control serum or abnormalities in the patient blood sample.

**TABLE 4-11.** Interpretation of results of Rh typing

**REACTIONS OF CELLS WITH:**

| Anti-D | Control Serum | Interpretation |
|---|---|---|
| + | 0 | Rh (D) positive |
| 0 | 0 | Rh (D) negative; confirm with weak D (D^u) test |
| + | + | Unable to interpret; repeat test using another method |

+ = agglutination
0 = no agglutination

### Procedural Notes

- Always follow manufacturers' instructions for the use of reagents.
- Identify patient and label slides and tubes accurately.
- Perform Rh (D) slide typing at 37°C, using a lighted, heated viewbox.
- Do not observe heated slides for more than two minutes before recording observations.
- Confirm negative Rh (D) slide typing with a tube test or a test for weak D (D^u).

### Safety Precautions

- Observe Universal and Standard Precautions when performing typing tests.
- Wear fluid-resistant, buttoned laboratory coat and other appropriate PPE.
- Discard all used supplies appropriately.
- Wipe work area with surface disinfectant frequently.

## LESSON REVIEW

1. What is the major antigen in the Rh system? *Anti D*
2. What circumstances must exist before anti-D antibody is produced by an individual?
3. What is the "weak D" antigen? *Ant D^u*
4. Explain how hemolytic disease of the newborn occurs.
5. Why is Rh D typing performed?
6. Why must D positive blood not be transfused into a D negative patient?
7. Define hemolytic disease of the newborn, immunization, and Rh (D) immune globulin.

## STUDENT ACTIVITIES

1. Reread the information on Rh typing.
2. Review the glossary terms.
3. Practice performing Rh typing on several blood samples as outlined on the Student Performance Guide, using the worksheet.

# Student Performance Guide

## LESSON 4-3 Immunohematology—Rh Typing

Name _____   Date _____

## INSTRUCTIONS

1. Practice performing Rh typing following the step-by-step procedure.
2. Demonstrate your understanding of this lesson by:
   a. Completing a written examination successfully, and
   b. Performing Rh typing satisfactorily for the instructor. All steps must be completed as listed on the instructor's Performance Check Sheet.

*Note:* Package insert should be consulted for specific instructions before test is performed.

## MATERIALS AND EQUIPMENT

- gloves
- hand disinfectant
- centrifuge
- test tube racks
- serological tubes, 13 x 75 mm
- physiological saline
- disposable plastic pipets
- clean microscope slides
- applicator sticks or stirrers
- anti-D serum (anti-Rh$_o$)
- Rh control solution
- blood specimen
- lighted viewbox
- Rh typing worksheet
- wax pencil
- stopwatch or timer
- surface disinfectant (10% chlorine bleach solution)
- biohazard container
- puncture-proof sharps container

## PROCEDURE

| Record in the comment section any problems encountered while practicing the procedure (or have a fellow student or the instructor evaluate your performance). | | | S = Satisfactory<br>U = Unsatisfactory |
|---|---|---|---|
| **You must:** | **S** | **U** | **Comments** |
| 1. Wash hands and put on gloves | | | |
| 2. Assemble equipment and materials | | | |
| 3. Turn on viewbox | | | |
| 4. Label two clean microscope slides "D" and "C" (control) | | | |
| 5. Place one drop of anti-D serum on the "D" slide | | | |
| 6. Place one drop of Rh control solution on the "C" slide | | | |

| You must: | S | U | Comments |
|---|---|---|---|
| 7. Place one large drop of well-mixed whole blood on each slide | | | |
| 8. Mix blood and anti-D well with an applicator stick, spreading the mixture over at least one-half of the slide | | | |
| 9. Repeat procedure for the control slide using a clean applicator stick | | | |
| 10. Place slides on the lighted viewbox and start timer | | | |
| 11. Tilt the viewbox slowly back and forth for two minutes | | | |
| 12. Observe the slides for agglutination at the end of two minutes | | | |
| 13. Record results on worksheet: agglutination = +; no agglutination = 0 | | | |
| 14. Determine the Rh type and record on worksheet | | | |
| 15. Repeat steps 4–14 on other blood samples, as directed by instructor | | | |
| 16. Perform tube typing on a specimen (or go to step 25) | | | |
| 17. Prepare a 2–5% suspension of the blood specimen by adding 19 drops of saline to one drop of well-mixed blood | | | |
| 18. Label two tubes "patient" and "control" | | | |
| 19. Add one drop of patient cell suspension to each labeled tube | | | |
| 20. Add one drop of anti-D to "patient" tube and one drop of control diluent to "control" tube | | | |
| 22. Mix contents of tubes and centrifuge for 30 seconds | | | |
| 23. Gently tap tubes to loosen cell pellets and observe for agglutination | | | |
| 24. Grade reactions and record results on worksheet. *Note:* absence of agglutination in patient tube requires a test for weak D before the patient can be definitively typed as D negative | | | |
| 25. Discard specimens, tubes, and slides in biohazard sharps container | | | |
| 26. Clean equipment and return to proper storage | | | |
| 27. Clean work area with surface disinfectant | | | |
| 28. Remove gloves and discard in biohazard container | | | |
| 29. Wash hands with hand disinfectant | | | |

*Evaluator Comments:*

Evaluator _____ Date _____

# Worksheet

## LESSON 4-3 Rh Typing

Name _____ Date _____

| Specimen I.D. | AGGLUTINATION RESULTS* | | INTERPRETATION** |
|---|---|---|---|
| | Anti-D | Control Diluent | Rh Type |
| _____ | _____ | _____ | _____ |
| _____ | _____ | _____ | _____ |
| _____ | _____ | _____ | _____ |
| _____ | _____ | _____ | _____ |
| _____ | _____ | _____ | _____ |

*Record results as:

0 = no agglutination

w+ = fine agglutinates, most cells not agglutinated

1+ = tiny clumps, cloudy background

2+ = several small clumps, clear background

3+ = several large clumps, clear background

4+ = 2-3 large clumps, clear background

**Record interpretation as:

Rh D positive or

Rh D negative

# Slide Test for Infectious Mononucleosis

## LESSON OBJECTIVES

**After studying this lesson, you should be able to:**

- *Name the cause of infectious mononucleosis.*
- *List five clinical symptoms of infectious mononucleosis.*
- *Name two types of tests performed to diagnose infectious mononucleosis.*
- *Perform a slide test for infectious mononucleosis.*
- *Interpret the results of a slide test for infectious mononucleosis.*
- *Define the glossary terms.*

## GLOSSARY

**Epstein-Barr virus (EBV)** / a virus that infects lymphocytes and is the cause of infectious mononucleosis

**heterophile antibodies** / antibodies that are increased in infectious mononucleosis

**lymphocytosis** / an increase above the normal number of lymphocytes in the blood

## INTRODUCTION

Infectious mononucleosis is commonly called "mono" or "kissing disease." It is a contagious viral disease that affects mostly the fifteen-to-twenty-five-year-old age group. The disease is caused by infection of B lymphocytes with the **Epstein-Barr virus (EBV)**, a member of the herpes group of viruses.

Infectious mononucleosis (IM) is accompanied by a variety of nonspecific symptoms that can mimic other diseases. Early diagnosis of IM is often based on laboratory test results. IM testing may also be done to follow the course of the disease.

The most common serological test for IM is the rapid slide test, which tests serum for the presence of heterophile antibodies. The slide test gives quick, reliable results and is simple to perform. Some test kits for IM are included in the list of CLIA-waived tests.

## DIAGNOSIS OF INFECTIOUS MONONUCLEOSIS

### Clinical Symptoms

Clinical symptoms of IM are non-specific. They include fatigue, fever, sore throat, weakness, headache, and swollen lymph nodes. Patients may have some or all of these symptoms. During the acute phase, patients may also have an enlarged spleen and liver. To aid in the diagnosis of IM, hematological and serological tests are used.

## Hematological Test for Infectious Mononucleosis

IM causes certain changes in the circulating lymphocytes that can be detected by a WBC count and evaluation of WBC morphology from a stained blood smear. Usually **lymphocytosis**, an increase in lymphocytes, occurs and large numbers (>20%) of the lymphocytes are atypical or reactive.

## Serological Test for Infectious Mononucleosis

Persons with IM produce antibodies called **heterophile antibodies** by the sixth to tenth day of the illness. Heterophile antibodies react with similar antigens in more than one species and are usually of the IgM class.

Detection of heterophile antibodies combined with the hematological and clinical findings provide the basis for diagnosing IM. The serological test is usually positive after the first week of illness. However, if test results are negative, the test should be repeated after a week if clinical symptoms are still present.

## SLIDE TESTS FOR INFECTIOUS MONONUCLEOSIS

The slide test is a rapid method of detecting heterophile antibodies in serum. The procedure is based on the agglutination of horse erythrocytes by the heterophile antibodies of IM. Since there are other antibodies in serum that will also react with horse erythrocytes, the patient's serum is reacted with absorbents to remove these other antibodies before the serum is reacted with the horse cells.

Several commercial kits are available to test for IM. Most kits are based on agglutination principles and are adaptations of the Davidsohn differential test for heterophile antibodies, a cumbersome time-consuming test. One-step immunoassay kits for IM are available. Examples of IM kits include the Color Slide®II Mononucleosis Test by Seradyn, the BBL® Monoslide™ Test by Becton Dickinson, the Monospot™ Slide Test by Meridian Diagnostics, the CMS Sure-Vue® Mono Kit, and MONO-Plus® WB by Wampole.

Serological test kits for IM usually provide all the necessary reagents, materials, and controls. The specimen tested can be a small sample of plasma, serum, or whole blood.

## PERFORMING THE SLIDE AGGLUTINATION TEST FOR IM

The procedure for detecting the heterophile antibodies of IM described in this lesson is the Monospot™ test by Meridian Diagnostics. Manufacturer's instructions for the kit should be strictly followed.

 ## Safety

Universal and Standard Precautions must be observed when performing serological tests. Gloves and other appropriate PPE must be used. Control sera made from human blood products must be treated as if potentially infectious. Used disposable test components must be discarded in appropriate biohazard containers.

> ## *Quality Assurance*
>
> Manufacturer's instructions for the kit being used must be followed. Reagents must be stored and used according to package inserts and should not be used beyond the expiration dates. Positive and negative serum controls provided with kits should be tested along with the patient sample to ensure that all reagents are reacting properly. Reagents from different kit manufacturers must not be interchanged. Reactions must be recorded and interpreted carefully, following the instructions in the package insert and the laboratory's procedure manual.

### Test Procedure

The test is performed using a glass slide that has two squares (I and II) etched on the slide. The slide is laid on a flat surface. The reagents are mixed thoroughly and a drop of indicator cells (horse erythrocytes) is added to a corner of each square using the capillary pipet provided. One drop of Reagent I is then placed in the center of square I and one drop of Reagent II is placed in the center of square II. One drop of serum is placed in the center of each square using the plastic pipet provided in the kit (Figure 4-14).

The serum and Reagent I are mixed using at least ten stirring motions with a clean applicator stick. The

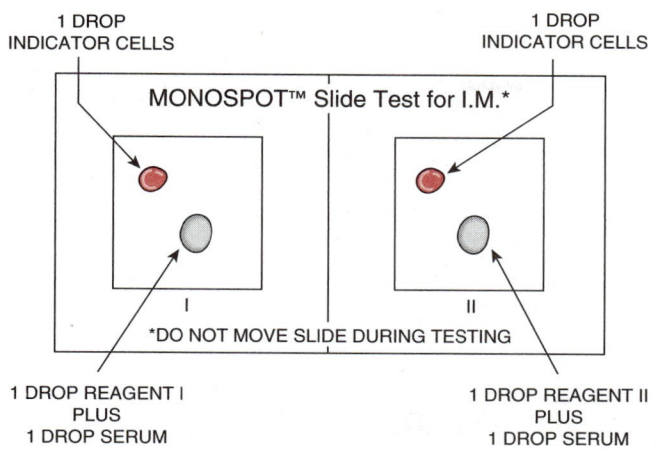

**FIGURE 4-14** Monospot™ slide with reagents added

**FIGURE 4-15** Mixing reagents on Monospot™ slide using applicator

indicator cells are then blended in with the mixture so the entire surface of the square is covered. The contents of square II are mixed in the same manner as square I (Figure 4-15).

A timer is started as soon as mixing is completed and the slide is observed for one minute for agglutination of the indicator (horse) cells. During this time, the slide should not be moved or picked up. At the end of one minute, the results are recorded and interpreted.

## Interpreting Results of Slide Test for IM

The presence or absence of heterophile antibodies of IM will be indicated by the presence or absence of agglutination, as indicated in Table 4-12.

The test is considered positive if agglutination is stronger on the left side of the slide (square I) than on the right side of the slide (square II). Any other pattern of agglutination or absence of agglutination is considered a negative test. Positive and negative control sera should give the appropriate reactions.

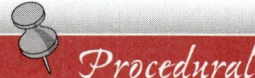

### Procedural Notes

- Follow manufacturer's directions for the kit being used.
- Use positive and negative control sera along with patient samples.
- Observe and interpret results carefully.

**Table 4-12.** Interpretation of results of Monospot™ test

| POSITIVE TEST | NEGATIVE TEST |
|---|---|
| Agglutination pattern is stronger on the left side of the slide (square I) than on the right side of the slide (square II) | A. Agglutination pattern is stronger on the right side of the slide (square II) than in square I<br><br>**or**<br><br>B. No agglutination appears in either square<br><br>**or**<br><br>C. Agglutination is equal in both squares of the slide |

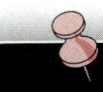

## Safety Precautions

- Follow Universal and Standard Precautions when performing serological tests.
- Discard all contaminated items in appropriate biohazard containers.
- Disinfect reusable materials before washing

5. What safety precautions should be followed in performing a slide test for IM? *use instr. in kit — α p.*

6. How soon after the disease begins will the serological test usually be positive? *6–10 days*

7. What is the function of horse erythrocytes in the slide test for IM?

8. What quality control measures must be performed with the slide test for IM? *cause IM*

9. Define Epstein-Barr virus, heterophile antibodies, and lymphocytosis.

## LESSON REVIEW

1. What causes infectious mononucleosis? *Epstein Barr virus*
2. What are the clinical symptoms of IM? *Lymph. enlarged*
3. What information can be gained from the hematological test? *> 20% larger of Lymp.*
4. What does the serological test detect? *slide test agglutination*

## STUDENT ACTIVITIES

1. Reread the information on the slide test for IM.
2. Review the glossary terms.
3. Practice performing the slide test for IM as outlined on the Student Performance Guide.

## *Student Performance Guide*

## **LESSON 4-4** Slide Test for Infectious Mononucleosis

Name _____ Date _____

 ### INSTRUCTIONS

1. Practice performing the slide test for IM following the step-by-step procedure.
2. Demonstrate your understanding of this lesson by:
   a. Completing a written examination successfully, and
   b. Performing the slide test for IM satisfactorily for the instructor. All steps must be completed as listed on the instructor's Performance Check Sheet.

*Note:* Procedure given is for Monospot™ test by Meridian Diagnostics. Package insert should be consulted before test is performed. If another kit is used, the manufacturer's instructions should be followed.

### MATERIALS AND EQUIPMENT

- gloves
- hand disinfectant
- test serum or plasma
- stopwatch or timer
- surface disinfectant (10% chlorine bleach solution)
- test kit for IM (kit should include instructions, slide, serum dispensers, stirrers, reagents, and controls)
- biohazard container

## PROCEDURE

Record in the comment section any problems encountered while practicing the procedure (or have a fellow student or the instructor evaluate your performance).

S = Satisfactory
U = Unsatisfactory

| You must: | S | U | Comments |
|---|---|---|---|
| 1. Wash hands and put on gloves | | | |
| 2. Assemble equipment and materials | | | |
| 3. Place the Monospot™ slide on a flat work surface | | | |
| 4. Mix the reagent vials several times by inversion | | | |
| 5. Fill the capillary pipet to the top mark with indicator cells:<br>  a. Place the rubber bulb on the end of the capillary pipet with the heavy black line<br>  b. Insert the pipet into the vial of indicator cells<br>  c. Allow the pipet to fill to the top mark by capillary action | | | |
| 6. Place your index finger over the hole in the bulb and squeeze gently to dispense one-half of the cells (10 µL) on a corner of square I of the slide (the level of the cells should now be at the lower mark on the pipet) | | | |

| You must: | S | U | Comments |
|---|---|---|---|
| 7. Deliver the remaining cells (10 μL) to a corner of square II | | | |
| 8. Place one drop of thoroughly mixed Reagent I in the center of square I | | | |
| 9. Place one drop of thoroughly mixed Reagent II in the center of square II | | | |
| 10. Add one drop of test serum to the center of each square using the disposable plastic pipet provided | | | |
| 11. Use a clean applicator stick to mix Reagent I with the serum using *at least ten* stirring motions without touching the indicator cells | | | |
| 12. Blend in the indicator cells in square I with the applicator stick using *no more than ten* stirring motions, and spreading the mixture over the entire surface of the square | | | |
| 13. Repeat steps 11–12 using Reagent II in square II, using a clean applicator stick | | | |
| 14. Start the timer after you have completed mixing of both squares | | | |
| 15. Do not pick up or move the slide | | | |
| 16. Observe both squares for agglutination at the end of one minute (no longer) without moving the slide or picking it up | | | |
| 17. Record the agglutination in each square and interpret the results: If the agglutination pattern is stronger in square I than in square II, the test is positive for the heterophile antibody of infectious mononucleosis. Any other combination of reactions is negative | | | |
| 18. Record test results as positive or negative | | | |
| 19. Repeat test procedure (steps 3–18) using positive and negative control sera | | | |
| 20. Discard contaminated materials in biohazard container | | | |
| 21. Dispose of specimen appropriately and disinfect reusable materials by soaking in 10% chlorine bleach solution for at least ten minutes. Wash and rinse thoroughly | | | |
| 22. Clean work area with surface disinfectant | | | |
| 23. Remove gloves and discard in biohazard container | | | |
| 24. Wash hands with hand disinfectant | | | |

*Evaluator Comments:*

Evaluator _____ Date _____

# Slide Test for Rheumatoid Factors

## LESSON OBJECTIVES

**After studying this lesson, you should be able to:**

- *Explain the significance of rheumatoid factors.*
- *Explain the reasons for performing the test for rheumatoid factors.*
- *Explain the principle of latex agglutination tests.*
- *Perform a qualitative latex agglutination test for rheumatoid factors.*
- *Perform a quantitative latex agglutination test for rheumatoid factors.*
- *Interpret the results of a latex agglutination test for rheumatoid factors.*
- *Define the glossary terms*

## GLOSSARY

**autoantibody** / an antibody directed against the self (one's own tissues)

**reciprocal** / inverse; one of a pair of numbers (as 2/3 and 3/2) that has a product of one

**rheumatoid arthritis (RA)** / a disease characterized by inflammation of the joints

**rheumatoid factors (RF)** / autoantibodies directed against human IgG that are often present in the serum of patients with rheumatoid arthritis

## INTRODUCTION

Arthritis, an inflammation of the joints, can occur in several diseases. Among these are gout, rheumatic fever, lupus, osteoarthritis, and **rheumatoid arthritis (RA)**. Several serological tests are available that aid in distinguishing rheumatoid arthritis from arthritis of other causes. Most of these tests are based on the detection of rheumatoid factors in the patient's serum using a latex agglutination method. This lesson describes a rapid slide test for the detection of rheumatoid factors.

## RHEUMATOID ARTHRITIS AND RHEUMATOID FACTORS

Between 75% and 85% of people with rheumatoid arthritis have elevated levels of **rheumatoid factors (RF)** in their serum. Rheumatoid factors are **autoantibodies**, usually of the IgM class, directed against human IgG. Rheumatoid factors are not usually elevated in other forms of arthritis. Because of this, the RF test is useful in diagnosing rheumatoid arthritis.

# PRINCIPLE OF SLIDE AGGLUTINATION TESTS FOR RHEUMATOID FACTORS

Most RF slide tests are modifications of a latex agglutination test developed by Singer and Plotz in 1956. In the RF test, small latex particles are coated with specially treated human immunoglobulin (IgG). When serum containing RF is mixed with the IgG-coated latex particles, the rheumatoid factors (which are autoantibodies) bind to the IgG and cause agglutination of the particles (Figure 4-16).

Commercial latex RF kits include the RFscan™ Latex Test by Becton Dickinson, SeraTest™ RF Latex Test by Seradyn, and CMS Sure-Vue® RF test. These kits provide the coated latex particles, positive and negative control sera, buffer, and other materials necessary to perform the tests. The Rheumaton® test by Wampole is a hemagglutination test that uses the agglutination of specially treated cells to detect RF.

# PERFORMING A QUALITATIVE TEST FOR RF

 **Safety**

Universal and Standard Precautions must be followed when performing all serological tests. Control sera produced from human blood products must be treated as if potentially infectious.

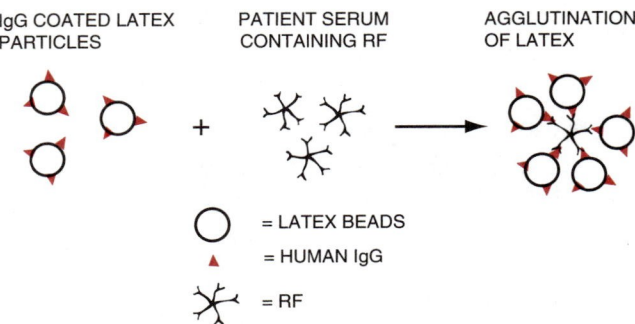

**FIGURE 4-16** Principle of latex agglutination test for rheumatoid factors. Rheumatoid factors in serum react with IgG-coated particles to cause agglutination.

by centrifugation. Some RF tests require that, before testing, the serum be diluted (usually 1:20) with a buffer included in the kit. This dilution is necessary because the serum of most normal individuals already has low levels of RF. Testing diluted serum assures that only significant levels of RF will be detected in the test.

## Test Procedure

To perform the test, one drop each of positive control serum, negative control serum, and (diluted) patient serum are placed in separate rings on a black glass, plastic, or cardboard slide (included in test kit). One drop of well-mixed latex reagent is dispensed into each ring. The latex reagent is then mixed with each serum using a clean stirrer or spreader for each. The mixtures are each spread over the entire surface of the ring. The slide is then rocked or rotated for the specified time (usually one to three minutes) and observed for agglutination under a bright light.

## Interpreting the Results of an RF Test

The ring containing the positive control serum should show agglutination. Agglutination appears as small white clumps against the black background of the slide (Figure 4-17). The negative control serum should have no agglutination. A negative reaction will appear as a milky white solution with no clumping in the test area (Figure 4-17).

Absence of agglutination with the patient serum indicates the level of rheumatoid factors is within normal range and is reported as "negative," "no agglutination seen," or, if diluted serum was used, "titer less than 20."

Presence of agglutination with the patient serum is considered a positive test and indicates a significantly elevated level of rheumatoid factors. A quantitative RF test should be performed on positive samples and the titer should be reported.

---

### Quality Assurance

For reliable test results, the manufacturer's instructions for the particular kit being used must be followed. Reagents from different manufacturers must not be interchanged. Storage recommendations must be followed and reagents should not be used beyond the expiration dates.

Positive and negative control sera provided with the kits must be run at the specified intervals and the results recorded. If controls do not give the expected reactions, patient specimens must not be tested until the problem has been identified and corrected.

---

## Specimen Collection and Preparation

Serum is the usual specimen for latex agglutination tests. This is obtained by collecting a clot tube from a venipuncture, and separating the serum from the cells

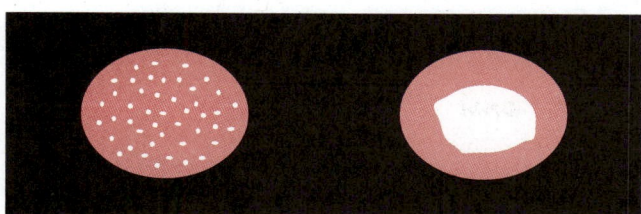

**POSITIVE**          **NEGATIVE**

POSITIVE = AGGLUTINATION (WHITE CLUMPS)
NEGATIVE = NO AGGLUTINATION
               (MILKY WHITE SOLUTION)

**FIGURE 4-17** Illustration of positive and negative reactions in the RF latex agglutination test.

If undiluted serum is tested and shows agglutination, the serum must be diluted 1:20 or serially diluted and reassayed. Test kits differ in sensitivity. For most test kits, only serum that is positive at a 1:20 (or higher) dilution can be considered positive for RF.

## Significance of Results

Diagnosis of rheumatoid arthritis should not be based on the RF test alone, since some other conditions, particularly inflammatory diseases, may also cause a positive RF test. Conversely, since only 75–85% of those with rheumatoid arthritis have increased levels of RF, *a negative test does not rule out the diagnosis of rheumatoid arthritis.*

Knowledge of the amount of RF present can be useful in monitoring the course of rheumatoid arthritis, since RF levels tend to parallel the patient's condition. Patients with active rheumatoid arthritis usually have higher RF levels than patients with inactive disease.

Higher-than-normal levels of RF can interfere with other types of laboratory assays, such as thyroid tests, causing false positive reactions.

## PERFORMING A QUANTITATIVE TEST FOR RF

A quantitative test for RF is performed by testing a series of dilutions of the patient's serum to determine the RF titer. The highest serum dilution showing agglutination (positive reaction) is recorded. The titer, which is the **reciprocal**, or inverse, of the highest dilution giving a positive result, is reported. For example: dilutions of 1:40, 1:80, and 1:160 were made from a serum that was positive in the qualitative test. When the dilutions were tested for RF, the 1:40 and 1:80 dilutions showed agglutination, and the 1:160 dilution was negative. The RF of this serum would be reported as a titer of 80 (the reciprocal of the 1:80 or 1/80 serum dilution).

### *Procedural Notes*

- ■ Follow manufacturer's instructions for the kit used.
- ■ Perform quantitative test if initial test for RF is positive.
- ■ Use good lighting to observe latex agglutination.
- ■ Run appropriate controls each time a patient sample is tested.
- ■ Do not reuse kit components, unless manufacturer's instructions allow.

### *Safety Precautions*

- ■ Observe Universal and Standard Precautions when performing assays.
- ■ Discard used materials in appropriate biohazard containers.
- ■ Handle controls and reagents produced from human products as if potentially infectious.

## LESSON REVIEW

1. What are rheumatoid factors?
2. An elevated level of RF is often associated with what disease?
3. Explain the principle of latex agglutination tests.
4. Describe the appearance of a positive test and a negative test.
5. What is the difference in a qualitative and quantitative agglutination test?
6. What is the significance of a positive RF slide agglutination test? Of a negative RF slide agglutination test?
7. Why is serum diluted before performing the RF test?
8. What is a titer?
9. Define autoantibody, reciprocal, rheumatoid arthritis, and rheumatoid factors.

## STUDENT ACTIVITIES

1. Reread the information on the slide test for RF.
2. Review the glossary terms.
3. Practice performing qualitative and quantitative slide agglutination tests for RF as outlined on the Student Performance Guide.

# *Student Performance Guide*

## **LESSON 4-5** Slide Test for Rheumatoid Factors

Name _____ Date _____

### ☣ INSTRUCTIONS

1. Practice performing the slide test for RF following the step-by-step procedure.
2. Demonstrate your understanding of this lesson by:
   a. Completing a written examination successfully, and
   b. Performing the slide test for RF satisfactorily for the instructor. All steps must be completed as listed on the instructor's Performance Check Sheet.

*Note:* Instructions given are general. The procedure should be modified to conform to the manufacturer's instructions for the kit being used.

### MATERIALS AND EQUIPMENT

- hand disinfectant
- gloves
- timer
- test tubes (13 x 75 mm)
- test tube rack
- serum samples
- pipets for delivering .05 mL (50 µL), 0.5 mL, 0.95 mL
- RF slide test kit that includes:
  RF latex reagent
  RF positive control serum
  RF negative control serum
  glycine diluent
  ringed black glass, plastic or cardboard disposable slide
  dispenser-spreaders
- surface disinfectant (10% chlorine bleach solution)
- biohazard container
- applicator sticks (if spreaders are not in kit)

### PROCEDURE

Record in the comment section any problems encountered while practicing the procedure (or have a fellow student or the instructor evaluate your performance).

S = Satisfactory
U = Unsatisfactory

| You must: | S | U | Comments |
|---|---|---|---|
| 1. Wash hands and put on gloves | | | |
| 2. Assemble equipment and materials | | | |
| 3. Allow all reagents to reach room temperature before performing test | | | |
| 4. Prepare a 1:20 dilution of the test serum:<br>a. Pipet 0.05 mL (50 µL) of serum into a 13 x 75 tube<br>b. Pipet 0.95 mL of glycine diluent into the tube and mix well | | | |
| 5. Dispense one drop of positive control serum into ring on slide | | | |

| You must: | S | U | Comments |
|---|---|---|---|
| 6. Dispense one drop of negative control serum into ring on slide | | | |
| 7. Dispense one drop of diluted patient serum (from step 4) into ring on slide using dispenser-spreader included in kit (save dispenser for mixing specimen) | | | |
| 8. Mix the RF latex reagent well by inversion | | | |
| 9. Dispense one drop of well-mixed RF latex reagent into each ring containing a control or test serum | | | |
| 10. Use the spreader end of the dispenser (used to dispense serum) to thoroughly mix serum with reagent, spreading the mixture over the entire surface of the ring. *Note:* Be sure to use a separate spreader-mixer for each serum or control sample. An applicator stick may be used if no spreaders are available. | | | |
| 11. Start timer and rock the slide in a figure-eight motion for the appropriate time (usually one to three minutes) to continue mixing | | | |
| 12. Observe the ringed areas for agglutination immediately at the end of the appropriate time period | | | |
| 13. Record the results of the controls and patient serum (agglutination = positive; no agglutination = negative or titer less than 20) | | | |
| 14. Perform the quantitative test (steps 15-18) if the patient sample is positive for agglutination; if it is negative, go to step 19 | | | |
| 15. Prepare a two-fold serial dilution of patient serum: a. Label five test tubes: 1 (1:40), 2 (1:80), 3 (1:160), 4 (1:320), and 5 (1:640) b. Pipet 0.5 mL of glycine diluent into each tube c. Pipet 0.5 mL of 1:20 dilution of patient serum (from qualitative test, step 4) into tube 1 (1:40) and mix contents of tube well d. Transfer 0.5 mL from tube 1 to tube 2 and mix well e. Transfer 0.5 mL from tube 2 to tube 3 and mix well f. Transfer 0.5 mL from tube 3 to tube 4 and mix well g. Transfer 0.5 mL from tube 4 to tube 5 and mix well | | | |
| 16. Use each dilution (tubes 1–5) as a separate test specimen and perform the agglutination test as in steps 5–13 | | | |
| 17. Record the results for each tube | | | |
| 18. Record the serum RF titer (the reciprocal of the highest dilution that shows agglutination) | | | |

| You must: | S | U | Comments |
|---|---|---|---|
| 19. Disinfect glass slide with 10% chlorine bleach solution for at least ten minutes and wash. Discard disposable slides into bio-hazard container | | | |
| 20. Return all reagents and materials to proper storage | | | |
| 21. Discard specimens and contaminated items appropriately | | | |
| 22. Clean and disinfect work area | | | |
| 23. Remove gloves and discard in biohazard container | | | |
| 24. Wash hands with hand disinfectant | | | |

*Evaluator Comments:*

Evaluator _____ Date _____

# Unit 5

# *Urinalysis*

**After studying this unit, you should be able to:**

- *Identify the organs of the urinary system.*
- *Identify the parts of the kidney and state the function of each part.*
- *Explain how urine is formed.*
- *Describe proper urine collection and preservation methods.*
- *Perform a physical examination of urine.*
- *Perform a chemical examination of urine.*
- *Identify components of urine sediment.*
- *Perform a microscopic examination of urine sediment.*
- *Explain how urinalysis results can give information about the status of a patient's health.*
- *Perform a urine pregnancy test.*

## UNIT OVERVIEW

Urine is examined as a part of most physical examinations. Urinalysis test results give the physician information useful in diagnosing disease or following a disease's course or treatment.

Routine urinalysis is one of the most frequently performed procedures in the medical laboratory. This procedure, in which tests are performed on one urine sample, is ordered often because urine is easily obtained and much information about the body's metabolism can be gained from the urinalysis results. Unit 5, Urinalysis, presents basic information about the urinary system, proper collection of urine specimens, methods of performing a routine urinalysis, and urine pregnancy tests.

Lesson 5-1 contains fundamental information about the anatomy of the urinary system organs, urine formation, and urine components. This information provides a foundation for understanding the importance of urine testing and urinalysis procedures and test results.

Lesson 5-2 describes routine and special urine-collection procedures and presents methods of preserving urine specimens. Lessons 5-3, 5-4, and 5-5 describe the tests that make up the three parts of the routine urinalysis procedure, the physical, chemical, and microscopic examinations of urine.

Lesson 5-6, Urine Pregnancy Tests, is included in this unit because these tests are often performed in the urinalysis section of the laboratory. Pregnancy test methods are based on immunological principles, discussed in Unit 4, Basic Immunology and Serology.

Changes occur in urine when kidney disease or other diseases are present. Urinalysis may be performed to check for certain metabolic end products that indicate particular diseases unrelated to the urinary system, or to observe physical, chemical, and microscopic characteristics that indicate disease of, or damage to, the urinary tract. Knowledge gained from studying this unit will demonstrate that urinalysis results can give the physician valuable information about a patient's health status.

# SUGGESTED READINGS AND REFERENCES

Addison, L. A. & Fischer, P. M. (1990). *The office laboratory*. Norwalk, CT: Appleton-Century-Crofts.

*Atlas of Urine Sediment*. (1993). Elkhart, IN: Miles, Inc., Diagnostics Division.

Baker, F. J., Silverton, R. E., & Pallister, C. J., Eds. (7th ed.). (1998). *Baker & Silverton's introduction to medical laboratory technology*. London: Butterworth-Heinemann Medical.

Barrett, J. T. (1998). *Microbiology and immunology concepts*. Philadelphia: Lippincott-Raven.

Barrett, J. T. (1991). *Medical immunology: text and review*. Philadelphia: F. A. Davis.

Flynn, J. C., Jr. & Whitlock, S. A. (1997). *Urinalysis: Delmar's clinical laboratory manual series*. Albany, NY: Delmar Publishers, Inc.

Free, H. M. (Ed.). (1996). *Modern urine chemistry*. Tarrytown, NY: Bayer Corp., Diagnostics Division.

Freeman, J. A. & Beeler, M. F. (2nd ed.). (1983). *Laboratory medicine: urinalysis and medical microscopy*. Philadelphia: Lea and Febiger.

Graff, L. (1992). *Handbook of routine urinalysis*. Philadelphia: Lippincott-Raven.

Henry, J. B. (Ed.). (19th ed.) (1996). *Clinical diagnosis & management by laboratory methods*. Philadelphia: W. B. Saunders Company.

McBride, L. J. (1998). *Textbook of urinalysis and body fluids: A clinical approach*. Philadelphia: Lippincott-Raven.

Package insert, ICON®II HCG, Beckman Coulter, Palo Alto, CA.

Package insert, KOVA® System for Standardized Urinalysis. Hycor Biomedical, Inc., Garden Grove, CA.

Ravel, R. (6th ed.). (1995). *Clinical laboratory medicine: Clinical application of laboratory data*. St. Louis: Mosby Yearbook.

Ringsrud, K. M. & Linne, J. J. (1995). *Urinalysis and body fluids: A colortext and atlas*. St. Louis: Mosby Yearbook.

Sacher, R. A. & McPherson, R. A. (10th ed.). (1991). *Widmann's clinical interpretation of laboratory tests*. Philadelphia: F. A. Davis Company.

Strasinger, S. K. (3rd ed.). (1994). *Urinalysis and body fluids*. Philadelphia: F. A. Davis Company.

Widman, F. K. & Itatani, C. A. (1998). *An introduction to clinical immunology and serology*. Philadelphia: F. A. Davis Company.

# Introduction to Urinalysis

## LESSON OBJECTIVES

After studying this lesson, you should be able to:

- *Identify the organs of the urinary system.*
- *Identify the parts of the kidney.*
- *State the functions of the parts of the kidney.*
- *Explain how urine is formed.*
- *Describe the composition of urine.*
- *List the three parts of a routine urinalysis.*
- *Explain the value of performing a routine urinalysis.*
- *List three kidney diseases that may cause abnormal urinalysis results.*
- *List three systemic diseases that may cause abnormal urinalysis results.*
- *Define the glossary terms.*

## GLOSSARY

**Bowman's capsule** / the portion of the nephron that receives the glomerular filtrate

**cortex** / the outer layer or portion of an organ

**cystitis** / inflammation of the urinary bladder

**distal convoluted tubule** / the portion of a renal tubule that empties into the collecting tubule

**diuresis** / output of abnormally large urine volume

**glomerular filtrate** / the fluid that passes from the blood into the nephron and from which urine is formed

**glomerulonephriti**s / inflammation of the glomeruli

**glomerulus (pl. glomeruli)** / a small bundle of capillaries that is the filtering portion of the nephron

**kidney** / the organ in which urine is formed

**loop of Henle** / the U-shaped portion of a renal tubule between its proximal and distal portions

**medulla** / the inner or central portion of an organ

**nephron** / the structural and functional unit of the kidney

**nephrotoxic** / toxic or destructive to kidney cells

**proximal convoluted tubule** / the portion of a renal tubule that collects the filtrate from Bowman's capsule

**pyelitis** / inflammation of the renal pelvis

**pyelonephritis** / inflammation of the kidney and the renal pelvis

**renal hilus** / the concavity in the kidney where nerves and vessels enter or exit

**renal pelvis** / the cavity in the kidney that receives urine from the renal tubules and the site where the ureter enters the kidney

**renal threshold** / the blood concentration above which a substance not normally excreted by the kidneys appears in urine

**tubular necrosis** / death of the tissue comprising the renal tubules

**ureter** / the tube carrying urine from the kidney to the urinary bladder

**urethra** / a canal through which urine is discharged from the urinary bladder

**urinary bladder** / an organ for the temporary storage of urine

**urine** / excretory fluid produced by the kidneys

**UTI** / urinary tract infection

## INTRODUCTION

The urinary system has a vital role in regulating many bodily processes. The formation and excretion of urine remove a variety of waste products from the body. These products, if not removed, can rapidly become toxic and cause death within a few days.

The kidneys, the primary functional organs of the urinary system, act like biological purification plants, filtering and cleansing the blood of harmful toxins, metabolic wastes, and excess ions, which then leave the body in the **urine**. Proper urinary system functioning is necessary to regulate blood volume, blood chemistry, acid-base balance, electrolyte concentrations, RBC production, and regulation of blood pressure.

To understand the relationship between the urinary system and health, a basic understanding of the structure and function of the urinary system is necessary.

## THE URINARY SYSTEM

The urinary system is an excretory system consisting of two kidneys, two ureters, the urinary bladder, and the urethra. The **kidneys** are the organs in which urine is formed. Humans have two kidneys, bean-shaped organs that lie on either side of the vertebral column. Connected to each kidney is a **ureter**, a funnel-shaped tube that carries urine from the kidney to the **urinary bladder**, where it is stored. The **urethra** is the canal through which urine is carried from the urinary bladder to the outside. Figure 5-1 is a diagram of the urinary system, showing the kidneys, ureters, urinary bladder, and urethra.

### Anatomy of the Kidneys

Each kidney is surrounded by a fibrous protective capsule. The **renal hilus** is the concave region of the kidney where blood vessels, lymphatic vessels, nerves, and the ureter enter or exit the kidney (Figure 5-1). Internally, the kidney has three major portions: the cortex, the medulla, and the renal pelvis (Figures 5-1 and 5-2). The **cortex** is the outermost layer of tissue, lying beneath the capsule. The **medulla** lies beneath the cortex and contains the renal pyramids, cone-shaped tissue masses. The renal columns are extensions of the renal cortex that separate the renal pyramids. Each pyramid and its associated cortical region make up a kidney lobe.

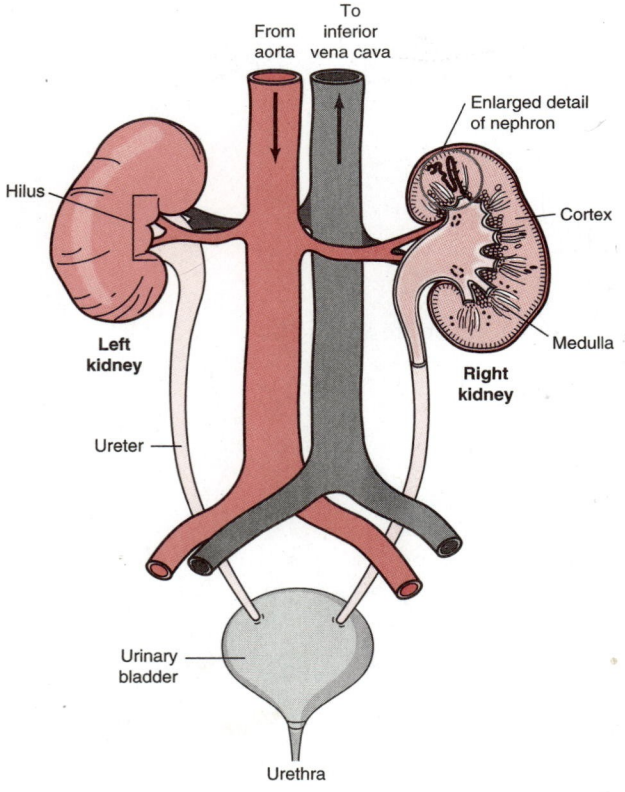

**FIGURE 5-1**  Organs of the urinary system

The **renal pelvis** is the funnel-shaped expansion of the upper (proximal) portion of the ureter.

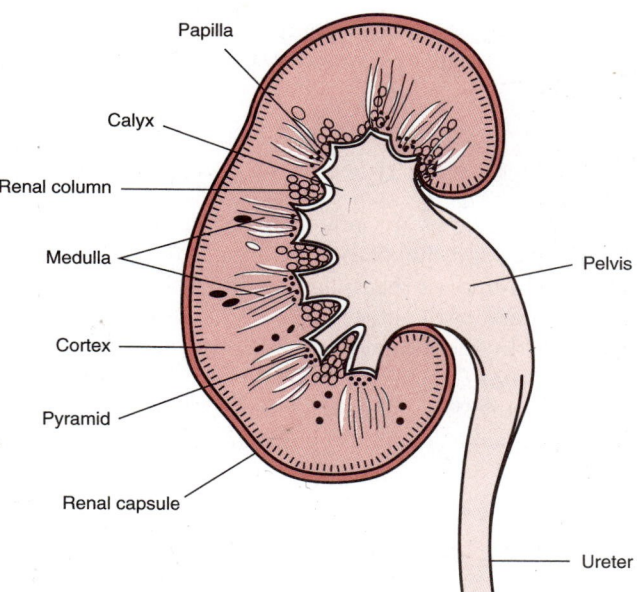

**FIGURE 5-2** Cross-section of the kidney

Labels: Papilla, Calyx, Renal column, Medulla, Cortex, Pyramid, Renal capsule, Pelvis, Ureter

## The Nephron

The functional unit in the kidneys is the **nephron** (Figure 5-3). Each kidney has approximately one million nephrons, each composed of a glomerulus and its associated renal tubule.

## The Glomerulus

The **glomerulus**, the filtering unit of the kidney, is composed of a bundle of blood capillary vessels (Figure 5-3). The glomeruli are located in the kidney cortex (Figure 5-1, arrow).

In the glomerulus, water and small molecules such as glucose, salt, and urea are filtered from (leave) the blood and pass into Bowman's capsule, while blood cells and larger molecules, such as proteins, remain within the capillary vessels (in the circulatory system). The fluid containing these molecules is called the **glomerular filtrate**. **Bowman's capsule** is the layer of cells surrounding each glomerulus that acts as a funnel to direct the filtrate into the renal tubule (Figure 5-3).

## The Renal Tubule

Each glomerulus is associated with a renal tubule. The glomerular filtrate passes through the renal tubule to be

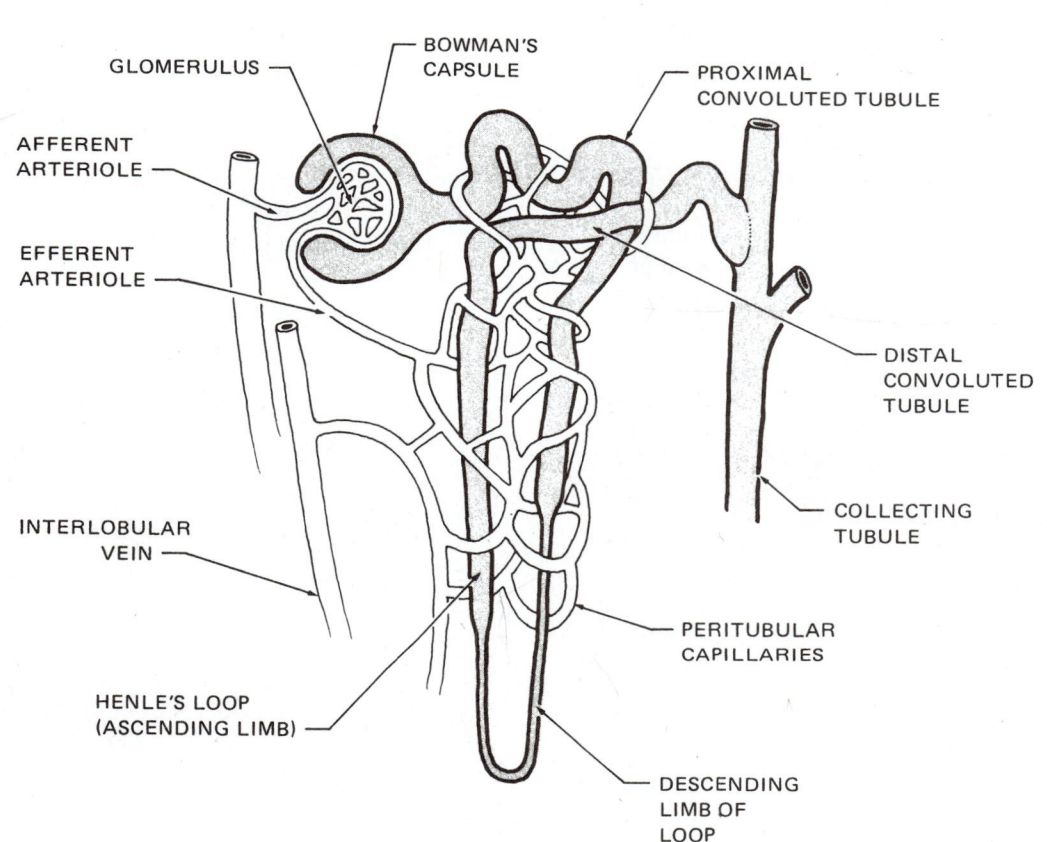

Labels: GLOMERULUS, BOWMAN'S CAPSULE, PROXIMAL CONVOLUTED TUBULE, AFFERENT ARTERIOLE, EFFERENT ARTERIOLE, DISTAL CONVOLUTED TUBULE, COLLECTING TUBULE, INTERLOBULAR VEIN, PERITUBULAR CAPILLARIES, HENLE'S LOOP (ASCENDING LIMB), DESCENDING LIMB OF LOOP

**FIGURE 5-3** The nephron

concentrated. The renal tubule has three major portions: (1) the **proximal convoluted tubule**, (2) the **loop of Henle**, and (3) the **distal convoluted tubule**, which empties into a collecting tubule (figure 5-3). The renal tubule is surrounded by blood capillaries (peritubular capillaries) and portions of the tubule may extend into the medulla of the kidney (Figure 5-1, arrow, and Figure 5-3).

## Urine Formation

In the tubules, substances such as vitamins, electrolytes, amino acids, and glucose are selectively reabsorbed from the filtrate. Most of the water passing through the glomeruli is reabsorbed, which produces a concentrated filtrate. Some tubular cells secrete substances such as potassium and hydrogen ions into the filtrate. The resulting concentrated fluid is **urine**, which passes into the collecting tubules, collects in the renal pelvis, and flows through the ureters into the urinary bladder.

The kidneys have an extremely high rate of blood flow. Approximately 1,200 milliliters of blood are cleansed of waste products each minute. As a result, approximately 180 liters of filtrate are formed daily by the glomeruli. After concentration in the tubules by selective reabsorption, this volume is reduced to approximately 1 to 2 liters of urine produced daily in a normal adult.

## Hormones That Affect Renal Function

Hormones that influence renal function include parathyroid hormone (PTH), aldosterone and antidiuretic hormone (ADH). Parathyroid hormone influences calcium reabsorption in the kidney tubules and works with vitamin D to regulate bone calcium. Aldosterone is a mineralocorticoid hormone that helps regulate electrolytes and promotes urinary potassium excretion. ADH, a hormone produced in the hypothalamus and also called vasopressin, regulates water reabsorption by the kidneys.

## Hormones Produced by the Kidney

While the kidneys are influenced by hormones such as ADH that are produced in other organs, the kidneys also produce hormones that influence physiologic processes in other parts of the body (Table 5-1). Three hormones produced by the kidneys are *erythropoietin, renin*, and *active vitamin $D_3$*. Erythropoietin stimulates RBC production in the bone marrow. Renin indirectly influences blood pressure. Vitamin $D_3$ helps in regulating bone calcium.

## CHARACTERISTICS OF URINE

The formation and excretion of urine is the principal way the body excretes water and gets rid of waste. Three processes are involved in urine formation:

- filtration of waste products, salts, and excess fluid from the blood,
- reabsorption of water and solutes from the filtrate, and
- secretion of ions and chemicals into the urine

Therefore, urine excretion provides a means of regulating the body's state of hydration and the blood concentration of ions such as sodium, potassium, and other electrolytes.

## Composition of Urine

Normal urine contains many substances. Approximately 95% of urine is water and the other 5% is solutes (Table 5-2). Urea, a breakdown product of amino acids, is the solute in highest concentration, followed by sodium. Other solutes include potassium, phosphate and sulfate ions, creatinine, and uric acid, as well as small amounts of calcium, magnesium, and bicarbonate ions.

**Table 5-1.** Hormones influencing or produced by the kidneys

| HORMONE | FUNCTION |
|---|---|
| **Hormones that influence kidney function** | |
| Aldosterone | Regulates electrolytes, especially potassium |
| Antidiuretic hormone | Regulates water reabsorption |
| Parathyroid hormone | Regulates calcium reabsorption |
| **Hormones produced by the kidneys** | |
| Erythropoietin | Stimulates red blood cell synthesis |
| Renin | Influences blood pressure |
| Active vitamin $D_3$ | Influences bone calcium levels |

**Table 5-2.** Some solutes found in normal urine

| | | | |
|---|---|---|---|
| Sodium | Magnesium | Urea | Creatinine |
| Potassium | Vitamins | Uric acid | Phosphorus |
| Chloride | Amino acids | Bile pigments | Calcium |

Urine composition changes depending on factors such as the time of day (diurnal changes) and the physical state, diet, and health of the individual. In some diseases, substances such as glucose, blood cells, protein, or bile pigments can be present in the urine. Abnormalities detected in urine alert doctors to possible disease and can aid in diagnosing and treating disease.

## Urine Volume

The amount of urine formed daily depends on age, water intake, metabolism, blood pressure, diet, hormone balance, and many other factors. Healthy adults excrete between one and two liters of urine per day. *Antidiuretic hormone* stimulates water reabsorption in the kidneys, thus creating a concentrated urine and decreasing urine output. *Diuretics* are substances that increase urinary output, and therefore dilute the urine. Caffeine and some hypertension medicines act as diuretics.

## Renal Threshold

Almost all components present in urine are also present in blood, but in different amounts. Most small molecules that enter the glomerular filtrate when blood is filtered, become reabsorbed into the blood as the filtrate passes through the tubules of the nephron. When the blood level of a substance becomes high enough to exceed the tubular reabsorption capacity, then the substance will be excreted in the urine. In those cases, the blood concentration is said to have exceeded the **renal threshold**. For example, the renal threshold of glucose is approximately 180 mg/dL. Blood glucose levels above this will cause glucose to be excreted in the urine. glucose = 180 mg/dL

## TESTS OF RENAL FUNCTION

A variety of tests can be performed on urine. Some are simple and rapid; others are complex and time-consuming. The procedures for performing the simplest urine test, the routine urinalysis, are given in Lessons 5-3, 5-4, and 5-5.

Abnormalities discovered during a routine urinalysis may lead the physician to request more specific tests of renal function. Serum tests for metabolites such as creatinine and blood urea nitrogen (BUN) are important in monitoring kidney function. Other tests used to assess renal function can be performed on twenty-four-hour urine specimens, such as the creatinine clearance test. Although the performance of clearance tests are beyond the scope of this text, the procedure for collecting twenty-four-hour urine specimens is covered in Lesson 5-2.

## DISEASES AFFECTING URINALYSIS RESULTS

The presence of disease can cause changes in the:

- amount of urine formed or excreted
- color of urine
- appearance of urine
- odor of urine
- cells present in urine
- chemical constituents in urine

Abnormal urinalysis results can be seen in (1) disorders of the urinary tract or (2) when disease in other parts of the body affects renal function or urine composition.

## Infections of the Urinary Tract  UTI = Urethra

Urine stored in the urinary bladder is normally sterile. Urinary tract infections (**UTI**) most commonly occur in the urethra. If left untreated, the infection may ascend to the bladder, causing **cystitis**. In severe cases, the kidney may become involved. **Pyelitis** is an inflammation of the renal pelvis; **pyelonephritis** is an inflammation of the kidney and renal pelvis. Both are usually caused by bacterial infections. Cystitis — Urethra & Bladder  Pyelitis — Kidney Renal Pelvis  Pyelonephritis — Kidney & Renal Pelvis

## Diseases of the Kidneys

Disease of the kidneys may cause a buildup of toxic  bacterial infect. products in the blood, such as urea, uric acid, and creatinine. If kidney function is suddenly lost, death will occur within a few days if treatment is not administered. One form of treatment is dialysis. In hemodialysis, blood is circulated outside the body, passed over a membrane to remove toxic waste products, and then returned to the body. Peritoneal dialysis removes toxic wastes by diffusion. Fluid is instilled into the peritoneal space and is periodically drained and replenished.

One healthy kidney is sufficient for life functions. This makes it possible for a living person to donate a kidney for transplant to a patient with incurable kidney disease.

Some common examples of kidney disease include glomerulonephritis, pyelonephritis, polycystic kidney disease, and tubular necrosis. **Glomerulonephritis** is an inflammation of the glomeruli, usually due to deposition of antibodies or immune complexes in the glomeruli, which results in damage to the tissue. These antibodies may be formed as a result of infection somewhere in the body or may be caused by autoimmune diseases. Diseases in which capillaries are damaged may cause glomerulonephritis, since the glomeruli are made of capillaries. In glomerulonephritis, protein and RBCs are usually present in the urine.

**Tubular necrosis** can occur when the blood supply to the kidney is diminished, or upon exposure to or ingestion of substances that are **nephrotoxic** (toxic to kidney cells). The capacity of the tubules to concentrate urine is affected in this condition. Polycystic kidney disease is an inherited condition in which glomerular function is lost due to formation of multiple cysts in the kidneys.

## Systemic Diseases with Abnormal Urinalysis Results

Some systemic diseases that may cause abnormal urinalysis results include diabetes mellitus, hypertension, atherosclerosis, and autoimmune diseases such as lupus erythematosus. Prolonged hypertension may cause kidney damage. Nephrotic syndrome, a condition usually associated with circulatory disorders and characterized by tissue edema, causes protein to appear in the urine. Malignancies arising in the urinary tract may cause obstruction, leading to abnormal urinalysis results, or may cause malignant cells to appear in the urine.

Tests such as the ones performed in the routine urinalysis provide an indication of an individual's metabolism and general state of health. A good understanding of kidney function and urine composition helps the laboratory worker understand and interpret routine urinalysis results.

## LESSON REVIEW

1. Name the organs of the urinary system.
2. Draw a kidney and label the parts.
3. What are the functions of the kidney?
4. Draw a glomerulus and label the parts. State the function associated with each part.
5. What components are in urine?
6. What are the three parts of a routine urinalysis?
7. List three hormones produced by the kidneys.
8. List three hormones that influence kidney function.
9. Name three kidney diseases that may cause abnormal urinalysis results.
10. Name three systemic diseases that may cause abnormal urinalysis results.
11. Define Bowman's capsule, cortex, cystitis, distal convoluted tubule, diuresis, glomerular filtrate, glomerulonephritis, glomerulus, kidney, loop of Henle, medulla, nephron, nephrotoxic, proximal convoluted tubule, pyelitis, pyelonephritis, renal hilus, renal pelvis, renal threshold, tubular necrosis, ureter, urethra, urinary bladder, urine, and UTI.

## STUDENT ACTIVITIES

1. Reread the introduction to urinalysis.
2. Review the glossary terms.
3. Research and report on a disease that might be discovered by an abnormal urinalysis result.

# Collection and Preservation of Urine

## LESSON OBJECTIVES

**After studying this lesson, you should be able to:**

- *Explain the importance of properly collecting urine specimens.*
- *List four types of urine specimens and explain when each might be required.*
- *State the normal twenty-four-hour urine volumes for adults, children, and newborns.*
- *Explain why a preservative is required for some urine specimens.*
- *Instruct male and female patients on how to collect a clean-catch urine specimen.*
- *Instruct male and female patients on how to collect a midstream urine specimen.*
- *Instruct a patient on how to collect a twenty-four-hour urine specimen.*
- *Explain how collecting urine specimens for drug screening differs from collecting specimens for routine urinalysis.*
- *Discuss the importance of quality assurance in urinalysis.*
- *Explain safety precautions that must be observed when handling urine specimens.*
- *Define the glossary terms.*

## GLOSSARY

**anuria** / complete failure of kidney function and suppression of urine production; absence of urine production

**clean-catch urine** / a midstream urine sample collected after the urethral opening and surrounding tissues have been cleansed

**midstream urine** / a urine sample collected in the middle of voiding

**nocturia** / excessive urination at night

**oliguria** / decreased production of urine

**polyuria** / excessive production of urine

**random urine specimen** / a urine specimen collected at any time, without regard to diet or time of day

## INTRODUCTION

Examining a patient's urine specimen can yield many results helpful to the physician in diagnosis and treatment. However, proper specimen collection is essential for the test results to be valid. Good quality assurance requires that specimens be collected with care to avoid contamination and to help prevent erroneous results. Proper handling and transport of the specimen after collection ensures that the laboratory receives a specimen of acceptable quality for testing.

## TYPES OF URINE SPECIMENS

The type of urine specimen required varies according to the type of test to be performed. Common types of urine specimens submitted for laboratory analysis are:

- random urine specimen
- fasting or first morning urine specimen
- clean-catch urine specimen
- timed urine specimen
- twenty-four-hour urine specimen

The *preferred* specimen for most routine urine testing is the first morning specimen. This specimen is normally more concentrated and usually has an acid pH that helps preserve any cells present. The first morning specimen can be used as a fasting specimen if it is collected before a patient has eaten.

Most specimens tested, however, are **random urine specimens**; that is, specimens obtained at any time during the day, without regard to food intake. Both first morning and random urine specimens should be collected by the midstream procedure. A **midstream urine** specimen is one in which the patient collects only the middle portion of the urine flow.

For certain tests, timed specimens may be required. For example, in one screening test for diabetes, urine collected post prandial (after eating) is tested for glucose.

Some quantitative urine tests require a twenty-four-hour urine specimen for testing. Protein, creatinine, urobilinogen, and calcium are examples of components that may be measured in twenty-four-hour urine specimens. These tests are performed primarily to check kidney function. The results obtained are quantitative and are expressed as units/twenty-four hours. These tests are usually performed in a large hospital or reference laboratory. Instructions for collecting 24-hour urine specimens are given in this lesson.

The **clean-catch urine** collection procedure, which is required when urine is to be cultured for microorganisms, is described in detail in this lesson.

(The procedure for urine culture is given in Lesson 7-6.) Occasionally, urine specimens for culture or routine analysis are collected by catheterization, a procedure not normally performed by laboratory personnel.

## HANDLING AND PRESERVING URINE SPECIMENS

 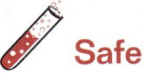 **Safety**

Universal and Standard Precautions must be observed by all personnel. All urine specimens must be in clean, non-leaking containers; otherwise, they should not be accepted for testing by laboratory personnel. Protective clothing such as gloves, protective face wear, and a buttoned, fluid-resistant laboratory coat should be worn when working with specimens. Splashes and the creation of aerosols must be avoided when pouring or discarding urine. Spills of urine must be wiped up with laboratory disinfectant. Sinks used for discarding urines should be flushed with water and disinfectant.

### *Quality Assurance*

Quality assurance must be considered in collecting, handling, and transporting urine specimens. Careful, complete instructions must be given to patients so they understand how to correctly collect the specimen. Written instructions must be understandable to all patients and should be available in non-English versions. Specimen labeling must be accurate and complete. Specimens must be delivered to the testing site as soon as possible after collection and tested within accepted time limits.

## Urine Specimen Containers

Several types of containers are available for collecting urine specimens. Random and first morning specimens may be collected in clean, lidded, disposable containers large enough to hold at least 50 mL. For clean-catch specimens, urine containers must be sterile (Figure 5-4). Large, opaque containers capable of holding four or more liters are provided to patients for collecting twenty-four-hour urine specimens (Figure 5-5). These containers may contain preservatives.

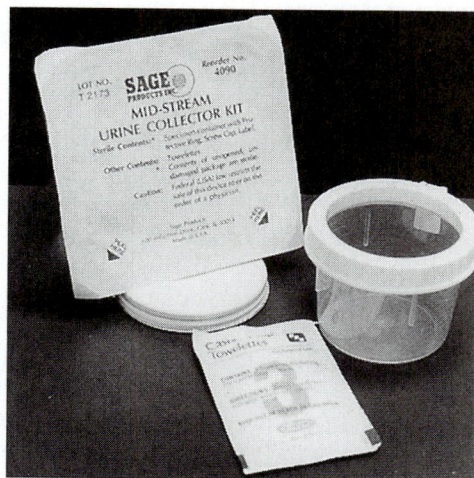

**FIGURE 5-4** Clean-catch urine collection kit

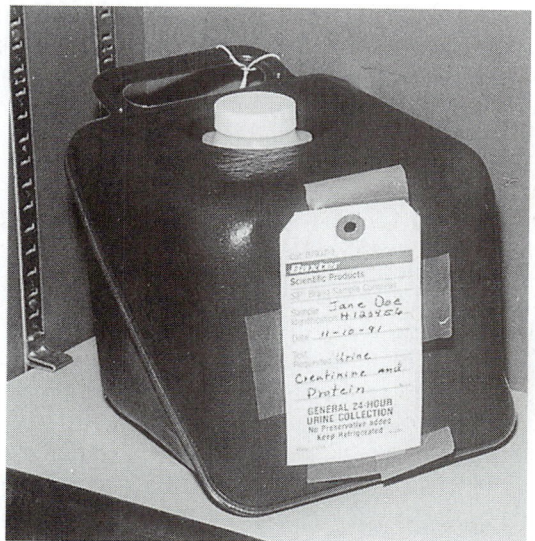

**FIGURE 5-5** One type of container used to collect a 24-hour urine specimen

## Labeling Urine Specimens

Urine specimens must be labeled clearly with the patient's name, as well as the date and time of collection. Labels should be on the container, not just on the lid.

## Refrigeration of Urine Specimens

The manner in which urine specimens are handled after collection can affect test results. If a urine specimen is allowed to sit at room temperature for an extended time, any bacteria present will multiply rapidly. This can change the urine pH and also cause the specimen to have an unpleasant, ammonia-like odor. A delay before testing can also increase the decomposition of **casts** and the cellular components of the specimen. To avoid specimen deterioration, urine specimens should be examined within one hour of voiding. If this is not possible, urine may be stored with a lid in the dark at 4–6°C for up to four hours.

## Preservation of Urine Specimens

Urine specimens that cannot be refrigerated or that have to be mailed or transported over a long distance may have preservatives added to them. The addition of a preservative will retard the growth of bacteria and slow the destruction or decomposition of other urine components. The preservative must be one that will not interfere with the tests that have been ordered. Some commonly used urine preservatives are hydrochloric acid (HCl), formalin, sodium carbonate, and boric acid (Table 5-3). Containers for twenty-four-hour urine specimens often have preservatives added before the urine is collected. No preservative of any kind should be added to urine for bacteriological culture.

## PROCEDURES FOR COLLECTING URINE SPECIMENS

## Collecting Midstream Urine Samples

Specimens for routine urinalysis should be collected by the midstream method. The patient should be instructed to begin voiding into the toilet and then to interrupt

**Table 5-3.** Common urine preservatives and their uses

| PRESERVATIVE | USE |
|---|---|
| Formalin | Preserves formed elements |
| HCl | Preserves for calcium and phosphorous tests |
| Sodium carbonate | Preserves porphyrins, urobilinogen |
| Boric acid | Preserves creatinine, uric acid, and glucose |
| Refrigeration | Barbiturates, drug abuse screen, protein |

the urine stream to collect only the middle portion of the urine stream in the specimen container. Using this method prevents contaminating the specimen with epithelial cells, microorganisms, or mucus from the urethra.

## Collecting Clean-catch Urine Samples

A clean-catch urine specimen is required if urine is to be cultured for bacteria. Most hospitals and physician offices provide the patient with a kit containing towelettes and a sterile disposable urine container (Figure 5-4). Male and female patients both should be instructed to carefully collect the urine specimen. Written instructions understandable to all patients must be available. They may be posted in the restroom near the toilet.

### Instructions to the Male Patient

The male patient should retract the penis foreskin (if not circumcised), using a towelette. A second towelette should be used to cleanse the urethral opening with a single stroke directed from the tip of the penis toward the ring of the glans. The towelette should then be discarded and the cleansing procedure repeated using two more towelettes.

The patient should begin to void into the toilet. The urine stream should be interrupted to collect only the middle portion of the urine flow in the supplied container.

After the specimen has been collected, the lid should be placed securely on the container. The patient should avoid touching the inside of both the container and the lid. The information on the label should then be completed and attached to the specimen container.

### Instructions to the Female Patient

The female patient should position herself comfortably on the toilet seat and swing one knee to the side as far as possible. She should spread the outer vulval folds (labia majora) using a towelette and wipe the inner side of one inner fold (labium minora) with a towelette, using a single stroke from front to back. The towelette should then be discarded and a second towelette used to repeat the procedure on the opposite side. A third towelette should be used to cleanse the urethral opening with a single front-to-back stroke.

The patient should then begin to void into the toilet. The urine stream should be interrupted to collect onl.y the middle portion of the urine flow in a container. Touching only the outside of the container and the lid, the patient should close the container securely. The information on the label should be completed and attached to the container. If the patient has vaginal discharge, a clean tampon should be inserted before collection to decrease the possibility of specimen contamination.

## Collecting A Twenty Four-Hour Urine Specimen

### Instructions to the Patient

The procedure for collecting a twenty-four-hour urine specimen must be followed carefully for the test results to be valid. The patient must be provided with written instructions describing the procedure to be followed (Figure 5-6). In addition, the laboratory must give the patient a collection container with any required preservative already added (Figure 5-5). The patient must be warned if the preservative can be harmful if spilled or splashed.

Twenty-four-hour urine specimens must contain all the urine produced by the patient in a twenty-four-hour period. Collection usually begins at a designated morning hour, for example 8 a.m. The patient should be instructed to empty his/her bladder by voiding into the toilet at 8 a.m. on the day collection begins. *This urine is not included in the twenty-four-hour collection.* The patient should be instructed to then collect all urine produced until 8 a.m. the following morning and transfer the urine to the twenty-four-hour container provided. At 8 a.m. on the day after collection began (twenty-four hours later), the patient should empty his/her bladder and add this urine to the twenty-four-hour container. The container should then be delivered to the laboratory.

### Measuring Urine Volume

When a routine urinalysis is performed, the volume of the specimen is usually not recorded. However, the vol-

---

Your physician has ordered a 24-hour urine test. Urine is usually collected from 8:00 A.M. one day until 8:00 A.M. the next day. It is important that you carefully follow these instructions:

1. To begin the collection, *void into the toilet* as usual, and note the time. (DO NOT SAVE THIS URINE.)
2. Collect the next urine specimen, and all urine after that for 24 hours, into a specimen cup and transfer to the special container. At 24 hours from the beginning of the test (the morning of the second day), empty the bladder and add this urine colleced to the 24-hour container.
3. Bring all the urine in the collection container to the laboratory the morning of the second day.

**FIGURE 5-6** Patient instruction card for collecting a 24-hour urine specimen

ume of a twenty-four-hour urine specimen must be carefully measured and recorded because the volume measurement is used in calculating the test results.

The specimen volume is measured using a large graduated cylinder and the urine is returned to its container. The total volume must be recorded on the specimen label and the accompanying requisition form.

### Reference Values for Urine Volumes

The normal volume of urine produced in twenty-four hours varies according to the age of the individual (Table 5-4). Infants and children produce smaller volumes than adults. The normal twenty-four-hour urine volume for newborns is 20-350 mL. By the age of one year, 300-600 mL is normal. For ten-year-olds, the volume may range from 750 to 1,500 mL in twenty-four hours. Normal adult urine volume is 750-2,000 mL in twenty-four hours, with 1,500 mL being average.

Urinary volume depends on various factors: fluid intake, diet, fluid lost in exhalation and perspiration, hormone levels, and the status of renal and cardiac functions. Excessive production of urine is called **polyuria**. **Oliguria** is insufficient production of urine and **anuria** is absence of urine production. The term **nocturia** refers to excessive production of urine at night.

## Collecting Urine Specimens for Drug Screens

Urine drug screens may be requested of participants in athletic events, job applicants, and suspected drug abusers. Although a random urine specimen is used, much documentation is required to guarantee the credibility of the collection procedure. Each laboratory that collects specimens for drug abuse screening must follow a detailed written protocol. Chain-of-custody must be documented; this is to safeguard against possible tampering and guarantee the specimen's integrity. Some

requirements likely to be included in a protocol for urine drug-screen collection are:

- photo identification and signed donor consent
- special collection kits provided to the donor by the laboratory
- bathroom inspection before and after collection, with a monitor outside during collection
- urine temperature measured and recorded
- specimen labeled in presence of donor, sealed in outer container, and secured under lock until picked up by testing agency

### Procedural Notes

- Be sure the patient understands the collection procedure for the test that has been ordered.
- Be sure the specimen is correctly labeled with patient's name, time and date of collection, and any other information required by the laboratory.
- Be sure the lid is kept on urine specimens until testing.
- Store urine specimens at 4-6°C for up to four hours if they cannot be tested within one hour of collection.
- Perform bacterial culture on clean-catch specimens *before* performing routine urinalysis.

| AGE | VOLUME (mL/24 HOURS) |
|---|---|
| Newborn | 20–350 |
| One year | 300–600 |
| Ten years | 750–1,500 |
| Adult | 750–2,000 |

**Table 5-4.** Normal 24-hour urine volumes

### Safety Precautions

- Use Universal and Standard Precautions when handling urine specimens.
- Use appropriate safeguards when handling urine preservatives.
- Wear gloves, protective face wear, and buttoned, fluid-resistant laboratory coat.
- Avoid creating splashes or aerosols when disposing of urine specimens.

## SUMMARY

Proper collection, labeling, handling, and storage of urine specimens are the first steps leading to reliable laboratory urine test results. To ensure the validity and quality of urinalysis results, the institution's procedures for urine collection must be strictly followed.

## LESSON REVIEW

1. Why is proper urine collection important?
2. How is a clean-catch urine sample collected?
3. When is a clean-catch urine sample required?
4. What is a midstream urine specimen?
5. Describe the procedure for collecting a twenty-four-hour urine specimen.
6. When is a urine preservative necessary?
7. Name three commonly used urine preservatives.
8. What is the major disadvantage of using preservatives in urine?
9. What is the normal twenty-four-hour urine volume for newborns? One-year-olds? Adults?
10. How may improper collection of urine affect urinalysis test results?
11. Why is the first morning specimen preferred for routine urinalysis?
12. How does collecting urine for drug screening differ from collecting urine for routine urinalysis?
13. Why might a twenty-four-hour urine test be ordered?
14. Define anuria, clean-catch urine, midstream urine, nocturia, oliguria, polyuria, and random urine specimen.

## STUDENT ACTIVITIES

1. Reread the information on urine collection and preservation.
2. Review the glossary terms.
3. Design patient instruction cards (for male and female patients) for collecting clean-catch urine specimens.
4. Practice giving instructions to male and female patients for obtaining clean-catch urine samples, using the patient instruction cards.
5. Practice instructing a patient on how to collect a twenty-four-hour urine specimen.

# Physical Examination of Urine

## LESSON OBJECTIVES

**After studying this lesson, you should be able to:**

- *Name the physical characteristics of urine evaluated during a routine urinalysis.*
- *List three causes of abnormal urine odor.*
- *Explain why normal urine is yellow.*
- *List three abnormal urine colors and give a cause for each.*
- *List two conditions that may affect the appearance or transparency of urine.*
- *Explain what determines urine's specific gravity.*
- *Demonstrate proper use of the urinometer and refractometer.*
- *Perform a physical examination of urine.*
- *Define the glossary terms.*

## GLOSSARY

**hematuria** / the presence of blood in the urine

**ketones** / a group of chemical substances produced during increased fat metabolism; ketone bodies

**melanin** / a dark pigment of skin, hair, and certain tumors

**myoglobin** / a pigmented protein found in muscle tissue

**opalescent** / having a milky iridescence

**porphyrins** / a group of pigments that are required for the synthesis of hemoglobin

**refractometer** / an instrument for measuring refraction

**specific gravity** / the ratio of the weight of a solution to the weight of an equal volume of distilled water; a measurement of density

**turbid** / having a cloudy appearance

**urinometer** / a float with a calibrated stem used for measuring specific gravity

**urochrome** / the yellow pigment that gives urine its color

## INTRODUCTION

A routine urinalysis consists of three parts: the physical, chemical, and microscopic examinations. Physical examination is the first part of the urinalysis and can provide the physician with useful information.

The physical examination of urine includes observing the color and appearance of the urine and measuring the specific gravity. This is the easiest and quickest part of a routine urinalysis and can be performed while the urine specimen is being prepared for other procedures. An example of a laboratory requisition form for a routine urinalysis is shown in Figure 5-7.

**Urinalysis Request Form**

Patient Name _____ Date _____

I.D. _____

Time Collected _____ ☐ a.m.   ☐ p.m.

Color (yellow-amber): _____

Transparency (clear): _____

Sp. Gravity (1.005-1.030) _____

pH (5.5-8.0) _____
Leukocytes (negative) _____
Nitrites (negative) _____
Protein (negative-trace) _____
Glucose (negative) _____
Ketones (negative) _____
Urobilinogen (0.2-1.0U) _____
Bilirubin (negative) _____
Blood (negative) _____

Microscopic
WBC (0-3 cells): _____
RBC (0-3 cells): _____
Epith cells (small # squamous): _____
Bacteria (none-trace): _____
Casts (none): _____
Crystals (none): _____
Mucus (none-trace): _____
Other: _____

Tech: _____
Date: _____
Time: _____

**FIGURE 5-7**   Example of laboratory requisition form for a routine urinalysis

# PHYSICAL CHARACTERISTICS OF URINE

## Urine Odor

Normal, recently voided urine has a characteristic aromatic and not unpleasant odor. Changes in urine odor may be due to disease, diet, or the presence of microorganisms. Although urine odor is not usually reported on the urinalysis form, it is a noticeable property that can alert the technologist to possible abnormalities or improper handling of the urine specimen.

The odor of urine from a patient with uncontrolled diabetes is described as fruity. This is because of the presence of **ketones**, products of fat metabolism. Other metabolic diseases may cause an unusual urine odor. Phenylketonuria (PKU), an inherited condition in which the amino acid phenylalanine is not metabolized, causes urine to have a mousy or musty odor. All newborns are tested for PKU because mental retardation will result if the condition is allowed to go untreated.

Maple syrup urine disease is a rare metabolic condition in which the urine has the odor of maple syrup. This condition is evident in the first weeks of life of affected infants.

If urine is allowed to remain unrefrigerated for a few hours, any bacteria present may break down urea to form ammonia; the resulting odor is similar to ammonia. A *freshly* voided sample of urine with a foul, pungent odor suggests urinary tract infection.

Foods such as garlic and asparagus can also produce an abnormal urine odor. Although urine odor may be striking in certain instances, it is not a reliable enough characteristic to use alone in diagnosing disease.

## Urine Color

The normal color of urine ranges from pale yellow, to straw, to amber. Variations in color may be caused by diet, medications, physical activity, and disease (Table 5-5). Urine color can sometimes provide a clue for diagnosing certain diseases or conditions.

### Yellow Urine

The pigment that produces the normal yellow-to-amber color of urine is **urochrome**. As the urine concentration varies, so will the color intensity. Dilute urine samples are pale; more concentrated urine samples are darker yellow or amber.

### Red Urine

The abnormal color seen most frequently in urine is red or red-brown. Cloudy red urine may be due to **hematuria**, the presence of blood. Clear red urine may be due to the presence of hemoglobin or **myoglobin**, a pigmented protein found in muscle tissue. RBCs, hemoglobin, or myoglobin may form a red-brown color in acidic urine. **Porphyrins** may cause the urine to be red or wine-red.

### Brown or Black Urine

Hemoglobin will become brown in acidic urine that has been standing. The formation of **melanin**, a dark pigment, will also cause urine to become dark or black on standing. This may occur in patients with advanced melanoma, a tumor of melanin-producing cells.

### Yellow-Brown or Green-Brown Urine

Bilirubin or bile pigments may cause urine to be dark yellow-brown or green-brown. These urines may have a yellow-green foam when shaken. Bilirubin may be present in the urine of patients with hepatitis. Since some organisms, such as the hepatitis virus, may be transmitted by urine, all urine specimens must be handled with caution to avoid exposing laboratory personnel to infectious organisms.

## Urine Appearance

Urine's appearance or transparency can give clues to possible problems. Clear urine usually has normal

**Table 5-5.** Table of abnormal urine colors and their causes

### COLORS CAUSED BY FOOD OR MEDICATIONS

| Color | Cause |
|---|---|
| Red | Beets, rhubarb (in alkaline urine) |
| Yellow-orange | Carrots, some antibiotics |
| Green, blue-green | Clorets, drugs such as amitryptiline |
| Brown-black | Methyldopa, metronidazole |

### COLORS CAUSED BY DISEASE STATES

| Color | Cause |
|---|---|
| Red, red-brown | RBCs, hemoglobin, myoglobin |
| Wine-red | Porphyrins |
| Brown-black | Melanin, homogentisic acid, hemoglobin (in acid urine) |
| Dark yellow-brown or green-brown | Bilirubin, bile pigments |

microscopic results; any abnormalities in a clear specimen are usually detected in the physical or chemical examination. The cause of a cloudy or turbid urine specimen usually becomes evident during the microscopic examination.

Fresh normal urine is usually clear immediately after voiding. As the urine reaches room temperature, or after refrigeration, it may become (turbid,) or cloudy. Depending on the pH of the urine, this cloudiness may be due to amorphous urates or phosphates (Table 5-6).

Turbidity or cloudiness in a freshly voided urine sample may be an indication of disease. Four common causes of turbid urine are WBCs, RBCs, epithelial cells, and bacteria. RBCs in urine give it a cloudy, red appearance. Mucus in the urine can also cause a cloudy appearance. Fats or lipids cause urine to appear **opalescent** (milky).

## Specific Gravity

The **specific gravity** of a solution is the ratio of the weight of the solution (urine) compared to the weight of an equal volume of distilled water at the same temperature. Stated another way, the specific gravity is the density of a solution compared to the density of distilled water, which is 1.000.

The specific gravity of urine indicates the concentration of substances such as urea, phosphates, chlorides, proteins, and sugars dissolved in the urine. The specific gravity is an indicator of renal tubular function; it is used to assess the ability of the kidneys to concentrate or reabsorb essential chemicals and water. Darker urine samples are usually more concentrated than pale

urine samples. Patients who are dehydrated may have highly concentrated urine with a high specific gravity.

# PERFORMING A PHYSICAL EXAM OF URINE

 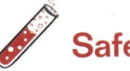 **Safety**

Universal and Standard Precautions must be observed when handling urine and all other body substances. Gloves and other PPE must be worn. Specimens can be poured down the sink, followed by water and disinfectant, but aerosol formation and splashes must be avoided. Equipment such as refractometers should be disinfected by placing a small amount of 10% chlorine bleach solution on the surface of the glass plate and cover and wiping dry.

---

### *Quality Assurance*

Only specimens that have been properly collected should be accepted by the laboratory for testing. Urines should be tested at room temperature after they have been well-mixed by gentle swirling. Refractometers and urinometers must be checked at specified intervals with distilled water (specific gravity 1.000) and control solutions, and the results documented.

---

## Specimen Collection

Physical characteristics are best observed by examining a urine sample immediately after voiding before the sample is refrigerated. If the urine cannot be examined within one hour after collection, it may be refrigerated at 4°C for up to four hours. Refrigerated specimens should be allowed to reach room temperature before the urinalysis is performed.

## Procedure for Physical Examination of Urine

The urine is mixed well by gentle swirling and a portion is poured into a clear container or tube. It is then observed for color and appearance. The specific gravity of the urine is measured and the urine is then kept for chemical and microscopic examination. The physical characteristics of normal urine are given in Table 5-7.

---

**Table 5-6.** Conditions affecting the appearance of normal and abnormal urines

### NORMAL URINES

| Appearance | Causes |
| --- | --- |
| Hazy | Mucus (females), talcum powder, squamous epithelial cells |
| Cloudy | Calcium oxalate, uric acid crystals, amorphous phosphates, amorphous urates |

### ABNORMAL URINES

| Appearance | Causes |
| --- | --- |
| Cloudy-red | Red blood cells |
| Turbid or cloudy | White blood cells, bacteria, yeasts, renal epithelial cells, lipids |
| Opalescent, milky | Fats, lipids |

**Table 5-7.** Physical characteristics of normal urine

| CHARACTERISTIC | NORMAL URINE |
| --- | --- |
| Appearance | Clear |
| Color | Straw to amber |
| Specific gravity | 1.005–1.030 |

## Appearance

The urine color is observed and recorded as pale or straw, yellow, amber, or other. The urine should be observed for clarity using a good light. Appearance is usually reported as clear, hazy, slightly cloudy, cloudy, turbid, or milky.

## Measurement of Specific Gravity

Specific gravity may be measured with a urinometer, refractometer, or reagent strip. The urinometer method requires 20–50 mL of urine, depending on the size of the urinometer. The refractometer method requires only a drop of urine. Measuring specific gravity with a reagent strip is performed with the chemical examination of urine (Lesson 5-4).

The specific gravity (sp. gr.) range of normal urine is 1.005–1.030, with most samples falling between 1.010 and 1.025 (Table 5-7). Specific gravity is highest in the first morning specimen, which is usually greater than 1.020.

***Urinometer Method.*** The urine is poured into a special cylinder and the **urinometer**, a weighted float with a calibrated stem, is placed in the urine with a slight spinning motion (Figure 5-8, left). The specific gravity is read from the float's stem at the urine's meniscus. The urinometer will float high in a concentrated sample (high sp. gr.) and will sink lower in a dilute sample (low sp. gr.). A disadvantage of this method is the large urine volume required for measurement.

***Refractometer Method.*** A **refractometer**, sometimes called a total solids meter (TS meter), measures specific gravity optically by measuring the refractive index of the urine. The refractive index is the ratio of the speed of light in air to light in a solution.

To use the refractometer, one drop of well-mixed urine is placed on the glass plate and the cover is gently closed (Figure 5-8, right). While viewing through the ocular, the specific gravity is read directly off a scale that converts refraction to specific gravity (Figure 5-9).

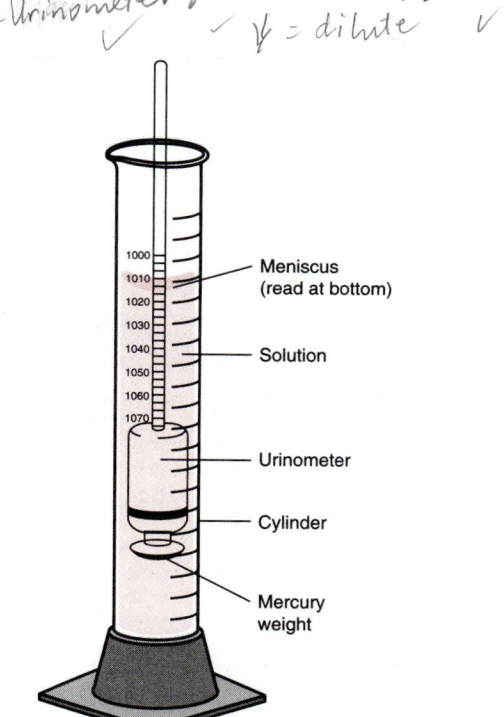
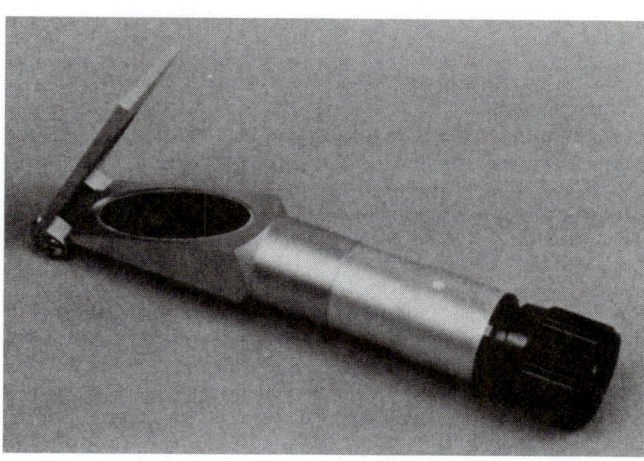

**FIGURE 5-8** Specific gravity measurement: left, urinometer; right, refractometer (Photo courtesy of John Estridge)

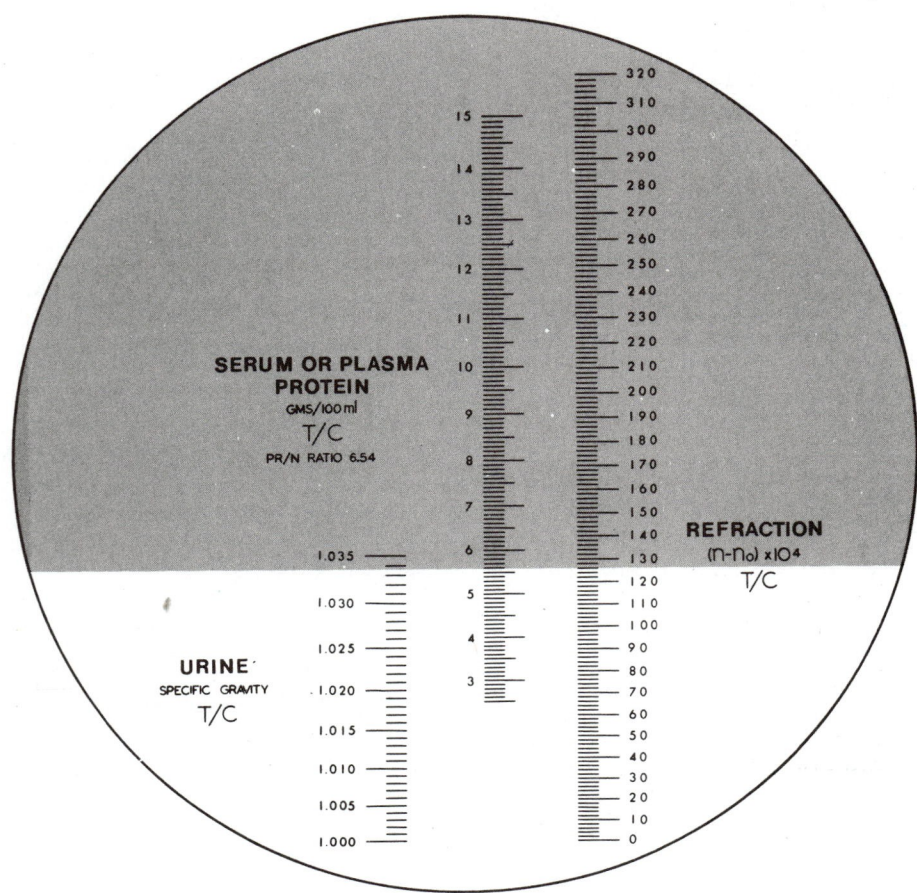

**FIGURE 5-9** Refractometer scale showing a specific gravity reading of 1.034. The small scale (lower left) is used to read the urine specific gravity (Photo courtesy of Leica, Inc., Buffalo, NY)

### Procedural Notes

- Test only properly collected specimens.
- Allow refrigerated specimens to reach room temperature before testing.
- Mix urine gently and thoroughly before making physical observations.
- Test refractometer or urinometer daily with distilled water and urine control solutions to check reliability.

### Safety Precautions

- Observe Universal and Standard Precautions when handling urine specimens and other body fluids.
- Wipe up all urine spills with surface disinfectant.
- Use appropriate exposure control methods when handling and discarding urine specimens to avoid potential exposure to infectious organisms.

## SUMMARY

Abnormalities in the physical characteristics of urine can provide significant clues to renal or metabolic disease. However, variations in characteristics such as color or appearance (transparency) do not always reflect pathologic changes. Sometimes these variations are caused by the handling of the specimen; for example, improper storage temperature or delay in examination. For best evaluation of the physical characteristics of urine, the sample should be examined immediately after voiding. The results of the physical examination of urine often confirm or explain chemical or microscopic results.

## LESSON REVIEW

1. What observations are included in the physical examination of urine? *color, odor, appearance sp. gr.*

2. What are some causes of abnormal urine odors? *disease*

3. What gives urine its normal color? *diet, medication, physical activity & disease*

4. Name four abnormal urine colors and list a possible cause for each. *Red = RBC → RBC present Y/Brown = Bilirubin Yellow = diluted*

5. What is the normal transparency of urine? *clear*

6. What are three causes of cloudy urine? *disease, WBC*

7. What is the normal specific gravity of urine? *1.005 - 1.030*

8. What kidney function is reflected by the specific gravity of urine? *Renal Tubule*

9. Define hematuria, ketones, melanin, myoglobin, opalescent, porphyrins, refractometer, specific gravity, turbid, urinometer, and urochrome. *— Produce normal → yellow color*

## STUDENT ACTIVITIES

1. Reread the information on physical examination of urine.

2. Review the glossary terms.

3. Obtain some urine samples. Compare the specific gravities of lighter-colored urines with those of darker-colored urines.

4. Divide a urine sample. Put one part in the refrigerator; place the other part on the counter at room temperature. Observe each for transparency changes and odor changes at the end of one hour, two hours, or more.

5. Practice performing physical examinations of several urine specimens as outlined on the Student Performance Guide, using the worksheet.

# Student Performance Guide

## LESSON 5-3 Physical Examination of Urine

Name _____ Date _____

## ☣ INSTRUCTIONS

1. Practice the procedure for performing a physical examination of urine following the step-by-step procedure and using the worksheet.
2. Demonstrate your understanding of this lesson by:
   a. Completing a written examination successfully, and
   b. Performing the procedure for the physical examination of urine satisfactorily for the instructor. All steps must be completed as listed on the instructor's Performance Check Sheet.

*Note:* Consult manufacturers' directions before using instruments or performing tests.

## MATERIALS AND EQUIPMENT

- gloves
- hand disinfectant
- puncture-proof container for sharps
- clear plastic conical centrifuge tubes
- test tube rack
- fresh urine sample
- dropping pipet
- refractometer or urinometer
- distilled water
- urinalysis report form or worksheet
- soft tissue or soft paper towels
- biohazard container
- 10% chlorine bleach solution or other surface disinfectant
- urine control solutions

## PROCEDURE

Record in the comment section any problems encountered while practicing the procedure (or have a fellow student or the instructor evaluate your performance).

S = Satisfactory
U = Unsatisfactory

| You must: | S | U | Comments |
|---|---|---|---|
| 1. Wash hands and put on gloves | | | |
| 2. Assemble equipment and materials | | | |
| 3. Obtain a fresh urine specimen. If specimen has been refrigerated, allow it to reach room temperature before proceeding with tests | | | |
| 4. Record the specimen identification on the worksheet (or report form) | | | |
| 5. Mix the urine gently by swirling and pour approximately 10 mL into a clear, conical centrifuge tube | | | |

| You must: | S | U | Comments |
|---|---|---|---|
| 6. Observe the color of the urine (straw, yellow, red, etc.) and record on the worksheet | | | |
| 7. Notice the odor of the urine. If unusual, record in comment section | | | |
| 8. Observe and record the appearance or transparency of the urine (clear, slightly cloudy, turbid) | | | |
| 9. Measure the specific gravity using both the refractometer and urinometer:<br>a. Refractometer<br>　(1) Place one drop of distilled water on the glass plate of the refractometer and close gently<br>　(2) Look through ocular and read the specific gravity from the scale. For water, the specific gravity should read 1.000. (If it does not, calibrate with the screwdriver provided with the refractometer)<br>　(3) Wipe the water from the glass plate, place one drop of urine control solution on the plate and close gently<br>　(4) Look through the ocular, read the specific gravity from the scale, and record the control value<br>　(5) Clean the glass plate with disinfectant and dry with a soft tissue<br>　(6) Repeat steps 9a3–9a5 with a urine specimen, recording result | | | |
| 　b. Urinometer<br>　(1) Pour 40–50 mL of distilled water into the glass cylinder (approximately three-fourths full)<br>　(2) Insert urinometer gently, with spinning motion<br>　(3) Read the specific gravity from the scale on the stem of the urinometer as it stops spinning and record (Specific gravity of water should be 1.000)<br>　(4) Rinse equipment and dry with laboratory tissue and repeat 9b1–9b3 with urine specimen, recording result | | | |
| 10. Discard urine sample properly (or save specimen for chemical examination, Lesson 5-4) | | | |
| 11. Disinfect and clean equipment and return to proper storage | | | |
| 12. Clean work area with disinfectant | | | |
| 13. Remove and discard gloves appropriately | | | |
| 14. Wash hands with hand disinfectant | | | |

*Evaluator Comments:*

Evaluator _____   Date _____

## *Worksheet*

## LESSON 5-3 Physical Examination of Urine

Name _____     Date _____

Specimen I.D. _____

| PHYSICAL EXAMINATION | OBSERVED RESULT | REFERENCE VALUES |
|---|---|---|

1. Appearance (transparency):

        _____ clear

        _____ hazy (slightly cloudy)

        _____ cloudy (turbid)

        _____ other

        describe _____

**REFERENCE VALUES**

clear

2. Color:     _____        straw to amber

3. Specific gravity:     _____        1.005–1.030

Comment: _____

_____

_____

_____

# Chemical Examination of Urine

## LESSON OBJECTIVES

**After studying this lesson, you should be able to:**

- *Name ten chemical tests routinely performed on urine and explain the principle of each.*
- *Give the reference values for the ten urine chemical tests.*
- *Explain the specimen requirement for the chemical examination of urine.*
- *Explain the importance and function of quality assurance procedures in the chemical examination of urine.*
- *Use a reagent strip for the chemical examination of urine and interpret the results.*
- *List a condition that may cause an abnormal result in each of the chemical tests routinely performed on urine.*
- *Perform four confirmatory chemical tests on urine.*
- *Discuss the safety precautions that must be observed in chemical testing of urine.*
- *Define the glossary terms.*

## GLOSSARY

**bilirubin** / a product formed in the liver from the breakdown of hemoglobin

**glycosuria** / glucose in the urine; glucosuria

**hematuria** / presence of blood in the urine

**ketonuria** / ketones in the urine

**proteinuria** / protein in the urine, usually albumin

**urobilinogen** / breakdown product of bilirubin formed by the action of intestinal bacteria

## INTRODUCTION

Several chemical tests may be performed quickly and easily on urine samples due to the development of reagent strip methodology. These tests are usually performed as part of a routine urinalysis. Chemical analyses usually include pH, protein, bilirubin, blood, nitrite, ketones, urobilinogen, glucose, leukocyte esterase, and sometimes specific gravity.

The results of chemical testing of urine provide information on the patient's carbohydrate metabolism, kidney and liver function, and acid-base balance. In some situations, the urine chemical test results can be critical to diagnosis. This lesson presents the principles and methods of chemical testing of urine using reagent strips. Procedures for performing confirmatory tests of some urine constituents are also given.

## METHODS OF CHEMICAL ANALYSIS OF URINE

Reagent strips are the most widely used technique of detecting chemicals in urine and are available in a variety of types. Two major manufacturers of urine reagent strips are Bayer Corporation (Multistix®) and Roche Diagnostics Corporation (Chemstrip®). Strips are available that test for substances such as glucose, ketones, or bilirubin or, one strip may contain as many as ten tests. When the chemical examination of urine is performed using reagent strips, it is a CLIA-waived test.

Other methods of chemical testing of urine are manual tests that singly measure each urine component. These are usually called confirmatory tests and are performed using a variety of methods.

## PRINCIPLES OF CHEMICAL TESTS BY REAGENT STRIP

Urine reagent strips, sometimes called dipsticks, are single-use plastic strips to which pads impregnated with various chemical reagents have been attached. When the strips are dipped into a urine specimen, the chemicals within the reagent pads react rapidly with substances in the urine to form color changes on the reagent pads (Figure 5-10).

In urinalysis, the reagent strips commonly used test up to ten parameters. Each manufacturer of reagent strips may use slightly different methods of detecting some of the urine components. Basic principles of the chemical reactions involved in each test on a strip are

discussed briefly in this section. However, the manufacturer's specific instructions must be consulted to determine the proper procedure for and the chemical principles of the test strip being used.

### pH

The pH is a measure of the degree of acidity or alkalinity of the urine. A pH below seven indicates an acid urine; a pH above seven indicates alkaline urine. The pH of urine may change with diet, medications, kidney disease, and metabolic diseases such as diabetes mellitus. Chemical indicators such as methyl red and bromthymol blue in the pH reagent pad form colors from yellow-orange for acid urine to green-blue in alkaline urine. Normal, freshly voided urine has a pH range of 5.5–8.0.

### Protein

The condition in which an increased amount of protein is present in the urine is called **proteinuria**. Proteinuria is an important indicator of renal disease, but can also be caused by other conditions, such as urinary tract infection. The reagent strip test for protein is based on the principle that proteins can alter the color of some acid-base indicator dyes without changing the pH. The protein reagent pad is buffered at an acid pH (3) with a dye such as tetrabromphenol blue. At the constant low pH, the development of any green color on the reagent pad is due to the presence of protein and is usually reported using a plus system (Neg, 1+, 2+, 3+, 4+). Colors range from yellow for negative to yellow-green or green for

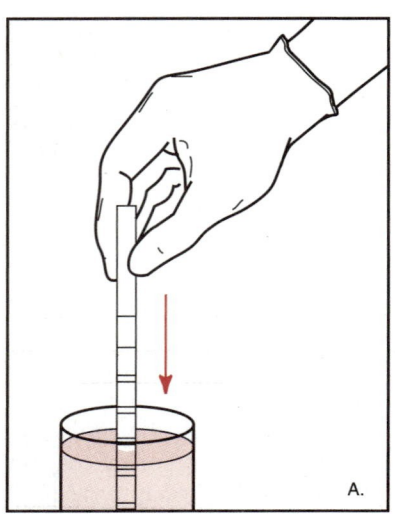 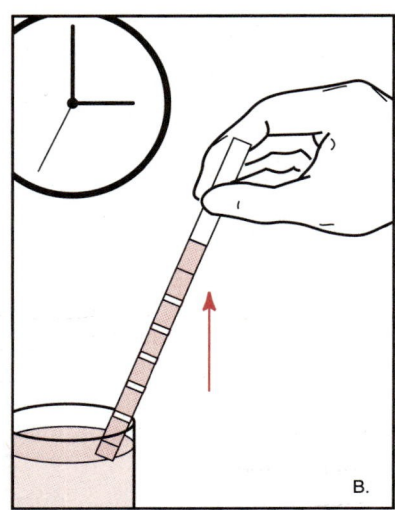 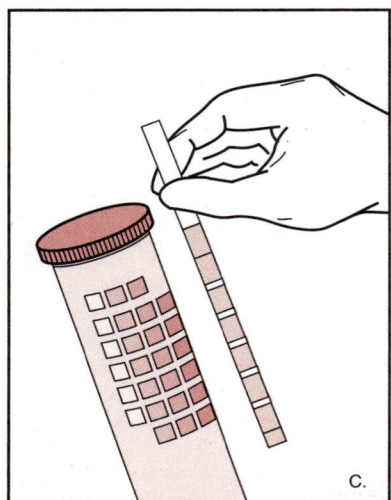

**FIGURE 5-10** Illustration of chemical testing of urine using reagent strips: (A) immerse test strip briefly in urine; (B) remove strip and begin timing; (C) read reactions at appropriate times and compare to a color chart

positive, depending on the amount of protein present. Normal urine is negative or contains just a trace of protein.

## Glucose

The presence of detectable glucose in urine is called **glycosuria**, which indicates that the blood glucose level has exceeded the renal threshold for glucose. This condition may occur in diabetes mellitus and in gestational diabetes. The reagent strip is specific for glucose. It uses the enzymes glucose oxidase and peroxidase plus a chromogen. The enzymes in the pad react with glucose in the urine to change the color of the reagent pad. The intensity of the color formed is proportional to the glucose concentration. Normal urine is negative for glucose by the reagent strip method.

## Ketones

When the body metabolizes fats incompletely, ketones such as acetoacetic acid are excreted in the urine. This condition is called **ketonuria**. Ketonuria may be present in uncontrolled diabetes and starvation or fasting states. The ketone test is based on the development of a light pink to maroon color when ketones react with sodium nitroferricyanide in the reagent pad. Since ketones evaporate at room temperature, urine should be kept tightly capped and refrigerated if it cannot be tested promptly. Normal urine is negative for ketones when tested by reagent strip.

## Bilirubin

**Bilirubin** is a hemoglobin breakdown product formed in the liver from senescent (old) RBCs. When bilirubin is present in urine, it may indicate conditions such as liver disease, bile duct obstruction, or hepatitis. The test for bilirubun is based on coupling bilirubin with a diazonium salt in the reagent pad to form a purple-brown color. Direct light causes decomposition of bilirubin. Therefore, specimens should be protected from light until testing is completed to avoid false negative results. Normal urine contains no detectable bilirubin by the reagent strip method.

## Blood

Presence of blood in the urine, **hematuria**, may indicate infection or trauma of the urinary tract or bleeding in the kidneys. Hemoglobin and RBCs may be detected by the formation of a color due to the peroxidase-like enzyme (in RBCs) reacting with chromogen and peroxide in the reagent pad. The resulting color ranges from orange through green to dark blue. Intact RBCs may cause a spotty appearance on the reagent pad. Myoglobin will also cause a positive reaction on the reagent strip. Normal urine is negative for blood by reagent strip method.

## Urobilinogen

**Urobilinogen** is a bilirubin degradation product that is formed by intestinal bacteria. It may be increased in hepatic disease or hemolytic disease. The urobilinogen reagent pad contains chemicals that react with urobilinogen to form a pink-red color, based on the Ehrlich aldehyde reaction. The reagent strip method can detect urobilinogen in concentrations as low as 0.1 EU (Ehrlich unit). Since urobilinogen is unstable in light and in acidic urine, negative results on routine specimens are not considered significant. The urobilinogen level is normally 0.1–1.0 EU per deciliter of urine.

## Nitrite

Gram-negative bacteria produce enzymes that convert urinary nitrate (a normal urine constituent) to nitrite. The nitrite produced reacts with chemicals in the nitrite reagent pad to form a pink color. A positive nitrite test is an indication of possible bacterial urinary tract infection (UTI). However, not all bacteria can convert nitrates, so a negative result is possible in the presence of infection. Examples of organisms that frequently cause UTI and cause a positive nitrite test are *Escherichia coli*, *Klebsiella*, *Proteus*, and *Pseudomonas*. Normal urine is negative for nitrite.

## Leukocyte Esterase

The presence of WBCs in urine may indicate infection or inflammation in the urinary tract. The esterase enzyme in granular WBCs reacts with chemicals in the leukocyte reagent pad to form a purple color. The color intensity is proportional to the number of leukocytes present. Normal urine is negative for leukocyte esterase.

## Specific Gravity

The specific gravity of the urine reflects the kidneys' ability to concentrate the urine. The specific gravity reagent pad contains an indicator that changes from blue-green to green to yellow-green depends the urine ion concentration. Specific gravity 1.000 and 1.030 can be measured. Alkali give a false low value and should be ch er method. The normal specific gravi 1.030.

## REFERENCE VALUES BY REAGENT STRIP

Normal urine, when tested with a reagent strip, is negative for glucose, ketone, bilirubin, bacteria (nitrite), leukocyte esterase, and blood (see Table 5-8). Normal urine may be negative for protein or contain a trace of protein. Normal, freshly voided urine usually has a pH of 5.5-8.0 and a specific gravity between 1.005 and 1.030.

Positive or abnormal results should be confirmed according to laboratory policy. Some laboratories retest with a single analyte reagent strip; others use confirmatory tests. Positive nitrite or leukocyte esterase tests should be confirmed microscopically by examining urine sediment for the presence of WBCs and/or bacteria.

## PERFORMING CHEMICAL TESTS BY REAGENT STRIP

Reagent strips are used once and discarded. Exact directions for the use of the strips and a color comparison chart are included with each vial. These instructions must be followed precisely for accurate results. The instructions also give information about causes of interference for each test on the strip. The technician should be familiar with these before performing the test and reporting results.

  **Safety**

Universal and Standard Precautions must be used in all urinalysis procedures. Since urine is a body fluid, all urine specimens must be considered potential biological hazards. Care must be taken to avoid spills, splashes, and creation of aerosols. Urine specimens often require more "handling" than other laboratory specimens, such as swirling to mix, pouring, etc. This means workers must be constantly vigilant to prevent being exposed to urines and must wear appropriate PPE.

### Quality Assurance

A good program of quality assurance ensures that the results from chemical analysis of urine are reliable. The program must encompass all procedures, from collecting specimens to reporting results. The specimen collection method is important, as is proper labeling of the specimen. Proper handling and storage of specimens before testing are essential to preventing deterioration of urine components.

The effectiveness of urine test materials such as reagent strips is validated by using urine chemistry controls. Examples of urine control solutions are Check-Stix® from Bayer Corporation and KOVA®-Trol™ from Hycor Biomedical, Inc. Urine controls should be run and results recorded at least once each shift (or day) that urine tests are performed, using commercial normal (negative), low abnormal, and high abnormal controls. In addition, controls must be run when a new vial of strips is opened, and any other time the technician has reason to question the strips' integrity. The results of these controls must be within the manufacturer's stated ranges before patient results can be reported.

When the control results are not within the specified ranges, the test should be repeated using a new reagent strip. If that result is also out of range, a strip from a new vial should be tested. Patient results should not be reported until the discrepancy's cause is identified.

Although reagent strip testing gives the appearance of being quick and easy, many factors must be kept in mind to assure the reported results are valid. Attention must be paid to individual manufacturer's directions for proper use, timing, storage, and interpretation of results, since these may vary with the brand of strip used. Strips must not be used after the expiration date.

Chemical testing of a urine specimen should be performed within one hour of collection. If the test cannot be performed within this time, the specimen may be refrigerated for up to four hours.

**Table 5-8.** Reference values for urine chemical tests using reagent strips

| SUBSTANCE TESTED | REFERENCE VALUE |
| --- | --- |
| pH | 5.5–8.0 |
| Protein | negative to trace |
| Glucose | negative |
| Ketone | negative |
| Bilirubin | negative |
| Blood | negative |
| Urobilinogen | 0.1–1.0 E.U./dL |
| Bacteria (nitrite) | negative |
| Leukocyte esterase | negative |
| Specific gravity | 1.005–1.030 |

Refrigerated specimens should be allowed to reach room temperature before testing. Specimens must be well mixed before using the reagent strip to be sure any solid constituents present, such as blood cells that settle out, will be exposed to the reagent pads. Because some urine constituents are volatile, labile, or light-sensitive, urine specimens should remain tightly covered until tested.

Since manual tests are interpreted using a color comparison chart included with the reagent strips or on the label of the reagent strip container, workers must pass a color blindness test before being allowed to perform urine strip tests.

## Manual Method

Testing is performed by quickly dipping a reagent strip into fresh, well-mixed urine. The excess urine is removed by touching the edge of the urine container with the strip as it is withdrawn from the urine. Timing of reactions should begin at this point. The edge of the strip should be quickly blotted on absorbent paper and the test areas observed at the manufacturer's specified time intervals. The color changes on the reagent pads must be visually compared to the color chart provided with the strips and the results recorded (Figure 5-10).

## Automated Strip Readers

Many laboratories use automated strip readers such as the Clinitek® analyzers by Bayer Corporation and the Chemstrip® line of urine analyzers by Roche Diagnostics Corporation (Figure 5-11). These readers contain reflectance spectophotometers that read the color changes and intensities from the reagent pads and print out the results. The reagent strip is dipped into the specimen by the technician, and the moistened strip is inserted into the instrument. The results are displayed on a lighted panel and may be printed out automatically. Use of these instruments eliminates technician error due to differences in timing or interpretation of colors.

Other tests are available as single analyte reagent strips, such as an hCG strip for pregnancy testing and a microalbumin strip for detecting minute quantities of protein in urine. These can be read visually by the technician or by using the strip reader.

## PERFORMING CONFIRMATORY TESTS ON URINE

Sometimes it may be necessary to measure chemicals in urine by a method other than reagent strip. These other methods are called confirmatory tests because their most common use is to confirm a positive (or negative) result obtained using the reagent strip.

Confirmatory tests are more time-consuming and require more reagents and equipment than the reagent strip method. Four of the most commonly performed confirmatory tests are those for protein, reducing sugars, ketone, and bilirubin.

  **SAFETY**

Universal and Standard Precautions must be observed when performing confirmatory tests on urine. In addition, some confirmatory tests present chemical hazards because they require the use of acids or caustic chemicals.

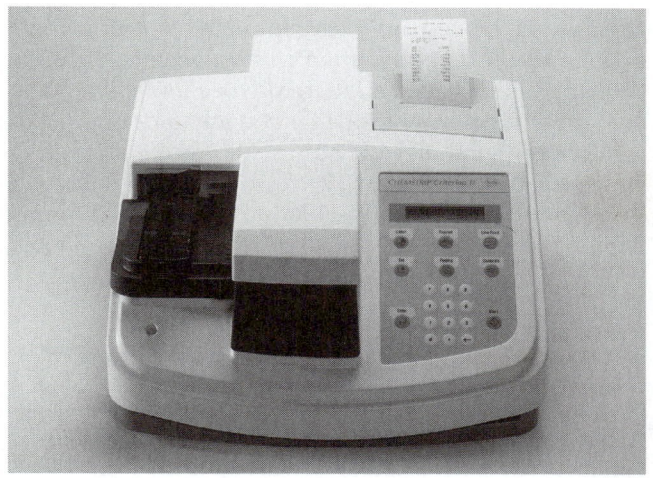

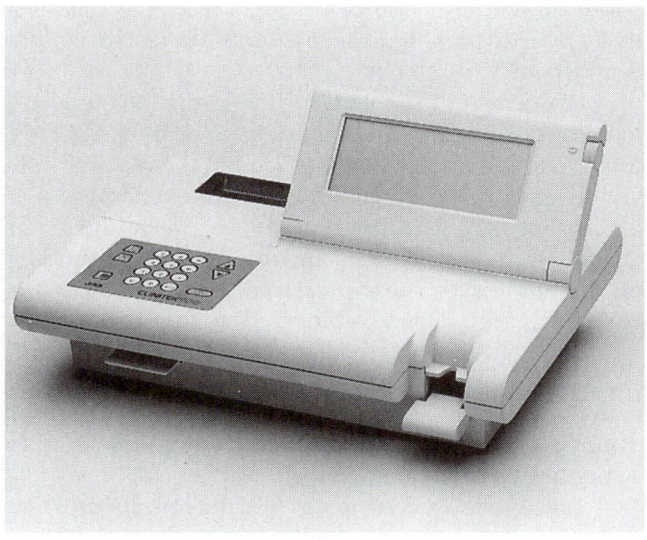

**FIGURE 5-11** Automated urine reagent strip readers. Top, Chemstrip® Mini UA; bottom, Clinitek® 100 (Photos courtesy of Roche Diagnostics Corp, Indianapolis, IN and Miles Laboratories, Elkhart, IN)

## Protein

Most simple confirmatory tests for urine protein involve treating a portion of the urine with an acid to cause the protein to precipitate and therefore become visible. The amount of precipitate formed is roughly proportional to the concentration of protein present. Precipitate is graded as negative, 1+ (turbid), 2+ (turbid with granulation), 3+ (granulation and flocculation), or 4+ (clumps). Acetic, nitric, and sulfosalicylic acids are commonly used.

## Reducing Sugars

A copper reduction test such as Clinitest® is the most common test performed to detect reducing sugars such as fructose, lactose, and galactose in urine. The test is based on the reduction of copper ions in the Clinitest® tablet by reducing sugars in the urine. Therefore, the test is not specific for glucose.

To perform the Clinitest®, five drops of urine and ten drops of water are added to a large heat-resistant test tube. The Clinitest® tablet is placed in the diluted urine and the color is observed while the tablet effervesces. If a reducing sugar is present in the urine, the color changes from blue to green and then orange, depending on the amount of sugar present. When the reaction is complete, the color is compared to the color chart included with the tablet vial and the results are recorded. The two-drop Clinitest® is performed in the same manner as the five-drop method except that two drops of urine are used and the color reaction is compared to a special two-drop color chart.

Since the Clinitest® is not specific for glucose, and a number of substances, such as penicillin, salicylates, and reducing sugars, may cause positive results, Clinitest® results should not be used as the sole basis for adjusting insulin dosage in diabetics.

## Ketone

The Acetest® is a test for ketones and is available in tablet form. The tablet test is based on the same principle as the reagent strip test. If ketones are present in urine, a drop of urine added to the tablet will produce a purple color. Serum or plasma may also be tested for the presence of ketones using Acetest® tablets. A strip such as Ketostix® or Ketodiastix® may also be used to confirm the presence of ketones.

## Bilirubin

The Ictotest® is a specific test for bilirubin and is four times as sensitive as the reagent strip method. The test uses a tablet and absorbent mat. A few drops of urine are placed on the mat, the tablet is placed on the moist area, and water is dropped on the tablet. If bilirubin is present, a purple color will develop on the mat within sixty seconds.

### Procedural Notes

- Collect and store urine specimens properly to ensure preservation of components such as bilirubin and ketones.
- Store reagents and reagent strips according to manufacturer's directions.
- Do not allow the pads of the reagent strips or the reagent tablets to touch anything other than the specimen tested.
- Test reagent strips with negative and positive controls on each day of use to be sure they are working properly.
- Observe and record color changes at the appropriate time intervals.

### Safety Precautions

- Use Universal and Standard Precautions when handling all urine specimens.
- Use care in performing the Clinitest® procedure because of the heat that is generated and the caustic nature of the reagent.
- Wipe up any spills promptly with surface disinfectant.
- Avoid creating aerosols or splashes when transferring or discarding urine specimens.

## LESSON REVIEW

*[handwritten: Leuk, keytone]*
*[handwritten: RBC, Bili, protein, nitrite, glucose, urobilinogen, sp. gr. PH]*

1. Name ten chemical tests routinely performed on urine using reagent strips.

2. Explain how a reagent strip is used. *[handwritten: dip in urine]*

3. What type of urine specimen is preferred for chemical testing? *[handwritten: random urine]*

4. Name four confirmatory tests performed on urine. *[handwritten: Protein, Sugar, keytone, Bili]*

5. For each of the following, name a condition that may cause an increase in the urine: protein, ketones, glucose, bilirubin, and nitrite. *[handwritten: Bili, amm]*

6. Name a method of measuring urine protein other than the reagent strip method. *[handwritten: spectrophotometers]*

7. Name a test that may be performed to detect a reducing sugar other than glucose. *[handwritten: Clinitest]*

8. Explain how quality control procedures are used in urine testing. *[handwritten: Uni V Stand]*

9. What is the advantage of using a urine strip reader? *[handwritten: test]*

10. How can collecting and handling specimens influence the results of chemical tests?

11. What safety precautions should be used when performing urine tests? *[handwritten: glucose, Bl Present, keytone]*

12. Define bilirubin, glycosuria, hematuria, ketonuria, proteinuria, and urobilinogen. *[handwritten: protein]*

## STUDENT ACTIVITIES

1. Reread the information on the chemical examination of urine.

2. Review the glossary terms.

3. Practice performing chemical examinations on several urine specimens as outlined on the Student Performance Guide, using the worksheet.

4. Compare the results of the physical examination of a urine sample with the chemical examination results. Are they as expected? If protein is present in a sample, is specific gravity high? If blood is positive on a reagent strip, was it detected in the physical examination?

*[handwritten:*
*Clinitest — Reducing sugar*
*Acetest — keytones*
*Ictotest — Bili]*

# Student Performance Guide

## LESSON 5-4 Chemical Examination of Urine

Name _____  Date _____

### INSTRUCTIONS

1. Practice the procedure for performing a chemical examination of urine following the step-by-step procedure.

2. Demonstrate your understanding of this lesson by:

   a. Completing a written examination successfully, and

   b. Performing the procedure for the chemical examination of urine satisfactorily for the instructor. All steps must be completed as listed on the instructor's Performance Check Sheet.

*Note:* Consult reagent package inserts for manufacturers' specific instructions before performing tests

### MATERIALS AND EQUIPMENT

- gloves
- hand disinfectant
- fresh urine samples
- urine control solutions (normal and abnormal)
- reagent strips with color chart
- paper towels or laboratory tissues
- stopwatch or timer
- reagent strip reader (optional)
- clear, conical graduated centrifuge tubes
- forceps
- centrifuge
- heat-resistant test tubes, 13 x 100 mm and 16 x 125 mm
- test tube clamp
- dropping pipets
- distilled water
- 20% sulfosalicylic acid (or 3%)
- Clinitest® tablets
- Acetest® tablets
- Ictotest® tablets and absorbent pads
- test tube racks
- worksheet
- urinalysis report forms
- 10% chlorine bleach solution or other surface disinfectant
- biohazard container
- protective eyewear
- puncture-proof sharps container

### PROCEDURE

Record in the comment section any problems encountered while practicing the procedure (or have a fellow student or the instructor evaluate your performance).

S = Satisfactory
U = Unsatisfactory

| You must: | S | U | Comments |
|---|---|---|---|
| 1. Wash hands with disinfectant and put on gloves | | | |
| 2. Assemble equipment and materials | | | |
| 3. Obtain urine specimen and urine control solutions. If specimen has been refrigerated, allow it to reach room temperature before proceeding | | | |

| You must: | S | U | Comments |
|---|---|---|---|
| 4. Perform reagent strip test:<br>  a. Dip reagent strip into urine sample, moistening all pads<br>  b. Remove strip from urine immediately and tap to remove excess urine; blot edge on absorbent paper towels.  Begin timing as strip is withdrawn from urine<br>  c. Observe reagent pads and compare colors to color chart at appropriate time intervals<br>  d. Record results on urinalysis worksheet<br>  e. Discard reagent strip into biohazard container<br>  f. Repeat 4a–4e using urine-control solution(s) | | | |
| 5. Perform sulfosalicylic acid test for protein (usually performed only if protein is positive by reagent strip method):<br>  a. Centrifuge 5 mL of urine<br>  b. Place 4 mL of clear supernatant (from 5a) into a test tube<br>  c. Add three drops of 20% sulfosalicylic acid (or add 4 mL of 3% sulfosalicylic acid)<br>  d. Mix thoroughly and estimate the amount of turbidity after ten minutes<br>  e. Record results on worksheet as negative, trace, 1+, 2+, 3+, or 4+ | | | |
| 6. Perform Clinitest® for reducing substances:<br>  a. Place a 16 x 125 mm test tube into a test-tube rack<br>  b. Place five drops of urine into the test tube<br>  c. Place ten drops of distilled water into the test tube<br>  d. Drop a Clinitest® reagent tablet into the urine-water mixture using forceps<br>  e. Observe color while allowing tablet to effervesce or boil until boiling stops and without touching the test tube<br>  f. Wait fifteen seconds, shake test tube gently using test tube clamp, and compare color to color chart (tube will be hot and opening should be pointed away from your face)<br>  g. Record results on worksheet as negative,  1/4%,  1/2%, 3/4%,  1%, or 2% or more<br>  h. Repeat 6a–6g using urine-control solution(s) | | | |
| 7. Perform Acetest® for ketones:<br>  a. Place an Acetest® tablet on a clean piece of white paper towel or filter paper<br>  b. Place one drop of urine on top of the tablet<br>  c. Compare color of tablet to color chart at thirty seconds<br>  d. Record results on worksheet as negative or positive<br>  e. Repeat 7a–7d using urine-control solution(s) | | | |

| You must: | S | U | Comments |
|---|---|---|---|
| 8. Perform Ictotest® for bilirubin:<br>a. Place ten drops of urine on an Ictotest® mat<br>b. Place an Ictotest® reagent tablet on the moistened area of the mat<br>c. Let two drops of water flow onto the tablet<br><br>*Note:* When elevated amounts of bilirubin are present in the urine specimen, a blue to purple color forms on the mat within sixty seconds. The rapidity of the color formation and the color intensity are proportional to the amount of bilirubin in the urine.  A pink or red color is a negative result<br>d. Record results on worksheet as negative or positive<br>e. Repeat 8a–8d using urine-control solutions | | | |
| 9. If available, retest the urine specimen using a reagent strip reader.  Compare the manual test results with those obtained with the strip reader | | | |
| 10. Dispose of urine specimen properly, avoiding splashes | | | |
| 11. Dispose of test tube contents properly, avoiding splashes | | | |
| 12. Clean equipment and return to proper storage | | | |
| 13. Clean work area with surface disinfectant | | | |
| 14. Remove gloves and discard into biohazard container | | | |
| 15. Wash hands with hand disinfectant | | | |

*Evaluator Comments:*

Evaluator _____ Date _____

*Worksheet*

# LESSON 5-4 Chemical Examination of Urine

Name _____  Date _____

Specimen I.D. _____

## Chemical Examination

**A. REAGENT STRIP**  **OBSERVED RESULT**

| | | REFERENCE VALUES |
|---|---|---|
| pH | _____ | 5.5-8.0 |
| Protein | _____ | negative, trace |
| Glucose | _____ | negative |
| Ketone | _____ | negative |
| Bilirubin | _____ | negative |
| Blood | _____ | negative |
| Urobilinogen | _____ | 0.1–1.0 EU/dL |
| Nitrite | _____ | negative |
| Leukocyte esterase | _____ | negative |
| Specific gravity | _____ | 1.005–1.030 |

## Confirmatory Test Results  (circle result)

**B.** Protein (sulfosalicylic acid)  negative  trace  1+  2+  3+  4+

Reducing substances (Clinitest®)  negative  1/4%  1/2%  3/4%  1%  2% or more

Ketones (Acetest®)  negative  positive

Bilirubin (Ictotest®)  negative  positive

Other _____  _____

# Microscopic Examination of Urine Sediment

## LESSON OBJECTIVES

After studying this lesson, you should be able to:

- *Describe the proper specimen to use for the microscopic examination of urine.*
- *Describe how to prepare urine sediment from a urine specimen.*
- *Name four types of cells that may be found in urine sediment.*
- *Name three types of casts that may appear in urine and explain how they are formed.*
- *List the reference values for RBCs, WBCs, casts, and bacteria in urine.*
- *List crystals that may occur in normal acid urine and in normal alkaline urine.*
- *List four abnormal crystals that may be seen in urine sediment.*
- *Identify cells, casts, crystals, and other sediment components in urine specimens or from visual aids.*
- *Prepare a slide for the microscopic examination of urine sediment.*
- *Perform a microscopic examination of urine sediment and identify the components.*
- *Report the results of a microscopic examination of urine sediment.*
- *Define the glossary terms.*

## GLOSSARY

**amorphous** / without definite shape

**cast** / in urinalysis, a protein matrix formed in the kidney tubules and washed out into the urine

**hyaline** / transparent, pale

**sediment** / solids that settle to the bottom of a liquid

**supernatant** / the clear liquid remaining at the top of a solution after centrifugation or settling out of solid substances

## INTRODUCTION

Microscopic examination of urine **sediment** is the third part of the routine urinalysis. In some laboratories, no microscopic examination is performed if the physical and chemical examinations are normal. However, microscopic examination may provide much helpful information. The examination may reveal infection, disease, or trauma in the urinary tract. In addition, certain results, such as the presence of abnormal crystals, may suggest a metabolic disorder.

# COMPONENTS OF URINE SEDIMENT

Urine **sediment** refers to the solids that settle to the bottom of the urine specimen after centrifugation or when urine is allowed to stand undisturbed. The components of urine sediment include blood and epithelial cells, crystals, **casts**, **amorphous** material, and microorganisms. These are identified through microscopic examination of the sediment, and the estimated numbers present are reported. Urine sediment is usually observed unstained, but stains such as Sedi-Stain® and KOVA® Stain may be used to aid in identifying components. (See Color Plates 18 to 30 for examples of some components of urine sediment.)

## Cells in Urine Sediment

### Blood Cells

Normal urine may contain a few blood cells. Blood cells are best identified using the high-power (40X) objective.

- RBCs—RBCs look like pale, light-refractive disks when viewed under high power (Figure 5-12 and Color Plates 18, 19, and 22). The presence of large numbers of RBCs in urine is called **hematuria** and is an abnormal condition indicating disease or trauma.

- WBCs—A few WBCs may be present in normal urine (Figure 5-13). The type usually present is the segmented neutrophil. WBCs in urine may be increased in UTIs. WBCs are slightly larger than RBCs, may appear granular, and have a visible nucleus (Color Plates 18 and 21).

### Epithelial Cells

Epithelial cells are constantly being sloughed off from the lining of the urinary tract. The epithelial cells appear large and flat, with distinct nuclei and much cytoplasm. These cells may be identified using the high-power (40X) objective. The cell most commonly seen is the squamous epithelial cell (Figure 5-14); less commonly

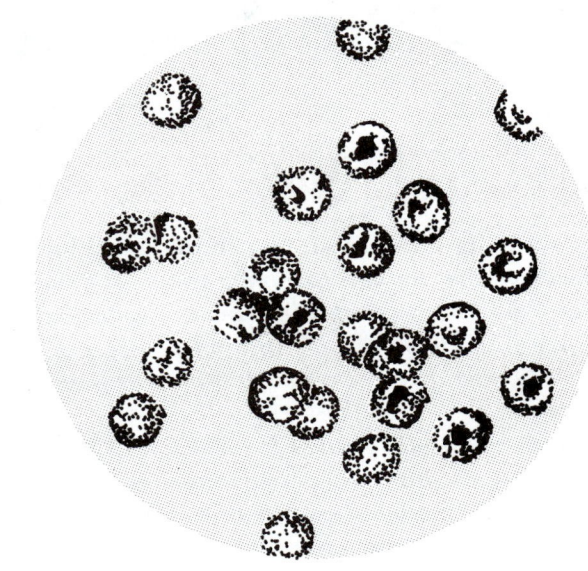

**FIGURE 5-13** WBCs in urine sediment

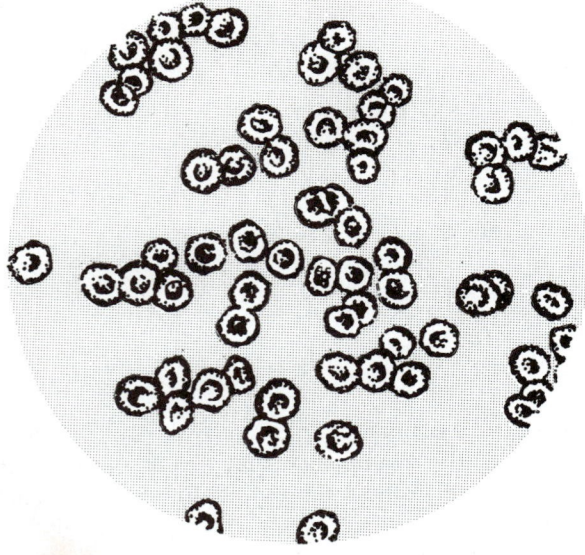

**FIGURE 5-12** RBCs in urine sediment

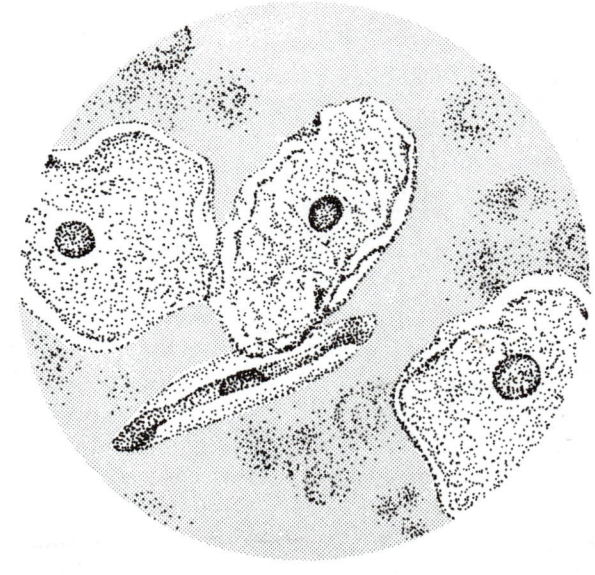

**FIGURE 5-14** Squamous epithelial cells

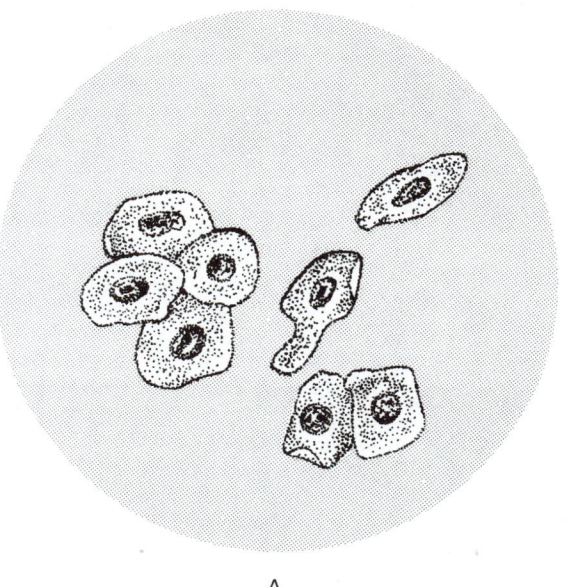

A.

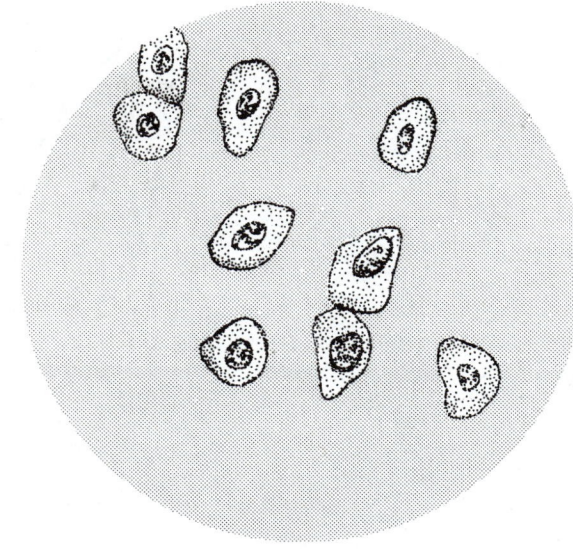

B.

**FIGURE 5-15** Bladder and renal tubular epithelial cells: (A) bladder epithelial cells and (B) renal tubular epithelial cells

seen are the smaller bladder and renal tubular cells (Figure 5-15). The latter may indicate renal disease if they are present in large numbers (Color Plates 18 and 19).

## Microorganisms

Microorganisms should not be present in properly collected, fresh, normal urine. The presence of large numbers of microorganisms indicates infection. Microorganisms are observed using the high-power (40X) objective.

■ Bacteria—Bacteria may appear as tiny round or rod-shaped structures. The rod-shaped bacteria are usually more noticeable because the round ones may resemble amorphous material (Figure 5-16).

■ Yeast—Yeast cells may be present in urine sediment. They are smaller than RBCs but may appear similar to them. Yeasts are ovoid and may be observed budding or in chains (Figure 5-17 and Color Plate 29). The most common yeast found is *Candida albicans*. To distinguish between yeasts and RBCs, one drop of dilute acetic acid is added to the urine sediment; RBCs will lyse and yeast will not.

■ Protozoa—*Trichomonas vaginalis* is the most frequently seen parasite in urine. It is a flagellated protozoan that may infect the genitourinary tract and is usually recognized in urine sediment because of its "twitching" movement (Figure 5-18 and Color Plate 28).

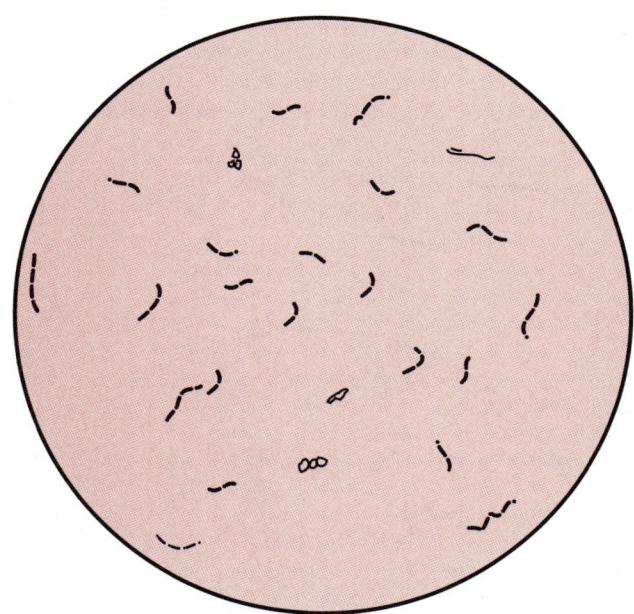

**FIGURE 5-16** Bacteria in urine sediment

## Spermatozoa

Spermatozoa may occasionally be observed in urine samples. They are easily recognized, have spherical heads and long thin tails, and may be motile (Figure 5-19). Spermatozoa should be reported following laboratory policy.

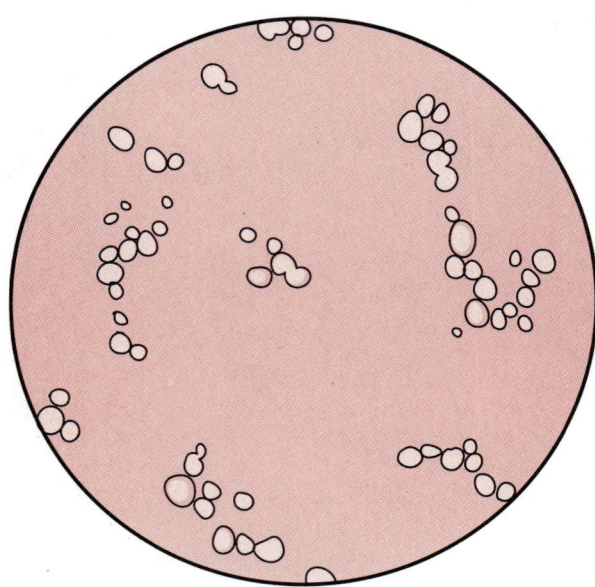

**FIGURE 5-17** Yeasts in urine sediment

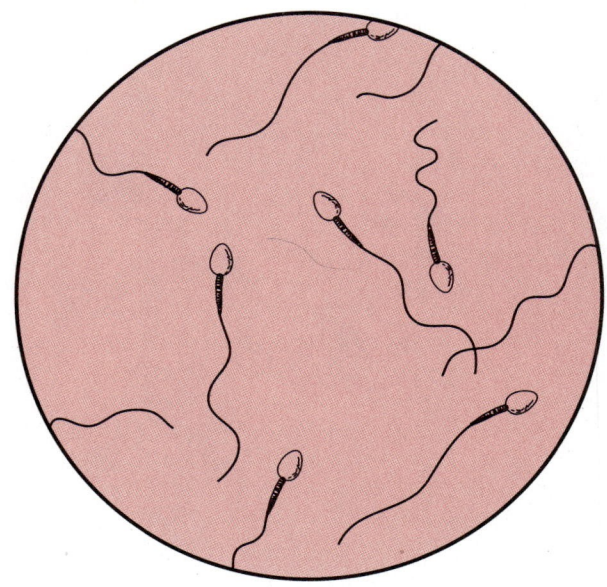

**FIGURE 5-19** Spermatozoa in urine sediment

## Casts in Urine Sediment

**Casts** are formed when protein accumulates and precipitates in the kidney tubules and is washed into the urine. They are called casts because they retain the form or shape of the tubule in which they formed.

The presence of casts in urine, other than an occasional 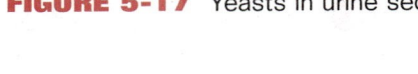hyaline cast, may indicate renal disease. Casts are

cylindrical, with rounded or flat ends, and are classified according to the substances observed in them (Figure 5-20). Some casts may trap cells or debris as they are formed and appear cellular or granular. Casts are counted using the low-power objective (10X) and low light, and classified using the high-power objective.

- Hyaline—Hyaline casts are occasionally found in normal urine. They are transparent, colorless cylinders and are best seen by reducing the light on the microscope and/or lowering the condenser (Color Plate 20).

- Granular—A granular cast contains remnants of disintegrated cells that appear as fine or coarse granules embedded in the protein (Color Plate 21).

- Cellular—Cellular casts may contain epithelial cells, RBCs, or WBCs embedded in the protein matrix (Color Plate 22).

- Waxy—waxy casts are broad, with an irregular outline.

## Crystals and Amorphous Deposits in Urine Sediments

A variety of crystals may be found in normal urine. The formation of crystals is influenced by pH, specific gravity, and urine temperature. Although most urine crystals have no clinical significance, there are some rare crystals that appear in urine because of certain metabolic disorders. Therefore, it is important to be able to recognize

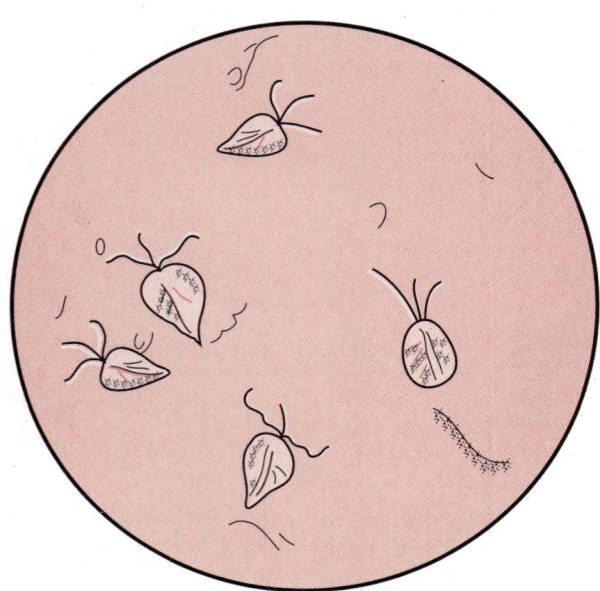

**FIGURE 5-18** Protozoa in urine sediment

# HEMATOLOGY

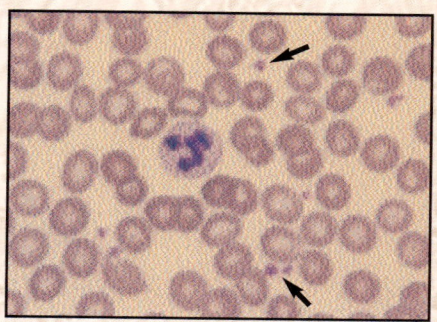

**PLATE 1**
Peripheral blood smear (Wright's stain) showing segmented neutrophil, erythrocytes and platelets (arrows)

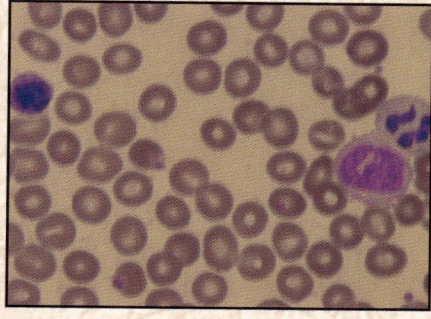

**PLATE 2**
Lymphocyte, monocyte and segmented neutrophil in peripheral blood (Wright's stain)

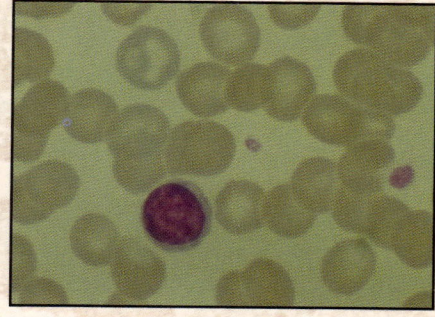

**PLATE 3**
Lymphocyte in peripheral blood

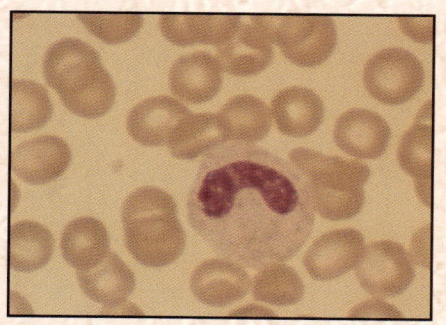

**PLATE 4**
Neutrophilic band in peripheral blood

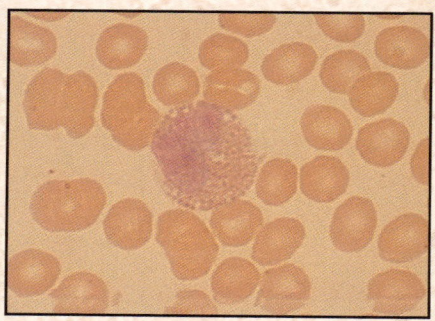

**PLATE 5**
Eosinophilic granulocyte in peripheral blood

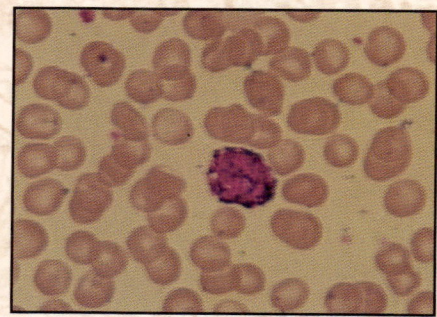

**PLATE 6**
Basophilic granulocyte in peripheral blood

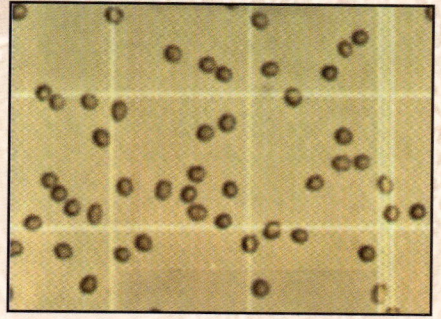

**PLATE 7**
Photomicrograph of erythrocytes as they appear on a hemacytometer (high power)

**PLATE 8**
Photomicrograph of leukocytes as they appear on a hemacytometer (low power)

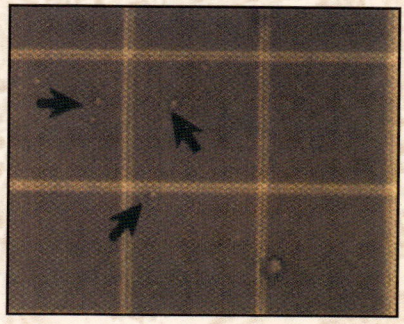

**PLATE 9**
Photomicrograph of platelets (arrows) as they appear on a hemacytometer (high power)

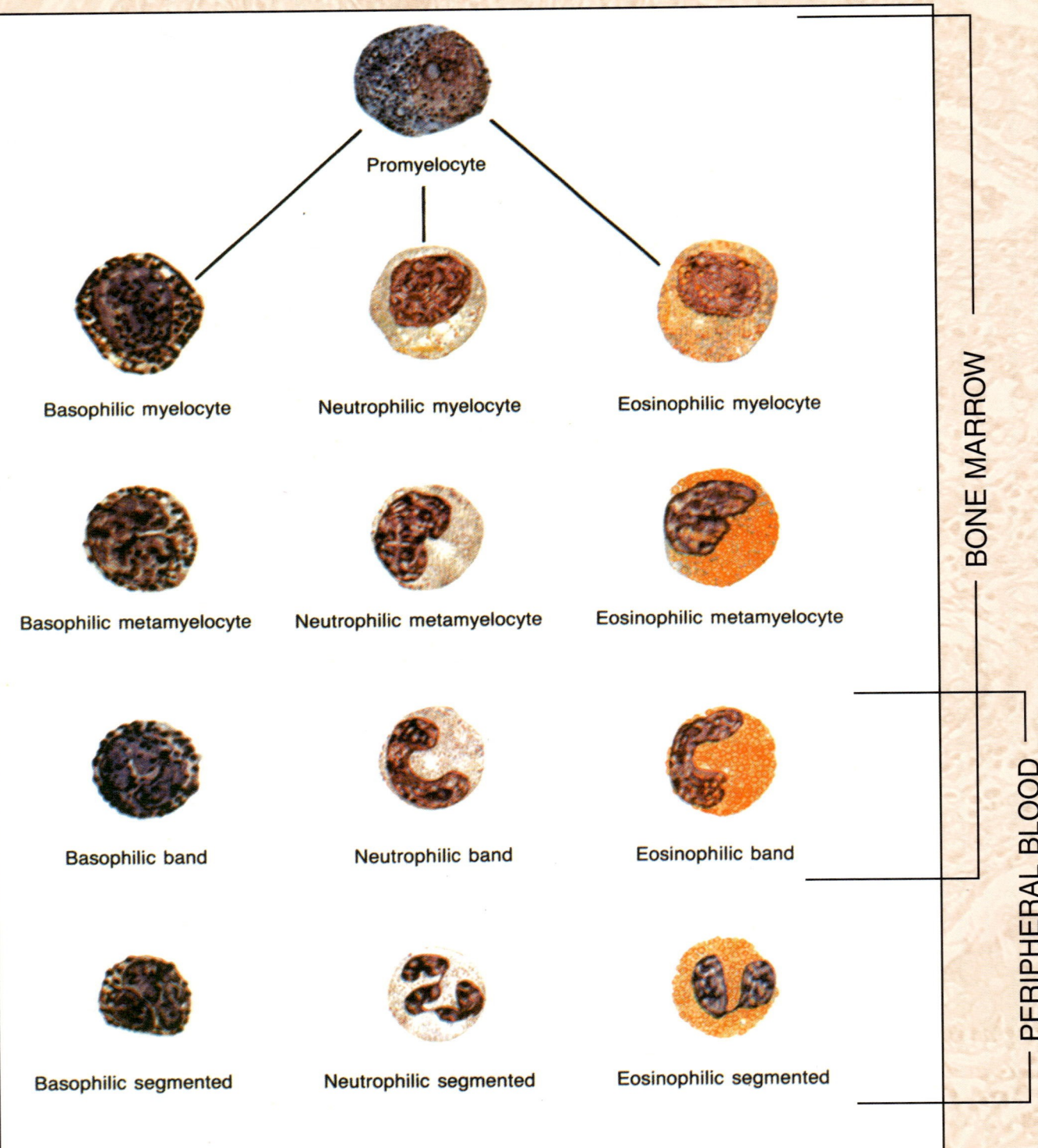

Promyelocyte

Basophilic myelocyte    Neutrophilic myelocyte    Eosinophilic myelocyte

Basophilic metamyelocyte    Neutrophilic metamyelocyte    Eosinophilic metamyelocyte

Basophilic band    Neutrophilic band    Eosinophilic band

Basophilic segmented    Neutrophilic segmented    Eosinophilic segmented

BONE MARROW

PERIPHERAL BLOOD

**PLATE 10**
Origin and development of the
granulocytic (myeloid) blood cells
(Courtesy Abbott Laboratories)

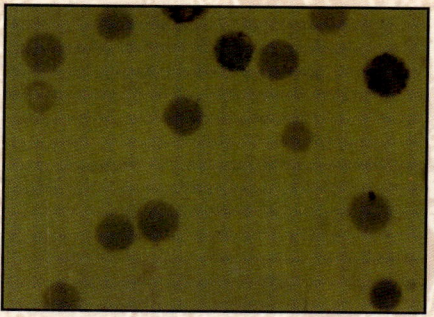

**PLATE 11**
Reticulocytes stained with New Methylene Blue (1OOOX)

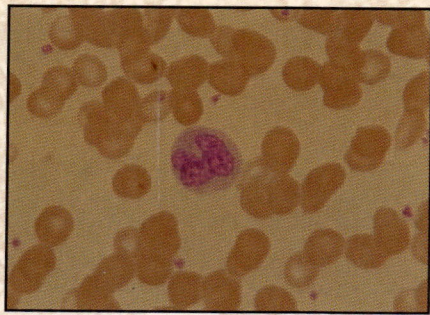

**PLATE 12**
Peripheral blood smear showing a monocyte, platelets, and rouleaux of red blood cells

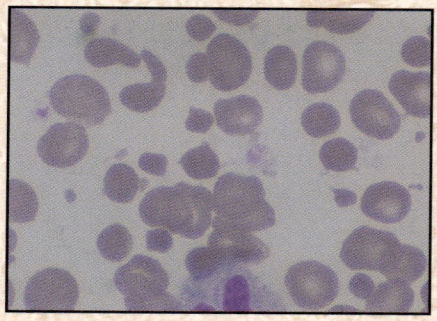

**PLATE 13**
Fragmented red blood cells (schizocytes) in peripheral blood of a burn patient

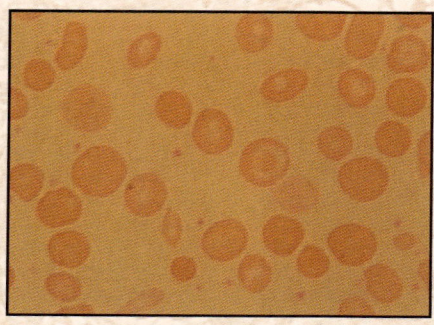

**PLATE 14**
Anisocytosis and poikilocytosis in peripheral blood of a patient with macrocytic anemia

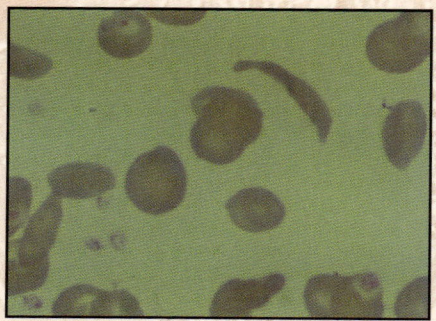

**PLATE 15**
Peripheral blood smear from a patient with sickle cell anemia, showing sickle-shaped red cells

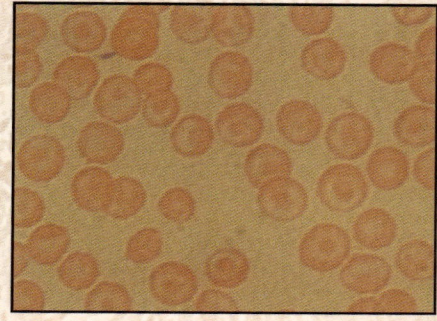

**PLATE 16**
Target cells in peripheral blood of a patient with a hemoglobinopathy

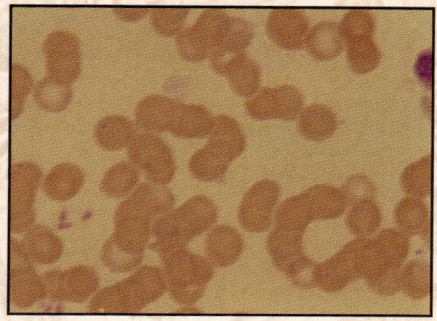

**PLATE 17**
Rouleaux formation in peripheral blood smear from a patient with multiple myeloma

# URINALYSIS

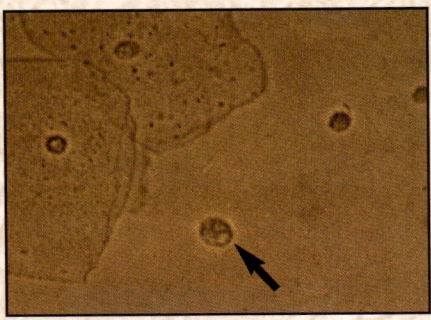

**PLATE 18**
Squamous epithelial cells, red
blood cells, and leukocyte (arrow)
in urine sediment

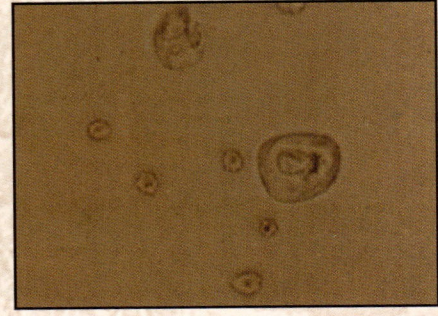

**PLATE 19**
Renal epithelial cell and red blood
cells in urine sediment

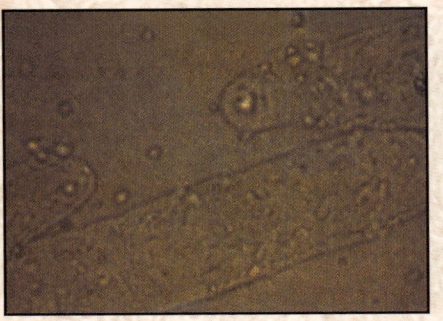

**PLATE 20**
Hyaline casts in urine sediment

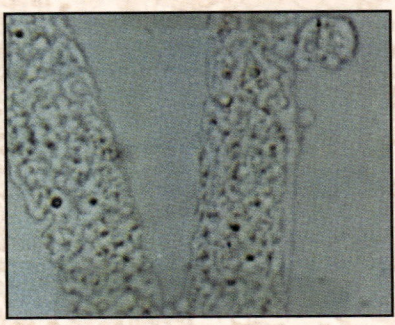

**PLATE 21**
Granular casts and a leukocyte

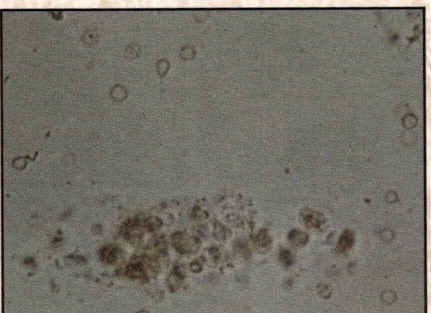

**PLATE 22**
A cellular cast and several red
blood cells

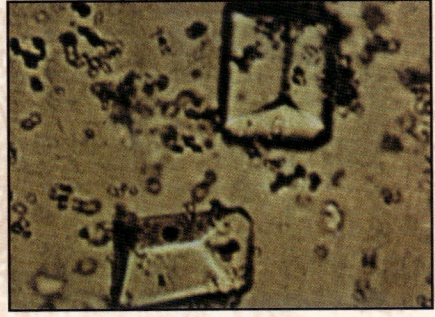

**PLATE 23**
Triple phosphate (ammonium magnesium phosphate) crystals and
amorphous phosphate crystals in
urine sediment

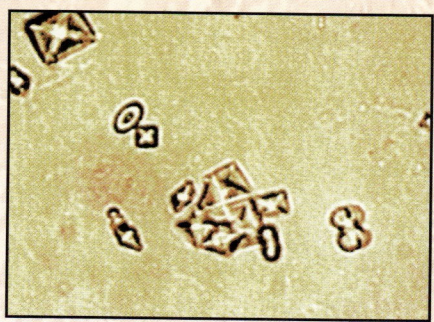

**PLATE 24**
Calcium oxalate crystals

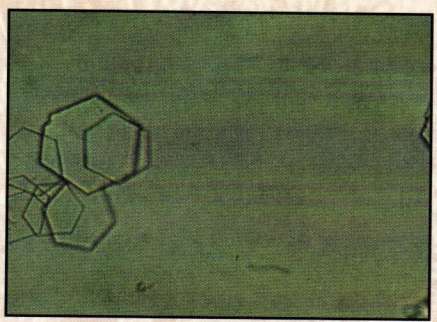

**PLATE 25**
Cystine crystals

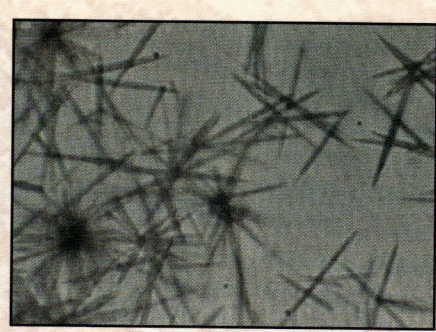

**PLATE 26**
Tyrosine crystals

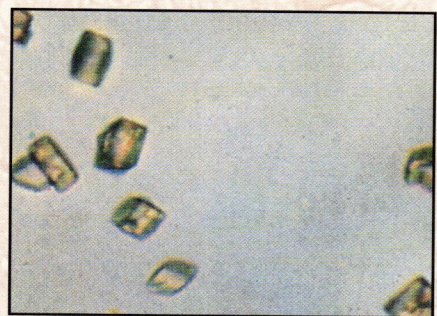

**PLATE 27**
Uric acid crystals

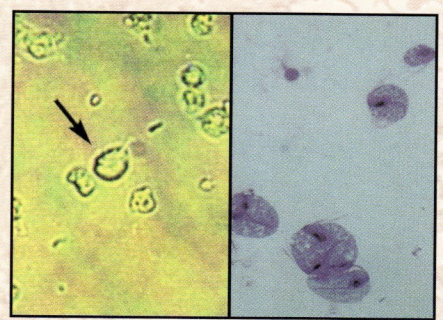

**PLATE 28**
*Trichomonas* (arrow) in unstained urine sediment (left) and stained *Trichomonas* (right)

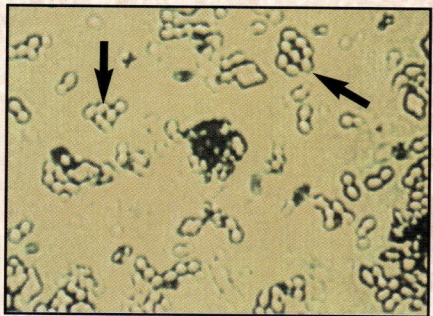

**PLATE 29**
Yeast cells (arrows) in urine sediment

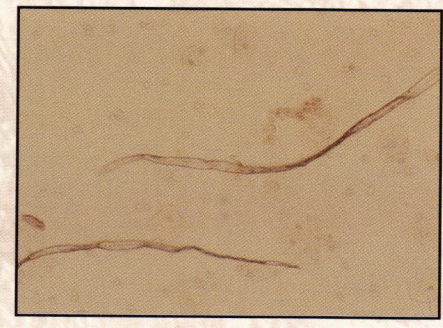

**PLATE 30**
Urine sediment containing fibers (artifacts)

# MICROBIOLOGY/PARASITOLOGY

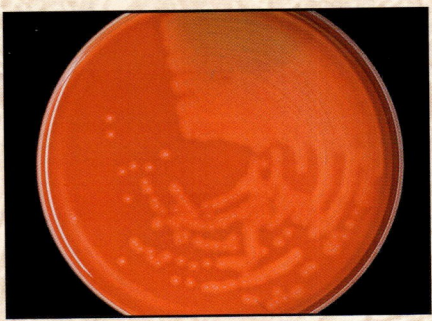

**PLATE 31**
Isolated bacterial colonies on a blood agar plate (Courtesy Becton Dickinson Microbiology Systems)

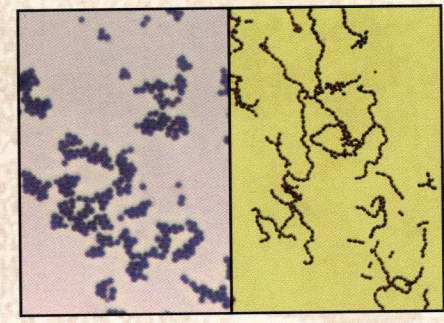

**PLATE 32**
Gram positive cocci. Left, *staphylococci* (clusters); right, *streptococci* (chains)

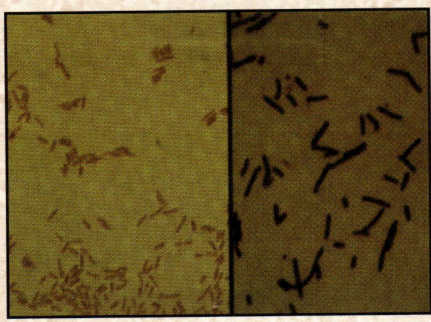

**PLATE 33**
Gram-stained *bacilli* (rods). Left, Gram negative rods; right, Gram positive rods

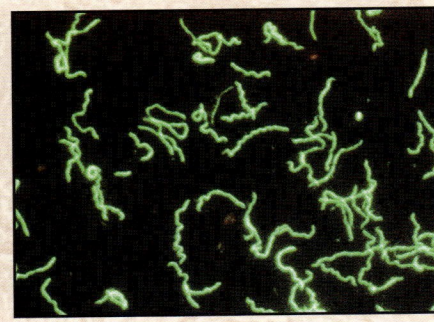

**PLATE 34**
Spirochetes. Immunofluorescence photomicrograph of the spirochete that causes Lyme disease, *Borrelia burgdorferi*

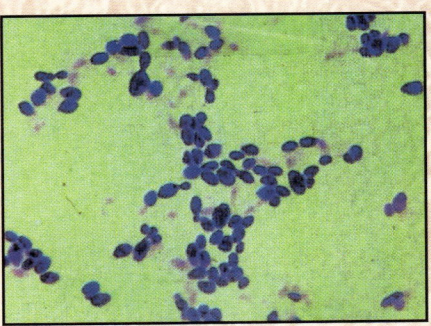

**PLATE 35**
Gram stain of *Candida albicans*, a common yeast

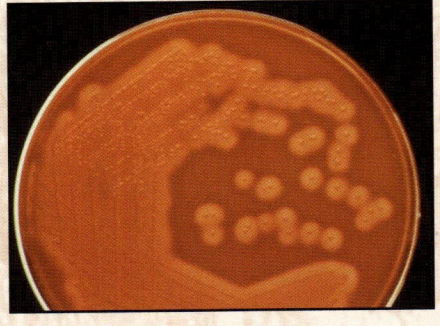

**PLATE 36**
Beta hemolytic *Streptococcus* growing on blood agar

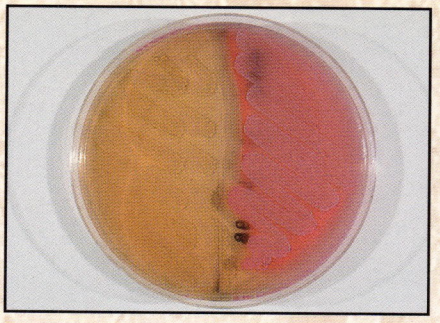

**PLATE 37**
*Salmonella* (left) and *Escherichia coli* (right) growing on MacConkey agar, a differential medium

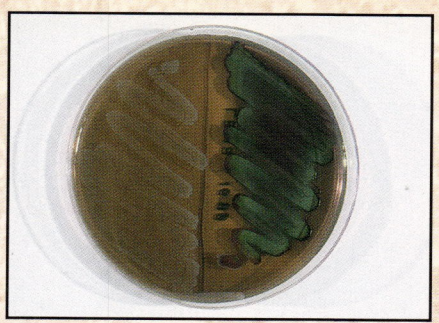

**PLATE 38**
*Salmonella* (left) and *E. coli* (right) growing on EMB, a selective and differential medium

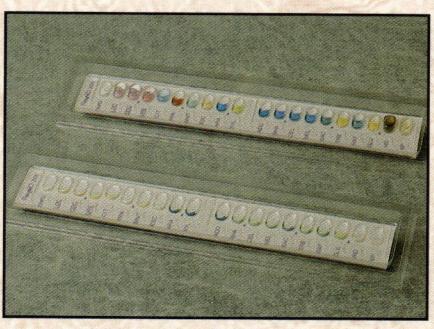

**PLATE 39**
API identification system for Gram negative bacilli

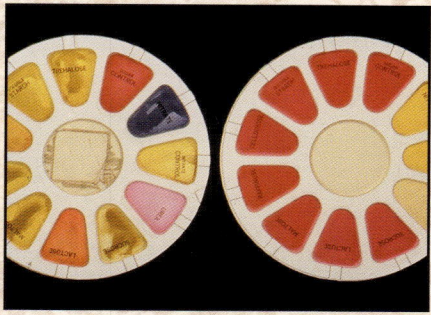

**PLATE 40**
Uni-Yeast-Tek® plates, for identification of yeasts (Courtesy Remel, Inc.)

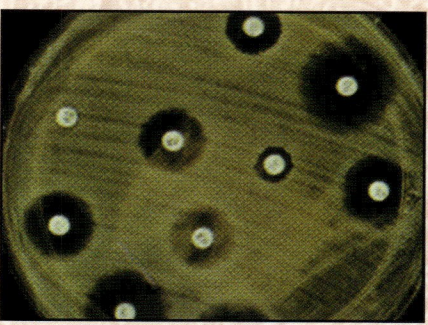

**PLATE 41**
Antibiotic susceptibility test plate

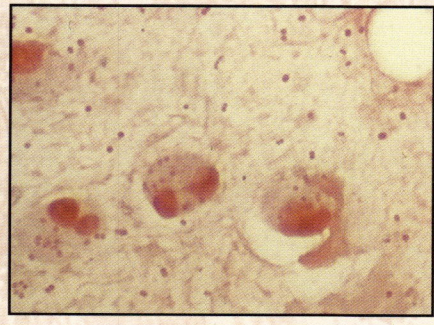

**PLATE 42**
Gram-stained smear of urethral discharge from a male, showing WBCs with intracellular Gram negative diplococci, morphologically resembling *Neiserria gonorrhoeae*

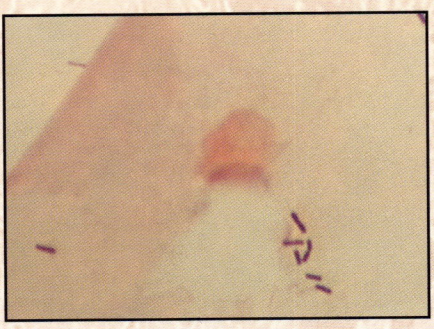

**PLATE 43**
Gram-stained vaginal smear showing Gram positive lactobacilli (normal flora)

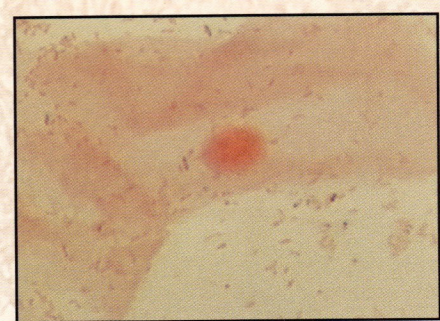

**PLATE 44**
Gram-stained vaginal smear from patient with bacterial vaginosis, showing "clue cells" with large numbers of small Gram-variable organisms, morphologically resembling *Gardnerella vaginalis*

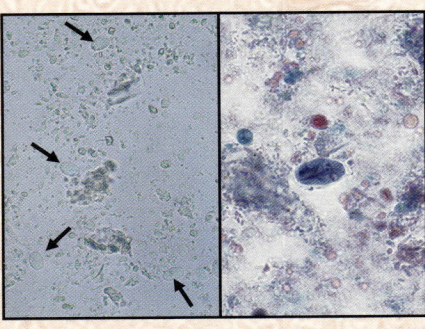

**PLATE 45**
*Giardia lamblia* cysts in fecal specimens. Left, wet prep (brightfield); right, trichrome-stained fecal smear

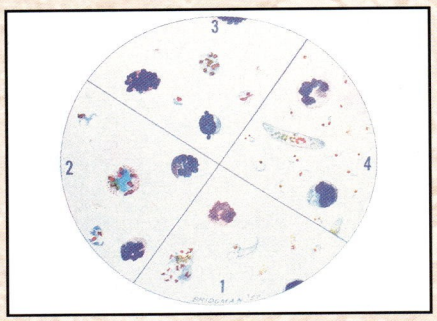

**PLATE 46**
Examples of malarial forms in thick smears. (1) *Plasmodium vivax*, (2) *Plasmodium ovale*, (3) *Plasmodium malariae*, (4) *Plasmodium falciparum*

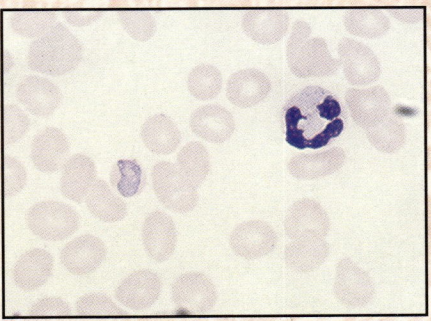

**PLATE 47**
*Plasmodium malariae*, banded schizont and a segmented neutrophil in peripheral blood

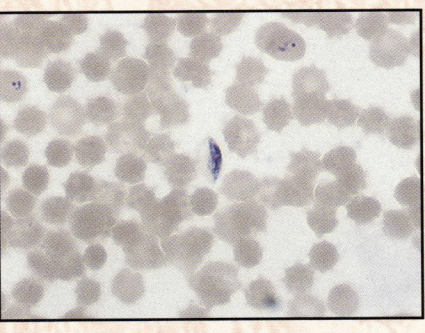

**PLATE 48**
*Plasmodium falciparum*, ring stages and gametocyte

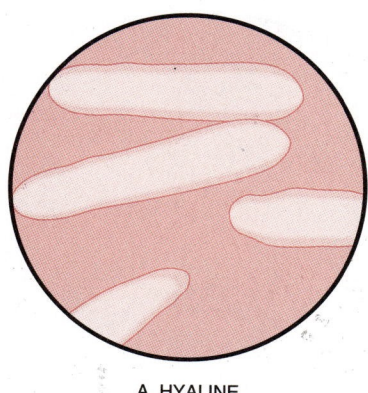

A. HYALINE

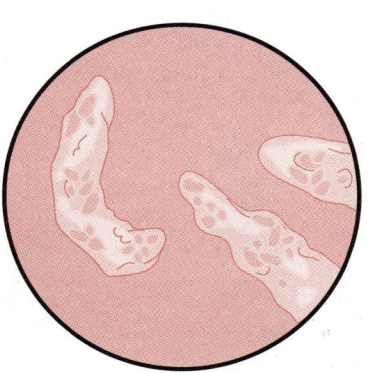

B. GRANULAR

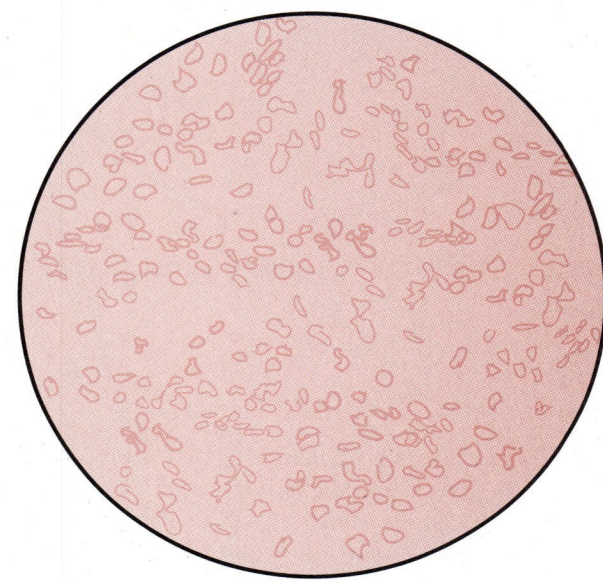

■ Amorphous urates—The amorphous urates may appear in urine as fine granules with no specific shape. Sediment may appear pink in the urine container but, under the microscope, will appear yellowish (Figure 5-21).

■ Uric acid—Uric acid may appear as yellow-brown crystals that can have a variety of shapes: irregular, rhombic, clusters, or rosettes (Figure 5-22, Color Plate 27). Uric acid crystals may be seen in the urine of patients with gout.

**FIGURE 5-21** Amorphous urates in urine sediment

C. CELLULAR

**FIGURE 5-20** Casts in urine sediment: (A) hyaline, (B) granular, and (C) cellular

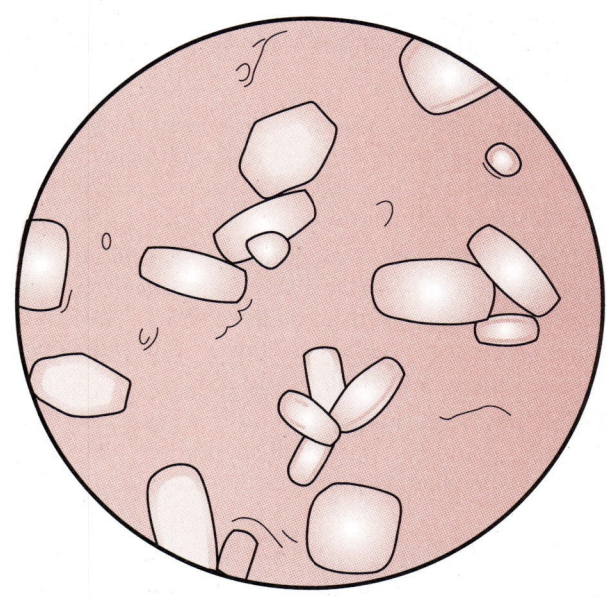

both normal and abnormal crystals. Crystals, when seen, should be identified and reported.

## Normal Crystals in Acid Urine

The normal crystals most commonly seen in acid urine are **amorphous** urates, uric acid, and calcium oxalate.

**FIGURE 5-22** Uric acid crystals in urine sediment

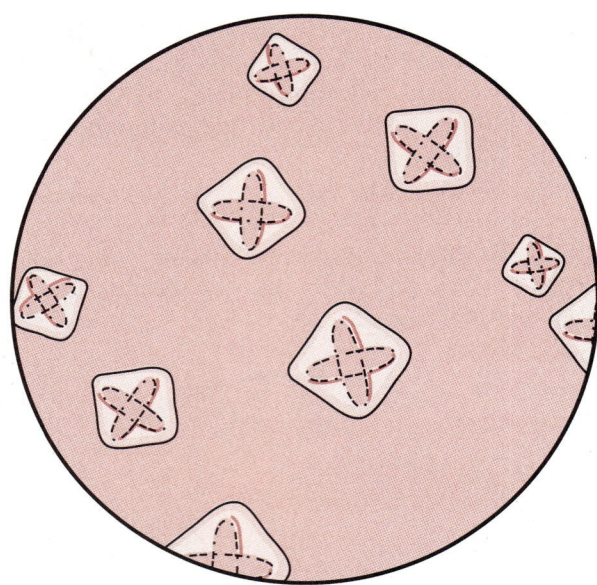

**FIGURE 5-23** Calcium oxalate crystals in urine sediment

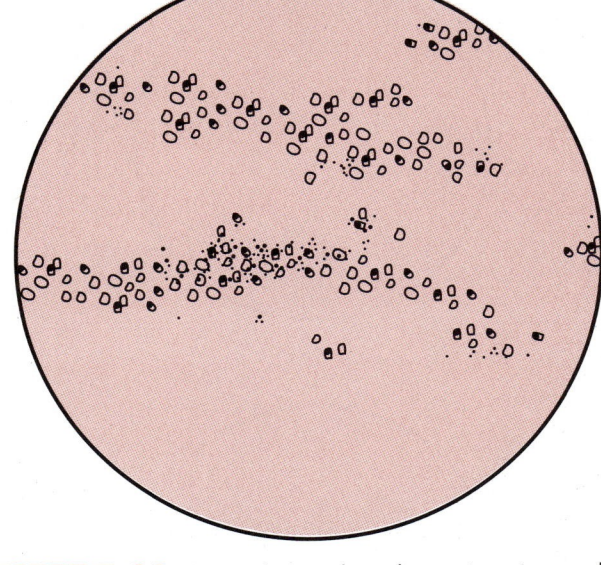

**FIGURE 5-24** Amorphous phosphates in urine sediment

- Calcium oxalate—Calcium oxalate forms colorless octahedral crystals that are refractile. They may look like "envelopes," having an X intersecting the crystal, and may vary in size (Figure 5-23 and Color Plate 24).

### Normal Crystals in Alkaline Urine

The normal crystals most commonly seen in alkaline urine are amorphous phosphates, triple phosphate, and calcium carbonate.

- Amorphous phosphates—Phosphates may appear as colorless, amorphous, granular particles in urine sediment. Amorphous phosphates are soluble in 10% acetic acid (Figure 5-24, Color Plate 23).
- Triple phosphate—Ammonium magnesium phosphate (triple phosphate) may form colorless, highly refractile prisms with three to six sides. The crystals are often described as having a coffin-lid appearance (Figure 5-25, Color Plate 23).
- Calcium carbonate—Calcium carbonate forms small, colorless, dumbbell-shaped or leaf-shaped crystals in alkaline urine (Figure 5-26).

### Abnormal Crystals in Urine

Abnormal crystals may be seen in the urine of patients with metabolic disease or after administration of drugs such as sulfonamides. Some rare crystals are cystine, tyrosine, leucine, cholesterol, and sulfonamide.

- Cystine—Cystine may form colorless, refractile, flat, hexagonal crystals, usually with unequal sides.

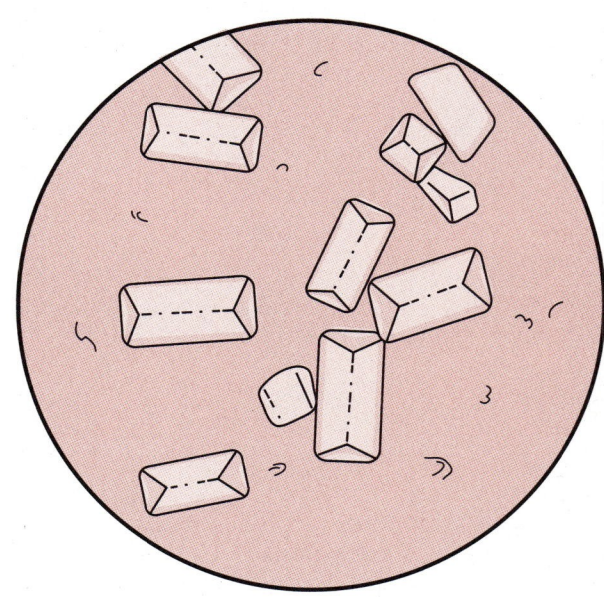

**FIGURE 5-25** Triple phosphate crystals in urine sediment

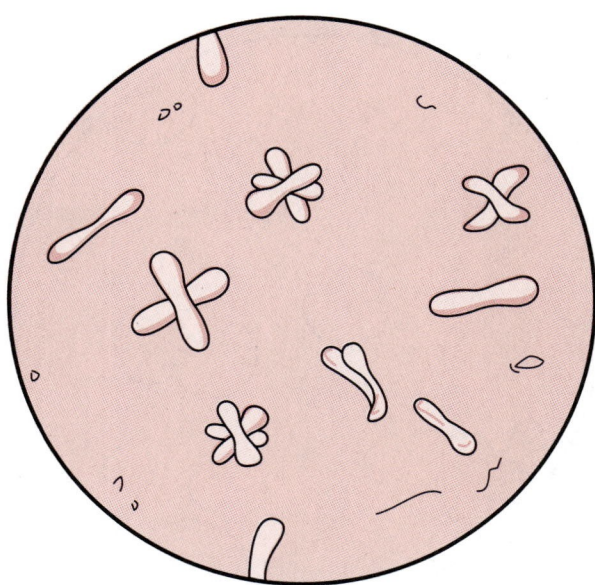

**FIGURE 5-26** Calcium carbonate crystals in urine sediment

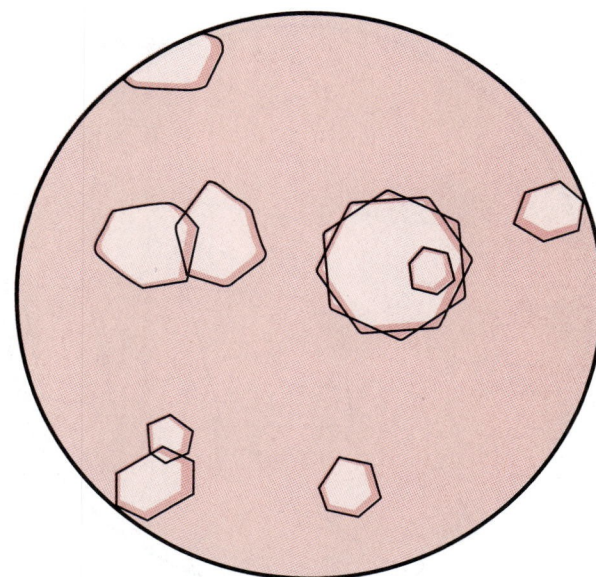

**FIGURE 5-27** Cystine crystals in urine sediment

Presence of these crystals in urine indicates disease such as *cystinuria* (Figure 5-27 and Color Plate 25).

- Tyrosine—Tyrosine forms fine needles arranged in sheaves. Presence of these crystals indicates liver disease or damage (Figure 5-28 and Color Plate 26).

- Leucine—Leucine crystals appear as oily spheres that may be yellow-brown in color and are refractive. Presence of these crystals in urine is an indication of liver disease or damage (Figure 5-29).

- Cholesterol—Cholesterol crystals are colorless, flat plates with notched corners. (Figure 5-30).

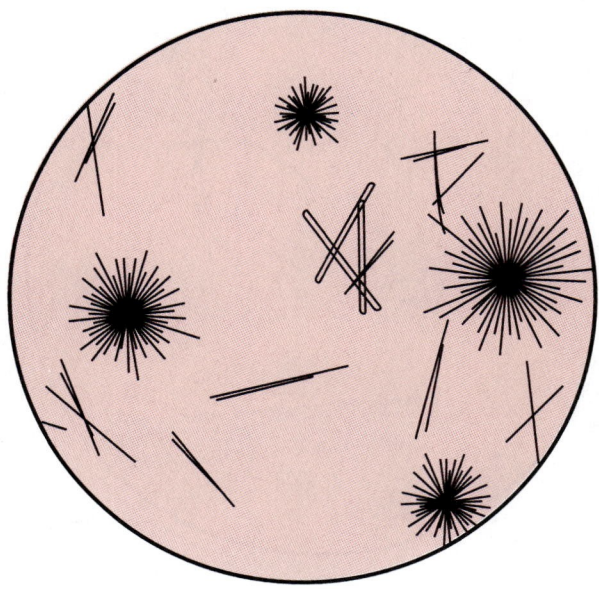

**FIGURE 5-28** Tyrosine crystals in urine sediment

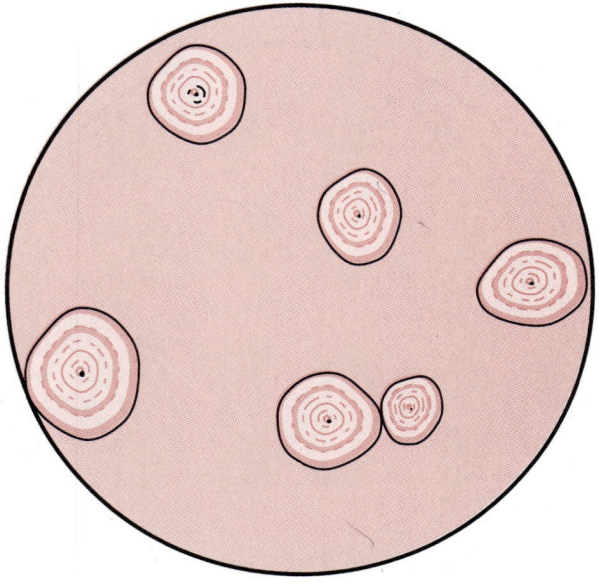

**FIGURE 5-29** Leucine crystals in urine sediment

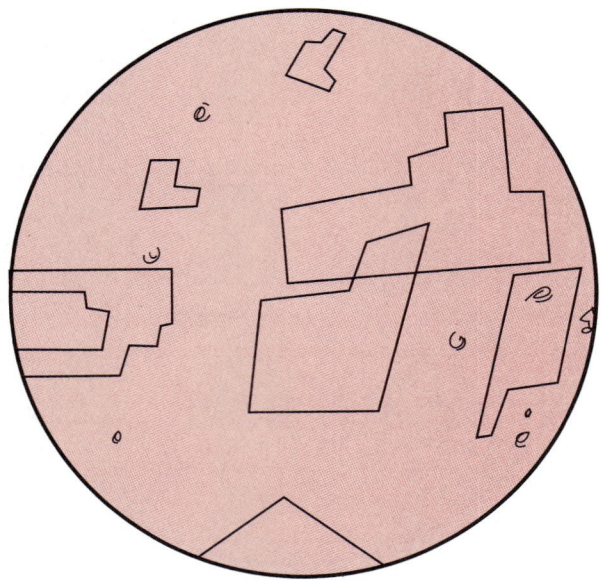

**FIGURE 5-30** Cholesterol crystals in urine sediment

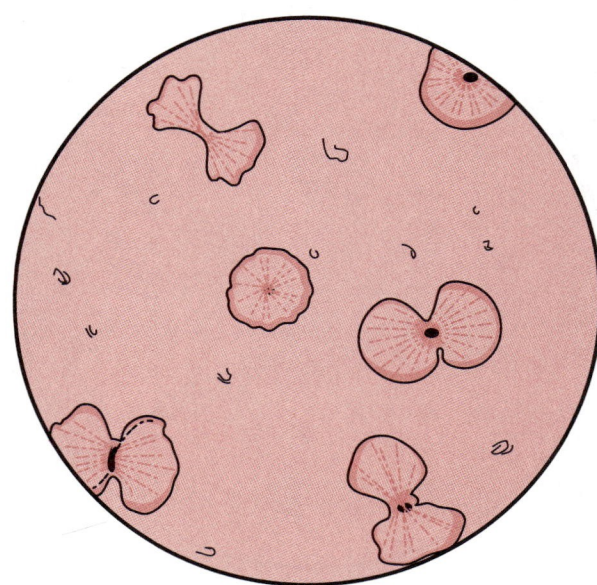

**FIGURE 5-31** Sulfonamide crystals in urine sediment

■ Sulfonamide—Sulfonamide crystals are rarely seen because of the increased solubility of sulfa drugs. When seen, these appear as bundles of needles with striations (Figure 5-31).

## Other Substances in Urine

Mucus threads (from the urinary tract lining) and contaminants such as fibers, hair, starch or talc granules, and oil droplets may sometimes appear in urine sediment (Color Plate 30). These substances must be recognized and should not be confused with clinically significant substances in the sediment. Mucus threads, when seen, are reported (Figure 5-32); contaminants or artifacts are not (Figure 5-33).

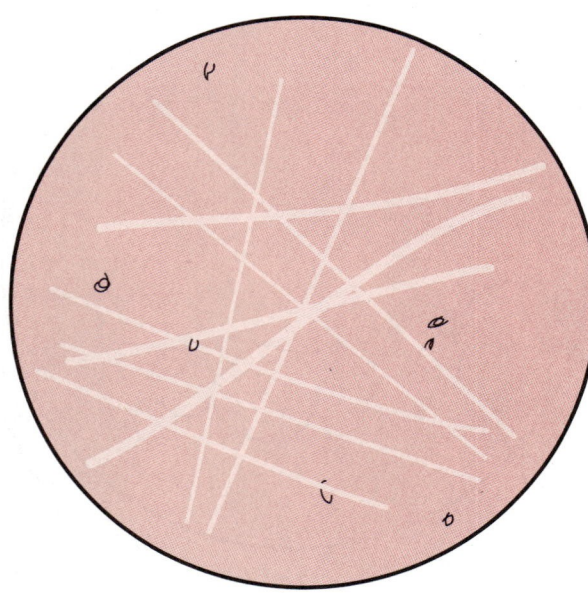

**FIGURE 5-32** Mucus threads in urine sediment

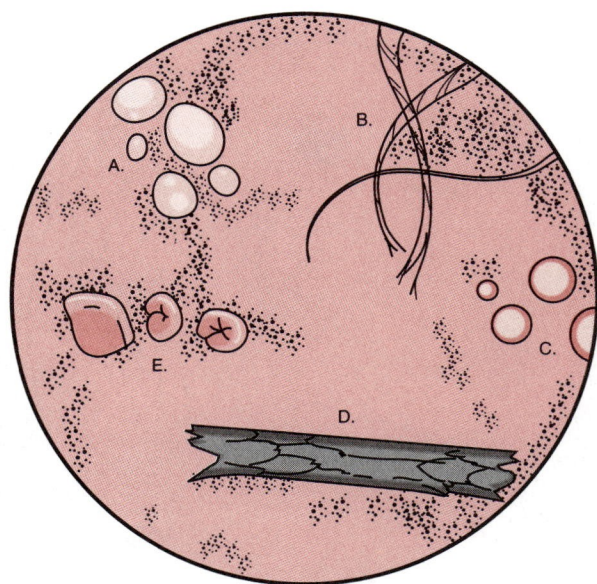

**FIGURE 5-33** Examples of artifacts that may be seen in urine sediment: (A) air bubbles, (B) fibers, (C) oil droplets, (D) hair, and (E) starch or talc granules

# MICROSCOPIC EXAMINATION OF URINE SEDIMENT

 ## Safety

Universal and Standard Precautions must be followed when preparing urine sediment for microscopic examination. Appropriate protective wear must be worn during specimen handling, preparation, and evaluation. Safety guidelines for the use of the centrifuge must be followed (see Lessons 1-5 and 1-8). Sediment slides must be discarded in a sharps container.

## Quality Assurance

Microscopic urine examination is an important procedure. The results may indicate infection, bleeding, abnormal crystals, or urinary tract disease. Controls for urine microscopy are difficult to make, since most components deteriorate rapidly. However, controls that contain stabilized red and white blood cells are available commercially. One example is KOVA®-Trol™ from Hycor. These controls may be used to check workers' recognition of blood cells in urine specimens. As with other control materials, each level of control should be tested a minimum of once per shift or day in which the tests are performed. All results of quality control testing must be documented.

## Specimen Collection and Handling

An early-morning urine specimen is preferred because the urine is usually more concentrated, which increases the chance of finding certain components. In addition, in dilute urines, the RBCs will be destroyed and the WBCs and epithelial cells may be damaged. This could cause the numbers of these components to appear falsely decreased.

All urine specimens should be examined as soon as possible to avoid cellular deterioration and multiplication of any bacteria present. To avoid contamination of the specimen with epithelial cells and microorganisms, a midstream specimen should be used.

## Preparing the Sediment for Microscopic Viewing

Several manufacturers have special systems for preparing and examining urine sediment that standardize the amount of sediment viewed to eliminate variation among workers. Examples of these are UriSystem® by Fisher Scientific, KOVA® System by Hycor Biomedical, and CenSlide® 2000 by StatSpin®, Inc. These systems ensure that a standard amount of urine is centrifuged and control the amount of sediment left for examination (Figures 5-34 and 5-35).

To obtain the sediment, pour 10 mL of well-mixed urine into a conical centrifuge tube. The tube of urine is centrifuged at 1500–2000 rpm (400 x g) for five minutes. The **supernatant** is then carefully poured off, leaving approximately 0.5 mL in the tube.

The sediment should be resuspended in the 0.5 mL of urine by gently tapping the tip of the conical tube. One drop of the mixture is removed either by disposable pipet or by the pipet provided with the kit. This drop is placed on a glass slide or into the special viewing chamber provided with the kit (Figure 5-35). If a microscope slide is used, the specimen should be covered with a coverglass. This forms a more uniform layer of sediment and makes it easier to count the components.

## Performing the Microscopic Examination

A drop of resuspended sediment is placed directly on a clean microscope slide and covered with a coverslip. The slide is first examined with the low-power objective (10X) and reduced light or lowered condenser to locate elements present in low numbers, such as casts. Ten to fifteen low-power fields (LPF) are scanned and the average number of casts per LPF is counted and recorded.

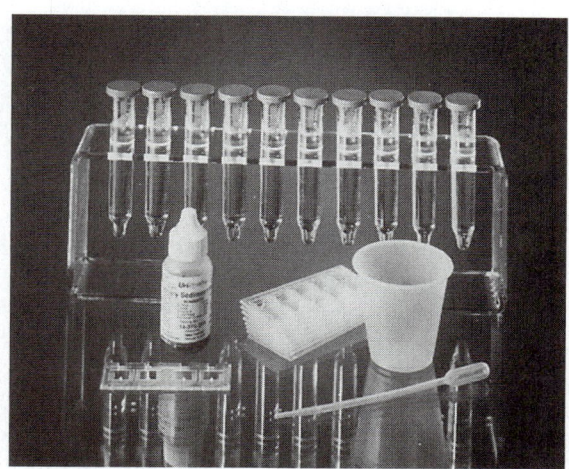

**FIGURE 5-34** UriSystem® standardized urinalysis system (Photo courtesy of Fisher Scientific)

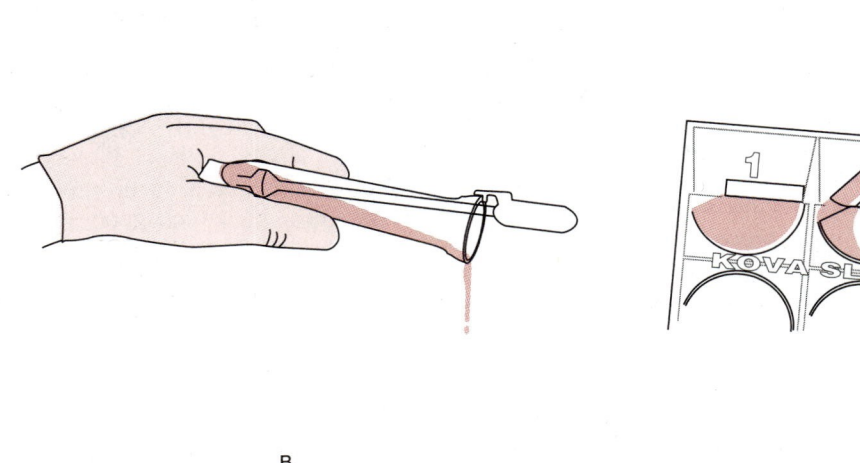

**FIGURE 5-35** Kova® System for standardized urinalysis: (A) inserting the pipet into a tube of centrifuged urine, (B) obtaining urine sediment by pouring off supernatant, and (C) loading the slide chamber using the special pipet

The high-power (40X) objective is used to identify RBCs, WBCs, epithelial cells, yeasts, bacteria, and crystals (ten to fifteen consecutive high-power fields should be scanned). The diaphragm of the microscope should be adjusted during scanning to obtain the proper amount of light. The average number of RBCs, WBCs, and epithelial cells per high-power field (HPF) is recorded. Table 5-9 lists the reference values for urine sediment. A phase-contrast microscope is very useful for viewing urine sediment.

Microorganisms such as yeasts (budding) and *Trichomonas* should be reported, if seen. Bacteria are usually reported only if large numbers are seen in a fresh urine sample that has been properly collected. (Bacteria are reported as neg, 1+, 2+, 3+, or 4+.)

Mucus threads and crystals should be reported, if seen, and crystals should be identified. Mucus is usually reported as negative, 1+, 2+, 3+, and 4+. Spermatozoa are reported according to laboratory policy.

## Method of Counting Sediment Components

The method of counting may differ among laboratories. Therefore, the method used should always be that of the laboratory where the test is being performed.

The counts for RBC, WBC, and epithelial cells represent an average of the number of cells seen in each of the ten high-power fields (HPF) scanned. The results may be reported as 0, rare, occasional, or a range such as 2–4 or 4–6.

The count for casts represents an average of the number of casts seen in each of the ten low-power fields (LPF) scanned. Casts should be categorized as hyaline, granular, or cellular. The method of reporting cast numbers is like that for cells.

**Table 5-9.** Reference values for components of urine sediment

| COMPONENT | REFERENCE VALUE |
|---|---|
| RBC/HPF | rare |
| WBC/HPF | 0–4 |
| Epith/HPF | occasional (may be higher in females) |
| Casts/LPF | occasional hyaline |
| Bacteria | negative |
| Mucus | negative to 2+ |
| Crystals | types present vary with pH (crystals such as cystine, leucine, tyrosine, and cholesterol are considered abnormal) |

## Automated Systems for Examining Urine Sediment

Systems are available that automate the steps in urinalysis, including counting and classifying components of urine sediment. An example is the IRIS (International Remote Imaging Systems, Inc.) family of instruments. In these systems, urines are loaded into a sample tray on the analyzer. Urine strips are wetted robotically and the color reaction is measured and recorded in a computer database. Portions of the urine specimens are then mixed with stain and the sample is passed through a video imaging system. The components' morphologies are compared to an image database and the results are saved to a disk. Technologists can review results on color-video displays before release to patient charts. Systems such as this require a large test volume to be cost-effective and are usually found only in large laboratories.

### Procedural Notes

- If a phase-contrast microscope is not available, adjust the light, iris diaphragm, and condenser of the microscope to give the best contrast of urine sediment.

- Use the fine adjustment to continually focus up and down to facilitate finding components, especially casts.

- Differentiate yeasts from RBCs by performing the acetic acid test.

### Safety Precautions

- Use Universal and Standard Precautions when handling urine samples to avoid potential exposure to infectious agents.

- Wipe the work area promptly with surface disinfectant if spills occur and when work is finished.

- Use proper safety procedures when operating the centrifuge.

- Avoid creating splashes or aerosols when pouring urine from the centrifuge tube and discarding specimen.

- Discard slides in a biohazard sharps container.

## LESSON REVIEW

1. What is the best type of urine specimen to use for microscopic examination of sediment?
2. How is urine sediment prepared for a microscopic examination?
3. Why are microscopic urine tests important?
4. What happens to cells in dilute urine samples?
5. What is the advantage of a standardized urine system such as the KOVA® System or UriSystem®?
6. Name four types of cells that may be seen in urine sediment.
7. Explain how casts are formed.
8. Name eight crystals that may be seen in urine sediment.
9. List the normal values for RBC, WBC, casts, and bacteria in urine sediment.
10. Define amorphous, cast, hyaline, sediment, and supernatant.

## STUDENT ACTIVITIES

1. Reread the information on microscopic examination of urine sediment.
2. Review the glossary terms.
3. Practice performing a microscopic examination on one or more urine specimens as outlined on the Student Performance Guide, using the worksheet. Practice identifying components of urine sediment using visuals provided by the instructor.
4. Compare the results of the examinations with results obtained by fellow students or the instructor.
5. Draw three components that were found in the urine sediments. Are they components of normal urine?

# Student Performance Guide

## LESSON 5-5 Microscopic Examination of Urine Sediment

Name _____ Date _____

### INSTRUCTIONS

1. Practice preparing and examining urine sediment following the step-by-step procedure.

2. Demonstrate your understanding of this lesson by:

   a. Completing a written examination successfully, and

   b. Performing the procedure for preparing and examining urine sediment satisfactorily for the instructor. All steps must be completed as listed on the instructor's Performance Check Sheet.

*Note:* Follow instructions on the package insert for the system being used

### MATERIALS AND EQUIPMENT

- gloves
- urine controls
- hand disinfectant
- fresh urine samples
- centrifuge
- microscope
- worksheet (urinalysis report form)
- 10–20% chlorine bleach solution or other surface disinfectant
- biohazard container
- puncture-proof biohazard container for sharp objects
- stopwatch or timer (if centrifuge lacks timer)
- visuals depicting various components of urine sediment or prepared slides of urinary sediment
- commercial standardized urine system or the following materials:
  – microscope slides
  – cover glasses
  – disposable pipets
  – conical graduated centrifuge tubes

### PROCEDURE

Record in the comment section any problems encountered while practicing the procedure (or have a fellow student or the instructor evaluate your performance).

S = Satisfactory
U = Unsatisfactory

| You must: | S | U | Comments |
|---|---|---|---|
| 1. Wash hands and put on gloves. Assemble equipment and materials | | | |
| 2. Practice microscopic identification of urine sediment using urine-control solutions | | | |
| 3. Obtain a urine sample | | | |
| 4. Pour 10–15 mL of well-mixed urine into a clean conical centrifuge tube (or tube from standardized system) | | | |

| You must: | S | U | Comments |
|---|---|---|---|
| 5.  Place filled tube in centrifuge, insert balance tube, and close lid (centrifuge must be balanced) | | | |
| 6.  Centrifuge at 1500–2000 rpm for five minutes | | | |
| 7.  Remove tube from centrifuge after rotor stops spinning | | | |
| 8.  Pour off supernatant urine, leaving approximately 0.5 mL of urine in tube (follow system instructions if applicable) | | | |
| 9.  Resuspend urine sediment by tapping the bottom of the tube | | | |
| 10.  Place one drop of resuspended urine onto a clean glass slide or into chamber provided with the system | | | |
| 11.  Place coverslip over drop of urine if using glass slide | | | |
| 12.  Place slide on microscope stage and focus using low-power (10X) objective and lowered condenser | | | |
| 13.  Scan ten to fifteen low-power fields, count the number of casts per field, and record the average | | | |
| 14.  Identify the type(s) of casts present and record | | | |
| 15.  Rotate the high-power (40X) objective into position (raise condenser if necessary) | | | |
| 16.  Scan ten to fifteen fields on high power | | | |
| 17.  Count the number of RBC, WBC, and epithelial cells per high-power field and record the average for each | | | |
| 18.  Observe the sample for the presence of microorganisms, crystals, or mucus, and record if present.  If crystals are present, identify type | | | |
| 19.  Complete the urinalysis report form or worksheet | | | |
| 20.  Discard specimen tube and pipet appropriately; avoid aerosol formation | | | |
| 21.  Discard slide in puncture-proof biohazard container | | | |
| 22.  Clean and return equipment to proper storage | | | |
| 23.  Clean work area with surface disinfectant | | | |
| 24.  Remove and discard gloves appropriately | | | |
| 25.  Wash hands with hand disinfectant | | | |
| 26.  Use unlabeled illustrations or pre-prepared slides of urine sediment provided by the instructor to identify components of sediment not seen on slides. | | | |

*Evaluator Comments:*

Evaluator _____   Date _____

## *Worksheet*

## **LESSON 5-5** Microscopic Examination of Urine

Name _____   Date _____

Specimen I.D. _____

**Microscopic Examination**

| | | **REFERENCE VALUE** |
|---|---|---|

WBC: _____ / HPF          0–4

RBC: _____ / HPF          rare

Epithelial cells: _____ / HPF          occasional (higher in females)

Casts: _____ / LPF          occasional, hyaline

    Type: _____

Yeasts: negative  1+  2+  3+  4+          negative

Bacteria: negative  1+  2+  3+  4+          negative

Mucus: negative  1+  2+  3+  4+          negative to 2+

Crystals: _____ none seen _____ present

    Type: _____

Other: _____

# *Routine Urinalysis Report Form*

## **LESSON 5-5** Microscopic Examination of Urine

Name _____     Date _____

Specimen I.D. _____

### 1. Physical Examination

| | | REFERENCE VALUES |
|---|---|---|

Transparency:　　　　_____ clear

　　　　　　　　　_____ hazy (slightly cloudy)

　　　　　　　　　_____ cloudy

Color:　　　　　　_____

Specific gravity:　_____

**REFERENCE VALUES**

clear

straw to amber

1.005–1.030

### 2. Chemical Examination

#### A. Reagent Strip

**REFERENCE VALUES**

| | | |
|---|---|---|
| pH | _____ | 5.5–8.0 |
| Protein | _____ | negative, trace |
| Glucose | _____ | negative |
| Ketone | _____ | negative |
| Bilirubin | _____ | negative |
| Blood | _____ | negative |
| Urobilinogen | _____ | 0.1–1.0 E.U./dL urine |
| Bacteria (nitrite) | _____ | negative |
| Leukocyte esterase | _____ | negative |

### B. Confirmatory Test Results (circle results)

| | | | | | | |
|---|---|---|---|---|---|---|
| Protein (sulfosalicylic acid): | negative | trace | 1+ | 2+ | 3+ | 4+ |
| Reducing substances (Clinitest®): | negative | 1/4% | 1/2% | 3/4% | 1% | 2% or more |
| Ketones (Acetest®): | negative | positive | | | | |
| Bilirubin (Ictotest®): | negative | positive | | | | |

## 3. Microscopic Examination

| | | REFERENCE VALUES |
|---|---|---|
| WBC: | _____ / HPF | 0-4 |
| RBC: | _____ / HPF | rare |
| Epithelial cells: | _____ / HPF | occasional (higher in females) |
| Casts: | _____ / LPF | occasional, hyaline |
| Type present: | _____ | |
| Crystals: | _____ none seen | |
| | _____ present | |
| | (type) _____ | |
| Amorphous deposits: | _____ none seen | |
| | _____ present | |
| Yeasts: (circle result) | negative  1+  2+  3+  4+ | negative |
| Bacteria: (circle result) | negative  1+  2+  3+  4+ | negative |
| Mucus: (circle result) | negative  1+  2+  3+  4+ | negative to 2+ |
| Other: (circle result) | _____ | |

Tech/Student _____    Date _____

# Urine Pregnancy Tests

## LESSON OBJECTIVES

**After studying this lesson, you should be able to:**

- *Name the hormone tested for in pregnancy tests.*
- *Name two types of specimens used in pregnancy tests.*
- *Name two common test methods for measuring hCG.*
- *Explain the principles of pregnancy tests.*
- *Perform a urine pregnancy test.*
- *Interpret the results of a urine pregnancy test.*
- *Name a cause of false-positive pregnancy tests.*
- *List safety precautions to observe when performing pregnancy tests.*
- *Define the glossary terms.*

## GLOSSARY

**agglutination inhibition** / interference with or prevention of agglutination

**EIA** / enzyme immunoassay

**hCG** / human chorionic gonadotropin, a hormone present in pregnancy; uterine chorionic gonadotropin (uCG)

## INTRODUCTION

Modern urine pregnancy tests are based on the detection of human chorionic gonadotropin (**hCG**) by immunological methods. HCG is a hormone produced by the placenta and is present in the serum and urine of pregnant women shortly after fertilization. It is sometimes called uterine chorionic gonadotropin, or uCG.

Many types of urine pregnancy tests are available. Several may be purchased in pharmacies or drug stores for in-home testing. Whether the kits are designed for home use or clinical use, they are based on the interaction of hCG in the specimen with anti-hCG, an antibody specific for the hormone. Manufacturers of pregnancy test kits have designed them to be sensitive and easy to perform and interpret, and to give rapid results. However, results of home tests should be confirmed by a laboratory using appropriate controls and by a physical exam.

## PRINCIPLES OF PREGNANCY TESTS

Pregnancy tests use antigen-antibody methods to detect hCG. A commercially prepared antibody to hCG (anti-hCG) is used to detect hCG (the antigen) in the patient specimen. The most commonly used pregnancy test kits are based on modified enzyme immunoassay (**EIA**) techniques.

## Enzyme Immunoassay Tests

Pregnancy tests that are modifications of enzyme immuno-assays (EIAs) are called solid-phase EIAs or membrane EIAs. (Principles of EIAs are also discussed in Lesson 4-1.) In the modified EIA tests, antibodies and other reagents are immobilized in an absorbent membrane, which is enclosed in a plastic test unit. When the specimen containing hCG is applied to the membrane, it migrates through it, contacting the various reagents and producing a colored reaction in the "result" area of the test unit (Figure 5-36). Examples of these types of pregnancy tests are Clearview™ hCG by Wampole Laboratories, Quick Vue® by Quidel, and ICON® II HCG distributed by Beckman Coulter.

## Agglutination Inhibition Tests

The first rapid tests for hCG were based on the principle of **agglutination inhibition**. The UCG-BETA slide test by Wampole Laboratories is an example of an agglutination inhibition pregnancy test. In these tests, the substance being tested for, if present, will inhibit the agglutination of specially coated particles in the test reagent. Therefore, *absence of agglutination is a positive test*. If the substance being tested for is not present, agglutination will occur and the test is interpreted as negative (Figure 5-37). Agglutination inhibition tests are being replaced by EIA methods in many laboratories because the EIA tests are easier to interpret and often have greater sensitivity.

## PERFORMING A URINE PREGNANCY TEST

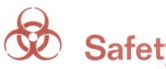 Safety

Universal and Standard Precautions must be observed when performing urine pregnancy tests. Care must be taken to avoid urine spills and splashes or the creation of aerosols. After testing, the specimen and used materials must be disposed of appropriately.

## Specimen Collection

Although, any urine specimen can be used for most hCG tests, the preferred specimen is the first urine voided in the morning because it usually has the highest hCG concentration. If the specimen cannot be tested immediately, it may be stored at 4°C for up to twenty-four hours. Either urine or serum may be used with some test kits; other kits use only one or the other. Serum is the specimen used for most quantitative hCG tests.

## Test Procedure: Modified Enzyme Immunoassay

EIAs for hCG vary in design, but have some features in common. Most have the reagents incorporated into an absorbent membrane within a self-contained test unit, which may look like a plastic slide, a reagent strip, or a test cylinder. Tests may require the addition of the urine specimen only or the addition of specimen and reagents to the test unit.

For most methods, the endpoint is the formation of a colored area on the membrane (Figures 5-36 and 5-38). Some manufacturers design the tests so the colored area forms a "+" or "−" to aid in test interpretation.

Bayer Corporation, a manufacturer of urine reagent strips, also makes an hCG strip. The strip is dipped in urine and the results are read visually or using the Clinitek®50 automated strip reader. This is a CLIA-waived test.

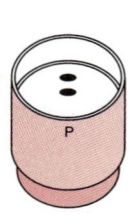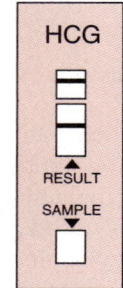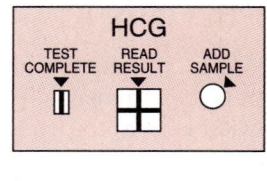

**FIGURE 5-36** Three examples of modified EIA pregnancy test kits

## POSITIVE PREGNANCY TEST:

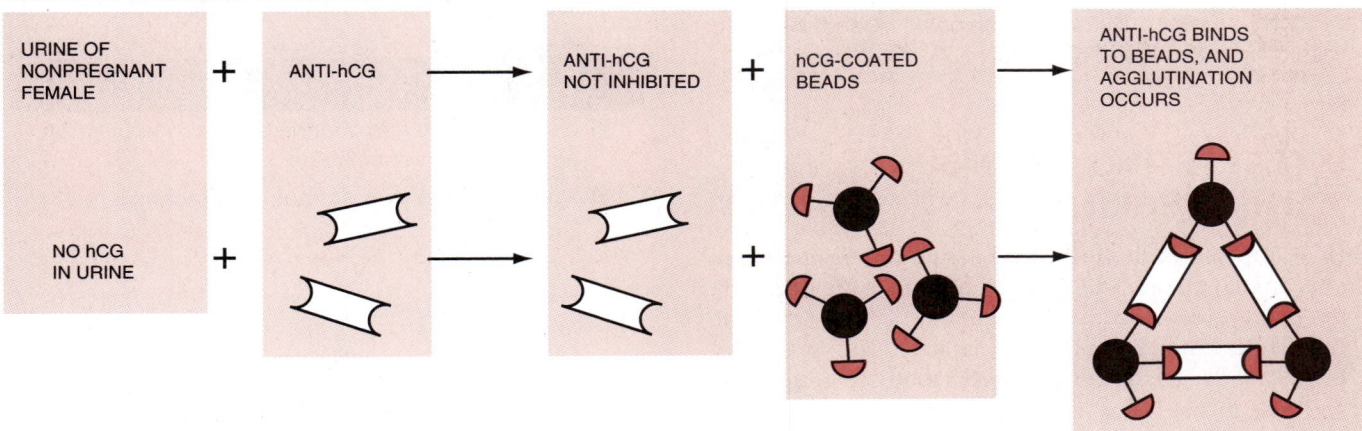

## NEGATIVE PREGNANCY TEST:

**FIGURE 5-37** Principle of agglutination inhibition test for hCG.

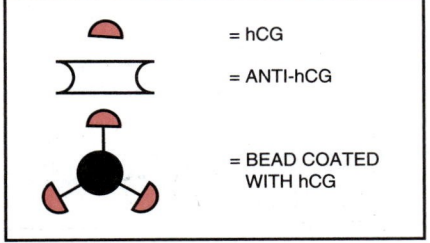

### ICON®II HCG Procedure

An example of a modified EIA for hCG is the ICON®II HCG. In this method, anti-hCG antibodies are immobilized in a membrane enclosed in a test cylinder. Urine is dispensed onto the membrane and any hCG in the urine binds to the antibody and becomes immobilized. A second anti-hCG antibody with enzyme attached is dispensed onto the membrane, incubated, and excess (unbound) antibody is washed away. A color developer is added and, after the appropriate time, the reaction is stopped. The test zone and reference zone are observed for blue color and the test is interpreted (Figure 5-38). The entire procedure requires only three minutes.

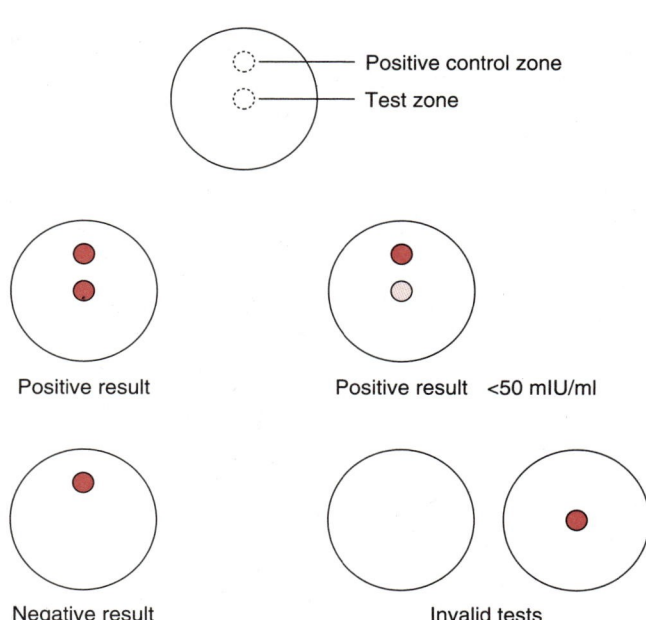

**FIGURE 5-38** Illustration of positive and negative results with ICON II® HCG test

## INTERPRETING PREGNANCY TESTS RESULTS

HCG appears in the urine and serum about one week after implantation. The level of hCG rises during early pregnancy, reaching levels greater than 100,000 mIU/mL (milli International Units per milliliter). The hCG level begins to decline about the third month of pregnancy, and disappears a few days after delivery. Many of the newer pregnancy tests are designed to detect hCG levels as low as 20 mIU/mL, and may be positive before a missed menstrual period.

Early in a pregnancy, urine hCG may be at undetectable levels, which may cause a false negative test result. Therefore, negative tests should be repeated after a few days to a week, if clinical symptoms still warrant. Patients with trophoblastic disease such as choriocarcinoma, or malignancies such as breast cancer or ovarian cancer, may have elevated hCG levels that cause false-positive pregnancy tests.

## USE OF PREGNANCY TESTS

Pregnancy tests are used when pregnancy is suspected and to rule out pregnancy before prescribing birth control pills, x-ray studies, chemotherapy, certain antibiotics or other drugs, and surgery. Quantitative pregnancy tests performed on serum are useful in diagnosing ectopic pregnancies, suspected spontaneous abortion, trophoblastic disease, and testicular tumors in males.

### Procedural Notes

- Keep urine specimens refrigerated and test within twenty-four hours.
- Store test kits at manufacturers' recommended temperatures.
- Do not use kits or controls after expiration date.
- Follow manufacturer's directions carefully for the kit being used.
- Use reagents only with the kit for which they were designed.
- Use appropriate control solutions to verify that test components are working properly.
- Interpret and report test results carefully.

### Safety Precautions

- Use Universal and Standard Precautions when handling urine specimens.
- Wipe up spills with surface disinfectant.

### LESSON REVIEW

1. What hormone is tested for in pregnancy tests?    *HCG*
2. What specimens are used for pregnancy tests?    *urine serum*
3. When will pregnancy tests be positive?    *no visible aggb*
4. List two principles of hCG tests. What is the minimum level of hCG detected by most test methods?
5. What may cause a false-positive test? What may cause a false-negative test?    *early pregnancy*
6. When does hCG first appear in pregnancy? When does it disappear?    *one week    3rd mth.*
7. What precautions must be observed in performing pregnancy tests?    *keep refrig.; use Univ. Stand. wipe up spills*
8. Define agglutination inhibition, EIA, and hCG.    *Enzyme Immunoassay = human chorionic Gonad*

### STUDENT ACTIVITIES

1. Reread the information on pregnancy tests.
2. Review the glossary terms.
3. Practice performing a pregnancy test as outlined in the Student Performance Guide.

# Student Performance Guide

## LESSON 5-6 Urine Pregnancy Tests

Name _____ Date _____

## ☣ INSTRUCTIONS

1. Practice performing an immunological test for pregnancy following the step-by-step procedure.
2. Demonstrate your understanding of this lesson by:
   a. Completing a written examination successfully, and
   b. Performing the pregnancy test procedure satisfactorily for the instructor. All steps must be completed as listed on the instructor's Performance Check Sheet.

*Note:* The procedures given are general. Always consult and follow the manufacturer's instructions for the kit being used.

## MATERIALS AND EQUIPMENT

■ gloves
■ hand disinfectant
■ urine specimen
■ stopwatch
■ surface disinfectant (10% chlorine bleach solution)
■ biohazard container
■ hCG negative urine control
■ hCG positive urine control
■ pregnancy test kit—EIA or slide test: pregnancy test kits should include slide or test unit, dispensers, reagents, etc.

## PROCEDURE

Record in the comment section any problems encountered while practicing the procedure (or have a fellow student or the instructor evaluate your performance).

S = Satisfactory
U = Unsatisfactory

| You must: | S | U | Comments |
|---|---|---|---|
| 1. Wash hands and put on gloves | | | |
| 2. Perform a modified EIA for hCG, following the manufacturer's instructions<br>a. Obtain test kit materials, reagents, and urine specimen<br>b. Apply urine to the test unit using the dispenser provided<br>c. Wait appropriate time interval (use stopwatch to time test)<br>d. Apply first reagent/antibody to test unit using dispenser provided<br>e. Rinse unreacted reagent from unit after appropriate time<br>f. Apply color reagent/substrate to test unit<br>g. Observe color development after appropriate time interval<br>h. Stop reaction<br>i. Record results. Always consult manufacturer's package insert to interpret test results<br>j. Repeat steps 2a–i using both positive and negative urine controls | | | |

| You must: | S | U | Comments |
|---|---|---|---|
| 3. Perform an agglutination inhibition test for hCG, following the manufacturer's instructions (if test is not available, go to step 4)<br>  a. Obtain slide test kit, reagents, and urine specimen<br>  b. Place one drop of antiserum in the center of the circled area of slide<br>  c. Dispense one drop of urine beside the drop of antiserum<br>  d. Mix urine and antiserum with stirrer provided<br>  e. Rock the slide in a figure-eight motion for the appropriate time, usually one to two minutes (use stopwatch to measure time)<br>  f. Apply one drop of well-mixed indicator particles to mixture on slide<br>  g. Mix indicator particles with antiserum-urine mixture and spread the mixture over the entire circled area of the slide using a stirrer<br>  h. Rock slide slowly in a figure-eight motion for the appropriate time (usually one to two minutes)<br>  i. Observe slide for agglutination at the end of the time interval and record the results (no agglutination = positive; agglutination = negative)<br>  j. Repeat steps 3a–3i using positive and negative urine controls | | | |
| 4. Disinfect reusable equipment by soaking in 10% chlorine bleach solution a minimum of ten minutes. Wash and rinse thoroughly | | | |
| 5. Discard disposable supplies in biohazard container | | | |
| 6. Dispose of specimen as instructed | | | |
| 7. Clean work area with surface disinfectant | | | |
| 8. Remove gloves and discard in biohazard container | | | |
| 9. Wash hands with hand disinfectant | | | |

*Evaluator Comments:*

Evaluator _____  Date _____

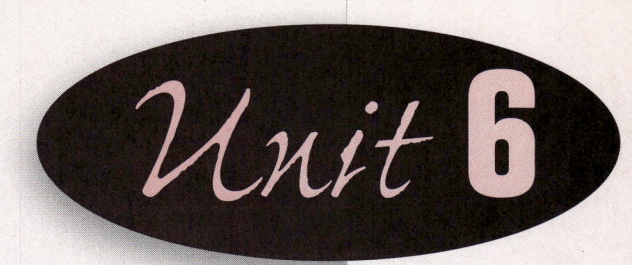

# *Basic Clinical Chemistry*

Unit 6

**After studying this unit, you should be able to:**
- *Discuss the importance of clinical chemistry.*
- *Identify fifteen clinical chemistry tests frequently performed and explain the significance of each.*
- *Explain the importance of properly collecting and handling specimens for clinical chemistry.*
- *Describe the principles of selected chemistry analyzers designed for use in smaller laboratories.*
- *Discuss the role of POCT in health care.*
- *Explain the principles of clinical chemistry tests for electrolytes.*
- *Explain the principles of clinical chemistry tests for cholesterol.*
- *Explain the principles of clinical chemistry tests for glucose.*

**UNIT** OVERVIEW

This unit is an introduction to some basic theories and principles of clinical chemistry. To understand the basis of the chemical tests discussed in this unit and the significance of test results, the student or health care worker must have a basic knowledge of human physiology. A short review of organ systems and functions may be appropriate before studying this unit.

Clinical chemistry is the branch of laboratory medicine that uses chemical analysis to study the level of various body constituents during health and disease. These chemical tests are usually performed on blood samples, but urine and other body fluids are also analyzed. The test results are used by the physician to diagnose disease, institute treatment, and follow the disease's progress. The physician may also use the results to counsel the patient in preventive medicine.

The study of body chemistry has a long history; as far back as Hippocrates, certain physicians emphasized chemical analysis in patient care. Early testing was performed on urine and feces because of the ease of collecting these specimens. These early tests were qualitative in nature in that they could only detect whether or not a constituent was present. As chemical analytical methods improved, it became possible to quantitate, or measure, how much of a substance was present. The results of analyses of some constituents performed by crude methods over 100 years ago compare very well with results obtained today using sophisticated methods.

The relationships between the values of certain components and the state of health or disease in the individual are examined in Lesson 6-1, which introduces clinical chemistry and in lessons dealing with specific tests, such as glucose, electrolytes, and cholesterol (Lessons 6-6, 6-7, and 6-8). Lesson 6-2 presents general information on specimen collecting and processing for clinical chemistry tests. Basic laboratory calculations and reagent preparation are discussed in Lesson 6-3.

The increase in testing in physician office laboratories (POLs) has resulted largely from the development of smaller, more diverse, affordable instruments that can perform a variety of tests. Lesson 6-4 presents the basic theory and operation of a few of these instruments. Lesson 6-5 discusses POCT, sometimes called bedside or near-patient testing. Since blood glucose (sugar) is one of the most frequently requested chemistry tests, Lesson 6-6 presents information about glucose metabolism and methods of glucose analysis. (Lesson 1-7, Quality Assurance in the Laboratory, should be reviewed before beginning this unit.)

The inclusion of specific instruments and methods in this unit does not imply endorsement by the authors. These instruments and methods were selected for inclusion because of the basic principles illustrated.

## SUGGESTED READINGS AND REFERENCES

Addison, L. A. & Fischer, P. M. (2nd ed.). (1990). *The office laboratory*. East Norwalk, CT: Appleton & Lange.

Baker, F. J., Silverton, R. E., & Pallister, C. J., Eds. (7th ed.). (1998). *Baker & Silverston's introduction to medical laboratory technology*. London: : Butterworth & Co., Ltd.

"Clinical Laboratory Improvement Act of 1988," *Federal Register*, vol. 7, no. 40, February 28, 1992.

Fischbach, F. T. (5th ed.). (1995). *A manual of laboratory diagnostic tests*. Philadelphia: Lippincott-Raven.

Henry, J. B., (Ed.). (19th ed.). (1996). *Clinical diagnosis & management by laboratory methods*. Philadelphia: W. B. Saunders Company.

Howanitz, J. H., & Howanitz, P. J. (Eds.) (1991). *Laboratory medicine—test selection and interpretation*. New York: Churchill Livingstone, Inc.

Kaplan, A., et al. (4th ed.). (1994). *Clinical chemistry: Interpretation and techniques*. Philadelphia: Williams & Wilkins.

Kovanda, B. M. (1998). *Point of care testing—capillary puncture*. Albany, NY: Delmar Publishers, Inc.

Ravel, R. (6th ed.). (1994). *Clinical laboratory medicine: Clinical application of laboratory data*. Chicago: Mosby Year Book.

Sacher, R. A., & McPherson, R. A. (11th ed.) (1999). *Widmann's clinical interpretation of laboratory tests*. Philadelphia: F. A. Davis Company.

Sigma Technical Bulletin, Procedure No. 352, *Sigma Diagnostics*, 1991.

Stewart, C. E., & Koepke, J. A. (1987). *Basic quality assurance practices for clinical laboratories*. Philadelphia: J. B. Lippincott Company.

Thomas, C. L., (Ed.). (16th ed.). (1989). *Taber's cyclopedic medical dictionary*. Philadelphia: F. A. Davis Company.

Tietz, N. W. (3rd ed.). (1987). *Fundamentals of clinical chemistry*. Philadelphia: W. B. Saunders Company.

Tietz, N. W. (1986). *Textbook of clinical chemistry*. Philadelphia: W. B. Saunders Company.

Tilton, R. C., et. al. (Eds.). (1992). *Clinical laboratory medicine*. St. Louis: Mosby-Yearbook.

Zilva, J. F., et al. (5th ed.). (1988). *Clinical chemistry in diagnosis and treatment*. London: Year Book Medical Publishers.

# Introduction to Clinical Chemistry

## LESSON OBJECTIVES

**After studying this lesson, you should be able to:**

- *List six body fluids tested in clinical chemistry.*
- *List fifteen constituents commonly assayed in a chemistry profile.*
- *Explain the significance or function of each of the constituents commonly included in a chemistry profile.*
- *List the normal or reference values for each of the constituents usually measured in a chemistry profile.*
- *Define the glossary terms.*

## GLOSSARY

**alanine aminotransferase (ALT)** / enzyme present in high concentration in liver and that is measured to assess liver function; SGPT

**albumins** / a homogeneous group of serum proteins made in the liver that help maintain osmotic balance

**alkaline phosphatase (ALP** or **AP)** / enzyme widely distributed in the body, especially in the liver and bone

**aspartate aminotransferase (AST)** / enzyme present in many tissues, including cardiac, muscle, and liver, that is measured to assess liver function; SGOT

**bilirubin** / product formed in the liver from the breakdown of hemoglobin

**BUN** / blood urea nitrogen; a test measuring urea in blood

**creatine kinase (CK)** / enzyme present in large amounts in brain tissue and heart and skeletal muscle that is measured to aid in diagnosing heart attack

**creatinine** / a breakdown product of creatine that is normally excreted in the urine

**electrolytes** / the cations and anions important in maintaining fluid and acid-base balance

**gamma glutamyl transferase (GGT)** / enzyme present in liver, kidney, pancreas, and prostate, that is measured to assess liver function

**globulins** / heterogeneous group of serum proteins with varied functions

**gout** / painful condition in which blood uric acid is elevated and urates precipitate in joints

**homeostasis** / tendency toward steady state or equilibrium of body processes

**hypercalcemia** / above-normal blood calcium levels

**hyperlipidemia** / excessive amount of fat in the blood

**hyperthyroidism** / excessive functional activity of the thyroid gland; excessive secretion of thyroid hormones

**hypoalbuminemia** / marked decrease in serum albumin concentration

**hypocalcemia** / below-normal blood calcium levels

**hypothyroidism** / thyroid function deficiency

**lactate dehydrogenase (LD** or **LDH)** / enzyme widely distributed in the body that is measured to assess liver function

**lipemic** / having a cloudy appearance due to excess lipid content

**lipids** / any one of a group of fats or fat-like substances

**thyroxine** / thyroid hormone, commonly called $T_4$

**triglycerides** / major storage form of lipids

**triiodothyronine** / one of the thyroid hormones, commonly called $T_3$

**uric acid** / breakdown product of nucleic acids

# INTRODUCTION

In a healthy body, chemical constituents are in a delicate balance, or equilibrium, and are influenced by both internal and external factors. This equilibrium or steady state is referred to as **homeostasis**.

Changes in concentration of a chemical constituent will usually trigger a reaction to bring concentration back to the equilibrium state. For example, when blood glucose levels rise after a meal, the pancreas releases insulin to bring the blood glucose concentration down to normal levels.

In the clinical chemistry laboratory, tests are performed on blood and other body fluids. These fluids are analyzed for the presence or absence of certain substances or for the level or amount of the substances. The tests may be for normal substances that have a biological function, nonfunctional metabolites or waste products, substances that indicate cell damage or disease, or drugs or toxic substances. The test results are then compared with normal, or reference, values, those found in a healthy body.

Physicians use the results of clinical chemistry tests to aid the diagnosing, treating, and preventing of disease. Interpretation of test results is based on understanding the physiological and biochemical processes occurring in health and in disease.

Test results must be reliable so the physician can have confidence in basing his or her diagnosis or treatment on test findings. Reliability is assured when specimens are collected, handled, and stored properly until tests can be performed; when specimens are analyzed using correct procedures and appropriate quality control measures; and when results are calculated and reported properly.

This lesson contains information about some routine clinical chemistry tests and the expected (reference) values of some commonly measured constituents.

# COMMONLY PERFORMED CLINICAL CHEMISTRY TESTS

Chemistry tests can be grouped into two basic categories—routine tests (tests that are frequently ordered) and special tests. Routine tests, such as glucose or creatinine, are useful in giving an overall view of the state of health, especially when used in combination with other tests. Because they can be performed quickly and in batches, their costs can be kept low.

Special chemistry tests, such as those measuring drug or hormone levels, are usually requested when a particular diagnosis is suspected or treatment must be monitored. These tests are usually more expensive, take longer to perform, and require special instruments or techniques.

## Chemistry Profiles

Most laboratories have a chemistry analyzer capable of performing chemistry profiles. A chemistry profile is a group of tests performed simultaneously on a patient specimen. The profile comprises a combination of tests designed to assess the patient's general condition. (An example of a laboratory requisition form for chemistry profiles is shown in Figure 6-1.) Tests usually included in a routine chemistry profile reflect the state of carbohydrate and lipid metabolism, and kidney, thyroid, liver, and cardiac function.

Clinical chemistry tests may also be grouped according to the biological system being studied. For example, laboratories may offer a liver profile, a group of tests designed to enable the physician to assess liver function, or a cardiac profile, a group of tests that aid in determining whether or not heart disease is present (Figure 6-1).

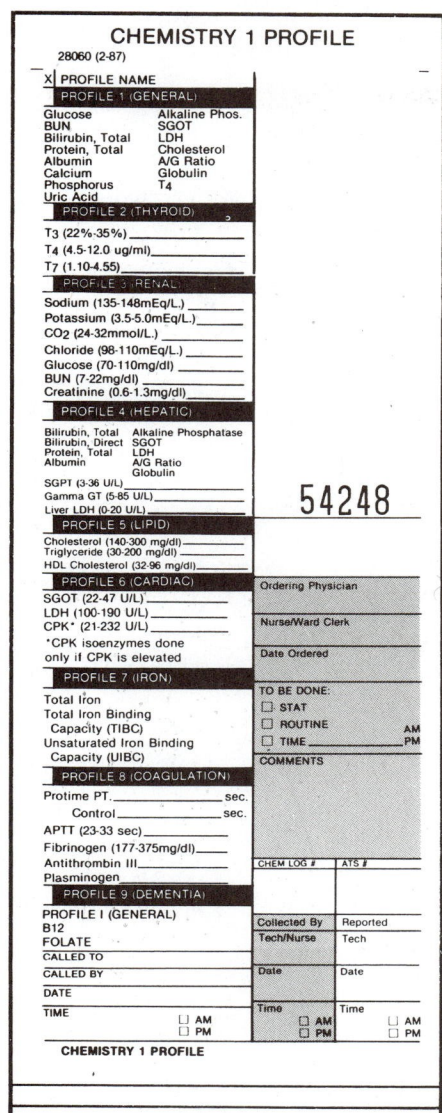

**CHEMISTRY 1 PROFILE**
28060 (2-87)

X PROFILE NAME
PROFILE 1 (GENERAL)

| | |
|---|---|
| Glucose | Alkaline Phos. |
| BUN | SGOT |
| Bilirubin, Total | LDH |
| Protein, Total | Cholesterol |
| Albumin | A/G Ratio |
| Calcium | Globulin |
| Phosphorus | T4 |
| Uric Acid | |

PROFILE 2 (THYROID)

T3 (22%-35%)
T4 (4.5-12.0 ug/ml)
T7 (1.10-4.55)

PROFILE 3 (RENAL)

Sodium (135-148mEq/L.)
Potassium (3.5-5.0mEq/L.)
CO2 (24-32mmol/L.)
Chloride (98-110mEq/L.)
Glucose (70-110mg/dl)
BUN (7-22mg/dl)
Creatinine (0.6-1.3mg/dl)

PROFILE 4 (HEPATIC)

| | |
|---|---|
| Bilirubin, Total | Alkaline Phosphatase |
| Bilirubin, Direct | SGOT |
| Protein, Total | LDH |
| Albumin | A/G Ratio |
| | Globulin |

SGPT (3-36 U/L)
Gamma GT (5-85 U/L)          **54248**
Liver LDH (0-20 U/L)

PROFILE 5 (LIPID)

Cholesterol (140-300 mg/dl)
Triglyceride (30-200 mg/dl)
HDL Cholesterol (32-96 mg/dl)

PROFILE 6 (CARDIAC)     Ordering Physician

SGOT (22-47 U/L)
LDH (100-190 U/L)       Nurse/Ward Clerk
CPK* (21-232 U/L)
*CPK isoenzymes done    Date Ordered
only if CPK is elevated

PROFILE 7 (IRON)     TO BE DONE:

Total Iron                  ☐ STAT
Total Iron Binding          ☐ ROUTINE      AM
  Capacity (TIBC)           ☐ TIME_____   PM
Unsaturated Iron Binding    COMMENTS
  Capacity (UIBC)

PROFILE 8 (COAGULATION)

Protime PT._____ sec.
      Control_____ sec.
APTT (23-33 sec)
Fibrinogen (177-375mg/dl)
Antithrombin III          CHEM LOG #    ATS #
Plasminogen

PROFILE 9 (DEMENTIA)

PROFILE I (GENERAL)
B12                    Collected By   Reported
FOLATE                 Tech/Nurse     Tech
CALLED TO
CALLED BY              Date           Date
DATE
TIME        ☐ AM      Time   ☐ AM    ☐ AM
            ☐ PM             ☐ PM    ☐ PM

**CHEMISTRY 1 PROFILE**

**FIGURE 6-1** One example of a laboratory requisition form for chemistry profiles

Analyzers used for chemistry profiles usually are capable of processing many patient samples per hour. This lesson lists some components commonly included in chemistry profiles, gives the normal or reference value for each component, and includes a brief description of the rationale for performing the test.

## Types of Specimens for Chemical Analysis

Fluids that may be submitted for chemical testing include blood and urine, and, less commonly, cerebro-spinal fluid (CSF), synovial, pleural, or pericardial fluids. Lesson 6-2 explains the proper methods of collecting and handling blood for routine chemical analysis. (Routine collection, handling, and chemical testing of urine is covered in Lessons 5-2 and 5-4. )

Fluids such as synovial, pericardial, or CSF are collected by the physician. The laboratory worker must always handle and store these specimens properly, as dictated by the tests to be performed.

Specimens for most chemistry tests require only routine handling, but some require special attention. It is important to know what tests will be performed on a specimen before collection so the specimen will be collected and processed appropriately.

## Units of Measure

Clinical chemistry test results are usually reported in metric units or SI units (International System of Nomenclature). Commonly used units are milligrams or micrograms per deciliter or per 100 mL (mg/dL or μg/dL), millimoles per liter (mmol/L), or, in the case of enzymes, enzyme activity units per liter (U/L).

## Reference (Normal) Values

The normal or reference value of a substance is determined by measuring the level of the substance in a portion of the general population. For instance, when establishing the reference range for a glucose test, a hospital may test 100 random samples from the nearby population and calculate the range of values. This range will be used for comparison to patient samples. (See Lesson 1-7 for a more complete explanation of quality control and reference ranges.)

The expected ranges of many substances differ according to the age or gender of the patient, the time of day, elapsed time after a meal, or drugs or medications a person may be taking. Reference ranges may also differ slightly for different methods of analysis and the population sample's geographical area. The reference values given in this lesson are those for an adult male using commonly accepted testing methodologies. Reference values for common chemical tests may be found in Table 6-1 and Appendix E.

## SUBSTANCES COMMONLY TESTED IN A CHEMISTRY PROFILE

### Protein

*Proteins* are essential components of cells and body fluids. They are formed from chains of amino acids; some

**Table 6-1.** Table of clinical chemistry reference values

| SUBSTANCE MEASURED | CONVENTIONAL UNITS | SI UNITS |
|---|---|---|
| Alanine aminotransferase (ALT) | 3–30 U/L | |
| Albumin | 3.8–5.0 g/dL | 38–50 g/L |
| Alkaline phosphatase (AP) | 20–130 U/L | |
| Aspartate aminotransferase (AST) | 6–33 U/L | |
| Bicarbonate ($HCO_3$) | 22–28 mEq/L | 22–28 mmol/L |
| Bilirubin (Total) | 0.1–1.2 mg/dL | 2–21 µmol/L |
| BUN | 8–18 mg/dL | 2.9–6.4 mmol/L |
| Calcium | 8.7–10.5 mg/dL | 2.18–2.63 mmol/L |
| Chloride | 98–108 mEq/L | 98–108 mmol/L |
| Cholesterol | 140–250 mg/dL (desirable level <200 mg/dL) | |
| Creatine kinase (CK) | 30–170 U/L | |
| Creatinine | 0.7–1.4 mg/dL | 62–125 µmol/L |
| Gamma glutamyl transferase (GGT) | 3–40 U/L | |
| Glucose | 70–110 mg/dL | 3.9–6.2 mmol/L |
| Iron | 65–165 µg/dL | 11.6–29.5 µmol/L |
| Lactate dehydrogenase (LD) | 125–290 U/L | |
| Phosphorus | 3.0–4.5 mg/dL | 0.96–1.44 mmol/L |
| Potassium | 3.5–5.4 mEq/L | 3.5–5.4 mmol/L |
| Sodium | 135–148 mEq/L | 135–148 mmol/L |
| $T_3$ | 60–160 ng/dL | 0.92–2.46 nmol/L |
| $T_4$ | 5.5–12.5 µg/dL | 72–163 nmol/L |
| Total protein | 6.0–8.0 g/dL | 60–80 g/L |
| Triglycerides | 10–190 mg/dL | 0.11–2.15 mmol/L |
| Uric acid | 3.5–7.5 mg/dL | 0.21–0.44 mmol/L |

amino acids are made by the body, while others must be provided by dietary protein.

Two major groups of serum proteins are the **albumins** and the **globulins**. Albumins comprise approximately 60% of total serum proteins, globulins about 40%.

The albumins are homogeneous in structure. They serve as transport proteins and help maintain fluid balance in the body.

The globulins are a heterogeneous group of molecules. Antibodies, blood coagulation proteins, enzymes, and proteins that transport iron are all serum globulins.

## Total Serum Protein

The total serum protein concentration is normally 6.0–8.0 g/dL, and represents the sum of many different proteins. Total protein values can provide information about the state of hydration, nutrition, and liver function, as most serum proteins are made in the liver. Protein is most commonly measured in serum, but it can also be measured in urine or CSF, where the concentration is normally low. Total serum protein may be measured chemically or using a refractometer.

## Albumin

The reference range for serum albumin is 3.8-5.0 g/dL. Albumin is synthesized in the liver. Decreased levels of albumin, or **hypoalbuminemia**, may occur in liver disease, starvation, impaired amino acid absorption, increased protein catabolism, and protein loss through the skin, kidneys, or gastrointestinal tract.

## A/G Ratio

Total serum protein and albumin are usually measured in a sample simultaneously and globulin is computed from the difference (total protein – albumin = globulin). A ratio of albumin to globulin (A/G ratio) may be computed and reported.

## Electrolytes

In clinical chemistry, the term electrolytes refers to the cations, *sodium* ($Na^+$) and *potassium* ($K^+$), and the anions, *chloride* ($Cl^-$) and *bicarbonate* ($HCO_3^-$). These four ions have a great effect on hydration, acid–base balance, and osmotic pressure, as well as pH and heart and muscle function. Electrolyte measurement is included in most routine chemistry profiles.

### Reference Ranges for Electrolytes

Sodium has the highest serum concentration of the electrolytes. The reference range for serum sodium is 135–148 mmol/L (mEq/L). The reference range for serum potassium is 3.5–5.4 mmol/L (mEq/L). Chloride is the anion with the highest serum concentration; the reference range for serum chloride is 98–108 mmol/L (mEq/L). The serum bicarbonate reference range is 22–28 mmol/L (mEq/L).

## Mineral Metabolism

Minerals are necessary for good health. Calcium, phosphorus (phosphate), and iron are examples of minerals often measured in chemistry profiles. Calcium and phosphorus are necessary for proper bone and tooth formation. Calcium is also required for blood coagulation. Iron is essential for hemoglobin production and is an integral component of some enzymes.

### Calcium

The reference range for serum calcium is 8.7–10.5 mg/dL (2.18–2.63 mmol/L). Of all the minerals in the body, calcium is present in the highest concentration. Approximately 99% of the body's calcium is in the skeleton bound in calcium complexes and is not metabolically active. Only unbound calcium ions are metabolically active.

Calcium is required for proper blood coagulation and for normal neuromuscular excitability. The calcium balance is influenced by vitamin $D_3$, parathyroid hormone, estrogen, and calcitonin. These hormones control dietary absorption of calcium, calcium excretion by the kidneys, and calcium movement in and out of bone.

**Hypercalcemia**, an increased level of calcium, occurs in parathyroidism, bone malignancies, hormone disorders, excessive vitamin $D_3$, and acidosis. It may cause deposits of calcium in soft organs, leading to complications such as kidney stones.

Decreased levels of calcium, or **hypocalcemia**, may be life-threatening and should be reported to the physician immediately. Extremely low levels may bring on increased muscle contraction, leading to tetany. Low calcium levels may be due to hypoparathyroidism, vitamin $D_3$ deficiency, poor absorption due to intestinal disease, and kidney disease.

### Phosphorus

The reference range for serum phosphorus is 3.0–4.5 mg/dL (0.96–1.44 mmol/L). Most phosphorus in the body is in the form of inorganic phosphate. Approximately 80% is in bone and the rest is mostly in high-energy compounds such as adenosine triphosphate (ATP). Phosphorus levels are influenced by calcium and certain hormones. Children have higher phosphorus levels than adults because they have higher levels of growth hormone.

### Iron

Serum iron is normally 65–165 µg/dL (11.6–29.5 µmol/L). Iron is essential for hemoglobin synthesis and synthesis of heme proteins. Iron is absorbed from dietary sources and is highly conserved by the body. In blood, iron is transported by *transferrin*, a serum protein. Iron levels differ with age, gender, and time of day, being higher in the A.M. than in the P.M.

Iron deficiency may lead to anemia. The deficiency may be due to insufficient iron in the diet, poor iron absorption, impaired release of stored iron, or increased iron loss due to bleeding. Serum iron levels may be elevated with hemolytic anemias, increased iron intake, or blocked synthesis of iron-containing compounds, such as occurs in lead poisoning.

## Kidney Function

Proper kidney function is necessary for water and electrolyte balance. The kidneys eliminate waste products, help maintain water and pH balance, and produce certain hormones. Substances are excreted into and reabsorbed from urine to help maintain homeostasis. The serum and plasma concentrations of some substances such as creatinine, BUN, and uric acid are altered in certain kidney diseases.

### Creatinine

The reference range for serum creatinine is 0.7–1.4 mg/dL (62–125 µmol/L). **Creatinine** is a waste product of creatine phosphate, a substance stored in muscle and used for energy. Creatinine is excreted by the kidney. When renal function is impaired, blood creatinine levels rise, but more than 50% of kidney function must be lost before this happens.

Creatinine levels are not affected by diet or hormone levels. Increases occur when there is impairment of urine formation or excretion, which occurs in renal disease, shock, water imbalance, or ureter blockage.

## BUN

The reference range for serum BUN is 8–18 mg/dL (2.9–6.4 mmol/L). In mammals, surplus amino acids are converted to urea and excreted by the kidneys. This surplus is measured as BUN, or blood urea nitrogen.

The BUN concentration is influenced by the amount of protein degraded, diet, hormones, and kidney function. Therefore, BUN level is not as good an indicator of kidney disease as is the creatinine level.

BUN levels may be low during starvation, pregnancy, and a low-protein diet. Increased BUN concentration may occur during a high-protein diet, after administration of steroids, and in kidney disease.

## Uric Acid

The reference range for serum uric acid is 3.5–7.5 mg/dL (0.21–0.44 mmol/L). Uric acid is formed from the breakdown of nucleic acids and is excreted by the kidneys. It has low solubility and tends to precipitate as uric acid crystals, or urates.

In kidney disease, uric acid concentration changes mirror changes in BUN and creatinine. However, uric acid measurement is principally used to diagnose and treat gout, a disease in which uric acid precipitates in tissues and joints, causing pain. Uric acid levels may also increase after massive radiation or chemotherapy because of increased cell destruction.

## Liver Function

The liver is both a secretory and excretory organ with numerous metabolic functions. The liver functions in carbohydrate metabolism, synthesizing glycogen from glucose. Almost all plasma proteins are made in the liver, including albumin, lipoproteins, blood coagulation proteins such as fibrinogen, and transport proteins. The liver is also important in lipid metabolism. In the liver, cholesterol is formed and degraded into bile acids, which emulsify fats so they can be absorbed.

The liver is a storage site for iron, glycogen, vitamins, and other substances. Other functions include destruction of old cells by phagocytosis and the detoxification of many substances.

Significant liver function must be lost or impaired before some laboratory tests show abnormality. Numerous tests are used to estimate liver function. Most are not specific for a particular disease, but only reflect liver tissue damage.

## Total Bilirubin

The reference range for serum bilirubin is 0.1–1.2 mg/dL (2.0–21.0 µmol/L). Bilirubin, a waste product from the breakdown of hemoglobin, is formed in the liver and excreted in the bile. As serum bilirubin levels are normally low, only increases in serum bilirubin are significant. Bilirubin concentration may be increased when there is excessive destruction of hemoglobin, such as in hemolytic anemias, impaired bilirubin processing, as in hepatitis, or impaired excretion by the liver, as in biliary obstruction. Bilirubin measurements are most helpful for diagnosis when both total and direct bilirubin are measured.

## Liver Enzymes

A rise in enzymes generally reflects injury to tissue, since most enzymes are intracellular. Some enzymes are widely distributed in many body tissues, whereas others are found in only a few tissues. The measurement of enzyme levels is not always specific for damage to a particular organ, but is most helpful when used with other tests, clinical symptoms, and patient history.

Enzymes used to assess liver function include alkaline phosphatase, lactate dehydrogenase, gamma glutamyl transferase, and the aminotransferases alanine aminotransferase and aspartate aminotransferase.

***Alkaline Phosphatase.*** Alkaline phosphatase (ALP or AP) is widely distributed in the body, especially in bone and the liver ducts. Serum AP levels may greatly increase with liver tumors and lesions, and may show a moderate increase with diseases such as hepatitis. Serum AP is normally 20–130 U/L.

***Aminotransferases.*** Liver tissue is rich in the aminotransferase enzymes. When liver cells are injured, these enzymes are released. Serum concentrations of these enzymes change with time, rising during acute liver disease and falling as recovery occurs. Generally, only one enzyme need be measured, as levels tend to mirror each other.

Alanine aminotransferase (ALT) was formerly called serum glutamic-pyruvic transaminase (GPT or SGPT). Levels are low in cardiac tissue and high in liver tissue. This enzyme usually rises higher than aspartate aminotransferase in liver disease, with moderate increases (up to 10 times normal) in cirrhosis, infections, or tumors, and increases up to 100 times normal in viral or toxic hepatitis. Serum concentration of ALT is normally 3–30 U/L.

Aspartate aminotransferase (AST) was formerly called serum glutamic oxaloacetic transaminase (GOT or SGOT). It is present in many tissues, particularly cardiac, muscle, and liver. It is elevated after myocardial infarction, as well as in liver disease. The serum concentration of AST normally is 6–33 U/L.

***Gamma Glutamyl Transferase.***   Serum GGT is normally 3-40 U/L. Gamma glutamyl transferase (GGT) is found in kidney, pancreas, liver, and prostate tissue.

GGT may be more helpful than AP in determining liver damage because GGT remains normal in bone disease, and is better than AST because it remains normal in muscle disorders. GGT measurement is often used to monitor recovery from hepatitis.

***Lactate Dehydrogenase.*** Serum LD is normally 125–290 U/L. **Lactate dehydrogenase (LD** or **LDH)** is widely distributed in tissue. The LD level increases in blood during liver disease and following myocardial infarction. Hemolysis of a blood sample will cause increased LD levels in the serum because of LD release from RBCs.

## Cardiac Function

The reference range for serum creatine kinase is 30–170 U/L. **Creatine kinase (CK)** is an enzyme measured to help diagnose myocardial infarction. CK is present in large amounts in muscle and the brain, but in small amounts in organs such as the liver and kidneys. Following heart attack, CK is released from the damaged heart muscle. The serum CK level peaks in about twenty-four hours, reaching five to eight times the upper limit of normal. It falls rapidly back to normal levels within three to four days. Serum CK levels also increase following skeletal muscle damage and brain injury.

## Lipid Metabolism

**Lipids** are synthesized in the body from dietary fats and oils that are broken down and reassembled. The most commonly measured lipids are cholesterol and triglycerides. These are of interest primarily because of their association with cardiovascular disease (CVD).

### Cholesterol

Cholesterol is present in all tissues, and serum concentrations tend to increase with age. Elevated cholesterol levels may increase the risk of coronary artery disease. It is now generally recommended that serum cholesterol levels be maintained below 200 mg/dL (reference range is 140–250 mg/dL).

### Triglycerides

Serum triglyceride reference levels range from 10–190 mg/dL (0.11–2.15 mmol/L). **Triglycerides** are the main form of lipid storage in humans, comprising approximately 95% of fat (adipose) tissue. Triglycerides are transported in the plasma bound to lipoproteins, complexes composed of lipid and protein. The group of lipoproteins called chylomicrons carry most of the plas-

ma triglycerides. Increased blood levels of triglycerides cause the plasma to have a milky appearance. Blood to be tested for triglycerides should be collected when the patient has been fasting for twelve to fourteen hours, such as in the morning before breakfast. **Hyperlipidemia** is the condition of having high blood levels of triglycerides.

## Carbohydrate Metabolism

### Glucose

The reference range for serum glucose is 70–110 mg/dL (3.9–6.2 mmol/L). Glucose metabolism is largely regulated by insulin, which is produced by the pancreas. It is also influenced by other hormones such as growth hormone, glucagon, and cortisol. Glucose is a commonly tested blood constituent.

## Thyroid Function

The thyroid gland synthesizes hormones that stimulate metabolism by increasing protein synthesis and oxygen consumption by the tissues. Thyroid hormones are synthesized from iodide and the amino acid tyrosine. In the blood, more than 99% of thyroid hormones are bound to serum proteins and are metabolically inactive. Many laboratory procedures are available to measure thyroid function. Chemistry profiles often include tests for the thyroid hormones **thyroxine** ($T_4$) and **triiodothyronine** ($T_3$).

### Thyroid Hormones

The reference range for total $T_4$ is 5.5–12.5 µg/dL, with the range differing slightly depending on the assay method. Thyroid hormones are usually measured by immunoassay methods. Graves' disease is an example of a disease caused by **hyperthyroidism**, excessive secretion of thyroid hormones. **Hypothyroidism**, decreased thyroid function, causes a condition called myxedema.

## LESS COMMONLY ORDERED CLINICAL CHEMISTRY TESTS

Dozens of available tests have not been mentioned here. Many are special tests that measure insulin, growth hormone, adrenocorticotropic hormone (ACTH), or follicle-stimulating hormone (FSH). Others measures vitamins or trace minerals, isoenzymes, or metabolic products. Such tests may require special specimen collection as well as special instruments and expertise. A clinical chemistry text should be consulted for more information.

## LESSON REVIEW

1. What are the two most commonly tested body fluids?

2. List three enzymes useful in diagnosing liver disease.

3. Give the reference ranges for fifteen constituents included in a chemistry profile. Explain the significance of variations from reference range for each constituent.

4. Name three tests that may be useful in diagnosing kidney disease.

5. What enzyme is most useful in diagnosing heart attack?

6. Name the four electrolytes in serum.

7. What are the two major types of plasma protein? What are their functions?

8. Define alanine aminotransferase, albumins, alkaline phosphatase, aspartate aminotransferase, bilirubin, BUN, creatine kinase, creatinine, electrolytes, gamma glutamyl transferase, globulins, gout, homeostasis, hypercalcemia, hyperlipidemia, hyperthyroidism, hypoalbuminemia, hypo-calcemia, hypokalemia, hyponatremia, hypothyroidism, lactate dehydrogenase, lipemic, lipids, thyroxine, triglycerides, triiodothyronine, and uric acid.

## STUDENT ACTIVITIES

1. Reread the information on introduction to clinical chemistry.

2. Review the glossary terms.

3. Ask what tests are included in chemistry profiles in a nearby hospital or laboratory. Find out the laboratory's reference ranges and compare them to those in this lesson.

4. Find out what special chemistry tests are performed in a nearby hospital or other large laboratory.

# Specimen Collection and Processing for Clinical Chemistry

## LESSON OBJECTIVES

**After studying this lesson, you should be able to:**

- *List six body fluids tested in clinical chemistry.*
- *Explain the importance of obtaining a quality specimen for clinical chemistry testing.*
- *Name five problems in blood specimen collection and processing that might cause erroneous test results.*
- *Explain safety rules that must be followed during specimen collection, handling, and processing.*
- *Define the glossary terms.*

## GLOSSARY

**anticoagulant** / a chemical that prevents blood coagulation

**diurnal** / having a daily cycle

**lipemic** / having a cloudy appearance due to excess lipid content

**plasma** / liquid portion of blood in which blood cells are suspended; the straw-colored liquid remaining after blood cells are removed from anticoagulated blood

**serum** / liquid obtained from blood that has been allowed to clot

## INTRODUCTION

The clinical chemistry department performs tests on blood and other body fluids, such as urine, cerebrospinal fluid (CSF), and pleural, synovial, or pericardial fluid. Collecting blood specimens for testing in the central laboratory is usually the laboratory's responsibility. Blood collection may be performed by laboratory technicians or phlebotomists.

Many tests are performed in the clinical chemistry laboratory. Special attention must be paid to the type of specimen required for each test and to processing the specimen before testing. Laboratory analyses can only give useful results if they are performed on a specimen that has been properly collected and maintained in an appropriate environment until the test is performed. This lesson describes procedures for collecting and processing blood specimens for clinical chemistry. Lesson 5-2 describes collection procedures for urine specimens. Other body fluids are usually collected by the physician. A review of venipuncture are capillary blood-collection procedures may be helpful before studying this lesson.

## *Quality Assurance*

The quality of the specimen is of utmost importance. Specific instructions for the type and volume of specimen required, the collection procedure, and the processing method are included in every laboratory's procedure manual for each test performed in that laboratory (or for which they collect a specimen). Table 6-2 gives examples of the uses of the various specimen-collection tubes.

Before a specimen is collected, the patient must be identified. Specimens must be labeled immediately after collection while the phlebotomist is still in the patient's presence. The label should include the patient's name and identification number, the date and time, and the phlebotomist's initials. Many laboratories now use bar-coded labels generated at the same time the test is requisitioned (Figure 6-2). Analyzers read the bar-code when the tube is inserted in the instrument and code the patient's identification to the test result, reducing transcribing errors.

The laboratory procedure manual includes a list of specific criteria that must be met for a specimen to be accepted for testing. Table 6-3 lists some of these criteria. Tests requiring special collection procedures will have additional criteria for acceptability. Failure to meet these criteria will cause the specimen to be rejected, necessitating another one being collected, which can be traumatic for the patient and is time-consuming for the laboratory. Therefore, every effort must be made to ensure that all requirements are met before collecting the specimen.

**Table 6-2.** Color codes of vacuum-collection tubes and their uses

| COLOR OF STOPPER | ANTICOAGULANT OR ADDITIVE | USED FOR: |
|---|---|---|
| Red | None | Serum; blood chemistries |
| Red/gray | None | Serum (separator tube); blood chemistries |
| Lavender | EDTA | Whole blood; hematology tests, blood banking |
| Green | Heparin | Whole blood; special analyses |
| Light blue | Buffered citrate | Coagulation studies |
| Black | Buffered sodium citrate | Westergren ESR |
| Gray | Glycolytic inhibitor | Glucose determination |

## TYPES OF BLOOD SPECIMENS FOR CHEMICAL ANALYSIS

Blood required for chemical analysis may be capillary, venous, or sometimes, arterial (for blood gas measurements). Some instruments and methods can use whole blood, serum, or plasma for testing; other instruments or methods may require one particular type of specimen, such as heparinized plasma.

**Table 6-3.** Examples of some criteria that must be met for a specimen to be acceptable for testing

- Label must be complete (name, date, time of collection, person collecting) and attached in the proper place
- Blood specimens must be free of hemolysis
- Anticoagulated blood specimens must be free of clots
- Specimens must be delivered to the laboratory within the specified amount of time after collection
- Outer surfaces of specimen containers must have no visible contamination
- Specimens must be stored properly until the time of testing
- Blood specimens cannot be drawn from a site above an intravenous line
- Specimens collected in anticoagulant must have the proper blood: anticoagulant ratio

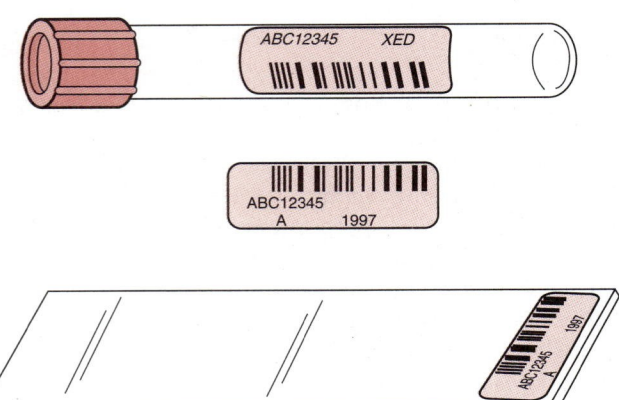

**FIGURE 6-2** Illustration of bar-coded specimen labels

## Serum, Plasma, and Whole Blood

Serum is the specimen used for most clinical chemistry tests. **Serum** is the fluid portion which remains after blood has been allowed to clot. It is obtained by collecting blood in a tube without anticoagulant, allowing the blood to clot, centrifuging the clotted sample, and removing the liquid (serum). Use of serum separator tubes containing a substance that forms a barrier between the serum and cells during centrifugation makes it easier to remove serum from the tube without disturbing the blood cells (Figure 6-3).

**Plasma** is obtained by removing the liquid portion of anticoagulated blood following centrifugation. When either plasma or serum are to be used for testing, the liquid must be removed from the blood's cellular portion as soon as possible after collection. This prevents the exchange of substances between the cellular and liquid portions, which could alter test results.

When whole blood is used, it may be capillary blood from a finger puncture or blood from a tube containing anticoagulant. Whole blood obtained by capillary puncture must be used immediately after collection. If testing is to be delayed, blood must be collected in an **anticoagulant**, such as heparin or EDTA, to prevent clotting. The tube of whole blood must be well mixed immediately before testing. (Detailed procedures for collecting blood by venipuncture and information on anticoagulants are given in Lesson 2-3.)

 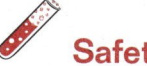 **Safety**

Accidental exposure to blood and body fluids is most likely to happen during collection and processing of specimens. Universal and Standard Precautions must be

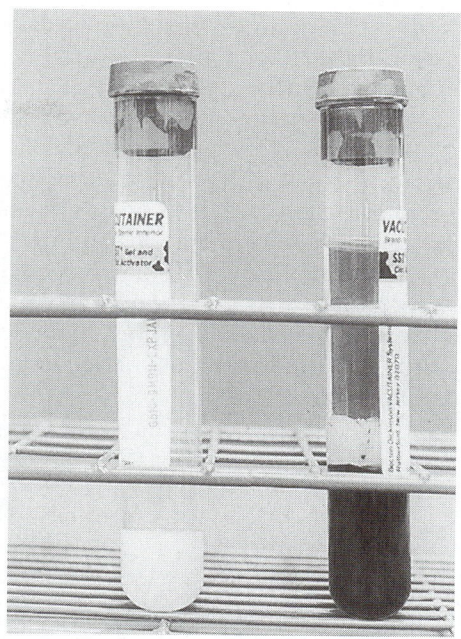

**FIGURE 6-3** Serum separator tubes

observed at all times. Appropriate PPE, including gloves, face protection, and a buttoned, fluid-resistant laboratory coat, should be worn. Frequent handwashing and changing of gloves are required.

Several safety collection devices are available, such as quick-release needles, needle-disposal containers, and needles that blunt on exit from the vein. Phlebotomy trays should be equipped with these devices (Figure 6-4) so that used needles can be immediately discarded.

Sometimes specimens must be collected from a patient who is suspected of being infectious. The phle-

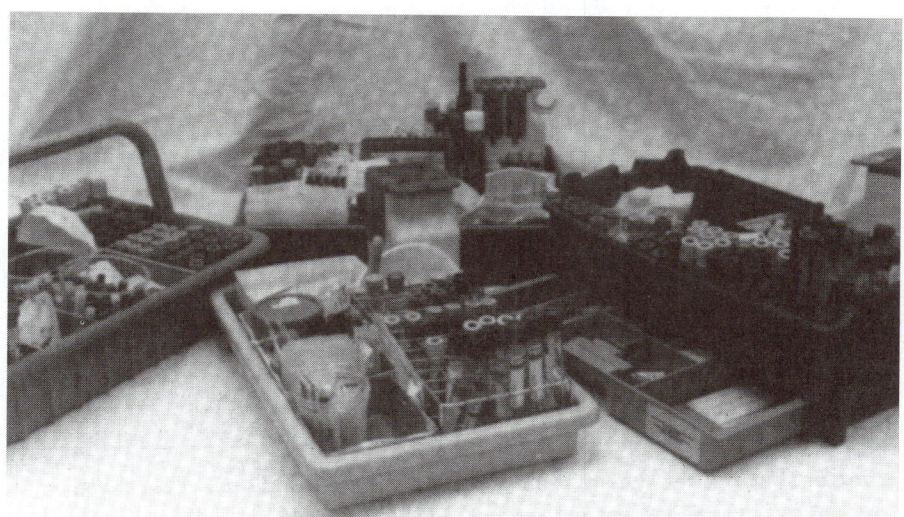

**FIGURE 6-4** Phlebotomy trays containing safety needles and disposal devices

botomist or technician must remain up-to-date on each Transmission-Based Precaution category. Lesson 7-2 discusses these in detail.

Uncapping vacuum tubes containing specimens presents the hazards of aerosol creation, splatters, and tube breakage. Several safety devices have been developed to eliminate these problems. Plastic vacuum tubes should be used whenever possible. Through-the-stopper samplers available on many analyzers and some sample-processing instruments prevent the aerosol potential created by uncapping tubes. Whenever possible, available safety devices must be incorporated into laboratory procedures.

# COLLECTING AND PROCESSING BLOOD SPECIMENS FOR CHEMICAL ANALYSIS

Collection procedures for capillary or venous blood should be followed as outlined in the laboratory's procedure manual. Strict attention must be paid to the specimen requirements for the test(s) ordered.

Special care must be used when collecting specimens from patients who are difficult to collect from, such as children and the elderly, to ensure that specimen qualitiy is not compromised. If a patient has an intravenous (IV) line, the specimen must be collected from a different arm or from a vessel below the IV insertion site.

## Effect of Specimen Collection Time on Chemical Constituents

Chemical constituent levels may be affected by meals, medication, or the time of day. Each laboratory test procedure contains specimen-collection and handling instructions that must be strictly adhered to.

Most blood constituents do not change significantly after eating, so blood used to test for these may be collected at any time. However, concentrations of constituents such as glucose, triglycerides, and cholesterol will change after eating, and specimens for these tests are usually collected when the patient is fasting, generally in the morning before breakfast.

Specimens collected from patients with lipid metabolism disorders or shortly after a patient has eaten may appear lipemic. Since **lipemic** serum or plasma is milky or cloudy, it may interfere with certain tests, particularly those that use colorimetry or spectrophotometry.

In some diseases, certain blood constituents follow patterns of increase or decrease that make the col-

lection time very important. For example, creatine kinase, an enzyme measured to detect heart attacks (myocardial infarctions), rises rapidly and falls back to normal levels in the three to four days following a heart attack. If this enzyme is not measured during this critical period, a heart attack may go undiagnosed.

**Diurnal** variation, changes with the time of day, can occur with certain blood constituents such as iron and corticosteroids. It is important, therefore, to note the collection time of specimens for these tests and to consider this when interpreting test results.

Some drug or medication blood levels will fluctuate depending on the dosage time. Some tests for therapeutic drug monitoring must be done at set intervals before or after administering medication.

## Specimen Transport

The specimen transport method is determined by the distance the specimen must travel and the type of transport systems available. POCT specimens require no transport, one of the benefits of bedside testing.

The phlebotomist or nursing staff may transport specimens to a nearby room or another floor or hospital wing for testing. Many hospitals have pneumatic tube systems for rapid transport of specimens to the central laboratory in special leak-proof, impact-resistant containers.

Sometimes couriers transport specimens to another laboratory, perhaps in a different city. Specimens may also be mailed to a reference laboratory for testing. Regardless of the transport methods used, specimens must be packaged in secure containers to protect carriers from contamination. They must also be transported in an environment that meets biosafety regulations and protects the quality of the specimen.

## Specimen Storage and Preservation

For most routine tests to be performed within one hour, the specimen may remain at room temperature until testing. However, if testing is to be delayed for a few hours, samples should be refrigerated at 4°C. Some tests involving certain enzymes require specimens to be frozen immediately after collection to prevent the loss of enzyme activity.

Most specimens may be stored in capped test or collection tubes until testing. However, certain specimens require special handling. For example, bilirubin is degraded by light, so specimens should be stored in a dark container.

## Problems Associated with Specimen Collection and Processing

Reliable test results can only be obtained if the technologist has a proper specimen to work with (Table 6-3). Improperly handled specimens may cause erroneous test results. Some problems to be avoided are:

### Hemolysis

Blood that is hemolyzed during collection (or processing) cannot be used for most analyses. The destroyed RBCs will release substances such as hemoglobin, enzymes (LD and AST), potassium (K) and other intracellular components into the serum, resulting in a sample that does not represent the patient's true status. Hemolysis may be caused by overcentrifugation, excessive turbulence of the sample (shaking, etc.), freezing of cells, forcing blood through the venipuncture needle, or poor venipuncture technique.

### Hemoconcentration

Hemoconcentration can occur if the tourniquet is left on too long (more than two minutes) during venipuncture. This causes blood stasis within the vein, resulting in some blood constituents being more concentrated than in properly flowing blood (Lesson 2-3).

### Overcentrifugation

Blood collected to obtain serum should remain undisturbed for twenty to thirty minutes, to allow clotting to occur. It is then centrifuged according to the laboratory procedure manual, usually for ten minutes at 1000 rpm. Serum should be separated from the cells as soon as possible. To obtain plasma, the anticoagulated specimen may be centrifuged immediately after collection. Serum and plasma must be removed from cells before freezing, since freezing will cause cell lysis.

### Evaporation

Specimens should remain capped until they are tested. Evaporation will occur in uncapped specimens, resulting in concentration of some constituents and gas escape or exchange, which may alter other values such as pH or bicarbonate ($HCO_3^-$) concentration.

### Microbial Contamination

Clean pipets or pipet tips should be used to transfer each sample. If reusable sample cups are used, they must be clean and dry to avoid contaminating or diluting the samples. Bacterial contamination of specimens must be avoided.

### Chemical Contamination

When multiple blood samples are obtained with a vacuum-collection system, the "order of draw" is important. Tubes for serum collection must be filled before those containing anticoagulant.

## SUMMARY

The first step in obtaining quality laboratory results is proper specimen collection. Specimen collection and processing must be done with care, with special attention paid to test requirements, the specimen quality, and safe practices.

## LESSON REVIEW

1. What are the most commonly tested body fluids?
2. Explain how to collect serum.
3. Explain how to collect plasma.
4. Explain the differences between serum and plasma.
5. What safety measures must be observed to avoid accidental needlesticks?
6. What PPE must be worn when collecting and processing specimens?
7. Name two types of tubes (stopper color) that can be used to collect serum.
8. How can the specimen collection time affect test results?
9. What can cause hemolysis of a specimen? How will test results be affected if hemolysis occurs?
10. Define anticoagulant, diurnal, lipemic, plasma, and serum.

## STUDENT ACTIVITIES

1. Reread the information on specimen collection and processing for clinical chemistry.
2. Review the glossary terms.
3. Visit a clinical laboratory and get information about the specimen-collection and processing section. Find out who is responsible for collecting, transporting, and processing specimens. Request permission to see the procedure manual that covers specimen collection.

# Laboratory Reagent Preparation and Calculations

## LESSON OBJECTIVES

**After studying this lesson, you should be able to:**

■ *Prepare laboratory solutions using proportion, ratios, and percentage.*
■ *State the formula for preparing a dilute solution from a concentrate.*
■ *Prepare a standard or control solution from a lyophilized sample.*
■ *Prepare serial dilutions.*
■ *Make conversions between the Fahrenheit and Celsius scales.*
■ *Define the glossary terms.*

## GLOSSARY

**Celsius scale** / temperature scale where the freezing point of water is 0° and the boiling point is 100°; indicated by "C"; also called centigrade

**Fahrenheit scale** / temperature scale where the freezing point of water is 32° and the boiling point is 212°; indicated by "F"

**gram-equivalent weight** / gram formula weight divided by the total positive charge (valence) of a molecule

**gram-formula weight** / weight in grams of the entity represented by a chemical formula

**lyophilize** / remove water from a frozen solution under vacuum; freeze-dry

**mole** / formula weight of a substance expressed in grams

**molar solution (M)** / solution containing one mole of solute per liter of solution

**normal solution (N)** / solution containing one gram-equivalent weight of a substance per liter of solution

**physiological saline** / 0.85% (0.15 M) sodium chloride solution

**proportion** / relationship in number or amount of one portion compared to another or to the whole

**ratio** / relationship in number or degree between two things

# INTRODUCTION

Although many laboratory reagents can be purchased in the required concentrations, sometimes reagents or solutions must be prepared in the laboratory. First though, it is important to understand some basic chemistry terms. The calculations involved are not difficult, but may require step-by-step clarification at first.

Math is also used to perform temperature conversions in the laboratory. Since the Celsius scale is used in laboratory work and the Fahrenheit scale is commonly used in the United States in everyday life, conversions between the scales are sometimes necessary.

# METHODS OF PREPARING LABORATORY SOLUTIONS

  **Safety**

Preparing laboratory reagents involves using chemicals and chemical solutions. Many chemicals are hazardous, presenting a danger to the technician because of their caustic or toxic properties. The chemical container label and MSDS information must be consulted before beginning any exercise. Appropriate PPE indicated must be used. Chemicals that produce fumes must be used only in a fume hood.

Pipet bulbs or automatic pipetters must be used to measure and dispense liquids. Mouth pipetting must *never* be done. When making serial dilutions of patient serum or reconstituting serum controls and standards, Universal and Standard Precautions must always be followed.

> ## *Quality Assurance*
>
> Many chemical solution preparations involve using pipets for measurement or transfer. Pipetting can create errors that affect results throughout several analyses. The correct pipet and tip must be used when using an automatic pipetter. Volume markings on beakers and Erlenmeyer flasks are only approximate; a volumetric flask must be used for accurate measuring or diluting.

# Common Reagents Prepared in the Laboratory

Several common laboratory solutions are easily prepared, such as the surface disinfectant, 10% chlorine bleach solution. **Physiological saline**, a 0.85% salt (sodium chloride) solution, is another. In addition, dilute acids are often prepared from concentrated acids.

Other solutions that may require laboratory preparation include controls and standards. These may be shipped as **lyophilized** reagents with all the liquid removed; they are rehydrated by adding either distilled water or a special diluting fluid provided by the manufacturer. Examples of lyophilized reagents include positive and negative controls for serology, and controls and standards for blood and urine chemistry tests. These must be rehydrated carefully, since the accuracy of patient results depends on them.

Whatever type of laboratory solution is being prepared, math is involved, either directly or indirectly. Solutions may be prepared by using proportion, ratios, or percentage. A solution's concentration may be indicated by its normality or molarity. Some serological procedures require serial dilutions.

## Using Proportion to Prepare Solutions

**Proportion** is used when reagents are prepared by adding a specific amount of one solution to a specific amount of another solution. An example is adding "two parts" (measures) of solution "A" to "three parts" of solution "B" to prepare the final reagent "C."

The formula to determine the volumes of "A" and "B" is:

$$\frac{C}{(A) + (B)} = V$$

where: C = Total volume of the final reagent
A = Total parts of solution A
B = Total parts of solution B
V = Volume of each part

An example of using proportion to prepare a reagent is shown in Figure 6-5.

Proportion can also be used to determine how much of a concentrate is required to prepare a dilute solution. A 0.1 N HCl solution can be made from a concentrated solution of HCl, such as a 1.0 N solution (Figure 6-6). The general formula is:

$$C_1 \times V_1 = C_2 \times V_2$$
$$\text{or}$$
$$V_1 = \frac{C_2 \times V_2}{C_1}$$

Where: $C_1$ = concentration of the solution of greater concentration
$V_1$ = volume required of the solution of greater concentration
$C_2$ = concentration of final (dilute) solution
$V_2$ = volume desired of final (dilute) solution

**Problem:** A buffer is made by adding 2 parts of "solution A" to 5 parts of "solution B." How much of solution A and solution B would be required to make 70 mL of the buffer?

**Formula:** $\dfrac{\text{Total volume required (C)}}{\text{parts of "A" + parts of "B"}} = \text{volume of one part (V)}$

**Solution:** $\dfrac{70\ \text{mL required}}{2\ \text{parts "A" + 5 parts "B"}} = \text{volume of one part}$

$\dfrac{70}{7} = 10\ \text{mL} = \text{volume of one part (V)}$

2 parts of solution "A" = $2 \times 10 = 20$ mL

5 parts of solution "B" = $5 \times 10 = 50$ mL

**Answer:** The buffer would be made by mixing 20 mL of solution A with 50 mL of solution B to give a total volume of 70 mL.

**FIGURE 6-5** Preparing a solution using proportion

**Problem:** Prepare 100 mL of 0.1 N HCl using 1.0 N HCl.

**Formula:** $C_1 \times V_1 = C_2 \times V_2$

**Solution:** $(1.0\ \text{N})\ (V_1) = (100\ \text{mL})\ (0.1\ \text{N})$

$V_1 = \dfrac{100\ \text{mL} \times 0.1}{10}$

$V_1 = 10\ \text{mL}$

**Answer:** 10 mL of 1.0 N HCl is added to 90 mL of $H_2O$ to make 100 mL of 0.1 N HCl solution.

**FIGURE 6-6** Using the formula $C_1 \times V_1 = C_2 \times V_2$ to prepare a solution

Solve for $V_1$, volume of concentrated solution needed to prepare the dilute solution

## Using Percentage to Prepare Solutions

### Weight/Volume (w/v) Percentage

The concentration of many laboratory solutions and reagents is expressed in percentage. Percentage solutions may be made by weighing out a specific amount of a solute (chemical) for each 100 mL of solvent (water or other liquid). This is called a *weight-to-volume (w/v) percentage*.

One example is the 0.85% physiological saline (NaCl) solution used for many serological and bacteriological procedures. One hundred milliliters of 0.85% saline is prepared by placing about 50 mL of distilled water into a 100 mL volumetric flask, adding 0.85 grams

NaCl, mixing, and then adding distilled water to the flask's fill line. Therefore, 100 mL of 0.85% saline solution contains 0.85 grams of NaCl. In a similar fashion, 500 mL of 0.85% saline could be prepared as shown in Figure 6-7.

### Volume/Volume (v/v) Percentage

Another type of percentage solution is called *volume-to-volume (v/v) percentage*, in which a certain volume of one liquid is added to a specific volume of another. One hundred milliliters of a 10% solution of bleach can be prepared by adding 10 mL of household bleach to 90 mL of water (Figure 6-8).

### Weight/Weight (w/w) Percentage

A percentage solution may also be prepared by weighing both the solute and the solvent. In this case, a 5% solution would require that five grams of a chemical be

---

**Problem:**    Prepare 500 mL of 0.85% saline.

**Solution:**    1. A 0.85% solution contains 0.85 g of the solute in every 100 mL of solution.
2. Therefore, to prepare 500 mL, 5 × 0.85 g, or 4.25 g, of sodium chloride (NaCl) must be used.
3. To prepare the solution:
   a. Weigh out 4.25 g of NaCl.
   b. Fill a 500 mL volumetric flask approximately half full with distilled water.
   c. Add 4.25 g of NaCl and swirl gently to dissolve.
   d. Add distilled water to the flask's fill line.

**FIGURE 6-7** Preparation of a weight-to-volume (w/v) percentage solution

---

**Problem:**    Prepare 500 mL of 10% bleach solution.

**Answer:**    1. A 10% solution of bleach contains 10 mL bleach (hypochlorite) per 100 mL of solution.
2. Therefore, 500 mL of solution would contain 50 mL of bleach (5 × 10 mL).
3. To prepare the solution:
   a. Place 450 mL of water into a flask or bottle.
   b. Add 50 mL of bleach.
   c. Carefully mix; label the container.

**FIGURE 6-8** Preparation of a volume-to-volume (v/v) percentage solution

---

added to about 90 mL of $H_2O$ and, with the flask on a balance, $H_2O$ added until the total weight is 100 grams. This type of percentage solution is rarely used.

## Using Ratios to Prepare Solutions

A **ratio** is the relationship in number or degree between two things. Dilutions, which are ratios, express the relationship between a part of a solution and the total solution. Dilutions are used frequently in the laboratory, especially in hematology and serology. One procedure for performing the WBC count requires that a 1-to-100 dilution of the blood sample be made to count the cells. This is accomplished by adding 0.02 mL of blood to 1.98 mL of diluent. The total volume is equal to 2.00 mL. The dilution factor of 100 is the relationship of 0.02 mL to the total volume of 2.00, expressed as a ratio of 1:100 (0.02:2.00) when expressed in whole numbers. It can also be called the 1:100 dilution.

## Preparing Normal and Molar Solutions

Chemical solution concentrations are usually expressed as normality (N) or molarity (M). A one **normal** (1 N) **solution** contains one **gram-equivalent weight** of the chemical (solute) per liter of solution. In aqueous solutions, the gram-equivalent weight is the formula weight in grams (**gram-formula weight**) divided by the total positive charge (valence) of the molecule. For example, NaOH has a formula weight of 39.99, which rounds off to 40. Sodium (Na) has 1+ charge (40/1 = 40). A 1 N solution contains 40 grams NaOH in one liter of water. The preparation of solutions using normality is illustrated in Figures 6-9 and 6-10.

Moles per liter (mol/L) is the term used to replace the older term, molarity (M). A **mole** of a pure compound is the formula weight of that compound expressed in grams. A solution containing one mole of a substance per liter is a one **molar solution**. To calculate the number of moles, divide the weight of chemical present by the formula weight of the chemical. For example, if one liter of solution contains 60 grams of NaOH (formula weight 40), the molarity is:

$$moles = \frac{60}{40}$$

$$moles = 1.5 \text{ or } 1.5 \text{ mol/L } (1.5 \text{ M})$$

## Preparing Serial Dilutions

Clinical laboratory workers often have to make serial dilutions of a serum sample to find the titer of a certain

> **Problem:** Prepare one liter of a 2 N solution of NaOH.
>
> **Answer:** A 1 N solution of NaOH contains one gram-equivalent weight of NaOH per liter of solution. The formula weight of NaOH is 40. The gram equivalent weight is also 40 since Na has a 1+ charge. Therefore, a 1 N solution of NaOH contains 40 grams/L.
>
> One liter of a 2 N solution contains 80 grams NaOH in one liter of solution.

**FIGURE 6-9** Preparation of a 2 N solution using a substance with a 1+ valence

> **Problem:** Prepare one liter of a 1 N solution of $Mg(OH)_2$.
>
> **Answer:** One liter of 1 N $Mg(OH)_2$ contains one gram-equivalent weight of $Mg(OH)_2$.
>
> $$\text{gram-equivalent weight} = \frac{\text{Formula weight Mg(OH)}_2}{2 \text{ (valence)}}$$
>
> $$\text{gram-equivalent weight} = \frac{58}{2} = 29$$
>
> Therefore, 29 grams $Mg(OH)_2$ is added to deionized or distilled water in a one-liter volumetric flask. After swirling to mix, water is added to the flask's fill line.

**FIGURE 6-10** Preparation of a 1N solution of Mg $(OH)_2$, a chemical that has a 2+ valence

component. The higher the dilution, the smaller the amount of the original sample and the larger the amount of diluent. This concept is sometimes difficult to understand; an example of setting up a serial dilution is illustrated in Figure 6-11.

Dilutions of serum are required for certain quantitative tests. The results for a quantitative pregnancy test or rheumatoid arthritis test are expressed in terms of the highest-dilution tube in which a reaction can be detected.

## MAKING MATHEMATICAL CONVERSIONS

### Temperature Conversions

Converting temperatures from Fahrenheit to Celsius, or vice versa, requires calculations. The temperature scale most widely used in clinical work is the **Celsius scale**. In this system, the freezing point of water is 0° and the

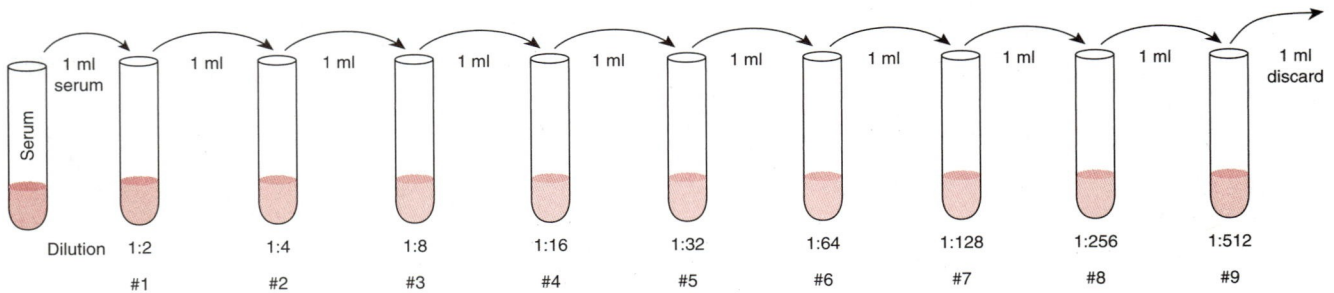

**FIGURE 6-11** Setting up a serial dilution

| | | | | | |
|---|---|---|---|---|---|
| **Problem A:** | Convert 98.6°F (normal body temperature) to Celsius (C) degrees. | | **Problem B:** | Convert 37°C to Fahrenheit (F) degrees. | |
| **Formula:** | $C = \dfrac{5}{9} (F - 32)$ | | **Formula:** | $F = \dfrac{9}{5} (C) + 32$ | |
| **Solution:** | $C = \dfrac{5}{9} (98.6 - 32)$ | | **Solution:** | $F = \dfrac{9}{5} (37) + 32$ | |
| | $C = \dfrac{5}{9} (66.6)$ | | | $F = 66.6 + 32$ | |
| | $C = 36.99$ or $37$ | | | $F = 98.6$ | |
| **Answer:** | 98.6°F is equal to 37°C | | **Answer:** | 37°C is equal to 98.6°F | |

**FIGURE 6-12** Examples of temperature conversions: (A) Fahrenheit temperature converted to Celsius, and (B) Celsius temperature converted to Fahrenheit

boiling point of water is 100°. Almost all reaction temperatures are expressed in Celsius.

The **Fahrenheit scale** is used widely for body temperature (98.6°F) and for weather reports. Although many books contain a temperature conversion table, laboratory workers may not always have access to this information. Two common conversions are body temperature (98.6°F to 37°C) and the freezing point of water (32°F to 0°C). Formulas for temperature conversion and an example of each are shown in Figure 6-12. A temperature conversion chart is given in Table 6-4.

## Converting Laboratory Results to SI Units

The International System of Units (SI) has been established for several years. However, some results continue to be reported in older conventional units. For example, in the United States, blood glucose is usually reported in mg/dL; the SI units are g/L or mmol/L (millimoles/L). The SI units for reporting RBC or WBC counts are cells/µL or cells/L, but counts are sometimes reported as cells/mm³. Examples of SI usage in labora-

### Table 6-4. Temperature conversion chart

| °F | = | °C | °F | = | °C | F | = | °C |
|---|---|---|---|---|---|---|---|---|
| 23 | | –5 | 101 | | 38.3 | 115 | | 46.1 |
| 32 | | 0 | 102 | | 38.9 | 116 | | 46.7 |
| 70 | | 21.1 | 103 | | 39.4 | 117 | | 47.2 |
| 75 | | 23.9 | 104 | | 40 | 118 | | 47.8 |
| 80 | | 26.7 | 105 | | 40.6 | 119 | | 48.3 |
| 85 | | 29.4 | 106 | | 41.1 | 120 | | 48.9 |
| 90 | | 32.2 | 107 | | 41.7 | 125 | | 51.7 |
| 95 | | 35 | 108 | | 42.2 | 130 | | 54.4 |
| 96 | | 35.6 | 109 | | 42.8 | 135 | | 57.2 |
| 97 | | 36.1 | 110 | | 43.3 | 140 | | 60 |
| 98 | | 36.7 | 111 | | 43.9 | 150 | | 65.6 |
| 98.6 | | 37 | 112 | | 44.4 | 212 | | 100 |
| 99 | | 37.2 | 113 | | 45 | 230 | | 110 |
| 100 | | 37.8 | 114 | | 45.6 | | | |

tory results and some equivalent terms are discussed in Lesson 1-4, The Metric System.

### Procedural Notes

- Weigh and mesure chemicals accurately to ensure good results.
- Pipet carefully, using the correct pipets and tips.
- Check mathematical calculations before proceeding with a task.
- Use the correct principles and formulas to make the required solution.

### Safety Precautions

- Observe Universal and Standard Precautions when handling standards and controls.
- Consult MSDS information for proper use of chemicals.
- Wear appropriate PPE.
- Clean all spills appropriately.
- Wipe work area with surface disinfectant.
- Wash hands with hand disinfectant.

## SUMMARY

Most instruments today operate using prepackaged reagents or reagents contained in the reaction cartridge or strip. However, sometimes reagent preparation, such as reconstitution of standards and controls, is necessary. Specimens may require dilution for accurate measurement of an analyte. General laboratory reagents such as alcohol solutions or buffers may be prepared. Dilute solutions may be prepared from concentrates. There-

fore the technician should be familiar with the principles involved in reagent preparation and pipetting techniques.

## LESSON REVIEW

1. Give an example of a percentage solution used in the laboratory.
2. Why are temperature conversions sometimes necessary?
3. Give the formula for converting degrees F to degrees C.
4. What is the dilution when one part is added to nine parts?
5. What are the two formulas used to solve proportion problems?
6. How is a 1% (v/v) solution prepared?
7. How is a 5% (w/v) solution prepared?
8. Explain how to prepare one liter of 1 N KOH (potassium hydroxide). Molecular weights are: K = 39, O = 16, H = 1.
9. Define Celsius scale, Fahrenheit scale, gram-equivalent weight, gram-formula weight, lyophilize, mole, molar solution, normal solution, physiological saline, proportion, and ratio.

## STUDENT ACTIVITIES

1. Reread the information on laboratory reagent preparation and calculations.
2. Review the glossary terms.
3. Find examples of temperature in Celsius degrees, percent solutions, and dilutions or ratios in a chemistry or similar textbook.
4. Practice preparing solutions and serial dilutions as directed by the instructor.
5. Practice the calculations for percentage solutions, proportions, and ratios using the worksheet.

# Worksheet

## LESSON 6-3 Laboratory Reagent Preparation and Calculations

Name _____  Date _____

1. A procedure calls for 200 mL of a 2% glucose solution. A 50% solution is available. How much of the 50% solution is needed? How would the solution be prepared?

2. A 1% solution of hydrochloric acid is required for a procedure. A 5% solution is available. How much of the 5% solution will be required to make 500 mL of a 1% solution?

3. A procedure calls for acetic acid and water, with the proportions being two parts acetic acid to three parts water. One hundred milliliters are needed. How much acetic acid and water are required?

4. One liter of 70% alcohol is needed. How much 95% alcohol is required to make the 70% solution?

5. Two hundred milliliters of 2% acetic acid are needed.  How many mL of 5% acetic acid are required to make the 2% solution?

6. How would one liter of a 10% solution of chlorine bleach be prepared?

7. Give the instructions for preparing  one liter of a 0.5N solution of Mg $(OH)_2$ (FW = 58; valence = 2).

8. How could  250 mL of a 4% solution of hydrochloric acid (HCl) be prepared from a 10% solution of HCl?

9. Give the instructions for preparing serial dilutions of a serum sample using 0.5 mL serum and 0.5 mL saline in each of five numbered tubes.

10. A 1-to-25 dilution of blood is required for a procedure. How is it prepared?

11. How could a 1:10 dilution of serum be prepared?

12. What is the dilution when 0.5 mL is diluted to a total of 100 mL?

13. If 0.5 mL of serum is added to 4.5 mL of saline, what is the dilution?

14. If 0.5 mL of blood is added to 9.5 mL of saline, what is the dilution?

# Chemistry Instrumentation in the Physician Office Laboratory

## LESSON OBJECTIVES

**After studying this lesson, you should be able to:**

- *Explain the major differences among the types of instruments used in small and large laboratories.*
- *Discuss the reasons for the increase in small laboratory testing.*
- *Discuss the principles of the spectrophotometer.*
- *Explain Beer's Law.*
- *Discuss the basic differences among discrete, solid-phase, and ion-selective analyzers.*
- *Explain the principle of discrete analyzers.*
- *Explain the principle of solid-phase analyzers.*
- *Explain the principle of ion-selective electrodes.*
- *Discuss the importance of instrument maintenance and quality control.*
- *Define the glossary terms.*

## GLOSSARY

**absorbance (A)** / a logarithmic expression of the amount of light absorbed by a substance containing colored molecules; optical density (O.D.)

**Beer's Law** / a mathematical relationship that demonstrates the linear relationship of concentration to absorbance and that forms the basis for spectrophotometric analysis

**centrifugal analysis** / a type of discrete chemical analysis in which the reagents and sample are mixed together by centrifugal action

**discrete analysis** / a method of analysis in which the assay procedure for each sample is performed in its own separate container within the instrument

**ion-selective electrode** / an electrode manufactured to respond to the concentration of a specific ion

**monochromator** / a device that isolates a narrow portion of the light spectrum

**percent transmittance (%T)** / the percentage of light that passes through a solution

**reflectance photometer** / an instrument that measures the light reflected from a colored reaction product

**solid-phase chemistry** / an analytical method in which the sample is added to a strip or slide containing, in dried form, all the reagents for the procedure

**spectrophotometer** / an instrument that measures intensities of light in different parts of the light spectrum

# INTRODUCTION

Automated instruments make it possible for clinical laboratory analyses to be performed in much less time than when done manually. When analysis time is reduced, the turnaround time (TAT), time elapsed between ordering a laboratory test and the physician receiving the results, is also usually reduced. Shortened TAT allows for more rapid diagnosis and treatment.

In general, results from automated methods are more precise and accurate than those from manual methods, since variation in technique is reduced. However, as with manually performed tests, good quality control must be maintained for instruments.

Analysis speed and the efficiency of running many patient samples at one time are especially important in larger laboratories, such as those in hospitals. These laboratories process hundreds of samples daily. The use of automation increases the productivity of these larger laboratories. However, automation also has a place in the smaller clinical laboratory and in physician office laboratories (POLs).

# CHOOSING AN INSTRUMENT FOR THE LABORATORY

Many points must be considered before purchasing an instrument for the laboratory. First, the decision must be made concerning which and how many tests need to be performed. This decision can be based on the types of patients who will be served and which test results would be most helpful to the physician. The price of purchasing the instrument versus leasing it should be compared. Other considerations are cost per test, ease of operation, and maintenance costs. The cost may be more than expected if an inexpensive instrument requires expensive reagents and supplies.

The most important factor in choosing an instrument is the quality of results. An instrument that produces unreliable results is detrimental to patient care.

# CURRENT TRENDS IN INSTRUMENTATION

Instrumentation technology is in a continuous state of change. Updated and improved instruments are constantly being brought to market. In the past, as the volume of testing increased, the major instrument manufacturers concentrated on developing larger and more diversified instruments designed to meet the needs of larger laboratories.

In the last two decades, however, a revolution has taken place in the technology of clinical laboratory instrumentation. Improved electronic and chemical technology have made it possible for manufacturers to drastically reduce the size of many instruments. These smaller instruments are well suited for the limited space in most POLs. Several instruments are available for patient home use, such as those for determining blood glucose. POCT volume has increased tremendously because their small size makes these instruments more portable.

This lesson presents just a few examples of instruments available for the smaller laboratory. The principles of each instrument are discussed, with examples provided of the tests each can perform.

The instruments featured in this lesson were chosen because they are in use in many laboratories. They were also chosen to present different principles of operation. *The inclusion of an instrument does not constitute an endorsement, just as omission of an instrument does not imply lack of endorsement.*

## Physician Office Laboratories (POLs)

The number of tests performed in POLs has increased in recent years. The availability of testing in the physician's office can be a benefit, especially to the very ill or elderly patient. Tests most often performed include complete blood counts, prothrombin time, blood glucose, and blood cholesterol. The tests performed are regulated by the Health Care Financing Administration (HCFA) and come under the Clinical Laboratory Improvement Amendments (CLIA) regulations. POLs are subject to inspection. The owner or director must obtain a copy of the CLIA regulations and implement them or hire a clinical consultant to assure compliance with the laws.

To be in compliance, laboratories are required to run quality control samples and keep records of the results. Since January 1994, laboratories have been required to enroll in proficiency testing programs, depending on the test complexity performed. If acceptable results are not obtained on proficiency samples, HCFA can prohibit the laboratory from performing certain tests until the deficiencies are corrected.

## Point-of-Care Testing (POCT)

One goal in critical care areas of the hospital is to cut down on the TAT for laboratory results. POCT enables the instrument to be near the patient, perhaps at his or her bedside. Tests usually performed are those for which the results may affect the patient's immediate well-being and treatment. These include blood glucose, blood urea nitrogen, blood gases, electrolytes, and coagulation tests.

Trained laboratory personnel or nursing staff may perform the tests, and testing is regulated by HCFA. Quality control samples must be run and records kept of the results. Proficiency testing by an approved agency must also be performed.

## SAFETY

Several potential hazards are present in operating, maintaining, and repairing laboratory instruments. Universal and Standard Precautions must be observed at all times. Instruments must be properly installed and grounded as recommended by the manufacturer to avoid electrical shocks. The outside case should never be removed except by a person trained in maintenance and repair. Removal of the case can expose wiring and other parts that could cause injury or death if touched. Dangling metal jewelry is especially dangerous, since it could inadvertently contact an electrical part.

Most chemical solutions used in analyses are hazardous. Workers should observe all label warnings to avoid poisoning, chemical burns, or other injury.

Workers should carefully follow instructions for operating and caring for battery-powered instruments, such as those used in POCT. The battery type must be the one recommended by the manufacturer. Used batteries must be disposed of properly.

## BASIC PRINCIPLES OF INSTRUMENTATION

Clinical laboratory instruments operate on various principles. However, the majority produce results by measuring the color of the end-product of a chemical reaction.

## Spectrophotometer

Spectrophotometers are used to determine the concentration of colored solutions. This determination is made by passing a narrow beam of light through a solution contained in a glass or plastic tube called a cuvette. The portion of light that passes through the colored solution is the **percent transmittance (%T)**. The light that does not pass through is absorbed by the colored solution and is measured as **absorbance (A)** units. The more concentrated the solution, the greater its absorbance and the less its transmittance (Figure 6-13). These solutions are said to follow **Beer's Law**; however, not all solutions follow Beer's Law.

Spectrophotometers vary in their external design, but the principles are the same, whether they stand alone or are included as part of an analyzer (Figure 6-14). A light source provides a beam of light that passes to a

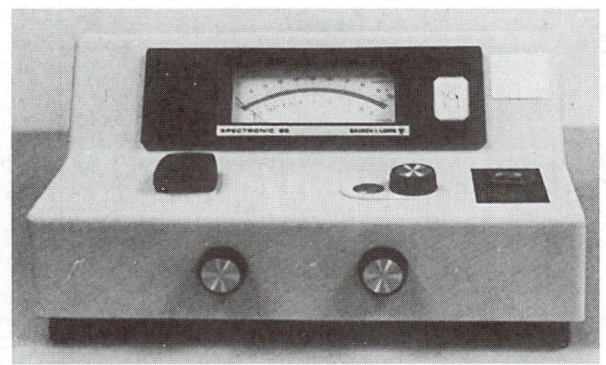

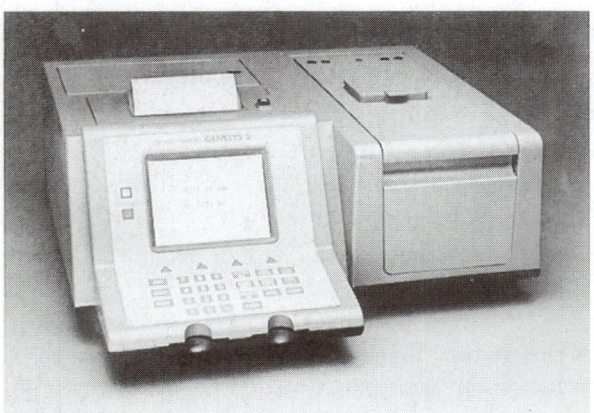

**FIGURE 6-14** Spectrophotometers: (top) Spectronic® 20 with galvanometer-type readout; and (bottom) SPECTRONIC® GENESYS™ 5UV/Visible Spectrophotometer with printer (Photo courtesy of Milton Roy Company, Analytical Products Division, Rochester, NY)

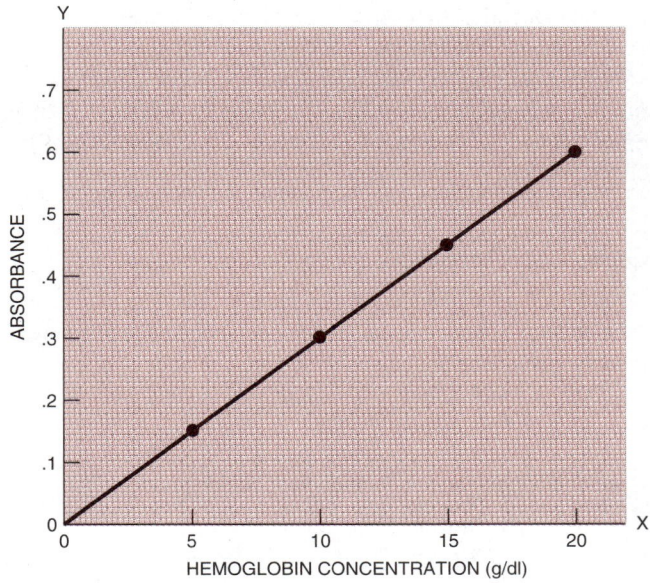

**FIGURE 6-13** Illustration of a standard curve showing absorbance vs. concentration

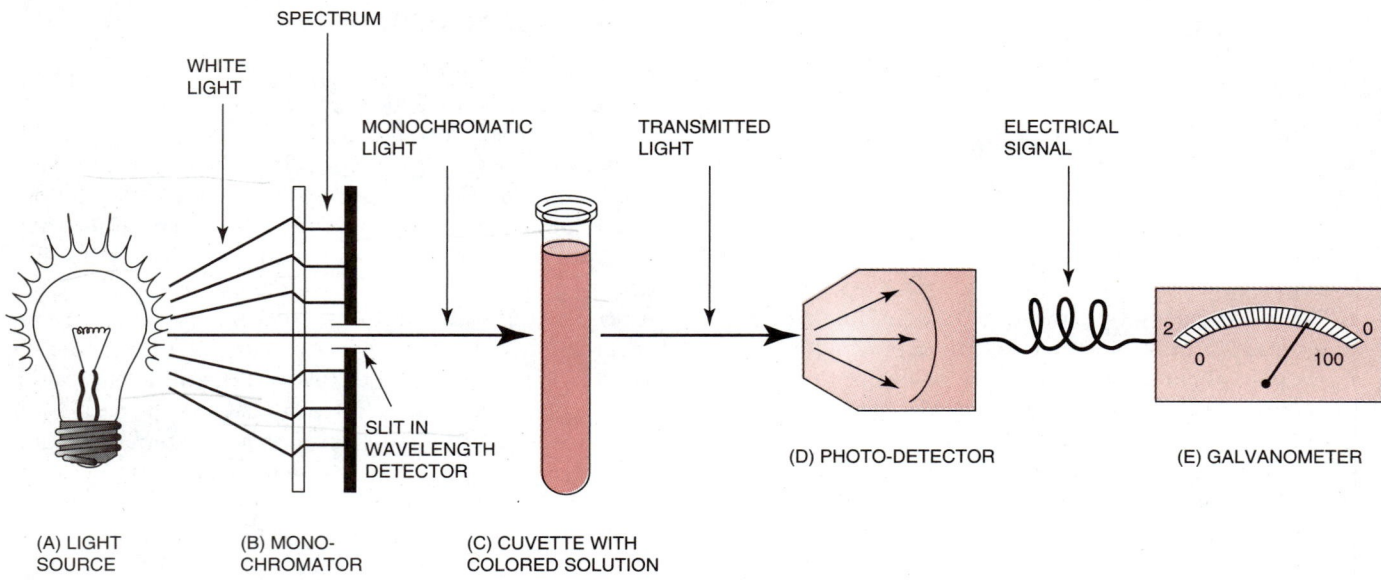

**FIGURE 6-15** ▶ Diagram of the internal parts of a spectrophotometer

**monochromator** with a diffraction grating that disperses the light into a spectrum. A narrow slit isolates a beam of monochromatic (one-wavelength) light selected by the operator according to the analysis being performed. The monochromatic light is directed through the tube of colored solution. The light that passes through is detected by a photoelectric cell that converts it to an electrical current which is measured and converted to a digital readout. This information can be displayed as either absorbance (A) or percent transmittance (%T) (Figure 6-15).

### Spectrophotometer Quality Control

Maintenance and quality control procedures must be performed on spectrophotometers at specified intervals according to the manufacturer's instructions. Some common quality control procedures include:

- The spectrophotometer should be checked for stray light before each use.
- Wavelength setting should be verified by using a didymium filter or holmium oxide glass that has maximum absorbance at a particular wavelength.
- Wavelength verification must be performed routinely, according to the manufacturer's instructions, and after any lamp adjustment.
- To ensure that spectrophotometer results are reliable, a standard curve must be constructed for each instrument at the beginning of each work day,

when new reagents are used, and after any repair or lamp replacement.
- Controls must be run with every set of determinations.

### Discrete Analysis

Most of the chemistry analyzers in smaller clinical laboratories use the principle of **discrete analysis**. The analyses are performed with each sample in its own container or packet. With this method, one sample cannot be affected by another sample. Two types of discrete analysis are centrifugal analysis and solid-phase chemistry.

### Centrifugal Analysis

Centrifugal analysis involves centrifugation of the samples within the instrument. During centrifugation, the patient sample and the test reagents are mixed together in the test packet. The final product is read by a spectrophotometer in the analyzer.

### Solid-Phase Chemistry

In solid-phase chemistry analyzers, the sample is added to a strip or slide that contains all the reagents for the analysis in dried form. The reagents are in multiple layers, with each layer having a specific function in the

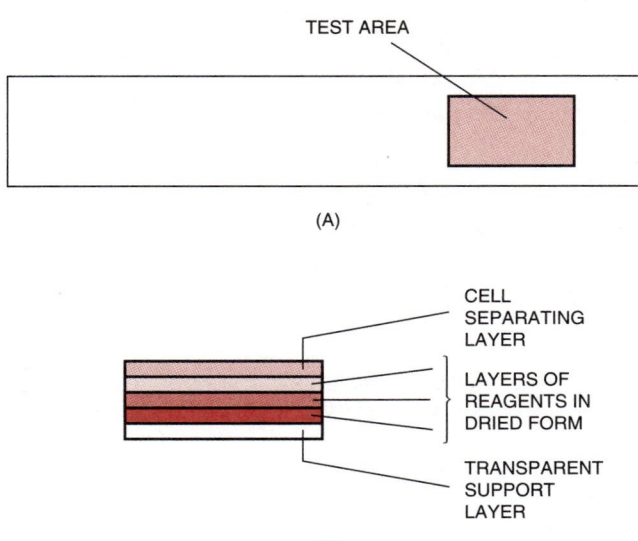

(A)

(B)

**FIGURE 6-16** Illustration of the composition of a solid-phase reagent strip: (A) top view of a strip, showing reagent test area; (B) expanded side view of a test area, showing the layers.

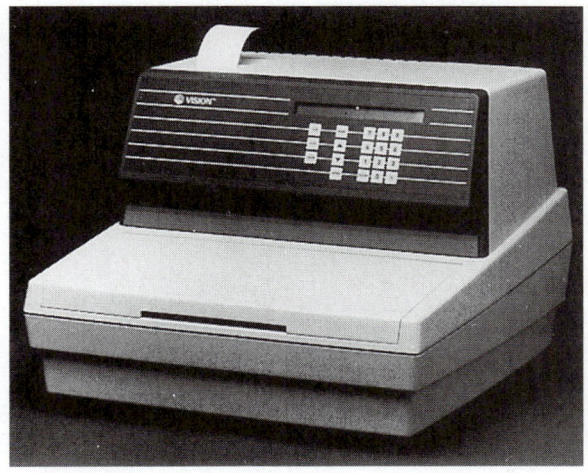

**FIGURE 6-17** The VISION™ System clinical chemistry analyzer (Photo courtesy of Abbott Laboratories)

reaction. The area of the strip or slide where the reagents are located is called the *test area or reagent pad*. (Figure 6-16).

Some reagent pads have the ability to filter RBCs out of whole blood, and allow only plasma to reach the reagents. The bottom support layer is transparent so the color of the reaction product can be read by the instrument.

## Ion-Selective Electrodes

The technology of **ion-selective electrodes** is being used in many clinical instruments. Each ion-selective electrode is manufactured to be responsive to a specific ion; for example, the sodium (Na+) electrode will measure only Na+ ions present in a solution or sample.

Two electrodes are used in an analysis. One electrode contains a known concentration of the ion to be measured and is called the *reference electrode*. The other electrode, which is responsive only to the ion being measured, is exposed to the unknown solution. The difference between the concentration of ions in the reference electrode and the ions in the unknown solution causes an electrical potential to develop. This potential across a membrane in the electrode is proportional to the difference between the two concentrations. A microprocessor converts this voltage into a number representing the concentration of the ion in the unknown solution.

## EXAMPLES OF INSTRUMENTS AND PRINCIPLES OF OPERATION

### Discrete Analyzers

#### Centrifugal Analysis

Abbott Laboratories markets the VISION™ System (Figure 6-17). The sample is added to a testpack containing all the reagents. Each testpack is specific for only one procedure, such as glucose or cholesterol measurement. Only two drops of sample are required for analysis. Serum, plasma, or whole blood may be used. The pack contains a cell-separating chamber to separate blood cells from a sample of whole blood, so that only the plasma takes part in the reaction.

After the sample is added, the testpack is placed into the instrument for analysis. During the reaction time, the testpack is centrifuged and rotated in various directions to force the sample and reagents together in sequenced chambers. A portion of the reaction takes place in each of the chambers. If heating or incubation time is needed for a particular test, the instrument provides it.

At the end of the reaction time, the instrument measures the absorbance of the final product. The built-in spectrophotometer measures the absorbance using a chamber of the testpack as a cuvette. The instrument displays the concentration of the substance being assayed.

The VISION™ System has the ability to perform analyses for more than twenty substances. Up to ten testpacks can be processed at the same time; however, each testpack analyzes only one substance. The time required for analysis is about eight minutes. Chemistries

**Table 6-5.** Examples of chemistry analyzers and their capabilities

| INSTRUMENT TYPE | EXAMPLE | TEST CAPABILITIES |
|---|---|---|
| Solid-phase chemistry | Ortho® DT60 II<br>Reflotron® Plus<br>HemoCue®<br>ProAct® Cholesterol System<br>Accu-Chek® meters | Several chemistry tests available; use dry reagent packs specific for each constituent |
| Discrete analysis (centrifugal) | VISION™ | Many chemistry tests available; each test requires a separate testpack |
| Ion-selective | Nova 14+<br>Nova Stat Profile™ Plus<br>Electrolyte Analyzer® II<br>i-STAT® | Measure electrolytes plus tests such as glucose, BUN, Hct |
| Combination discrete analysis and ion-selective | COBAS MIRA® | $Na^+$, $K^+$, $Cl^-$ plus testpacks for a variety of chemistry tests |

available include glucose, total cholesterol, high-density lipoprotein (HDL) and low-density lipoprotein (LDL) cholesterol, creatinine, aspartate aminotransferase (AST), and alanine aminotransferase (ALT). Hematology testpacks are also available (see Table 6-5).

## Solid-Phase Analyzers

***Ortho® DT60 II.*** Several manufacturers offer solid-phase analyzers, such as the Ortho® DT60, that are especially suitable for small laboratories. Each test procedure is contained on a separate slide specific for that analysis.

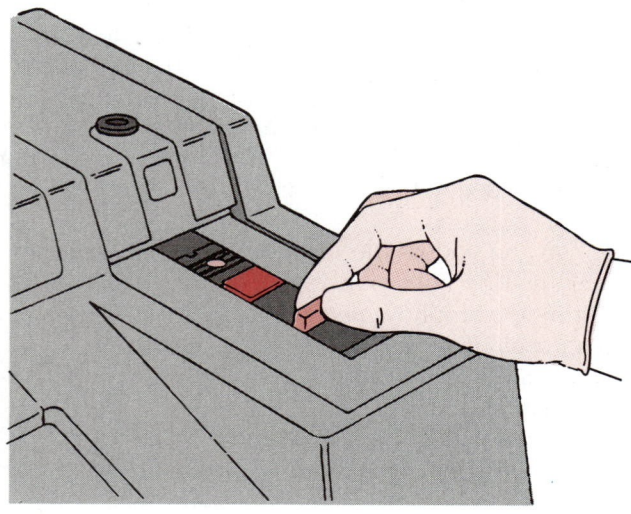

**FIGURE 6-18** Illustration of insertion of the sample card into a dry-slide technology chemistry analyzer

To perform the analysis, the appropriate slide is chosen for the test to be performed. If the slide has been refrigerated, it must be warmed to room temperature before it is used. The slide is placed in the sample drawer of the instrument (Figure 6-18), which reads a magnetic code on the slide to determine which procedure to perform.

The patient sample is drawn into a pipet provided with the system. The pipet tip is inserted into an opening on top of the instrument and 10 µL are dispensed onto the test slide. The colored product produced by the reaction is automatically measured by a reflectance photometer inside the instrument. A **reflectance photometer** measures the light that a colored product reflects onto a light detector. The instrument converts this information into concentration.

The Ortho® DT60 II performs more than thirty different test procedures. These include blood glucose, blood total cholesterol, and cholesterol fractions. Other tests available are creatinine, bilirubin, amylase, and hemoglobin. The instrument can complete approximately sixty-five tests per hour.

Various modules are available that permit testing for sodium, potassium, chloride, and carbon dioxide ($CO_2$). An additional module adds the ability to analyze constituents such as AST, ALT, and creatine kinase (CK).

***Reflotron®.*** The Reflotron® is distributed by Roche Diagnostics Corp. (Figure 6-19). This instrument has been a popular choice for POLs or other small laboratories. It requires only 30 µL of whole blood, plasma, or serum.

The reagents required for each test are already on the strip in dried form. These strips are called reagent

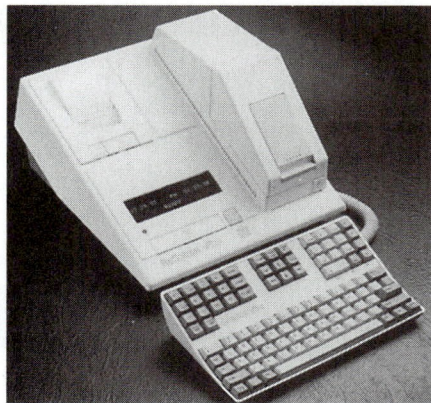

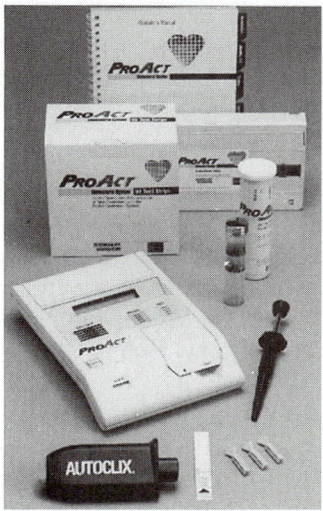

**FIGURE 6-19** Chemistry analyzers suitable for small laboratories: (Top) Reflotron Plus® and (bottom) ProAct® Cholesterol System (Photos courtesy of Boehringer Mannheim Corp.)

tabs. The reagent tabs for different analyses are kept in separate vials and protected by a foil covering.

To perform a test, the appropriate reagent tab is chosen and the foil is removed. The sample is drawn up into the Reflotron® pipet and dispensed onto the reagent pad. The tab must be inserted into the instrument within fifteen seconds of applying the sample. The instrument reads the magnetic code to determine which analysis to perform. Confirmation of the analysis selected is displayed on the screen.

The time required for most analyses is 180 seconds (three minutes). The time is counted down on the digital display screen of the instrument. The absorbance of the colored reaction product is read by reflectance photometry. The instrument converts the photometer reading into mg/dL (conventional units) or mmol/L (SI units).

Two additional instruments manufactured by this company are the ProAct™ and the Accu-Chek® meters.

The ProAct™ is the size of a large book and is used for measuring total cholesterol. The Accu-Chek® meters analyze blood for glucose and can be used at home by diabetic patients. (See Table 6-5.)

## Ion-Selective Electrodes

### Electrolyte Analyzer® II

The Electrolyte Analyzer® II, manufactured by Ionetics, Inc., is an ion-selective analyzer used to determine sodium ($Na^+$) and potassium ($K^+$) levels. The system consists of a reference electrode and two ion-selective electrodes, one for $Na^+$ and a second for $K^+$. The system can analyze whole blood, plasma, or serum. However, the electrodes function longer if whole blood is not used. The anticoagulant used to prevent clotting must not contain either $Na^+$ or $K^+$ because they are being measured in the patient sample; therefore, heparin is the usual anticoagulant.

The Electrolyte Analyzer® II is a convenient size and will fit on top of many other small analyzers to save counter space. The instrument is used in emergency rooms, physician's offices, and other small laboratories.

### Nova 12+ Analyzer

Nova Biomedical manufactures several analyzers suitable for use in smaller laboratories and in critical care areas. The Nova 12+ has a test menu that includes $Na^+$, $K^+$, chloride ($Cl^-$), glucose, BUN, and hematocrit. It can analyze more than fifty samples per hour and requires about 200 μL of whole blood, serum, plasma, or urine. Other models are available that offer various combinations of procedures, including lithium analysis (Figure 6-20). The small size of this series of analyzers is made possible because of the compact size of the electrodes.

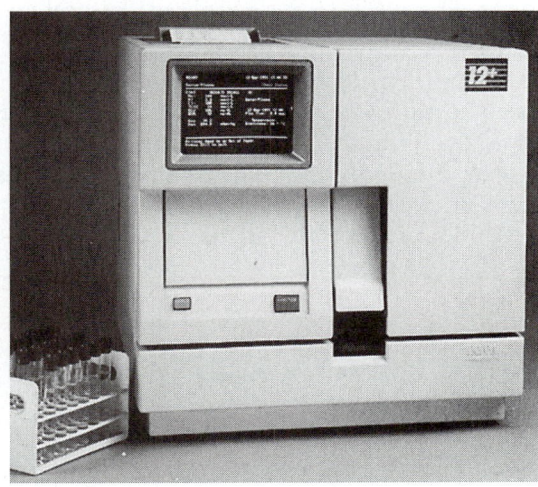

**FIGURE 6-20** The Nova 12+ clinical chemistry analyzer (Photo courtesy of Nova Biomedical, Waltham, MA)

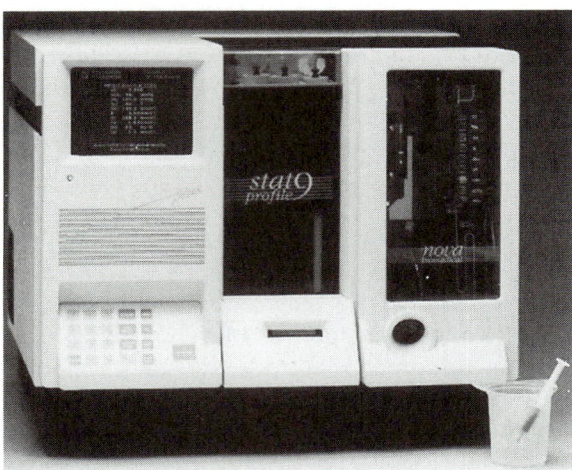

**FIGURE 6-21** The Nova Stat Profile™ Plus (Photo courtesy of Nova Biomedical, Waltham, MA)

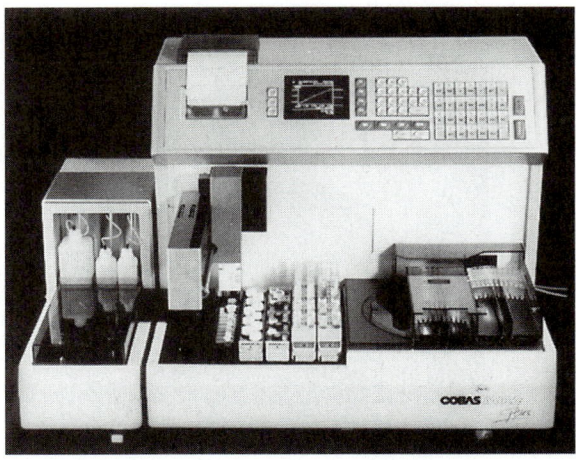

**FIGURE 6-22** The COBAS MIRA® Plus Analyzer (Photo courtesy of Roche Diagnostics Corporation, Branchburg, NJ)

Nova Biomedical also markets a line of analyzers to be used in POCT areas such as emergency rooms. This series is called the Stat Profile™ Plus. The instruments in the series can perform different combinations of blood gas, electrolyte, and hematocrit analyses (Figure 6-21).

## COBAS MIRA®

The COBAS MIRA® Plus Analyzer, manufactured by Roche Diagnostics Corporation (Figure 6-22), is a combination of a discrete centrifugal analyzer and ion-selective electrode analyzer. With the optional ion-selective electrode module, $Na^+$, $K^+$, and $Cl^-$ ions can be measured directly. The instrument can process from ninety to 132 samples per hour, depending on the combinations of tests chosen. Tests can be performed without removing the cap on the tube of blood if the optional COBAS Tip Server is used. This means the operator can insert samples into the instrument without being exposed to potentially infectious blood samples. In addition, this instrument has a menu of more than 100 other test procedures, including routine chemistries and drug abuse assays. (See Table 6-5).

ular instrument must be consulted. The reagent strips, slides, or electrodes from one analyzer should never be used on another analyzer. Also, as new modules or accessories become available, the laboratory professional must become familiar with their operation, care, and maintenance.

The instrument manufacturers discussed in this lesson have quality control products available for use with each instrument. These include calibrator solutions and control sera with known normal and abnormal values. Specific quality control information for some of the analyzers is given below.

## Discrete Analyzers

### The VISION™ System

Quality control materials for the VISION™ System are available from the manufacturer, Abbott Laboratories. These can be charted in the laboratory's daily quality control program. In addition, the laboratory may subscribe to an Abbott program in which control samples are sent to the laboratory four times a year. These are analyzed and the results sent to the manufacturer. If the results are within two standard deviations ($2s$) of the manufacturer's acceptable value(s), the laboratory receives a certificate verifying the success. If the results are not within specifications, a technical representative will be sent to the laboratory to help review their procedures and check the instrument's operation.

The manufacturer's operating manual for the instrument must be consulted for maintenance proce-

### Quality Assurance

Most chemistry analyzers are capable of providing reliable results for the constituents being measured. However, certain maintenance and upkeep procedures must be performed on a regular basis if the analyses' results are to be credible.

Although many instruments operate on similar principles, the manufacturer's protocol for each partic-

dures. A notebook or log containing a record of all maintenance and repair must be kept.

### Reflotron®

Controls are available from Roche Diagnostics Corp. for the Reflotron®, the ProAct™, and other instruments it markets. Two levels of controls, normal and abnormal, are included in a set. The control samples are applied to the test tabs and analyzed in the same manner as patient samples. If a control value is out of range, prescribed cleaning instructions should be followed, and the test repeated using controls with a different lot number. The company's technical service department must be called if the values are still out of range after cleaning the instrument and repeating the control tests.

Maintenance procedures are outlined in the operating manuals. Records must be kept of all instrument repair and maintenance procedures.

## Ion-Selective Electrodes

Quality control samples for ion-selective electrode instruments are analyzed like patient samples. Reconstituted lyophilized control sera may be used, if they have assay values for ion-selective electrode instruments. If the instrument is run only a few times a day, a set of controls may need to be included in each run.

A regular program of maintenance must be performed. The electrodes require special care to avoid error in results. The electrodes should be rinsed immediately after use to prevent the blood sample from drying on them; rinsing may be automatically performed by the instrument. The electrodes must be stored in the special solution provided. Each electrode has an expiration date and must not be used after that date.

### SUMMARY

Using chemistry analyzers in smaller laboratories or POLs can be a real convenience for the patient and physician. Many chemistry analyzers are available. Factors to consider in choosing one include the number and kinds of tests to be performed and the patient population. Purchase price, ease of operation, and maintenance requirements also should be considered, along with reagent costs. In addition, current users of instruments being considered should be contacted to discuss reliability, accuracy and precision, and quality of technical support. Training sessions offered by the manufacturer or distributor should be attended if possible or, preferably, a representative may come to the laboratory to train everyone who will be using the instrument.

Quality assurance program must be maintained for each instrument.

### Procedural Notes

- Always read the operating manual before using an instrument.
- Understand the quality control and maintenance requirements of the instrument.
- Never use reagents or supplies for one instrument in another.
- Call the manufacturer's technical service department if a problem cannot be resolved.
- Attend training sessions offered by the instrument manufacturer.

### Safety Precautions

- Follow Universal and Standard Precautions when using, maintaining, and repairing instruments.
- Always read the manufacturer's operating manual before using or attempting to repair an instrument.

### LESSON REVIEW

1. Explain why small laboratories might use different types of instruments than large laboratories.
2. Discuss the reasons for increased testing in POLs.
3. What are the basic differences among solid-phase, discrete, and ion-selective analyzers?
4. How do solid-phase analyzers operate?
5. What is the principle of the ion-selective methods?
6. Discuss the principles of spectrophotometers.
7. Discuss the importance of a regular maintenance program.
8. Discuss the importance of a quality control program.
9. Define absorbance, Beer's Law, centrifugal analysis, discrete analysis, ion-selective electrode, mono-

chromator, percent transmittance, reflectance photometer, solid-phase chemistry, and spectrophotometer.

## STUDENT ACTIVITIES

1. Reread the information on chemistry instrumentation in the POL.
2. Review the glossary terms.
3. Tour a small laboratory to observe some instruments in operation.
4. Using the information from this lesson and an instrument available in the laboratory, complete the worksheet at the end of this lesson.

# *Worksheet*

## **LESSON 6-4** Chemistry Instrumentation in the Physician Office Laboratory

Name _____    Date _____

**Part A.**  Answer the following questions:

1. What types of technologies are used in most clinical chemistry analyzers?

2. How do the requirements for a POL instrument differ from those for an instrument in a large hospital laboratory?

3. What is the advantage of an instrument that can analyze a whole blood sample instead of only serum or plasma?

4. List five procedural notes to follow when an instrument is being used for analysis.

5. Why would the information in a maintenance logbook be important when a problem arises with an instrument?

**Part B.**  Read the manufacturer's operatoring manual (or laboratory procedure manual) for an instrument available in the laboratory and answer the following questions:

7. What is the name of the instrument? _____

8. Does this instrument use solid-phase, discrete, or ion-selective electrode technology? _____

9. If the instrument does not fit into any of these categories, what type of technology is involved? _____

10. List two test procedures that can be performed using this instrument. _____ _____

11. How does the worker "tell" the instrument which test procedure is to be performed?

12. How are control solutions used with this instrument?

13. Has a Levey-Jennings chart been constructed for the procedures run on this instrument? _____ Are values plotted daily? _____

14. Is plasma, serum, or whole blood used for the analyses performed on this instrument? _____

15. Are maintenance and repair records kept in a logbook? _____

16. List in order the steps for performing a glucose (or other) analysis using this instrument.

# Point-of-Care Testing

## LESSON OBJECTIVES

**After studying this lesson, you should be able to:**

- *Explain what is meant by point-of-care testing (POCT).*
- *List three benefits of POCT.*
- *Name the health care professionals who are part of the POCT team.*
- *Explain why quality assurance compliance is important in POCT.*
- *List five test procedures performed as POC Tests.*
- *Name three common POCT sites.*

## INTRODUCTION

Testing at the point of care is a way of bringing laboratory testing to the patient, rather than sending patients or patient specimens to the laboratory. POCT has been made possible in part by the development of small, portable analyzers that give rapid test results. These analyzers are easy to use, give reproducible results, and require little maintenance.

POCT began when blood glucose monitors were developed for home use by diabetics. No special expertise was required to operate these first monitors and the glucose test could be performed using a drop of capillary blood. Patients could have daily access to rapid test results and could use these results for adjusting their insulin dosage, diet, or activity levels.

In the 1990s, technological advances in instrument design mushroomed. Today, numerous small, sophisticated, but easy-to-use analyzers are available that can perform hematology, urinalysis, coagulation, chemistry, microbiology, and immunological tests. These analyzers are being used in a variety of settings to provide rapid laboratory testing.

In addition, rapid immunological and serological tests that require no instrument have been developed and are used at the point of care. Some of these, such as pregnancy tests kits, are also available over the counter.

## BENEFITS OF POCT

The immediate benefit of near-patient, or POC, testing is that laboratory test results can be obtained sooner, decreasing turnaround time (TAT). This benefits patients, health care workers, and the health care system (Table 6-6). Patients can receive required therapy more quickly, which can be especially important for critically ill patients.

Another benefit is that these testing methods are less traumatic, requiring only a drop or two of capillary blood. Patients also feel a greater sense of participation in their own care, usually learning of the test results immediately, since the test is performed in their presence.

POCT programs in hospitals may lead to shorter hospital stays, due to the rapid availability of test results. The potential for errors is also decreased because the specimen need not be labeled, transported to the laboratory, or processed before testing—all opportunities for mishandling, mislabeling, or degrading a sample. POCT provides increased communication

### Table 6-6. Benefits of POCT programs

Improved TAT of test results

Increased patient participation in health care

Less traumatic testing method

Smaller specimen required

Shorter hospital stays

More rapid therapy intervention

Improved cooperation and communication among all members of health care team

Reduced errors in specimen handling and processing

Reduced need for specimen transport

and cooperation among the laboratory, nursing services, and patients, enhancing the quality of care.

## WHO IS INVOLVED IN POCT?

Good POCT programs require a multidisciplinary team effort among laboratory, nursing, and physician or hospital medical staff (Table 6-7). Nurses, medical assistants, emergency medical technicians, licensed practical nurses, or physicians may perform testing that has been traditionally done by laboratory personnel. The laboratory's usual role in POCT is to provide technical assistance, data management, quality assurance, compliance monitoring, and personnel training.

## POCT SITES

POCT programs are varied. Hospital POCT programs are usually geared toward providing rapid service to critically ill patients in intensive and critical care units, emergency rooms, surgical suites, and cardiac units. These patients' outcomes may depend on rapid test results that allow therapies to be instituted more rapidly.

POCT is also used in POLs, nursing homes, screening centers, blood donation centers, physical examinations for insurance or employment, and homes. In these settings, rapid results are usually not critical to patient immediate care, but on-site testing saves time and costs for the patient, as well as the health care provider.

### Hospital POCT

Hospital POCT programs are designed to provide rapid results for the critically ill patient whose condition will benefit from rapid action by the medical team. An example of a hospital POCT program is using bedside analyzers that measure glucose, clotting time, and electrolytes in the emergency room, intensive care unit, and operating room. These analyzers are calibrated and maintained by laboratory personnel, who provide procedure manuals and technical assistance, train nursing staff, and assess the training. A POCT coordinator is responsible for reviewing and analyzing QC data, ensuring compliance with accreditation agencies, coordinating staff training, and serving as a liaison between the nursing service and the laboratory.

When a critical need arises for stat test results, the instruments are used by nursing personnel to perform the test, obtaining results in a matter of minutes (Figure 6-23). The test results are immediately charted and therapy is instituted.

### Non-Hospital POCT Programs

POCT programs outside the hospital setting have a different purpose. POCT programs in POLs, nursing

| **Table 6-7.** Departments and agencies involved in decision-making in POCT programs | |
| --- | --- |
| clinical laboratory | infection control |
| nursing staff | safety officer |
| medical staff | regulatory agencies |
| administration | |

homes, health screening stations, and homes are designed to provide a small menu of laboratory tests in a convenient, cost-effective, and efficient way. These tests are important in preventive medicine and can be used to screen for anemia, cardiovascular disease risk, and kidney disease, as well as to monitor and provide information for managing oral anticoagulant therapy or conditions such as diabetes.

An example of a non-hospital POCT program is a one-day cholesterol screening program at a mall. People are encouraged to come by and have a rapid cholesterol test and heart attack risk assessment. Volunteer health care personnel perform rapid cholesterol tests on capillary blood using a portable cholesterol analyzer. Maintenance, calibration, and quality control of these analyzers are performed at the central laboratory facility by laboratory personnel before and after the screening

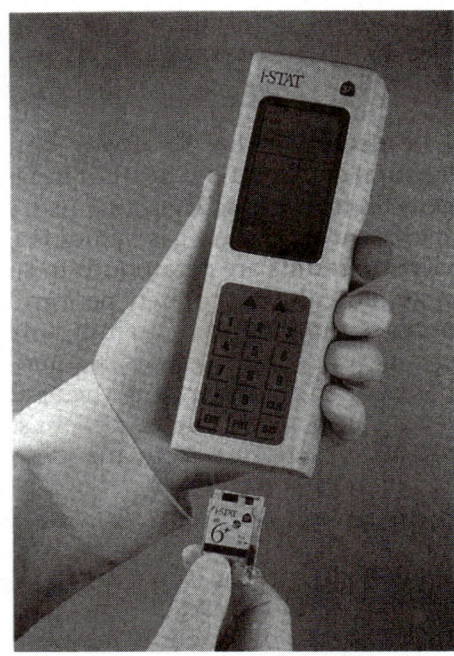

**FIGURE 6-23** The i-STAT® portable clinical analyzer provides rapid test results in POCT programs (Courtesy of Abbott Laboratories, Inc.)

event. Minimal quality control procedures are then required during the screening period. Cholesterol results are given on the spot so the people tested can decide whether or not to consult their physician.

Another example of a non-hospital POCT program is a POL that offers tests such as hemoglobin, blood glucose, urine dipstick, and prothrombin time. These rapid tests can be performed by medical assistants or nursing staff before the patient sees the physician. The results are available for the physician to use in making decisions concerning further patient treatment or follow-up. This is much more efficient than sending patients to a laboratory for tests, waiting for the results, and calling or having the patients come back later to learn their test results.

Most POLs use CLIA-waived analyzers that require few routine maintenance and quality control procedures. However, procedure manuals and documentation of maintenance and quality control procedures are required, even though they may be minimal compared to those for more complex analyzers. A laboratory professional may be employed as a consultant to provide periodic review of procedures and technical assistance when needed.

## FACTORS TO CONSIDER IN ESTABLISHING A POCT PROGRAM

The primary impetus behind establishing a POCT program should be to enhance the quality of patient health care. POCT programs are not useful if test results are unreliable or not evaluated or acted upon quickly. The health care facility must maintain a high-quality program, meet all regulatory requirements, and train and assess testing personnel. Factors that must be considered in establishing a POCT program will differ somewhat depending on the setting. However, the following are issues that must be addressed in all POCT programs.

### Compliance with Regulatory Guidelines

The primary law that regulates POCT is CLIA '88. This law describes the standards that must be met for all testing procedures used in diagnosing and treating human disease. To receive federal Medicare and Medicaid funds, laboratories must obtain a CLIA certificate granting permission to perform certain tests.

  **Safety**

OSHA and CDC guidelines must be followed to prevent exposure of health care personnel and patients to chemical, physical, and biological hazards. Written safe-

ty rules that encompass Universal and Standard Precautions must be included in all procedure manuals and must be followed rigorously.

### Quality Assurance

A POCT program must be able to provide accurate, reliable test results. This is assured by having a comprehensive quality assurance program in place. Quality assurance includes procedures that ensure the quality of the test procedure from beginning (test requisition) to end (interpretation and reporting of results). Instrument calibration, up-to-date procedure manuals, testing of control sera or reagents, participation in a proficiency testing program, comprehensive documentation, and employee training and assessment are all part of a quality assurance program. Central laboratories that operate POCT sites must also assure that the values obtained at the POCT sites are equivalent to the values obtained in the central laboratory.

### Training and Assessment

Depending on the type of POCT program, personnel may be trained by the laboratory or by a technical representative of the instrument manufacturer. Testing personnel must be trained and their competence verified before they can be permitted to test patient specimens. Periodic review and documentation of personnel performance is required. Participation in a proficiency testing program is one method of assessing performance.

### Technical Support

Laboratories running POCT programs must either have a director on site or employ a qualified laboratory consultant who is available to provide technical assistance. Technical support is also available through the instrument manufacturers, usually through a hotline or local service representative.

### Data Management

Data management at POCT sites may be simple or complex. In a POL, test results are usually written directly on the patient's chart or an instrument printout is inserted into the chart. In a hospital POCT program, the data management system may be sophisticated. Testing personnel may have bar-coded badges that allow access to an analyzer. In this way, only personnel who have proven competency in performing the procedure can operate the instrument. The analyzers may also be linked directly to the laboratory information system (LIS) and with results transferred electronically to the lab as soon as they are generated.

## SUMMARY

Although POCT is not called for in all situations, it can be an important component of health care. Careful studies must be done to determine if a POCT program should be implemented and what the scope of the program should be. Improved patient care should be the most important goal. POCT programs must be constantly monitored to ensure they are achieving their goal and that test results are of the highest quality.

Many test procedures have been adapted to POCT use (Table 6-8). Some provide important data useful in acute care facilities, such as electrolyte analysis, activated clotting time assay, troponin assay for heart attack assessment, and arterial blood gases. Others are more useful in health-screening situations or physician offices. These include hemoglobin, urine dipstick, rapid strep tests, pregnancy tests, prothrombin time, and fecal occult blood tests.

### Table 6-8. Tests commonly performed at POCT sites

Hematology
  hemoglobin
  hematocrit
Coagulation
  activated clotting time
  prothrombin time
  activated partial thromboplastin time
Chemistry
  cholesterol
  electrolytes
  blood glucose
  cardiac troponin
  blood gases
  fecal occult blood test
  blood urea nitrogen (BUN)
  creatinine
  hemoglobin $A_{1c}$
Urinalysis
  urine dipstick
  pregnancy test
  microalbumin
Microbiology—rapid immunological-based tests
  rapid strep test
  test for infectious mononucleosis

## LESSON REVIEW

1. What is the primary factor to consider when establishing a POCT program?
2. Name five departments that participate in managing POCT programs.
3. What technological developments have made POCT possible?
4. Explain how hospital POCT programs differ from non-hospital programs.
5. Name two hematological tests often performed at point of care.
6. Name four chemistry tests often performed at point of care.
7. Discuss the importance of quality assurance in POCT programs.
8. Name the primary law that regulates POCT.
9. What safety precautions must be observed when performing POCT?

## STUDENT ACTIVITIES

1. Review the information on POCT.
2. Inquire about a POCT program in a hospital near you. Find out what tests are performed, who performs them, and how quality assurance is accomplished. Note POCT programs that may be in place in your community and comment on the benefits they provide.

# Measuring Blood Glucose

## LESSON OBJECTIVES

**After studying this lesson, you should be able to:**

- *Explain the function of glucose in the body.*
- *Describe factors that affect blood glucose levels.*
- *Name two disorders of glucose metabolism.*
- *Explain the collection method for blood glucose specimens.*
- *Explain the principles of glucose test methods.*
- *Explain the purpose of a postprandial glucose test.*
- *Explain how a glucose tolerance test is performed.*
- *Give the reference values for fasting blood glucose, two-hour postprandial glucose, and glucose tolerance tests.*
- *Discuss the importance of quality control when measuring glucose.*
- *Perform a blood glucose measurement using a glucose analyzer.*
- *Discuss safety precautions that must be observed when performing glucose tests.*
- *Define the glossary terms.*

## GLOSSARY

**chromogen** / substance that becomes colored when it undergoes a chemical change

**diabetes mellitus** / a disorder of carbohydrate metabolism characterized by a state of hyperglycemia due to insulin deficiency

**glucagon** / pancreatic hormone that increases blood glucose concentration by promoting the conversion of glycogen to glucose

**glucose dehydrogenase** / enzyme used in glucose analytical methods that converts glucose to gluconolactone

**glucose oxidase** / enzyme used in many glucose analytical methods that converts glucose to gluconic acid

**glucose tolerance test (GTT)** / analyzing blood glucose at timed intervals following ingestion of a standard glucose dose; oral glucose tolerance test (OGTT)

**glycogen** / storage form of glucose found in high concentration in the liver

**glycolysis** / energy production as a result of the metabolic breakdown of glucose

**glycosuria** / glucose in the urine; glucosuria

**hexokinase** / enzyme used in glucose analytical methods that converts glucose to glucose-6-phosphate

**hyperglycemia** / blood glucose concentration above normal

**hypoglycemia** / blood glucose concentration below normal

**insulin** / pancreatic hormone essential for proper metabolism of blood glucose and maintenance of blood glucose levels.

**peroxidase** / enzyme that converts hydrogen peroxide to water and oxygen

**postprandial** / after eating

**renal threshold** / blood concentration above which a substance not normally excreted by the kidneys appears in the urine

## INTRODUCTION

Glucose, the major carbohydrate in blood, is used for energy by the body's cells. Measuring blood (or serum) glucose is one of the most frequently performed clinical chemistry tests.

Two types of disorders of glucose metabolism are (1) **diabetes mellitus**, in which there is increased blood glucose, or **hyperglycemia**, and (2) **hypoglycemia**, (decreased blood glucose), as may be seen in deficiencies of adrenocorticotropic hormone (ACTH) or growth hormone.

The glucose test is most often used to aid in diagnosing and managing diabetes, or in managing hypoglycemia. This lesson presents information about glucose metabolism, diagnosis and management of diabetes, and methods of glucose analysis.

## MECHANISMS REGULATING BLOOD GLUCOSE LEVELS

Although the body has many enzymatic pathways that use glucose, hormones keep blood glucose within a fairly narrow range. **Insulin**, a hormone produced by the pancreas, *lowers* blood glucose by increasing glucose up-take by body cells and increasing the rate of **glycolysis**. Glycolysis is a cellular process that produces energy by the metabolic breakdown of glucose. Insulin also increases the rate of conversion of glucose to **glycogen**, the short-term storage form of glucose.

Hormones such as growth hormone, epinephrine, cortisol, and **glucagon** act in a variety of ways to *increase* blood glucose concentration. These hormones are sometimes called insulin antagonists, because their action is opposite to the action of insulin.

## DIAGNOSTIC TESTS FOR DIABETES AND HYPOGLYCEMIA

Tests used to diagnose diabetes and hypoglycemia are fasting blood glucose, two-hour postprandial glucose, and the oral **glucose tolerance test (GTT)**.

## Fasting Blood Glucose

A fasting blood glucose is performed on a blood sample taken when the patient has not eaten for a specified period of time. A fasting specimen is usually obtained before breakfast after the patient has gone without food since the previous evening's meal. Fasting periods may be as short as six hours or as long as fourteen hours.

## Two-Hour Postprandial Glucose

A two-hour **postprandial** test is a measurement of glucose two hours after the patient has eaten. Postprandial tests are most reliable if the patient is tested following a standard glucose dose (50–100 g) rather than a random meal.

## Glucose Tolerance Test

In the glucose tolerance test, the patient's fasting glucose level is measured. The patient is given a standard dose of glucose (usually a liquid) to ingest. The blood glucose is then measured at set intervals for two to three hours following ingestion of the glucose.

In the past, a typical GTT would include the fasting assay and glucose measurements again at thirty minutes, one hour, two hours, and three hours after the glucose dose. However, it has been found that diabetes can often be diagnosed by using just two glucose measurements; the fasting blood glucose and a glucose measurement two hours after the glucose dose ingestion. Hypoglycemia diagnosis may require testing at more frequent intervals for five to six hours following ingestion of the glucose dose. Patients undergoing GTT should be monitored carefully for adverse reactions.

Urine samples may be collected and tested for glucose at the same times blood is taken for the GTT. Glucose is normally reabsorbed from the glomerular filtrate by the kidney tubules, so the blood glucose level must be elevated before it exceeds the kidney's capacity to reabsorb. The blood glucose concentration above which glucose can be detected in urine is called the

**Table 6–9.** Glucose reference values*

| TEST | GLUCOSE CONCENTRATION | |
| --- | --- | --- |
| | mg/dL | mmol/L (SI) |
| Fasting | | |
|    Serum | 70–110 | 3.9–6.1 |
|    Whole blood | 60–100 | 3.3–5.6 |
| Two-hour postprandial | ≤110 | ≤6.1 |
| Glucose tolerance (oral, serum) | | |
|    Fasting | 70–110 | 3.9–6.1 |
|    1 hour | 20–50 above fasting | 1.1–2.8 above fasting |
|    2 hour | fasting level or below | fasting level or below |
|    3 hour | fasting level or below | fasting level or below |

* Values vary slightly among laboratories, depending on test method used

**renal threshold** for glucose, and is normally approximately 160–180 mg/dL. The presence of glucose in urine, **glycosuria**, may be an indication of diabetes mellitus.

## GLUCOSE REFERENCE VALUES

### Normal Fasting Glucose Values

The normal or reference value for serum or plasma glucose following an overnight fast is 70–110 mg/dL. Whole blood glucose reference values are slightly lower. Traditionally, fasting glucose levels above 120 mg/dL have been interpreted to indicate hyperglycemia. However, the American Diabetic Association (ADA) recently recommended a cutoff of 126 mg/dL for the upper normal reference range.

### Two-Hour Postprandial Glucose Values

The blood glucose level should be less than 110 mg/dL two hours postprandial. Patients with two-hour postprandial levels above 110 mg/dL should receive further testing (Table 6-9).

### Glucose Tolerance Test Reference Values

In a GTT, a person with normal glucose metabolism would have a normal fasting glucose level (70–110 mg/dL), a one-hour level of 90–160 mg/dL, and two- and three-hour levels at or below the fasting level.

Values outside these ranges may indicate a problem with carbohydrate metabolism.

## CRITICAL GLUCOSE VALUES

Generally, a patient is considered to be hypoglycemic if his or her blood glucose level falls below 50 mg/dL. Abnormally low glucose levels must be reported immediately so appropriate action can be taken. Hypoglycemic patients may experience fainting, weakness, confusion, or lack of coordination, and may lapse into unconsciousness if left untreated.

Extremely high blood glucose levels pose the danger of diabetic coma and require immediate treatment to reduce the levels. Glucose levels over 400 mg/dL are considered dangerously high. Symptoms of hyperglycemia include confusion, lethargy, extreme thirst, weak pulse, dry skin, and nausea.

Each laboratory must establish the critical glucose values that require immediate action. For example, values below 40 mg/dL or above 400 mg/dL usually require physician notification. Table 6-10 lists examples of critical (action) glucose values and symptoms of hypoglycemia and hyperglycemia.

## DIABETES MANAGEMENT

Good diabetes management is important for preventing or delaying microvascular complications. Meters for patient use in monitoring blood glucose levels were first introduced in the 1970s. Since then, the meters' accura-

**Table 6-10.** Critical glucose values and symptoms that may accompany them

| HYPOGLYCEMIA <40 mg/dL | HYPERGLYCEMIA >400 mg/dL |
| --- | --- |
| faintness | confusion |
| weakness | coma |
| hunger | nausea |
| diaphoresis | intense thirst |
| visual disturbances | ketoacidosis |
| palsy | dry flushed skin |
| confusion | weak pulse |
| personality changes | |

*Note: Patient may not experience all symptoms*

cy, precision, and ease of use have improved. It is recommended that all diabetic patients use a home glucose monitoring system regularly.

The patient's ability to keep blood glucose levels within acceptable ranges can be assessed by periodic measurement of hemoglobin $A_{1c}$, also called glycated or glycosylated hemoglobin. This is hemoglobin produced when glucose molecules become attached to hemoglobin during periods of high blood glucose. Hemoglobin $A_{1c}$ values less than 7% indicate good glucose management; higher values indicate poorer management. The Bayer DCA® 2000 test for Hemoglobin $A_{1c}$ is CLIA waived.

# PRINCIPLES OF GLUCOSE ANALYSIS

Most glucose testing methods use the enzymes **glucose oxidase**, **hexokinase**, or **glucose dehydrogenase** to measure glucose concentration. These enzyme tests are simple, quick, specific for glucose, and have been adapted for use in many types of glucose analyzers. In general, tests that use hexokinase or glucose dehydrogenase are more specific and have less interferences than those using glucose oxidase.

## Glucose Oxidase Method

The glucose oxidase method of analysis is a two-step reaction. In the first part of the reaction, glucose is converted to gluconic acid and hydrogen peroxide ($H_2O_2$) in the presence of glucose oxidase and oxygen. The resulting concentrations of gluconic acid and $H_2O_2$ are proportional to the amount of glucose originally pres-

ent. In the second part of the reaction, in the presence of the **peroxidase** enzyme and a **chromogen**, the $H_2O_2$ is converted to water ($H_2O$) and the chromogen produces a color:

(1) $\text{Glucose} + H_2O + O_2 \xrightarrow{\text{Glucose Oxidase}} \text{Gluconic acid} + H_2O_2$

(2) $H_2O_2 + \text{Chromogen} \xrightarrow{\text{Peroxidase}} 2\,H_2O + \text{Color formation}$

The color intensity is proportional to the amount of $H_2O_2$ (and thus the amount of glucose) and can be measured using a spectrophotometer or reflectance photometer.

## Hexokinase Method

The hexokinase method is also a two-step reaction. This method has advantages over the glucose oxidase method, primarily because fewer substances interfere and it uses safer reagents. In the first step, hexokinase, in the presence of adenosine triphosphate (ATP), adds a phosphate to glucose to form glucose-6-phosphate (G6P). In the second step, G6P in the presence of nicotinamide adenine diphosphate (NADP) and the enzyme glucose-6-phosphate dehydrogenase (G6PD) is converted to 6-phosphogluconate (6PG) with the production of reduced nicotinamide adenine diphosphate (NADPH):

(1) $\text{Glucose} + ATP \xrightarrow{\text{Hexokinase}} G6P + ADP$

(2) $G6P + NADP \xrightarrow{\text{G6PD}} 6PG + NADPH$

NADPH absorbs ultraviolet light at 340 nm. This absorbance can be measured using a spectrophotometer. The increase in absorbance due to NADPH in the solution is proportional to the glucose concentration in the original reaction.

## Glucose Dehydrogenase (GDH) Method

Glucose meters such as the HemoCue® and Accu-Chek® use the enzyme glucose dehydrogenase to measure glucose, a method having few interferences. The HemoCue® system uses a reagent containing three enzymes: mutarotase, glucose dehydrogenase, and diaphorase. The reagent also contains NAD and MTT, a color reagent. The reaction of glucose with the reagents and enzymes causes the formation of gluconolactone, NADH, and MTTH, which has a blue color; the intensity of the color is proportional to the glucose concentration and is read by the HemoCue® photometer.

The Accu-Chek® meters also use conversion of glucose to gluconolactone by glucose dehydrogenase to measure glucose concentrations. However, these meters measure the current produced in the reaction, rather than a colored end product.

## METHODS OF GLUCOSE ANALYSIS

Glucose concentrations may be measured using manual methods or automated methods.

### Manual Glucose Analysis Methods

Manual glucose analysis methods require adding a serum or plasma sample to a test tube containing glucose reagent (enzyme and chromogen) and allowing a reaction to occur. The color formed is measured using a spectrophotometer and compared to a set of standards measured in the same way.

### Automated Glucose Analysis Methods

Many types of glucose analyzers are available. Some measure only glucose and are simple to use. Others measure glucose as part of a profile and may require more expertise.

Several types of glucose analyzers are suitable for POLs. Many of these operate on the principle of reflectance photometry or spectrophotometry and use adaptations of enzymatic glucose analysis methods. Examples are the REFLOTRON®, VISION™, and Hemo-Cue® Blood Glucose Analyzer (Figure 6-24).

Several small, inexpensive, handheld glucose meters are available for home use by diabetics. Examples of these are the Accu-Chek® analyzers by Roche Diagnostics Corp., the ONE TOUCH® meters by Lifescan Inc., and the Glucometer® family of glucose meters by Bayer Corporation (Figure 6-25). Similar models are also available for POCT or POLs. All these analyzers are designed to be easy to use and give rapid results.

## PERFORMING BLOOD GLUCOSE MEASUREMENTS

  **Safety**

Universal and Standard Precautions must be followed when performing blood glucose measurements. Appropriate PPE must be worn when obtaining the blood specimen and performing the test. All test materials must be discarded in appropriate biohazard containers.

### *Quality Assurance*

The manufacturer's instructions must be followed for the particular analyzer used. It is important to use consistent, proper technique to avoid variations in results. Glucose controls purchased from instrument manufacturers should be used to check instrument performance. Test materials, such as reagent strips or cuvettes, made for a particular instrument must be used only with that instrument.

Control tests and calibration checks must be performed daily before patient samples are run and any time results are questionable. Control tests let the technician know that test strips, cuvettes or cartridges, and the instrument are working properly.

Control tests use solutions of known glucose concentrations that react similarly to blood when used with the test cuvette or strip. The controls are available in normal, low, and high concentrations and are used in the same manner as a blood sample.

When control tests are performed, the results on the display screen must be recorded and compared to the values printed on the control bottle or package insert. If the results are within the given range, the patient test may be run. If not, the controls must be repeated using new test strips, being certain that correct technique is used. If the controls are still out of the given range, the strips may be defective and a new lot should be tested. If the new lot of strips gives out-of-range results, the instrument may have a problem and the operating manual should be consulted. Patient samples must not be run until the instrument and strips are working properly, as indicated by the control results. A log of control test results must be kept. In this way, any deterioration of the test system will be noted early so corrective action can be taken.

### Specimen Collection

Glucose measurement can be performed on whole blood, plasma, serum, urine, or cerebrospinal fluid. If serum or plasma is used, it must be separated from the blood cells as soon as possible after collection. Blood cells metabolize glucose and, if left in contact with serum or plasma, may rapidly lower the specimen's glucose concentration. Failure to separate serum or plasma from cells may cause a false low glucose value.

If whole blood glucose is to be measured, the test should be performed immediately following capillary puncture, or on blood collected in a suitable anticoagu-

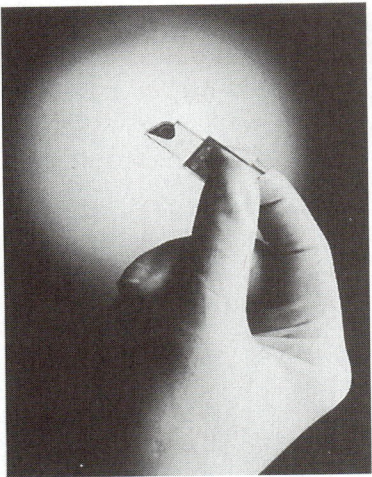 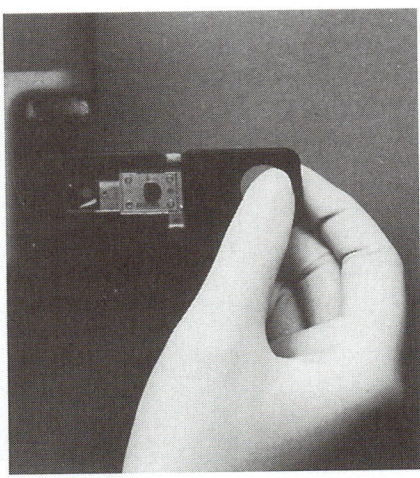 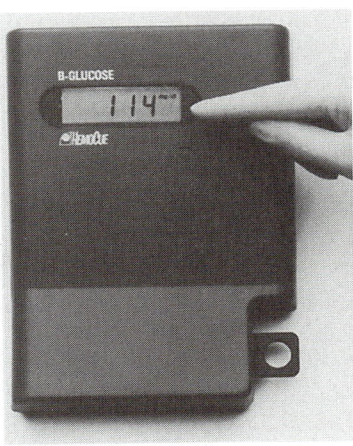

**FIGURE 6-24** HemoCue® Blood-Glucose system: left, blood specimen is drawn up automatically into the glucose microcuvette; center, the microcuvette is inserted into its holder and pushed into the photometer; and, right, the glucose concentration is displayed in mg/dL after 45–240 seconds (Photo courtesy of HemoCue®, Inc.)

lant, such as EDTA or heparin. The anticoagulant must be one that will not interfere with the glucose analysis method being used.

The laboratory requisition will specify whether the specimen may be a random specimen or must be fasting.

## The HemoCue® Blood-Glucose System

The HemoCue® Blood-Glucose system consists of a compact photometer and disposable clear microcuvettes that contain the glucose enzyme reagent (Figure 6-24). The self-filling microcuvette automatically draws up 5 uL of blood from a capillary puncture into its reaction chamber (Figure 6-24, left). The microcuvette is then placed in the holder and pushed into the photometer (Figure 6-24, center). The glucose concentration in mg/dL or mmol/L is displayed in 45-240 seconds (Figure 6-24, right). This system is ideal for POLs and POCT because of its calibration stability and the minimal operator training required. Data management programs are available with this analyzer.

## Reflectance Photometers

Several glucose analyzers based on reflectance photometry operate similarly to each other. The Reflotron® and Glucometer® are examples of reflectance photometer analyzers. Blood from a fingerstick, serum, or plasma is applied to the reagent area of a test strip. The glucose in the sample reacts with the reagents in the pad(s), caus-

ing a color to form. The more glucose present in the sample, the darker or more intense the color. At the appropriate time, the strip is inserted into the test chamber and light is directed on to the test area. The amount of light reflected from the colored test area is measured by the photometer and converted to a digital readout showing the glucose concentration in mg/dL or mmol/L. Most instruments give results in one to three minutes. *Instructions included with the test strips must be carefully followed for reliable test results.*

## Accu-Chek® Glucose Meters

The Accu-Chek® Advantage is a glucose meter that uses the principle of biamperometry. The center of the test strip contains a target area for applying the blood specimen and the end of the strip inserted into the meter contains electrodes. The glucose dehydrogenase enzyme within the test strip reacts with glucose in the blood specimen to form gluconolactone, causing release of electrons. The glucose meter is able to detect voltage changes that result from the electrons released in this reaction and convert this electrical signal to a readout of glucose concentration.

Accu-Chek® glucose meters (Figure 6-25) can be used in a glucose test system module that allows data storage and retrieval and interfaces with the hospital computer system (Figure 6-26). Quality control data can also be stored in the system's memory. Special codes or coded strips can be used to limit use of the instrument to qualified testing personnel.

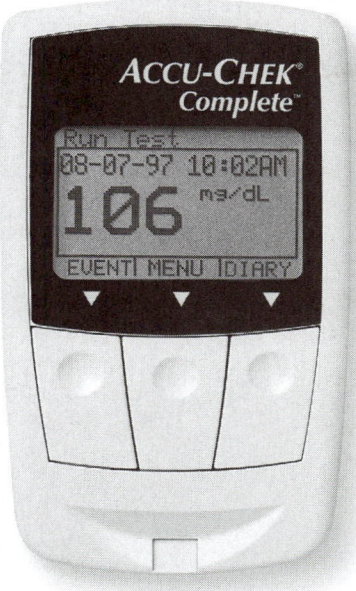

**FIGURE 6-25** Accu-Chek® Complete glucose meter (Photo courtesy of Boehringer Mannheim Corp.)

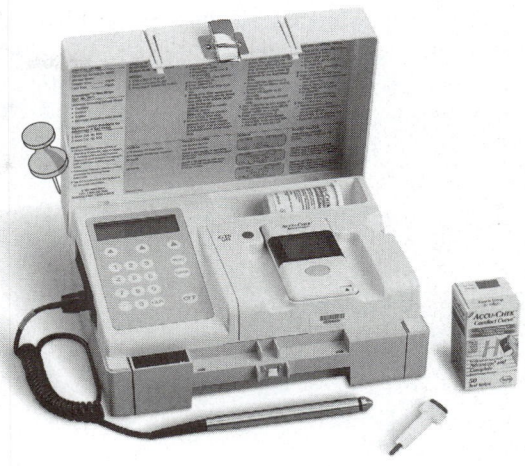

**FIGURE 6-26** Example of glucose-monitoring system workstation used in POCT sites. Features include automatic data storage of patient test results, storage of quality control data, and hospital computer system interface capabilities. (Courtesy of Roche Diagnostics Corp.)

## Procedural Notes

- Follow manufacturers' directions for the instrument and reagents used.
- Use appropriate controls and calibrators and record the results on the quality control log sheets.
- Use a specimen appropriate for the test method.
- Be sure all reagents and test packs or strips are used before their expiration dates.

## Safety Precautions

- Follow Universal and Standard Precautions when performing glucose measurements.
- Clean and disinfect the instrument before returning it to storage.

## LESSON REVIEW

1. How are glucose levels controlled?

2. What is a storage form of glucose?

3. What are two major types of glucose metabolism disorders?

4. Why must serum or plasma be separated from cells immediately following collection if the specimen is to be tested for glucose?

5. What is a two-hour postprandial glucose test?

6. What are the reference values for glucose?

7. Explain how a glucose tolerance test is performed. What would normal results be?

8. Explain the glucose oxidase and hexokinase methods of analyzing glucose. What end product is measured in the glucose oxidase method? In the hexokinase method?

9. What is the purpose of running controls on glucose analyzers?

10. Explain the glucose dehydrogenase method of glucose analysis.

11. Define chromogen, diabetes mellitus, glucagon, glucose dehydrogenase, glucose oxidase, glucose tolerance test, glycogen, glycolysis, glycosuria, hexokinase, hyperglycemia, hypoglycemia, insulin, peroxidase, postprandial, and renal threshold.

1. Reread the information on measuring blood glucose.
2. Review the glossary terms.
3. Practice performing a glucose measurement using a glucose analyzer as outlined on the Student Performance Guide, using the worksheet.

# *Student Performance Guide*

## **LESSON 6-6** Measuring Blood Glucose

Name _____ Date _____

### ☣ INSTRUCTIONS

1. Practice the procedure for measuring glucose using a glucose analyzer and following the step-by-step procedure.
2. Demonstrate your understanding of this lesson by:
   a. Completing a written examination successfully, and
   b. Using the glucose analyzer to measure glucose satisfactorily for the instructor. All steps must be completed as listed on the instructor's Performance Check Sheet.

### MATERIALS AND EQUIPMENT

- gloves
- glucose meter such as HemoCue®, Accu-Chek®, or Glucometer®
- test strips, cuvettes, or cartridges for glucose meter
- control solutions for glucose meter
- soft laboratory tissue
- capillary puncture materials
- hand disinfectant
- surface disinfectant (10% chlorine bleach solution)
- biohazard container
- worksheet
- 70% alcohol and cotton balls, or alcohol swabs
- micropipetter 0–100 µL, (optional depending on analyzer used)
- puncture-proof sharps container

*Note:* The following is a general procedure for using a glucose analyzer or glucose meter. Consult the procedure manual for the instrument used and package inserts for specific instructions.

### PROCEDURE

Record in the comment section any problems encountered while practicing the procedure (or have a fellow student or the instructor evaluate your performance).

S = Satisfactory
U = Unsatisfactory

| You must: | S | U | Comments |
|---|---|---|---|
| 1. Review operating instructions for the glucose analyzer | | | |
| 2. Wash hands and put on gloves | | | |
| 3. Assemble materials and supplies | | | |
| 4. Record instrument name, control ranges, control lot #, and test strip lot # on the worksheet | | | |
| 5. Measure blood glucose using the Accu-Chek® Advantage by following steps 5a–5h (For the HemoCue®, skip to step 6; for other meter, go to step 7):<br>a. Perform quality control check:<br>  (1) Turn on the meter. Check that code on display matches code on test strip vial | | | |

| You must: | S | U | Comments |
|---|---|---|---|
| (2) Insert "Chek Strip" into monitor<br>(3) Note that "OK" appears if monitor is functioning properly<br>(4) Remove Chek Strip and return it to storage<br>(5) Insert a test strip into the meter when the test strip symbol flashes (within thirty seconds). Wait until the display indicates it is ready for the specimen (display will read "L1")<br>(6) Apply one drop of Level 1 control to the target area on the test strip<br>(7) Record the displayed value on the quality control log. Verify that control solution is within acceptable range (Display will read "OK")<br>(8) Discard used test strip<br>(9) When "L2" appears on display, insert a new strip into meter. Repeat steps 5a6–5a8 using Level 2 control<br>b. When meter indicates it is ready, insert a new test strip<br>c. Perform capillary puncture on patient<br>d. Hold finger over test strip and apply one large hanging drop of blood to target area on strip, being certain that entire area is covered with blood<br>e. Read the patient's glucose value from the meter and record<br>f. Discard the test strip in biohazard container<br>g. Turn off the meter and return it to storage | | | |
| 6. Perform a blood glucose measurement using the HemoCue® following steps 6a-6k:<br>a. Turn on the meter<br>b. Insert the control cuvette into the meter. Check to see that instrument is calibrated.<br>c. Fill a cuvette with a glucose control solution following the manufacturer's directions<br>d. Place the cuvette in the carrier and gently push it into the HemoCue®. Read the value displayed and record on quality control log. Verify that control solution is within acceptable range<br>e. Discard cuvette<br>f. Obtain a new cuvette<br>g. Perform capillary puncture on patient<br>h. Fill the cuvette from the capillary puncture. Do not allow air bubbles into the cuvette<br>i. Place the cuvette in the carrier and gently push it into the HemoCue®<br>j. Read the patient's glucose value from the display and record<br>k. Discard the cuvette in a biohazard container<br>l. Turn off the meter, wipe it with disinfectant, if necessary, and return it to storage | | | |
| 7. Perform a blood glucose measurement using a glucose meter:<br>a. Perform quality control check following manufacturer's instructions<br>b. Perform capillary puncture on patient | | | |

| You must: | S | U | Comments |
|---|---|---|---|
| c. Apply blood to test strip or cartridge and insert into meter according to manufacturer's instructions<br>d. Read the patient's glucose value from the meter and record<br>e. Discard the test strip in biohazàrd container<br>f. Turn off the meter and return it to storage | | | |
| 8. Discard used capillary puncture materials in appropriate bio-hazard containers | | | |
| 9. Disinfect work area with surface disinfectant | | | |
| 10. Remove and discard gloves in biohazard container and wash hands with hand disinfectant. | | | |

*Evaluator Comments:*

Evaluator _____ Date _____

## *Worksheet*

### LESSON 6-6 Measuring Blood Glucose

Name _____  Date _____

1. Instrument Name: _____
2. Control test:  Record lot numbers and acceptable ranges of glucose controls and reagent test unit.  Record results of control test(s).  If test(s) is within range, mark acceptable (A); if not, mark unacceptable (U).

Test Unit Lot # _____

**Glucose Controls**

|  | Lot No. | Acceptable Range | Control Results | A | U |
|---|---|---|---|---|---|
| Normal | _____ | _____ | _____ | _____ | _____ |
| Low | _____ | _____ | _____ | _____ | _____ |
| High | _____ | _____ | _____ | _____ | _____ |

Action taken if control test is unacceptable: _____

_____

_____

3. Patient test:  Record the results below and compare with the normal range given.

| Patient I.D. | Test Result | Reference Range (whole blood) |
|---|---|---|
| _____ | _____ | 60-100 mg/dL |
| _____ | _____ | |
| _____ | _____ | |
| _____ | _____ | |

# Measuring Electrolytes

## LESSON OBJECTIVES

**After studying this lesson, you should be able to:**

- *Name the major cations and anions in body fluids.*
- *Name the four electrolytes routinely tested for.*
- *Name the major intracellular electrolyte.*
- *List the major extracellular electrolytes.*
- *Give the electrolyte reference ranges.*
- *Measure electrolytes using an analyzer.*
- *Describe safety precautions that must be observed when performing clinical chemistry tests.*
- *Define the glossary terms.*

## GLOSSARY

**acidosis** / abnormal condition in which blood pH falls below 7.35

**alkalosis** / abnormal condition in which blood pH rises above 7.45

**hyperkalemia** / blood potassium levels above normal

**hypernatremia** / blood sodium levels above normal

**hypokalemia** / blood potassium levels below normal

**hyponatremia** / blood sodium levels below normal

**osmolality** / measure indicating the number of dissolved solids in a fluid, usually serum or urine

## INTRODUCTION

Ions in body fluids are called electrolytes. Major ions include the positively charged cations, sodium, potassium, calcium, and magnesium, and the negatively charged anions, chloride, bicarbonate, and phosphate. However, a request for laboratory electrolyte measurement usually means the physician wants serum levels of four electrolytes measured—sodium ($Na^+$), potassium ($K^+$), chloride ($Cl^-$), and bicarbonate ($HCO_3^-$).

Proper electrolyte balance within the body's fluid compartments is essential to normal cellular functions. Electrolyte concentrations in body fluids are maintained within narrow ranges. The factors contributing to balanced electrolyte concentrations are complex. Homeostatic mechanisms regulate the distribution of fluid and ions within various body compartments, as well as their excretion.

Electrolyte imbalances occur when the serum concentration of an electrolyte is either too high or too low, affecting all organs and body systems. These imbalances can be life-threatening if not brought under control. Therefore, electrolyte measurement is often ordered as a STAT test and is included in many hospital POCT programs.

This lesson provides a brief introduction to the functions of the four major electrolytes and to methods of measurement. Other ions such as calcium and phosphorus are discussed in Lesson 6-1.

# FUNCTION AND IMPORTANCE OF ELECTROLYTES

Changes in electrolyte balance affect the function of all organ systems. In general, sodium affects osmolality of blood, and therefore influences body water distribution, blood volume, blood pressure, and fluid retention or loss. Potassium is important in maintaining normal muscular activity in the heart and skeletal muscle through transmission of electrical impulses. Bicarbonate, produced from carbon dioxide ($CO_2$) formation during cellular metabolism, is important in maintaining blood pH.

# ELECTROLYTE REFERENCE RANGES AND CLINICAL SIGNIFICANCE

Electrolyte concentrations are expressed either in millimoles per liter (mmol/L), which are SI units, or as milliequivalents per liter (mEq/L). Since one mEq equals one mmol for monovalent ions such as electrolytes, the numerical value of an electrolyte is the same regardless of the units used. Reference ranges for serum electrolytes are given in Table 6-11.

The electrolytes are distributed unequally between the intracellular (inside the cell) and extracellular (outside the cell) spaces (Figure 6-27). In some illnesses, the normal water and electrolyte balance is altered because of sudden fluid loss due to vomiting, diarrhea, or excessive urination. Such sudden imbalances can be harmful.

As shown in Figure 6-27, potassium is the major intracellular cation, whereas sodium is the major extracellular cation. Chloride and bicarbonate are in low concentrations inside the cells and in higher concentrations outside cells.

## Sodium

The reference range for serum sodium is 135–148 mmol/L (mEq/L). Sodium has an important influence on osmotic concentration and determines the extracellular fluid volume. Water moves back and forth across cell membranes to maintain proper sodium balance; rapid shifts in the water volume in cells can damage or destroy cells. Sodium concentration is influenced by aldosterone levels and kidney function.

**Hypernatremia**, increased concentration of sodium, occurs in dehydration, hyperadrenalism (Cushing's disease), and diabetes insipidus (a deficiency of antidiuretic hormone). **Hyponatremia**, decreased concentration of sodium, occurs in severe diarrhea, acidosis of diabetes mellitus, decreased aldosterone secretion (Addison's disease), and renal disease in which there is poor ion exchange in the tubules.

## Potassium

The reference range for serum potassium is 3.5–5.4 mmol/L (mEq/L). Potassium is excreted by the kidney. Abnormally high or low levels of potassium should be reported immediately to the physician because levels outside normal limits can affect muscle function, particularly in the heart.

**Hyperkalemia**, increased serum potassium, can occur when potassium leaves cells rapidly, and may occur in anoxia and acidosis. Increased potassium levels cause a decrease in muscle function, and may occur in decreased aldosterone secretion, circulatory failure (shock), and renal failure. **Hypokalemia**, decreased serum potassium, may be due to decreased intake of potassium, increased levels of aldosterone, or increased loss of potassium due to vomiting, diarrhea, or use of diuretics.

**Table 6-11.** Reference values for serum electrolytes

| ELECTROLYTE | REFERENCE RANGE mmol/L (mEq/L) |
|---|---|
| sodium ($Na^+$) | 135–148 |
| potassium ($K^+$) | 3.8–5.5 |
| chloride ($Cl^-$) | 98–108 |
| bicarbonate (total $CO_2$) | 22–28 |

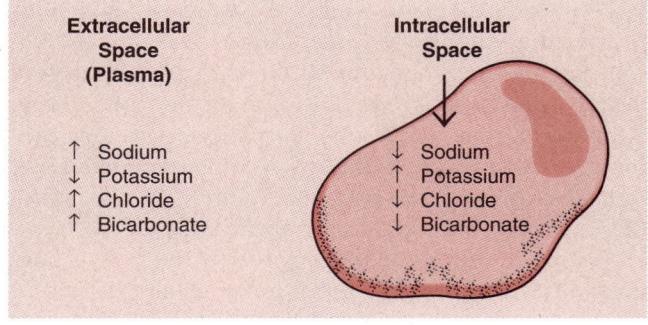

**FIGURE 6-27** Relative intracellular and extracellular electrolyte concentrations

## Chloride

Chloride is the anion with the highest extracellular concentration; the reference range for serum is 98–108 mmol/L (mEq/L). Chloride concentration varies inversely with bicarbonate ($HCO_3^-$). The concentration of chloride will increase in dehydration or in loss of $CO_2$ by hyperventilation (respiratory alkalosis). Decreased chloride concentration may occur in acidosis caused by uncontrolled diabetes, renal disease, and excessive vomiting.

## Bicarbonate (CO$_2$ Content)

The bicarbonate anion is part of the blood buffer system that helps maintain a normal blood pH of 7.4; it is usually measured as total $CO_2$. The reference range for serum is 22–28 mmol/L (mEq/L). Carbon dioxide ($CO_2$) is constantly generated by metabolic processes. Combining of $CO_2$ and water ($H_2O$) creates carbonic acid ($H_2CO_3^-$), which is converted to hydrogen ion (H+) and bicarbonate:

$$H_2O + CO_2 \longrightarrow H_2CO_3 \longrightarrow H^+ + HCO_3^-$$

When the ratio of bicarbonate anion to carbonic acid changes, the pH changes. **Acidosis** occurs when the pH falls below 7.35 and may be caused by decreased $HCO_3^-$ concentrations. **Alkalosis**, caused by increased $HCO_3^-$ concentrations, occurs when the pH is greater than 7.45.

The bicarbonate concentration is affected rapidly by changes in respiration, the body's way of eliminating $CO_2$. Changes in lung function, such as pneumonia, or central nervous system (CNS) depression or stimulation due to drugs, will affect $HCO_3^-$ concentrations. Concentration changes may also occur in diabetic ketosis and renal failure.

## Anion Gap

The anion gap (AG) is a mathematical calculation of the difference between the cation concentrations (sodium and potassium) and anion concentrations (chloride and bicarbonate) routinely measured in the electrolyte test. The cations not measured in the electrolyte test are calcium and magnesium; these average 7 mmol/L. The anions not measured in the electrolyte test are phosphate, sulfate, and anions of organic acids; these average 24 mmol/L.

The anion gap is calculated by the following formula:

$$([NA^+] + [K^+]) - ([Cl^-] + [HCO_3^-]) = AG \ (mmol/L)$$

The normal anion gap is 10-17 mmol/L. If the sum of measured anions subtracted from the sum of measured cations is greater than 17 (mmol/L), this indicates an increase in unmeasured anions. Conditions that could cause this are acidosis, diabetic ketosis, starvation, or uremia. The anion gap calculation is useful for quality control of electrolyte laboratory results.

# METHODS OF MEASURING ELECTROLYTES

In the past, sodium and potassium were measured by atomic absorption spectrophotometry or flame photometry. Chloride was measured by titration or colorimetry, and $CO_2$ by manometry or colorimetry. Most analyzers today use ion-selective electrodes and $PCO_2$ electrodes that can be incorporated in compact instruments suitable for use in small laboratories (Figure 6-28). These analyzers can test serum, plasma, or whole blood, depending on their design. Principles of ion-selective electrodes are discussed in Lesson 6-4, Instrumentation in the POL.

 **Safety**

Universal and Standard Precautions must be observed when performing any laboratory test using blood or other body substances. Gloves and other appropriate PPE must be worn when obtaining the blood specimen and performing the test. Used test cartridges must be discarded in appropriate biohazard containers.

*Quality Assurance*

Manufacturer's instructions must be followed for the instrument used. All performance checks must be performed and documented as outlined in the procedure manual. Test cartridges or cassettes must be tested with abnormal and normal control sera or calibrators at required intervals. Patient specimens should be run only after all quality control procedures have been successfully performed.

## i-STAT® Portable Clinical Analyzer

The i-STAT® Portable Clinical Analyzer, distributed by Abbott Laboratories, is an example of an instrument used in POCT at critical care sites. It is a hand-held analyzer with a test menu that includes sodium, potassium, chloride, and bicarbonate, as well as glucose, BUN, calcium, pH, hemoglobin, and hematocrit. Several parame-

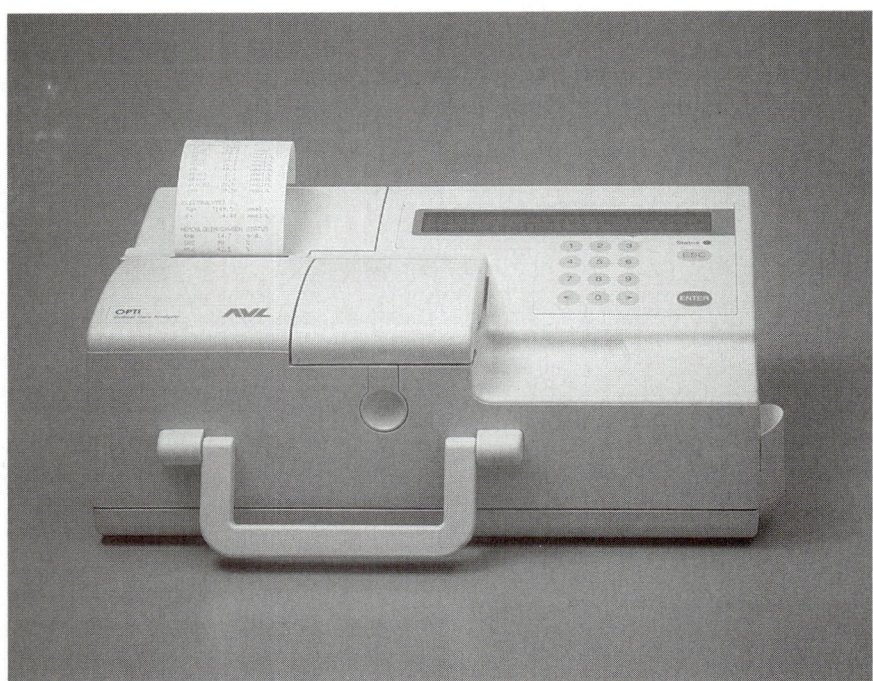

**FIGURE 6-28** Example of small chemistry analyzer that can measure electrolytes

ters can be measured at one time using a sample size of only two or three drops of blood easily obtained from a capillary puncture and directly applied to a test cartridge. Test results are available within two to three minutes.

Electrolyte levels are measured by applying the patient's specimen to a single-use cartridge that also contains a calibration solution. The calibrator and the patient specimen are passed over miniaturized ion-specific electrodes within the cartridge that detect and measure the various electrolytes and correlate the results to values obtained with serum or plasma. Procedural checks within the instrument monitor the cartridge performance and user technique. Quality control cartridges inserted in the instrument monitor the electrical sensors. The i-STAT® also contains data management capabilities that simplify reporting patient results and maintaining quality control records.

## Other POCT Electrolyte Analyzers

### GEM® Premier Plus

Instrumentation Laboratory's GEM® Premier Plus is a blood gas and electrolyte analyzer useful in POCT sites such as intensive care units, emergency rooms, and sur-

gery suites. The analyzer can also measure hematocrit and perform coagulation tests. A computerized data management system allows central management of information generated by all units.

### IRMA® SL Blood Analysis System

The IRMA SL Blood Analysis System by Diametrics Medical is a bedside system that tests for blood gases, electrolytes, hematocrit, BUN, and blood glucose. The analyzer also measures $Na^+$, $K^+$, and $Cl^-$ and calculates $HCO_3^-$.

### OPTI® Critical Care Analyzer™

The OPTI® Critical Care Analyzer™ by AVL Scientific has single-use cassettes to measure up to eight different parameters, including some calculated parameters (Figure 6-28). The instrument operates on the principle of optical fluorescence. Tests available include blood gases (pH, oxygen saturation), hemoglobin, and electrolytes. The analyzer standardizes sample introduction. Whole blood, serum, or plasma may be used and sampling can be done directly from syringes and capillary tubes.

## Nova 16 Analyzer

The Nova 16 Analyzer provides a chemistry profile containing the tests most frequently ordered in STAT chemistries. It is small enough to be portable on a cart and is useful both in intensive care units in large hospitals or in POLs. Most tests are performed using ion-selective electrodes and biosensors within the instrument. These electrodes are self-cleaning and essentially maintenance-free. The instrument aspirates the patient sample with an automatic sampling probe and completes an eight-test profile in eighty-five seconds. Only three drops of whole blood, serum, plasma, or urine are required to measure eight analytes.

### Procedural Notes

- Follow manufacturer's guidelines for proper specimen collection.
- Run appropriate normal and abnormal control sera or calibrators as required.
- Follow instrument manufacturer's operating instructions.

### Safety Precautions

- Follow Universal and Standard Precautions when handling specimens for chemical analysis.
- Discard all contaminated materials in appropriate biohazard containers.

## LESSON REVIEW

1. Name the four electrolytes commonly tested for. Give the reference ranges for each.
2. Which electrolyte is important in pH balance?
3. Which electrolyte is most important in maintaining fluid balance?
4. Which electrolyte is in highest concentration in the intracellular fluids?
5. What is the importance of potassium in the body?
6. What kind of blood specimens can be used to measure electrolytes?
7. Name four conditions that could cause electrolyte imbalance.
8. By what method are electrolytes measured in the newest analyzers?
9. What is the anion gap?
10. Define acidosis, alkalosis, hyperkalemia, hypernatremia, hypokalemia, hyponatremia, and osmolality.

## STUDENT ACTIVITIES

1. Reread the information on measuring electrolytes.
2. Review the glossary terms.
3. Perform measurement of electrolytes as outlined on the Student Performance Guide.

## *Student Performance Guide*

## **LESSON 6-7** Measuring Electrolytes

Name _____ Date _____

### INSTRUCTIONS

1. Practice measuring electrolytes using an analyzer and following the step-by-step procedure.
2. Demonstrate your understanding of this lesson by:
   a. Completing a written examination successfully, and
   b. Performing the procedure for measuring electrolytes as directed by the instructor. All steps must be completed as listed on the instructor's Performance Check Sheet.

*Note:* The following is a general procedure for measuring electrolytes. The manufacturers' instructions for the specific methods or instruments being used must be consulted and carefully followed.

### MATERIALS AND EQUIPMENT

- gloves
- serum or plasma specimens
- blood-collection equipment for:
  syringe venipuncture
  vacuum-tube venipuncture
  capillary puncture
- i-STAT® analyzer or other small analyzer capable of measuring electrolytes, including test cartridges and necessary controls
- quality control charts
- surface disinfectant
- biohazard container
- biohazard sharps container

### PROCEDURE

Record in the comment section any problems encountered while practicing the procedure (or have a fellow student or the instructor evaluate your performance).

S = Satisfactory
U = Unsatisfactory

| You must: | S | U | Comments |
|---|---|---|---|
| 1. Assemble equipment and materials | | | |
| 2. Wash hands and put on gloves | | | |
| 3. Turn on instrument | | | |
| 4. Perform quality control checks as directed by manufacturer and record results on quality control chart | | | |
| 5. Obtain test cartridge or cassette | | | |
| 6. Perform capillary puncture (or use previously obtained blood specimen) | | | |

| You must: | S | U | Comments |
|---|---|---|---|
| 7.　Apply blood specimen to test cartridge | | | |
| 8.　Insert cartridge into instrument | | | |
| 9.　Read and record test results | | | |
| 10.　Discard test cartridge in biohazard container | | | |
| 11.　Turn off instrument and store according to manufacturer's directions | | | |
| 12.　Discard all capillary puncture materials appropriately | | | |
| 13.　Clean work surface with surface disinfectant | | | |
| 14.　Remove and discard gloves and wash hands with hand disinfectant | | | |

*Evaluator Comments:*

Evaluator _____ Date _____

# *Measuring Blood Cholesterol*

## LESSON OBJECTIVES

**After studying this lesson, you should be able to:**

- *Explain the functions of cholesterol in the body.*
- *Give the mean values for total cholesterol for males and females in each age group.*
- *Discuss the dangers of elevated cholesterol levels.*
- *Explain the importance of high-density lipoprotein (HDL) and low-density lipoprotein (LDL) cholesterol.*
- *Give the mean values for HDL cholesterol for males and females in each age group.*
- *Explain how the risk factor for heart disease can be calculated from the HDL and LDL cholesterol values.*
- *Explain the principle of enzymatic cholesterol measurement methods.*
- *Perform a cholesterol determination.*
- *Define the glossary terms.*

## GLOSSARY

**atherosclerosis** / condition in which lipids, calcium, and other substances deposit on the inner surface of the arteries

**endogenous** / produced within; growing from within

**enzyme** / protein that causes or accelerates changes in other substances without being changed itself

**exogenous** / originating from the outside

**HDL cholesterol** / high-density lipoprotein fraction of total blood cholesterol

**LDL cholesterol** / low-density lipoprotein fraction of total blood cholesterol

**myocardial infarction (MI)** / heart attack caused by obstruction of the blood supply to or within the heart

## INTRODUCTION

Measuring the total blood cholesterol level, along with the levels of cholesterol fractions, has become commonplace as the important role of cholesterol in coronary artery disease and other atherosclerotic conditions has become apparent. The level of cholesterol, its fractions, and other blood lipids may be included in a chemistry profile, or ordered as a lipid profile.

Many people know their "cholesterol number" and are aware of food especially high or low in choles-terol. Although most people have the test performed in a POL or reference laboratory, cholesterol screening is often offered through health fairs and by employers, pharmacies, or others. Blood bank organizations such as the Red Cross often measure the total cholesterol level and report it to the donor. Increased interest in and availability of blood cholesterol testing is a responsible reaction to knowing the importance of controlling blood cholesterol levels.

This lesson presents basic information about the biological function of cholesterol, sources of choles-

447

terol, and the relationship of blood cholesterol levels to health. Both manual and automated methods of measuring blood, serum, and plasma cholesterol levels are introduced.

## BIOLOGICAL ROLE OF CHOLESTEROL

Cholesterol, a lipid sterol, is an important component of all body tissues. It is a major constituent of all mammalian cell membranes, except those in RBCs. Since lipids have limited solubility in water, they help the cellular membrane control the flow of water-soluble substances in and out of the cell. A relatively large amount of cholesterol is located in the skin, where it protects against the absorption of water-soluble substances. It also aids in protecting against damaging chemical agents, such as acids, and excessive water evaporation from the skin.

Another major function of cholesterol is to serve as a precursor to bile salts and steroid hormones. The sex hormones, adrenal steroids, and bile salts are synthesized from cholesterol in specific cells of the ovaries, testes, adrenal gland, and liver. The chemical structure of cholesterol is shown in Figure 6-29.

### Sources of Cholesterol

Everyone eats at least some cholesterol. This dietary cholesterol is called **exogenous** cholesterol and is found in animal fats and egg yolks. People who eat a rich, fatty diet may develop dangerously increased blood cholesterol levels. Certain body tissues, especially the liver, can synthesize cholesterol; this is called **endogenous** cholesterol.

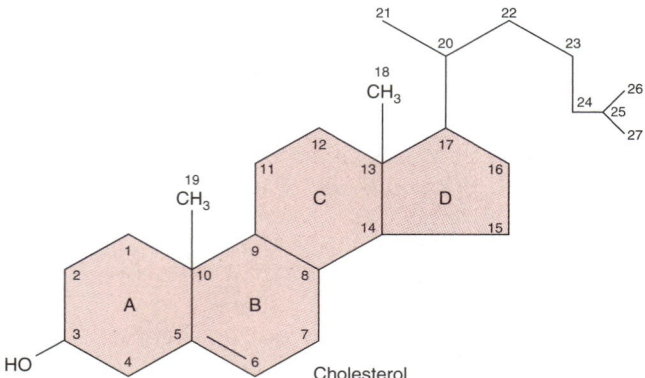

**FIGURE 6-29** Structure of the cholesterol molecule

## RISKS ASSOCIATED WITH INCREASED BLOOD CHOLESTEROL

When blood cholesterol levels remain elevated, a condition known as **atherosclerosis** may occur in which fat accumulates on the inner walls of blood vessels, narrowing the vessel opening. These deposits are especially likely to form on any damaged surface of the vessel wall. Although other fats (lipids) are found in these deposits, the major portion is cholesterol. Once these deposits form, their rough edges may cause blood clots to develop. These clots can either damage the area they are in or travel to smaller vessels in vital organs such as the brain, heart, kidneys, or liver, and cut off the blood supply to these organs. The result may be stroke, heart attack, damage to other organs, or disease of the blood vessels themselves.

## BLOOD CHOLESTEROL: TOTAL CHOLESTEROL, HDL, AND LDL

In the past, blood cholesterol was reported only as total cholesterol. Now it is more meaningful to measure total cholesterol and the fractions of cholesterol. The two fractions commonly measured are called high-density lipoprotein (**HDL**) cholesterol and low-density lipoprotein (**LDL**) cholesterol. Some experts believe that HDL or LDL levels are genetically determined.

HDL transports cholesterol from the tissues to the liver to be broken down, mostly into bile acids. Because of this, HDL is called "good" cholesterol. LDL transports cholesterol to the tissues to be deposited as fat. LDL is sometimes referred to as "bad" cholesterol.

If the total cholesterol concentration is elevated in a patient, the physician can use the HDL and LDL values to aid in determining the heart attack risk factor of the elevated cholesterol. Other factors, such as smoking and lack of exercise, also influence the risk.

### Reference Values for Cholesterol

At birth, serum cholesterol ranges from about 50 mg/dL to 100 mg/dL. At one month, the levels approach 100 to 230 mg/dL and remain at those levels until the age of 20 or 21 years. Cholesterol levels for adults are affected by age, diet, and gender. Even the patient's posture at collection can effect results. Studies have shown that cholesterol values increase 10-20% in the nonresting patient compared to the resting patient. Estrogen seems to lower cholesterol levels, since in post-menopausal women the cholesterol level tends to increase.

Typical cholesterol values by age group are shown in Table 6-12. *These are not the recommended levels.* Organizations such as the American Heart

**Table 6–12.** Reference values for total blood cholesterol

| AGE (years) | RANGE* mg/dL | MALES mg/dL | FEMALES mg/dL |
|---|---|---|---|
| 0-19 | 120-230 | — | — |
| 20-29 | 120-240 | 235 | 220 |
| 30-39 | 140-270 | 265 | 240 |
| 40-49 | 150-310 | 280 | 265 |
| 50-59 | 160-330 | 300 | 320 |

\* The upper limits of ranges are not necessarily the desired levels, but represent levels found in the U.S. population.

**Table 6–13.** Reference ranges for HDL and LDL cholesterol

| Age (years) | HDL | | LDL |
| | Male Range mg/dL | Female Range mg/dL | Male and Female mg/dL |
|---|---|---|---|
| 0-19 | 30-65 | 30-70 | 50-170 |
| 20-29 | 30-65 | 36-78 | 60-170 |
| 30-39 | 30-59 | 33-77 | 70-190 |
| 40-49 | 25-61 | 40-81 | 80-190 |
| 50-75 | 29-72 | 38-91 | 80-210 |

Association and the National Cholesterol Education Program recommend total cholesterol be kept below 200 mg/dL. Cholesterol of 240 mg/dL or above is considered to present a high risk of heart disease. Cholesterol levels between 200 and 239 mg/dL are considered borderline. Typical values for HDL and LDL are shown in Table 6-13.

## DETERMINING THE HEART ATTACK RISK FACTOR

To determine the heart attack risk factor, the physician uses the LDL/HDL ratio. The smaller the ratio, the less the risk factor. When HDL is above the average value, it may reduce the risk of **myocardial infarction**, a type of heart attack, by as much as one-third.

As an example, a forty-five-year-old male (patient one) with an LDL level of 80 mg/dL and an HDL of 59 mg/dL would have a lower risk of heart attack than a second male (patient two) of the same age and identical LDL level, but an HDL of 30 mg/dL. The risk factor (RF) is calculated by dividing the LDL by the HDL (RF = LDL/HDL). A low number means the risk of heart attack is decreased.

Patient one: $\dfrac{\text{LDL}}{\text{HDL}} = \text{RF}$

$\dfrac{80 \text{ mg/dL}}{59 \text{ mg/dL}} = 1.3$

Patient two: $\dfrac{\text{LDL}}{\text{HDL}} = \text{RF}$

$\dfrac{80 \text{ mg/dL}}{30 \text{ mg/dL}} = 2.7$

Therefore, in this comparison, patient one has a lower risk factor for heart attack than patient two.

## PERFORMING CHOLESTEROL TESTS

  **Safety**

The specimen for measuring the blood cholesterol level can be serum, heparinized plasma, or whole blood. Universal and Standard Precautions must always be followed when handling patient samples and controls and standards. Appropriate PPE must be used. Blood-collection supplies, such as lancets or needles, must be discarded in the biohazard sharps container. Reagent strips, test packs, alcohol swabs, and other supplies used in the test must be discarded in biohazard waste containers.

*Quality Assurance*

When a patient has a blood cholesterol test performed, the result is used to guide the physician. If the value is elevated, the physician may prescribe medication, exercise, or diet change, or some combination of these. The correct type of specimen must be collected for the analytical method being used.

Manufacturers of both manual and automated methods of cholesterol determination provide calibrators (if necessary to the method) and controls. The controls are analyzed along with the patient samples. In the automated reagent strip methods, the liquid control is applied to a new strip in the same manner as a patient sample and is then analyzed in the instrument. This checks the reliability of the reagent strips, the function of the instrument and the worker's technique. If the control assay results are not within acceptable limits, the patient results cannot be reported until the problem is found and corrected.

## Cholesterol Test Methods

The serum cholesterol level can be determined in the laboratory using either chemical or enzyme methods. Techniques for measuring total serum cholesterol have been used for decades, but efficient, easy methods for measuring HDL and LDL cholesterol have been available only since about 1980.

The enzymatic methods for testing cholesterol and its fractions are simpler, and use safer chemicals than the nonenzyme (chemical) methods. Several enzymatic kits that use serum, whole blood, or plasma are available commercially. The enzymatic methods have also been adapted to automated instruments.

## Manual Methods for Measuring Cholesterol

Several enzymatic methods are available for determining total cholesterol and HDL and LDL fractions. The different methods' principle is similar. The reactions described here are in Procedure No. 352 from Sigma Diagnostics®.

### The Sigma Method

Cholesterol is separated from the other constituents in the sample by an **enzyme**, cholesterol esterase. A second enzyme, cholesterol oxidase, oxidizes the cholesterol released in the previous reaction, producing a ketone (cholestenone) plus hydrogen peroxide ($H_2O_2$). The hydrogen peroxide produced is then coupled with the chromagen, 4- aminoantipyrine, and p-hydroxybenzenesulfonate in the presence of peroxidase. A quinoneimine dye whose absorbance can be measured at 500 nm is the end product of the reaction. The intensity of the dye color is proportional to the concentration of cholesterol in the sample. The reactions are as follows:

$$\text{Cholesterol esters} + H_2O \xrightarrow[\text{Esterase}]{\text{Cholesterol}} \text{Cholesterol} + \text{Fatty acids}$$
(in patient sample)

$$\text{Cholesterol} + O_2 \xrightarrow[\text{Oxidase}]{\text{Cholesterol}} \text{cholest-4-en-3-one} + H_2O_2$$

$$2\,H_2O_2 + \text{4-aminoantipyrine} + \text{p-hydroxybenzenesulfonate}$$

$$\xrightarrow{\text{Peroxidase}} \text{Quinoneimine dye} + 4\,H_2O$$

The preferred specimen for this procedure is either serum or heparinized plasma. Plasma collected in other anticoagulants such as oxalate, citrate, or EDTA yields slightly lower total cholesterol values.

All of the reactants necessary to perform the test are contained in one reagent called Cholesterol Reagent, which is reconstituted by adding deionized water just before use.

A series of tubes is set up for Blank, Calibrator, Control, and Sample. The reagent is warmed to the assay temperature. One milliliter of reagent is added to each tube in the series. The test specimens—Blank (10 μL of deionized water), Calibrator, Control, and Sample—are added to appropriately labeled tubes. The tubes are then mixed by gentle inversion, using Parafilm® to cover the tops. All the tubes are incubated for the appropriate time for the selected incubation temperature. The absorbance of each tube is read at 500 nm within thirty minutes after incubation is completed. The concentration of cholesterol is calculated using the following formula:

$$\text{Serum cholesterol (mg/dL)} = \frac{A_{TEST} - A_{BLANK}}{A_{CALIBRATOR} - A_{BLANK}} \times \text{Calibrator (mg/dL)}$$

For example, a test serum was assayed for total cholesterol concentration by the described procedure, and the following absorbance values were obtained:

$$A_{BLANK} = 0.022$$
$$A_{TEST} = 0.325$$
$$A_{CALIBRATOR} = 0.310$$

$$\text{Serum cholesterol (mg/dL)} = \frac{A_{TEST} - A_{BLANK}}{A_{CAL} - A_{BLANK}} \times \text{Cal (mg/dL)}$$

$$\text{Serum cholesterol (mg/dL)} = \frac{0.325 - 0.022}{0.310 - 0.022} \times 200^*$$

$$= 210 \text{ mg/dL}$$

\* Concentration (mg/dL) of cholesterol in calibrator

The total serum cholesterol of this sample is 210 mg/dL.

The instructions are accompanied by a list of materials required, calibration instructions, and quality control information. It is important to always read the procedure bulletin that accompanies the assay kit being used, since procedures are periodically modified.

### Determination of HDL Cholesterol

Some cholesterol kits also can assay the HDL fraction of cholesterol. To determine the serum HDL, lipoproteins other than HDL are precipitated with a precipitating reagent, and the sample is centrifuged. The liquid portion (supernatant) contains the HDL fraction of cholesterol. This supernatant is used as the sample in cholesterol measurement methods. In this case, the dye color is proportional to the amount of HDL cholesterol in the serum.

## Automated Methods for Measuring Cholesterol

The most popular automated methods for measuring cholesterol are based on the same principles as the enzymatic manual methods. However, many of these automated methods are simple to perform and take much less time to complete than the manual methods.

### Solid-phase Reagent Strip Methods

The majority of the automated methods used in small laboratories use *solid-phase reagent strips*. All the reagents needed for the test reactions are embedded in a reagent pad on the plastic strip. As in the manual method, the reaction is enzymatic, and uses the same enzymes. Examples of such instruments are the Reflotron® and Accu-Chek® Instant Plus by Roche Diagnostics Corporation.

To perform the test, the worker selects the appropriate strip for cholesterol. A drop of whole blood, serum, or plasma is placed directly on the test area (reagent pad). If whole blood is being used, the cellular elements of the blood are removed by a special layer in the pad. The plasma is absorbed into the pad and mixes with the reagents.

The strip must be placed in the instrument within a specified time after sample application. A magnetic code on the back of the strip signals the instrument as to which test is to be performed. The instrument then displays this information in the read-out area and the worker can confirm that the correct test strip is being used.

A reflectance photometer detects color changes in the reagent pad. The reaction proceeds for the required time, usually about three minutes. The instrument then displays the result in the read-out area. The simplicity, short time requirement, and option of using a drop of whole blood from a fingerstick make this a very desirable test method for POLs.

### Cholestech L*D*X®

Another compact instrument that can perform a lipid profile, plus glucose determination, is marketed by Cholestech Corporation (Figure 6-30). The Cholestech L*D*X® System can be used to screen for risk of coronary disease in corporate wellness programs or community health screens.

A capillary blood sample is collected and added to the sample well of the test cassette. Each cassette contains the reagents for a specific analysis, such as total cholesterol, or total cholesterol and HDL. The test cassette is inserted into the analyzer and the result is ready in less than five minutes.

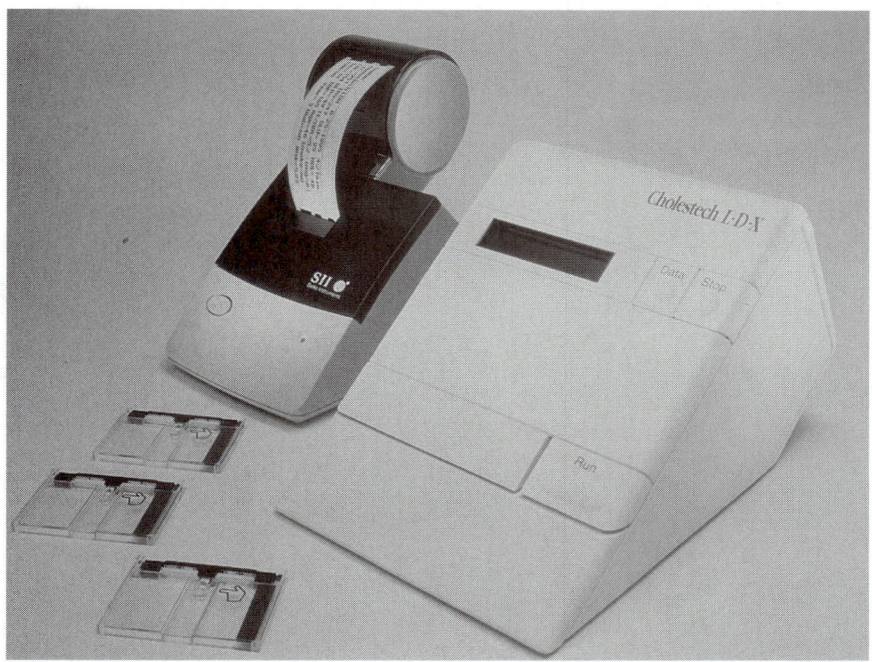

**FIGURE 6-30** Cholestech L*D*X® cholesterol analyzer (Photo courtesy of Cholestech Corporation, Hayward, CA)

## Procedural Notes

- Use test kits or reagent strips only with the instruments for which they are intended.
- Follow manufacturer's instructions exactly.
- Pipet accurately to ensure good results.

## Safety Precautions

- Observe Universal and Standard Precautions when working with blood samples and standard and control solutions.
- Discard used sharps in a biohazard sharps container.
- Dispose of all biohazard waste in a biohazard container.
- Wipe work area with surface disinfectant when work is finished.
- Wash hands with hand disinfectant.

## LESSON REVIEW

1. What are the functions of cholesterol in the body?
2. What are the dangers of an elevated serum cholesterol?

3. Why are HDL and LDL cholesterol levels important?
4. What are the normal reference values for total cholesterol for males and females in the age groups 20-29 and 40-49?
5. Give the mean HDL cholesterol reference values for males and females in the 40–49-year-old age range.
6. How is the risk factor for heart disease calculated using HDL and LDL cholesterol values?
7. Explain the principles of the enzymatic cholesterol measurement methods.
8. Explain how to perform a manual cholesterol determination.
9. Define atherosclerosis, endogenous, enzyme, exogenous, HDL cholesterol, LDL cholesterol, and myocardial infarction.

## STUDENT ACTIVITIES

1. Reread the information on measuring blood cholesterol.
2. Review the glossary terms.
3. If cholesterol screening is offered in your community, ask which method of analysis is being used.
4. If possible, determine which instruments are used in some local POLs.
5. Review the general instructions for performing an automated cholesterol test.
6. Practice performing a cholesterol determination as outlined in the Student Performance Guide, using whichever method is available.

# *Student Performance Guide*

## **LESSON 6-8** Measuring Blood Cholesterol

Name _____ Date _____

## INSTRUCTIONS

1. Practice the procedure for measuring blood cholesterol following the step-by-step procedure.
2. Demonstrate your understanding of this lesson by:
   a. Completing a written examination successfully, and
   b. Performing the procedure for measuring blood cholesterol satisfactorily for the instructor. All steps must be completed as listed on the instructor's Performance Check Sheet.

*Note:* The following procedure is a general procedure for measuring cholesterol using Sigma Diagnostics® Procedure No. 352. Consult the manufacturer's instructions for the specific method being used.

## MATERIALS AND EQUIPMENT

- gloves
- blood-collecting equipment
- hand disinfectant
- spectrophotometer
- commercial kit for manual determination of cholesterol (or use an instrument, following all of the manufacturer's instructions)
- serum controls and cholesterol standards
- marking pencil
- test tubes (13 x 100 mm)
- test tube rack
- cuvettes for spectrophotometer
- laboratory tissue
- Parafilm®
- calculator (optional)
- pipetter with disposable tips
- water bath at 30°C or 37°C (optional)
- surface disinfectant (10% chlorine bleach solution)
- biohazard container
- instrument for performing cholesterol determination, including test materials, controls, and standards
- Levey-Jennings chart
- biohazard sharps container

## PROCEDURE

Record in the comment section any problems encountered while practicing the procedure (or have a fellow student or the instructor evaluate your performance).

S = Satisfactory
U = Unsatisfactory

| You must: | S | U | Comments |
|---|---|---|---|
| 1. Assemble equipment and materials | | | |
| 2. Wash hands and put on gloves | | | |
| 3. Obtain blood sample from the patient, either by fingerstick or venipuncture, depending on the type of sample required | | | |

| You must: | S | U | Comments |
|---|---|---|---|
| 4. Perform either method a or b:<br>   a. Manual method (Sigma Diagnostics® Procedure No. 352)<br>     (1) Prepare Cholesterol Reagent according to instructions<br>     (2) Turn on spectrophotometer and set wavelength to 500 nm<br>     (3) Set the absorbance reading to zero using water as the blank (reference)<br>     (4) If using spectrophotometer with temperature-controlled cuvette compartment, set temperature to 37°C, or the assay may be performed at ambient (room) temperature, or using a water bath at 30° or 37°C<br>     (5) Label cuvettes or test tubes for Blank, Calibrator, Control, and Sample<br>     (6) Warm reagent to the temperature being used for the assay<br>     (7) Pipet 1.0 mL of reagent into each of the prepared tubes<br>     (8) Add 0.01 mL (10 μL) deionized water to the Blank<br>     (9) Add 10 μL of Calibrator, Control, and Sample to the appropriately labeled tubes. Cover tubes with Parafilm® and mix tubes by gentle inversion<br>   (10) Incubate tubes or cuvettes for five minutes at 37°C or ten minutes at 25–30°C<br>   (11) Read and record absorbances of all tubes at 500 nm. Complete the readings within thirty minutes after the end of incubation time<br>   (12) Calculate total cholesterol in sample and control, using the absorbance formula (below). Record the results<br><br>$$\text{Serum cholesterol (mg/dL)} = \frac{A_{TEST} - A_{BLANK}}{A_{CALIBRATOR} - A_{BLANK}} \times \text{Calibrator (mg/dL)}$$ | | | |
|    b. Automated method (general)<br>     (1) Turn on the instrument<br>     (2) Wash hands and put on gloves<br>     (3) Prepare any control or calibrator reagents<br>     (4) Run appropriate controls or calibrator samples<br>     (5) Obtain correct patient specimen<br>     (6) Choose appropriate test strip or pack for cholesterol determination<br>     (7) Add patient sample to test system<br>     (8) Insert strip or pack in instrument<br>     (9) Ensure that correct test is being performed<br>   (10) Wait for results to be displayed or printed out<br>   (11) Record results | | | |
| 5. For each method, add the control values to a Levey-Jennings chart | | | |
| 6. If the method is in control, report patient values | | | |
| 7. Disinfect and clean reusable equipment | | | |

| You must: | S | U | Comments |
|---|---|---|---|
| 8. Dispose of contaminated materials in biohazard container or sharps container | | | |
| 9. Wipe work area with surface disinfectant | | | |
| 10. Turn instrument "OFF" (or leave as manual instructs) | | | |
| 11. Remove gloves and discard in biohazard container | | | |
| 12. Wash hands with hand disinfectant | | | |

*Evaluator Comments:*

Evaluator _____ Date _____

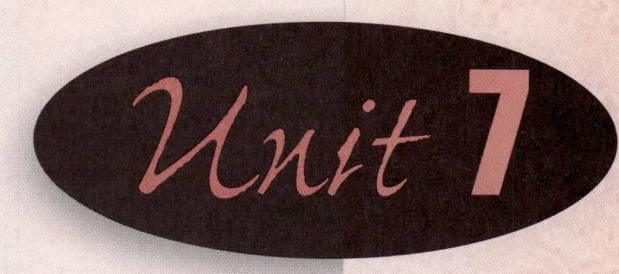

# Unit 7

# Basic Clinical Microbiology

Unit 7

## UNIT OBJECTIVES

**After studying this unit, you should be able to:**

- *Discuss the organisms included in the study of microbiology.*
- *Discuss the types of diseases caused by the different groups of microorganisms.*
- *Explain why organisms are classified as pathogens, opportunistic pathogens, or normal flora.*
- *Explain Standard Precautions and Transmission-Based Precautions.*
- *Discuss basic techniques and media used in bacteriology.*
- *Prepare, stain, and microscopically observe bacterial smears.*
- *Describe the three basic types of bacterial morphology.*
- *Discuss growth requirements of some common bacteria.*
- *Perform a throat culture and a rapid test for Group A Streptococcus.*
- *Perform a urine culture, colony count, and antibiotic susceptibility test.*
- *Explain the importance of laboratory testing for sexually transmitted diseases.*
- *Discuss laboratory test methods used to detect sexually transmitted diseases.*
- *Explain the importance and use of the fecal occult blood test.*

## UNIT OVERVIEW

Unit 7 is an introduction to clinical microbiology, including the microorganisms that cause disease and some of the laboratory tests to detect them. The clinical laboratory's microbiology department isolates and identifies medically important bacteria, viruses, fungi, and parasites. Although several test methods are presented in this unit, the emphasis is on those suitable for the smaller laboratory or physician's office. The majority of this work is bacteriology; however, advances in technology are providing more tests for virology and parasitology.

Lesson 7-1 concentrates on history, background information, terminology, and knowledge about the different groups of organisms in microbiology and the diseases they cause. Infection control and the new

CDC categories of Transmission-Based Precautions are discussed in Lesson 7-2. In Lesson 7-3, growth requirements of various bacteria are presented, along with instructions on using the inoculating loop. The differences in primary, selective, and indicator media are described, as well as their uses. Safety in the microbiology laboratory and use of aseptic technique are emphasized.

The stained bacterial smear is important in identifying an organism. Lesson 7-4 details how to prepare a smear, perform a Gram stain, and examine the smear microscopically for Gram stain reaction and morphology.

Rapid tests for Group A *Streptococcus*, which causes strep throat, are performed many times a day in most laboratories. A throat culture may also be performed if the rapid test is negative. The procedures to perform these two tests are given in Lesson 7-5.

Lesson 7-6 describes how to perform a urine culture, colony count, and antibiotic susceptibility test. Urine cultures are among the most frequently performed laboratory tests. They can be performed in the small laboratory as long as quality control measures are followed and qualified personnel are available.

Lesson 7-7 discusses sexually transmitted diseases (STDs) and the types of STD diagnostic tests available, including those suitable for the small laboratory.

The fecal occult blood test, discussed in Lesson 7-8, is used to screen for colorectal cancer. This test is often performed in the microbiology department.

## SUGGESTED READINGS AND REFERENCES

Baron, E. J., Peterson, L. R., & Finegold, S. M. (9th ed.). (1996). *Bailey & Scott's diagnostic microbiology*. St. Louis: C. V. Mosby Company.

Becan-McBride, K., & Ross, D. L. (1988). *Essentials for the small laboratory and physician's office*. Chicago: Year Book Medical Publishers, Inc.

Black, J. G. (3rd ed.). (1996). *Microbiology principles and applications*. Upper Saddle River, NJ: Prentice Hall.

Collins, C. H. (Ed.). (1988). *Safety in clinical and biomedical laboratories*. London: Chapman and Hall.

Greenwood, D., Slack, R., & Peutherer, J. (Eds.). (14th ed.). (1992). *Medical microbiology: A guide to microbial infections: Pathogenesis, immunity, laboratory diagnosis and control*. Edinburgh: Churchill Livingstone.

Henry, J. B. (Ed.). (19th ed.). (1996). *Clinical diagnosis and management by laboratory methods*. Philadelphia: W. B. Saunders Company.

Holt, J. G. (Ed.). (1984). *The shorter Bergey's manual of determinative bacteriology*. Baltimore: The Williams and Wilkins Company.

Hoawanitz, J. H. & Howanitz, P. J. (Eds.). (1991). *Laboratory medicine: Test selection and interpretation*. New York: Churchill Livingstone.

Jorgensen, J. H. (Ed.). (1987). *Automation in clinical microbiology*. Boca Raton, FL: CRC Press, Inc.

Kleger, B., et al. (Eds.). (1989). *Rapid methods in clinical microbiology: Present status and future trends*. New York: Plenum Publishing.

Koneman, E. W., et al. (4th ed.). (1992). *Color atlas and textbook of diagnostic microbiology*. Philadelphia: J. B. Lippincott.

Manufacturer's package insert, ColoScreen®. Helena Laboratories, Beaumont, TX.

Manufacturer's package insert, Hemoccult® and Hemoccult SENSA®. Beckman Coulter, Palo Alto, CA.

Marshall, J. (1993). *Fundamental skills for the clinical laboratory professional*. Albany, NY: Delmar Publishers, Inc.

O'Leary, W. (1989). *Practical handbook of microbiology*. Boca Raton, FL: CRC Press.

Rayburn, S. R. (1990). *The foundations of laboratory safety: A guide for the biomedical laboratory*. New York: Springer-Verlag.

Shimeld, L.A. & Rodgers, A. T. (1999). *Essentials of diagnostic microbiology*. Albany, NY: Delmar Publishers, Inc.

Stokes, E. J. & Ridgeway, G. L. (1987). *Clinical microbiology*. Baltimore: Edward Arnold.

Tenover, F. C. (1989). *DNA probes for infectious diseases*. Boca Raton, FL: Boca Raton Press, Inc.

# Introduction to Clinical Microbiology

## LESSON OBJECTIVES

**After studying this lesson, you should be able to:**

- *List the fields of study included in microbiology.*
- *Describe the microbiology department's organization in small and large laboratories.*
- *Discuss the differences among normal flora, pathogens, and opportunistic pathogens.*
- *Explain how infection occurs.*
- *Discuss the three basic shapes of bacteria.*
- *Explain the importance of correct specimen collection.*
- *Discuss seven methods used to help identify bacteria.*
- *Discuss common diagnostic methods used in virology, mycology, and parasitology.*
- *Define the glossary terms.*

## GLOSSARY

**aerobic** / requiring oxygen

**anaerobic** / growing only in the absence of oxygen

**antibiotic susceptibility testing** / determining the susceptibility of microorganisms to specific antibiotics

**bacillus** / rod-shaped bacterium

**coccus** / spherical bacterium

**colony** / defined mass of bacteria assumed to have grown from a single organism

**communicable** / able to be transmitted directly or indirectly from one individual to another

**culture** / growth of microorganisms in a special medium; the process of growing microorganisms in the laboratory

**DNA** / nucleic acid found primarily in the nucleus of all living cells that carries genetic information; deoxyribonucleic acid

**fastidious organism** / organism that requires special nutritional factors to survive

**fission** / asexual reproduction of a microorganism

**formalin** / solution of formaldehyde used as a fixative or preservative

**gram-negative** / designation for bacteria that lose the crystal violet (purple stain) and retain the safranin (red stain) in the Gram stain procedure

**gram-positive** / designation for bacteria that retain the crystal violet (purple stain) in the Gram stain procedure

**Gram stain** / differential stain used to classify bacteria

**host** / organism from which a parasite obtains nutrients and in which some or part of the parasite's life cycle is carried out

**hyphae** / filaments of mold that make up the mycelium

**immunoassay** / diagnostic method using antigen-antibody reactions

**infection** / pathological condition caused by growth of microorganisms in the host

**medium** / substance used to provide nutrients for growing microorganisms

**minimum inhibitory concentration (MIC)** / minimum concentration of an antibiotic required to inhibit the growth of a microorganism

**mycelium** / mass of hyphae that makes up the vegetative body of molds

**mycosis** / infection caused by fungi

**normal flora** / microorganisms normally present at a specific site

**opportunistic pathogen** / microorganism that causes disease in the host only when normal defense mechanisms are impaired or absent

**pathogen** / organism or agent capable of causing disease in a host

**progeny** / offspring or descendants

**RNA** / nucleic acid found in all living cells that is important in protein synthesis; ribonucleic acid

**spirochetes** / motile bacteria with a helical or spiral shape

**zone of inhibition** / in the antibiotic susceptibility test, the area around an antibiotic disk that contains no bacterial growth

## INTRODUCTION

Microbiology is the study of living organisms of microscopic size. Louis Pasteur first used the term in the 1860s. However, microorganisms were first observed in 1675 by Antony van Leeuwenhoek, a Dutchman. The term "microbe" was introduced in 1878 to refer to these organisms. At present the term "microorganism" is common usage.

All living things are classified according to international rules of nomenclature. Species of organisms are given two part names, according to the rules of the binomial system of nomenclature. The first part is the name of the *genus* to which the organism belongs and is written with the first letter capitalized. The second, uncapitalized name is the *specific epithet*. It is never used without the genus name (or genus abbreviation) preceding it. The scientific names of organisms are always in italics in print or underlined when hand-written.

Clinical microbiology encompasses the study of viruses, fungi, bacteria, and parasites. Included are tests to isolate and identify these microorganisms. Table 7-1 lists the organism group and terms used to describe their study.

In a large hospital laboratory or reference laboratory, each of these specialties might be in a separate department. However, a small laboratory may have a single microbiology department responsible for bacteriology, virology, parasitology, and mycology testing.

In the physician office laboratory (POL), only the less complicated procedures are performed; the majority of these are usually bacteriology tests. Most parasitology, virology, and mycology specimens are sent to a reference laboratory for testing.

## BACTERIOLOGY
### Characteristics of Bacteria

Bacteria are a large, diverse group of single-celled microorganisms. They usually multiply by **fission**, a process in which the parent body divides into two identical independent cells. A bacterium is a single organism. When many bacteria grow from a single organism they form a **colony**.

**Table 7-1.** Groups of microorganisms and the terms used for their study

| MICROORGANISM | TERM |
| --- | --- |
| Bacteria | Bacteriology |
| Viruses | Virology |
| Fungi and yeast | Mycology |
| Parasites | Parasitology |

## Bacterial Morphology

Bacteria can be divided into three general groups by their morphology, or shape. The three types are **coccus** (round), **bacillus** (rod), and **spirochete** (spiral) (Figure 7-1 and Color Plates 32, 33, and 34). Certain kinds of cocci occur in pairs and are called diplococci. Some bacilli are filamentous, meaning they form multi-celled, branching patterns.

## Gram Stain Reactions

The **Gram stain** is a procedure that stains bacteria differentially according to the composition of their cell walls. A Gram stain is performed by applying crystal violet, Gram's iodine, a decolorizer, and a counterstain, safranin, to a bacterial smear. The complete procedure is described in Lesson 7-4. Certain bacteria retain the crystal violet. These appear blue-purple and are called **gram-positive**. The bacteria that do not retain the crystal violet stain pink-red with the safranin. They are called **gram-negative** (See Color Plates 32 and 33).

## CLINICAL BACTERIOLOGY

Clinical bacteriology laboratories deal with the isolation and identification of bacterial **pathogens**, those bacteria

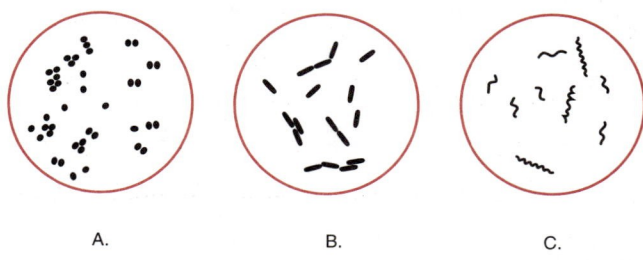

A.       B.       C.

**FIGURE 7-1** Three morphological types of bacteria: (A) cocci and diplococci, (B) bacilli, and (C) spirochetes

capable of causing disease. Bacterial pathogens cause disease by overcoming the body's normal defenses and invading the tissues. The damage is caused by their growth in tissues or by the toxins they produce. This invasion is called infection. Diseases spread from person to person are called infectious or **communicable** diseases.

Pathogens make up only a small portion of the total population of bacteria. Most microorganisms are free-living, in soil or water. Some are natural inhabitants of the human body and are thus part of **normal flora**. Microorganisms that invade the body and cause illness only when the body's immune defenses are impaired or absent are called **opportunistic pathogens**.

The work of the bacteriology laboratory is to isolate the organism that has infected the patient. Once it has been isolated, the organism is subjected to various tests to help identify it. The next step is **antibiotic susceptibility testing** to determine which antibiotic will be most effective in treating the patient.

## Bacteriological Procedures in the Small Laboratory

Procedures performed in a small laboratory or POL usually include throat cultures or rapid strep tests, urine cultures, and, occasionally, *Neisseria gonorrhoeae* testing. The organism(s) in the specimen is grown, isolated, and either identified on site, or sent to a reference laboratory.

## Specimen Collection for Bacteriology

The results of culture, growing an organism on a special **medium** in the laboratory, are only as reliable as the method used to collect the specimen. In addition, growth requirements of different organisms must be considered, such as moisture, temperature, oxygen, $CO_2$, and essential nutrients. Organisms sensitive to drying must be put into a transport medium immediately after collection to prevent loss of viability. Bacteria that require a specialized medium to grow and multiply are called **fastidious** bacteria. **Aerobic** bacteria grow only in the presence of oxygen, **anaerobic** bacteria live and grow in the absence of oxygen, and some bacteria have enhanced growth in 5-10% $CO_2$. Examples of some common bacteria and their growth requirements are shown in Table 7-2.

When specimens are collected, the microorganism's growth requirements must be considered. No matter how good the specimen, if an anaerobic organism is kept in an aerobic atmosphere while being transported

**Table 7-2.** Examples of some common bacteria and their growth requirements

| ORGANISM | DISEASE | MEDIUM | OXYGEN REQUIREMENTS |
|---|---|---|---|
| *Streptococcus* | Strep throat | Blood agar | $\downarrow O_2$, $\uparrow CO_2$ |
| *Neisseria gonorrhoeae* | Gonorrhea | Chocolate agar, modified Thayer-Martin (MTM) | $\downarrow O_2$, $\uparrow CO_2$ |
| *Staphylococcus* | Infections, boils | Blood agar | $O_2$ |
| *Escherichia coli* | Urinary tract infections | Blood agar, eosin methylene blue (EMB) MacConkey's (MAC) | $O_2$ |

to the reference laboratory, it will probably not survive. A special anaerobic transport system must be used.

*Neisseria gonorrhoeae*, the causative agent of the sexually transmitted disease (STD) gonorrhea, requires a special medium and an atmosphere of reduced oxygen and increased $CO_2$. Therefore, the specimen must be collected from the patient and immediately placed on the special medium in a reduced-oxygen and increased $CO_2$ atmosphere.

## Specimens Commonly Sent to Reference Laboratories

Laboratory personnel sending bacterial specimens to a reference laboratory must be familiar with the transport media the reference laboratory provides. The reference laboratory should provide a procedure manual that explains how and when to use the various microbiology transport systems. Wound cultures, blood cultures, and sputum samples are usually sent to reference laboratories. Sputum samples are examined for the presence of *Mycobacterium*, which causes tuberculosis. Since the organism is hazardous, only well-trained personnel in specially equipped laboratories work with these specimens.

## Identifying Bacteria

Test methods used by reference laboratories to aid in bacterial identification include microscopic morphology, colony appearance, Gram and other stain reactions, biochemical reactions, gene probes, and antibody reactions (Table 7-3). Four common types of media that help isolate and identify bacteria are shown in Table 7-4.

## Antibiotic Susceptibility Testing

Once the microorganism causing the patient's infection has been identified, antibiotic susceptibility must be determined. This may be accomplished by measuring the **zone of inhibition** around each antibiotic disk, which is the Bauer-Kirby method, or by finding the **minimum inhibitory concentration (MIC)** of various antibiotics.

The Bauer-Kirby method is performed on the solid surface of a special medium called Mueller-Hinton. This nonautomated procedure is interpreted visually. The MIC is determined by growing the organism in a special welled plate. Dilutions of various antibiotics are added

**Table 7-3.** Test methods used to help identify bacteria

Microscopic appearance
Colonial morphology
Selective or indicating media
Gram and other stains
Biochemical reactions
Gene probes
Antibody reactions

**Table 7-4.** Four common types of media used to isolate and identify bacteria

| MEDIUM | USE |
|---|---|
| 5% Sheep's blood agar (BA) | Supports growth of most gram-positive and gram-negative organisms, demonstrates hemolysis |
| Eosin methylene blue (EMB) | Supports growth of gram-negative organisms, inhibits gram-positive organisms, inhibits Proteus motility, demonstrates lactose and sucrose use |
| "Chocolate" agar | Provides heme to fastidious organisms (Neisseria) |
| Thayer-Martin (TM) and modified Thayer-Martin (MTM) | Chocolate agar with antibiotics added to suppress normal flora and contaminants |

to the growth wells. The minimum antibiotic amount that inhibits the organism's growth is determined by instrumentation and is used as a guide to antibiotic dosage.

Bacteriology is an important part of the clinical laboratory. Isolating and identifying the organism causing a patient's illness is the first step in determining proper treatment. Although certain bacteria are usually found in particular infections, this is not always true; the technician should never eliminate testing for a particular organism just because it is not usually involved in that type of infection.

## PARASITOLOGY

Clinical parasitology involves studying and identifying parasites, the diseases they cause, and the disease treatments. Parasites live in, on, or at the expense of another organism, called the **host** organism. Parasites may be unicellular or multicellular. They may be present in the blood, bone marrow, intestinal tract, liver, spleen, skin, hair, or any organ system. Table 7-5 lists specimens required to detect some common parasites. Commonly encountered parasites in the United States are intestinal, blood, and urogenital parasites and lice.

Tests for parasitic infection are not usually performed in smaller laboratories; instead, the specimens are sent to hospital, state, or reference laboratories for identification. For malaria detection, thick and thin blood smears must be prepared for the reference laboratory. Tests usually performed in small laboratories include the cellophane tape test for pinworm and wet preps for a urogenital parasite, *Trichomonas vaginalis* (Figure 7-2).

### Detection of Common Intestinal Parasites

Roundworms, flukes, and hookworms, all of which are "helminths," are common intestinal parasites. In addi-

tion, single-celled protozoa with amoeba forms are sometimes found. Stool specimens are examined for ova and parasites (O & P). The ova (eggs) may be detected in roundworm, hookworm, pinworm and tapeworm infections. Larvae (immature forms) or adults of some helminths may also be found. When protozoan parasites are suspected, the specimen is examined for cysts (nonmotile forms) and trophozoites (motile forms).

***Preserving and Transporting Specimens.*** To be examined for parasites, stool specimens must be placed in special solutions to preserve them. The reference laboratory should provide either a one- or two-vial collection kit. The one-vial kit has a vial containing a preservative, PVA (polyvinyl alcohol). The two-vial kit consists of one PVA vial and one **formalin** vial.

***Stool Examination for Parasites.*** The O & P examination has traditionally consisted of three parts: a direct smear, a concentration, and a stained smear. The *direct smear* for microscopic detection of protozoan motility requires a fresh stool specimen (Table 7-5). The *concentration* is for protozoan cysts and helminth eggs and larvae. The *stained smear* is for identifying and confirming intestinal protozoa. **Immunoassays** are also available to detect certain parasitic infections.

To diagnose parasitic infections, the physician must recognize the symptoms and request the appropriate tests. Patients infected with parasites often have eosinophilia, which will show up as an increased per-

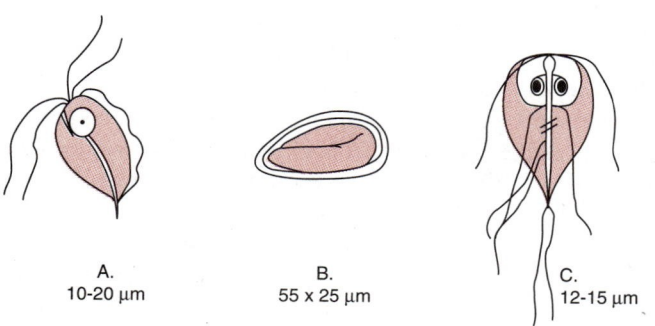

A.
10–20 µm

B.
55 x 25 µm

C.
12–15 µm

**FIGURE 7-2** Examples of three common parasites: (A) *Trichomonas*, (B) pinworm egg, and (C) *Giardia*

**Table 7-5.** The types of specimens required for parasite detection

| ORGANISM | SPECIMEN |
|---|---|
| *Trichomonas vaginalis* | Urine, vaginal secretions, urethral discharge, prostatic secretions |
| *Entamoeba histolytica* | Feces |
| *Giardia lamblia* | Feces |
| *Cryptosporidium parvum* | Feces |
| *Enterobius vermicularis* (pinworm) | Cellophane tape prep |
| *Necator americanus* (hookworm) | Feces |
| *Plasmodium* (malarial parasite) | Blood |

centage in the differential count and increased absolute number of eosinophils in the complete blood count (CBC). One stool specimen a day must be collected for three separate days to increase the probability of detecting a parasite.

## Detection of *Trichomonas Vaginalis*

The urogenital parasite, *Trichomonas vaginalis,* may be detected in urine, vaginal or urethral discharge, or prostatic secretions (Table 7-5). It may be visible by microscopic examination of secretions in a coverslip preparation or in a well-slide. *Trichomonas* is recognized by its characteristic "twitching" motility.

## Detecting Blood and Tissue Parasites

In the United States, only a few organisms infect blood or other tissues. Worldwide, the most common blood parasite is the malarial parasite, *Plasmodium.* Blood parasites are discovered and identified by microscopically examining stained blood smears. Specimens for blood and tissue parasites are usually sent to a reference laboratory. More information on malaria and other parasitic diseases can be found in Unit 8.

## VIROLOGY

Virology is the study of viruses and the diseases they cause. Common viruses that cause disease are influenza (flu), rubella, mumps, rubeola (red measles), Epstein-Barr (infectious mononucleosis), and herpes (Table 7-6). As a group, viruses are the most common cause of human infectious diseases. Some are known to cause cancer.

Viruses are not considered living cells and can only replicate by invading a cell. Once inside the cell, they cause the cell's replication processes to make more virus **progeny**, or offspring.

Each virus consists of a nucleic acid *core* and a protein coat called a *capsid.* Some have an additional component called an *envelope.* Living organisms contain both DNA and RNA, but a virus has only one or the other. **DNA** is the nucleic acid, found primarily in chromosomes, that carries genetic information. RNA is a nucleic acid responsible for protein synthesis. Viruses are much smaller than microorganisms (30 nm to 300 nm) and cannot be seen with a light microscope; therefore, electron microscopes are used to study them (Figure 7-3).

**Table 7-6.** Common viruses, their abbreviations or acronyms, and the diseases they cause

| VIRUS | ABBREVIATION OR ACRONYM | DISEASE |
|---|---|---|
| Herpes simplex virus, type 1 | HSV-1 | Cold sores, fever blisters |
| Herpes simplex virus, type 2 | HSV-2 | Genital herpes |
| Epstein-Barr virus | EBV | Infectious mononucleosis |
| Human papilloma virus | HPV | Warts and tumors of genital tract |
| Hepatitis B virus | HBV | Hepatitis B |
| Hepatitis C virus | HCV | Hepatitis C |
| Rhinoviruses | — | Common cold |
| Influenza A,B,C | "Flu" | Influenza |
| Rubella virus | — | Rubella (German measles, three-day measles) |
| Human immuno-deficiency virus | HIV | Acquired immuno-deficiency syndrome (AIDS) |
| Measles virus | — | Rubeola (red measles) |

## Diagnostic Testing in Virology

Interest in diagnostic clinical virology has increased dramatically because of the demand for more rapid diagnosis of human immunodeficiency virus (HIV) and human papilloma virus (HPV). In addition, increasing cases of hepatitis B and C, which can be chronic or fatal diseases, have helped motivate development of improved laboratory tests for viral infection.

The standard method for isolating and identifying viruses has been cell culture, which is performed in large microbiology departments and in reference laboratories. Patient serum can also be tested for viral antibodies using the ELISA (enzyme-linked immunosorbent assay) technique, usually now referred to as EIA. Table 7-7 lists the basic approaches to clinical virology testing.

Smaller laboratories do not have the personnel and resources to perform most viral testing. However, they may often collect and send specimens to the reference laboratory. A procedure manual listing available

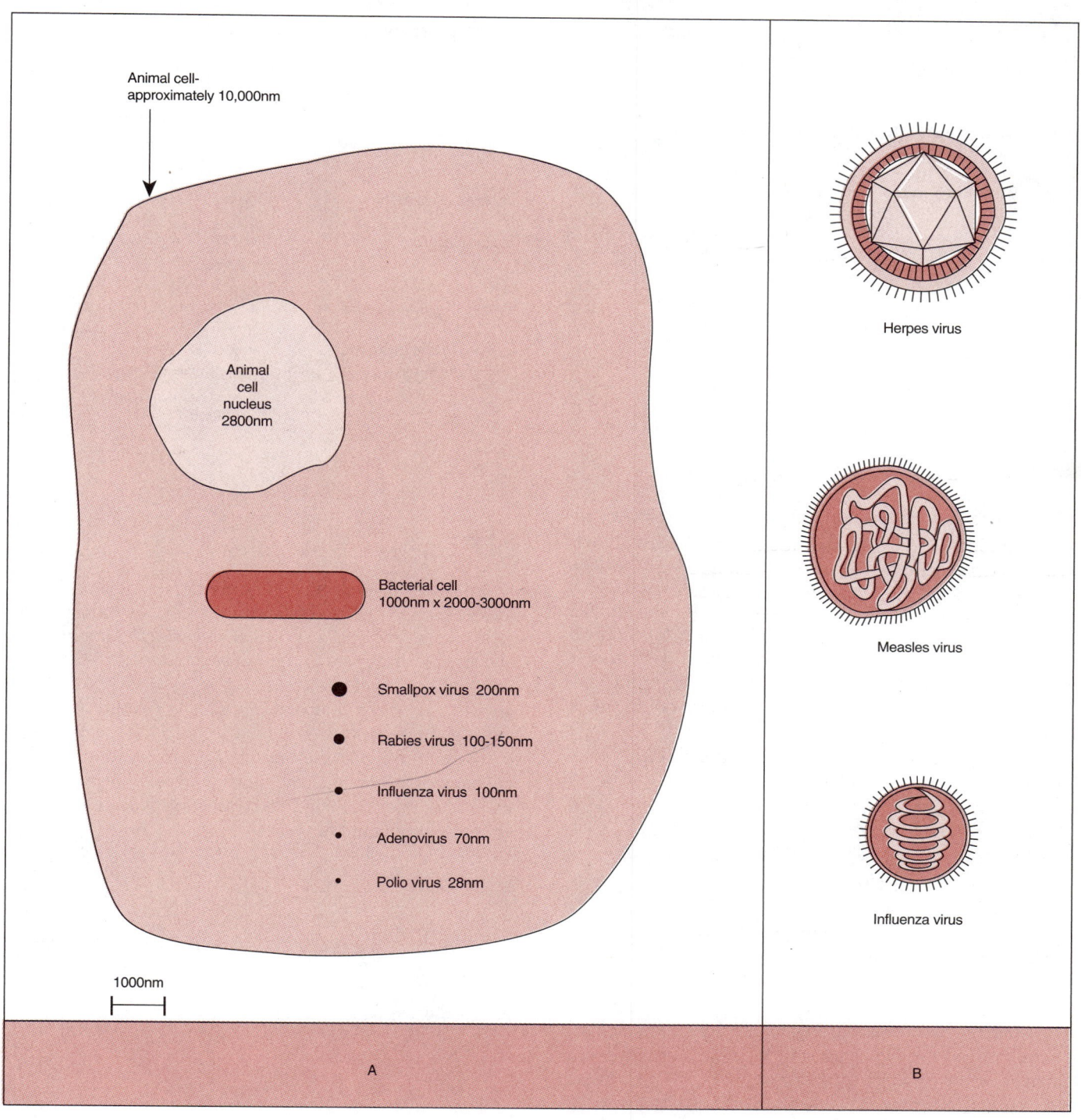

**FIGURE 7-3** Sizes and morphologies of viruses: (A) relative sizes of viruses compared to a bacterial cell and an animal cell; (B) illustration of the morphology of three common viruses (adapted from Brock, T.D., & Brock, K.M. (1973). *Basic microbiology and applications*. Englewood Cliffs, NJ: Prentice-Hall, Inc.)

**Table 7-7.** Basic approaches to detecting viruses

1. **Cell culture:** isolating and identifying the viruses in cell culture

2. **Direct detection:** detecting the viral antigen in a clinical specimen

3. **Serodiagnosis:** detecting antibodies to the virus

**Table 7-8.** Some common fungi and the diseases they cause

| ORGANISM | DISEASE |
| --- | --- |
| *Tinea* species | Ringworm (dermatomycosis) |
| *Candida* | Thrush, vaginal infections (candidiasis) |
| *Malassezia furfur* | Pityriasis versicolor |
| *Coccidioides immitis* | Coccidioidomycosis (Valley fever) |
| *Histoplasma capsulatum* | Histoplasmosis |
| *Aspergillus, Candida,* and *Cryptococcus* | Involved in systemic infections (especially in immunocompromised patients) |

tests, collection methods, and transport media should be provided by the reference laboratory.

## Diagnostic Kits for Virology

Diagnostic kits to test for several common viruses include latex slide agglutination tests for rubella and immunoassays to detect herpes simplex, influenza, rubella, and certain other viruses. Many of these kits are suitable for use in the smaller laboratory. A screening test called the Torch test is often requested during pregnancy. The letters T,R,C,H represent *Toxoplasma*, Rubella, Cytomegalovirus, and Herpes. Being infected with any one of these during pregnancy could injure the fetus.

T = Toxoplasma
R = Rubella
C = Cytomegalovirus
H = Herpes

## MYCOLOGY

Mycology is the study of fungi, a diverse group of microorganisms that exist in mold or yeast form. Most fungi are found in soil and on decaying plant matter. Of 250,000 known fungal species, only about 180 are considered capable of causing disease.

Infection caused by fungi is called mycosis. The mycosis incidence is related to the degree of exposure to fungi in living conditions, occupation, and leisure activities, and to immune status. Table 7-8 lists some fungi and the diseases they cause.

Most pathogenic fungi can infect any exposed individual. Two important examples are *Histoplasma capsulatum* and *Coccidioides immitis*. Others, such as *Candida* and *Aspergillus*, are opportunistic pathogens; they ordinarily cause disease only in immunosuppressed (compromised) patients, such as those with AIDS.

## Characteristics of Molds

Molds have branching filaments called **hyphae** that make up the vegetative structure, the **mycelium**. They reproduce by forming spores (Figure 7-4). Most molds are aerobic and grow in the range of 22–30°C. They will grow on the usual bacteriological media; however, their growth is so slow that bacteria usually overgrow them. One of the best-known media to select for growth of pathogenic fungi is Sabouraud's dextrose agar, which contains dextrose, maltose, and peptones. In addition, antibiotics may be included to inhibit growth of bacteria and nonpathogenic fungi.

Sabourads ʒconsist dextrose dextrose maltose peptones.

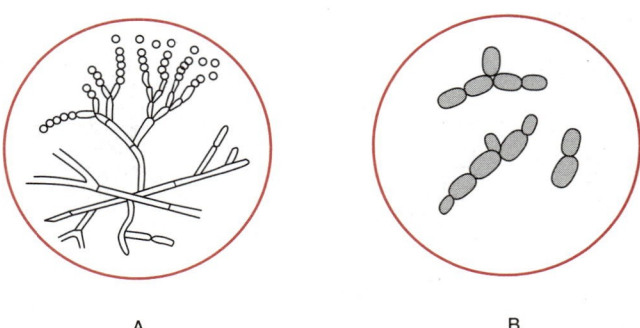

A.  B.

**FIGURE 7-4** Reproductive methods of molds and yeasts: (A) molds producing spores and (B) budding yeasts

**Table 7-9.** A simplified scheme for identifying molds and yeasts

| ORGANISM | GROWTH MEDIUM | METHOD OF IDENTIFICATION |
|---|---|---|
| Molds | Sabouraud's 22–27°C agar | Macroscopic and microscopic appearance; |
| Yeasts | Blood agar 37°C | Fermentation of sugars, using carbon or nitrogen compounds |

## Characteristics of Yeast

The most common form of yeast is a unicellular (one-celled) egg shape. Yeasts usually reproduce by budding instead of forming spores (Figure 7-4 and Color Plate 35). There are about 350 known species of yeasts. Yeasts are used in fermentation processes, including those for beer and wine production and leavening of bread.

Although many yeasts are useful for industrial purposes, some yeasts are pathogenic. *Candida* species (usually *C. albicans*) infects the mucous membranes of the mouth and vagina. *Malassezia furfur* causes a skin infection called pityriasis versicolor. In the majority of patients yeast infections are superficial.

Since yeast infections are usually superficial, they can be identified by examining or culturing skin scrapings or nail clippings. Specimens are cultured on Sabouraud's dextrose agar. Yeasts grow best with an abundant supply of oxygen and grow satisfactorily on common bacteriological media. *C. albicans* can be identified by the development of pseudohyphae in a test called the "germ tube test."

## Identifying Fungi

Identification techniques for fungi depend on whether the organism is a mold or a yeast. Molds are largely identified by macroscopic and microscopic study of their morphology and the spores they produce. Yeast identification depends on the results of biochemical reactions. The Uni-Yeast-Tek system identifies yeasts based on their ability to ferment certain sugars (Color Plate 40). Table 7-9 gives a simplified scheme for identifying molds and yeasts.

### SUMMARY

Microbiology is the study of a wide variety of organisms, some helpful to man and some harmful. These organisms are named in a systematic way using international rules, so that scientists all over the world use the same nomenclature.

Humans have conquered many diseases caused by microorganisms, mainly because of the discovery and use of antibiotics. However, we frequently hear of a new disease or discovery of a "new microorganism." Microorganisms can undergo rapid genetic change. An animal pathogen may become pathogenic to humans. A microorganism may become resistant to antibiotics. These discoveries lead to more microbiology research in academic institutions and pharmaceutical and research laboratories.

Each discovery causes a trickle-down effect in clinical laboratories. Eventually, if the organism is a pathogen, test methods are developed to detect it or antibodies to it. At the same time, methods to detect more commonplace causes of disease are always being improved and more automated methods are being introduced in the microbiology laboratory.

### LESSON REVIEW

1. When was the term "microbiology" first used?

2. List the areas of study encompassed by microbiology.

3. What are the organizational differences between a small and large microbiology laboratory?

4. What is meant by the term "normal flora?"

5. What is a pathogen? An opportunistic pathogen?

6. How does infection occur?

7. Describe the three morphological types of bacteria.

8. What is a Gram stain?

9. What are the two morphological forms of fungi?

10. What is the difference between aerobic and anaerobic bacteria?

11. List the microbiological tests usually performed in a small laboratory.

12. How are viruses different from microorganisms? Name three viral diseases.

13. What type of specimen is required to detect malaria? To detect *Giardia*?

14. List seven test methods used to help identify bacteria.

15. Define aerobic, anaerobic, antibiotic susceptibility testing, bacillus. coccus, colony, communicable, culture, DNA, fastidious organism, fission, formalin, gram negative, gram positive, Gram stain, host, hyphae, immunoassay, infection, medium, minimum inhibitory concentration, mycelium, mycosis, normal flora, opportunistic pathogen, pathogen, progeny, RNA, spirochetes, and zone of inhibition.

## STUDENT ACTIVITIES

1. Reread the introduction to clinical microbiology.
2. Review the glossary terms.
3. Visit a microbiology laboratory in the community. Inquire about the laboratory's organization. Find out what types of tests are performed in the laboratory and which tests are sent to reference laboratories.

# Infection Control and Transmission-Based Precautions

## LESSON OBJECTIVES

**After studying this lesson, you should be able to:**

- *Discuss the role of the hospital's infection control department.*
- *Explain why isolation techniques are used.*
- *List the three types of Transmission-Based Precautions and explain the basis for each classification.*
- *Demonstrate proper handwashing technique.*
- *Demonstrate proper gowning technique.*
- *Demonstrate the proper method of putting on a mask.*
- *Demonstrate proper gloving technique.*
- *Demonstrate proper removal and disposal of mask, gown, and gloves.*
- *List five rules for preventing exposure to blood and body fluids.*
- *Define the glossary terms.*

## GLOSSARY

**Airborne Precautions** / a CDC isolation category designed to prevent transmission of infectious diseases such as pulmonary tuberculosis, rubeola (measles), and varicella (chickenpox)

**carrier** / person who harbors an organism, has no symptoms or signs of disease, but is capable of spreading the organism to others

**Contact Precautions** / CDC isolation category designed to prevent transmission of diseases spread by close or direct contact

**Droplet Precautions** / CDC isolation category designed to prevent transmission of diseases spread through the air over short distances

**fomites** / inanimate objects, such as bed rails, linens, or eating utensils, that may be contaminated with infectious organisms and serve as a means of their transmission

**infection** / pathological condition caused by growth of microorganisms in the host

**isolation** / practice of limiting the movement and social contact of a patient who is potentially infectious or who must be protected from exposure to infectious agents

**microorganism** / single-celled microscopic organism

**nonpathogenic** / not normally causing disease in a healthy individual

**nosocomial infection** / infection acquired in a hospital or health care facility

**pathogen** / organism or agent capable of causing disease in a host

**protective isolation** / reverse isolation; an isolation category designed to protect highly susceptible patients from exposure to infectious agents

**Standard Precautions** / set of CDC safety procedures designed to protect patients and health
care workers from infectious agents

## INTRODUCTION

The hospital's infection control department monitors contagious diseases and prevents their spread. This department also sets standards to ensure patients do not acquire infections while in the hospital. This can be accomplished by setting guidelines for managing patients who are contagious or who are highly suscepti-ble to infection (have little resistance or immunity).

Every health care institution has an infection con-trol program based on regulations and recommenda-tions of agencies such as the Centers for Disease Control and Prevention (CDC), the Joint Commission for Accreditation of Healthcare Organizations (JCAHO), the Association for Practitioners in Infection Control (APIC), and state regulatory agencies. One control method is **isolation**, which includes separating the patient from other patients and limiting visitor and staff contact with that patient.

This lesson provides general guidelines for isola-tion precautions for laboratory workers such as phle-botomists or other personnel who must obtain blood from the patient in isolation, and who normally have only limited patient exposure. The student or worker must be sure to follow the particular institution's rules and guidelines. Other texts should be consulted for guidelines for nursing personnel, who have more extensive patient contact.

## CAUSES OF INFECTION

**Microorganisms** are single-celled microscopic organ-isms present in the environment and in and on the human body. These organisms include bacteria, viruses, protozoa, and fungi. Most microorganisms are **non-pathogenic**, meaning they do not normally cause dis-ease in a healthy individual. Microbes capable of causing disease are called **pathogens**.

**Infection** occurs when the body is invaded by a pathogenic agent that may, under favorable conditions, multiply and cause disease. Three components must be present for infection to occur: (1) a source of microor-ganisms; (2) a susceptible person or host; and (3) a method of microorganism transmission from the source to the susceptible host. The source may be an infected person or animal, the environment, or **fomites** (con-taminated objects). The transmission method may be direct contact; inhaling dust or droplets containing microorganisms or air droplets produced by coughing or sneezing; exposure to infectious body fluids; ingest-ing contaminated water or food; or vectors such as insects (Table 7-10).

Infections usually cause symptoms such as fever, redness, fluid accumulation, or pain. However, infec-tions may also be present in a person who feels well and has no symptoms. This person may be a **carrier**, a source of infection for others.

A small percentage (approximately 5-10%) of hos-pitalized patients in the United States develop **nosoco-mial infections**, infections acquired while in the hospital, through contact with infected personnel, visi-tors, or contaminated equipment.

## ISOLATION CATEGORIES

Historically, each institution developed isolation proce-dures appropriate for its patient population, taking into consideration newly emerging diseases. In 1992, CDC issued Universal Precautions to assist health care providers in reducing the risk of contracting or transmit-ting infectious diseases, particularly AIDS and hepatitis B.

In 1996, changes were made in these rules and also in isolation procedures, and **Standard Pre-cautions** were issued to augment and synthesize the

**Table 7-10.** Methods of infection transmission

Direct contact
Inhalating droplets produced by coughing or sneezing
Inhalating dust particles containing microorganisms
Exposure to infectious body fluids
Ingesting contaminated food or water
Exposure to disease vectors such as insects or rodents

**Table 7-11.** List of current CDC Transmission-Based Precautions and former isolation categories

| CURRENT TRANSMISSION-BASED PRECAUTIONS | FORMER ISOLATION CATEGORIES |
|---|---|
| Droplet Precautions* | Contact isolation |
| Airborne Precautions* | Respiratory isolation |
| Contact Precautions* | Acid-fast bacillus (AFB) isolation |
| | Complete or strict isolation |
| | Reverse or protective isolation |
| *Used in addition to Standard Precautions | |

Universal Precautions and the techniques known as body substance isolation (BSI). Standard Precautions represent the most current and comprehensive approach to protecting all health care providers, patients, and visitors from acquiring infectious diseases.

In addition, CDC has simplified isolation procedures by reducing the five categories of isolation to three categories of *precautions*, classified by the routes of transmission of disease: (1) **Droplet Precautions**, (2) **Contact Precautions**, and (3) **Airborne Precautions** (Table 7-11). Standard Precautions are always used; Transmission-Based Precautions are used in addition to Standard Precautions.

The former isolation classification scheme included: (1) contact isolation, (2) respiratory isolation, (3) acid-fast bacillus (AFB) isolation, and (4) strict or complete isolation, plus enteric precautions and drainage secretion precautions. A comparison of the current and former categories is shown in Table 7-11.

## Contact Precautions

Contact Precautions are used when patients have diseases spread primarily by close or direct contact (Table 7-12). The patient should be in a private room, if possible. This category is intended to protect health care workers against infection from contact with infective material from, for example, a wound or fecal material. Exposure could occur if the patient is incontinent, or has diarrhea, an ileostomy, a colostomy, or wound drainage not contained by a dressing. Since surfaces and items in the room may be contaminated, the health care worker must wear gloves and gown and remove both before leaving the room to avoid transferring organisms outside the room. After glove removal, hands must be washed with an antimicrobial agent. Contaminated materials must be discarded in biohazard containers for disposal or disinfection. All Standard Precautions must also be observed (Figure 7-5).

## Droplet Precautions

Droplet Precautions are used when patients are infected with organisms easily transmitted through the air over short distances. Examples include mumps, pertussis (whooping cough), meningococcal pneumonia, and meningitis (Table 7-12). These patients should be in pri-

**Table 7-12.** Types of transmission-Based Precautions and examples of illnesses and disease agents that require them (adapted from CDC)

**Standard Precautions**
Use for all patients

**Airborne Precautions**
Use in addition to Standard Precautions for illnesses transmitted by airborne droplet nuclei. Examples:
measles
tuberculosis
varicella

**Droplet Precautions**
Use in addition to Standard Precautions for illnesses transmitted by large-particle droplets. Examples:

| | |
|---|---|
| Diphtheria | *Mycoplasma* pneumonia |
| Pertussis | Pneumonic plague |
| Invasive *Hemophilus* influenzae | Adenovirus |
| | Influenza |
| Invasive *Neisseria* meningitidis | Influenza |
| | Rubella |
| Mumps | Parvovirus B19 |
| Streptococcal pharyngitis | |

**Contact Precautions**
Use in addition to Standard Precautions for illnesses transmitted by direct contact. Examples:

| | |
|---|---|
| Wound infections | Enteric infections |
| Respiratory syncytial virus | Skin infections |
| Colonization with multidrug-resistant bacteria | |
| Viral hemorragic infections | |

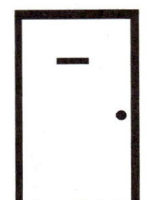

**CONTACT PRECAUTIONS**
**(in addition to Standard Precautions)**
**VISITORS: Report to nurse before entering.**

### Patient Placement
**Private room**, if possible. Cohort if private room is not available.

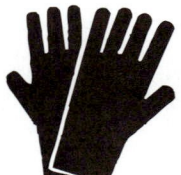

### Gloves
Wear gloves when entering patient room.
**Change** gloves.after having contact with infective material that may contain high concentrations of microorganisms (fecal material and wound drainage).
**Remove** gloves before leaving patient room.

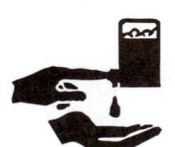

### Wash
Wash hands with an **antimicrobial** agent immediately after glove removal. After glove removal and handwashing, ensure that hands do not touch potentially contaminated environmental surfaces or items in the patient's room to avoid transfer of microorganisms to other patients or environments.

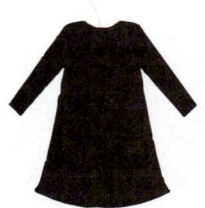

### Gown
Wear gown when **entering** patient room if you anticipate that your clothing will have substantial contact with the patient, environmental surfaces, or items in the patient's room, or if the patient is **incontinent**, or has **diarrhea**, an **ileostomy**, a **colostomy**, or **wound drainage** not contained by a dressing. **Remove** gown before leaving the patient's environment and ensure that clothing does not contact potentially contaminated environmental surfaces to avoid transfer of microorganisms to other patients or environments.

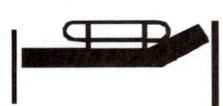

### Patient Transport
Limit transport of patient to essential purposes only. During transport, ensure that precautions are maintained to minimize the risk of transmission of microorganisms to other patients and contamination of environmental surfaces and equipment.

### Patient-Care Equipment
Dedicate the use of noncritical patient-care equipment to a single patient. If common equipment is used, clean and disinfect between patients.

**FIGURE 7-5A** Contact Precautions, one category of Transmission-Based Precautions (Courtesy of Brevis Corp.)

vate rooms, if possible. Masks are required for those who come within three feet of the patient or upon entering the room, since the infectious agents are readily spread by the patient's coughing or sneezing, a major mode of transmission for respiratory infections. Gloves and gown are required since Standard Precautions must also be observed. See Figure 7-5B for graphics illustrating PPE.

## Airborne Precautions

Airborne Precautions are used when a patient is known or suspected of being infected with microorganisms transmitted by airborne route (Table 7-12). Persons entering the room of a patient with known or suspected infectious pulmonary tuberculosis must wear an N95 respirator. In addition, susceptible personnel should not enter rooms of patients known or suspected to have measles (rubeola) or chickenpox (varicella) unless an immune caregiver is not available. Susceptible persons must wear the N95 respirator if they enter the room. The patient must be in a private room with negative air pressure, six to twelve air changes per hour. and discharge of air outside or through a HEPA filter. In addition, caregivers must observe Standard Precautions (Figure 7-5C).

## DROPLET PRECAUTIONS
### (in addition to Standard Precautions)
### VISITORS: Report to nurse before entering.

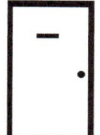

**Patient Placement**
**Private room**, if possible. Cohort or maintain spatial separation of 3 feet from other patients or visitors if private room is not available.

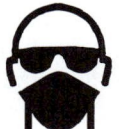

**Mask**
Wear mask when working within 3 feet of patient (or upon entering room).

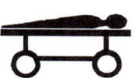

**Patient Transport**
Limit transport of patient from room to essential purposes only. Use **surgical mask** on patient during transport.

**FIGURE 7-5B** Droplet Precautions, one category of Transmission-Based Precautions. (Courtesy of Brevis Corp.)

## AIRBORNE PRECAUTIONS
### (in addition to Standard Precautions)
### VISITORS: Report to nurse before entering.

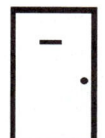

**Patient Placement**
Use **Private room**, that has:
   Monitored negative air pressure
   6 to 12 air changes per hour,
   Discharge of air outdoors or HEPA filtration if recirculated.
**Keep room door closed and patient in room.**

**Respiratory Protection**
Wear an **N95 respirator** when entering the room of a patient with known or suspected infectious pulmonary **tuberculosis**.
**Susceptible** persons should not enter the room of patients known or suspected to have **measles** (rubeola) or **varicella** (chickenpox) if other immune caregivers are available. If susceptible persons must enter, they should wear an **N95 respirator**. (Respirator or surgical mask not required if immune to measles and varicella.)

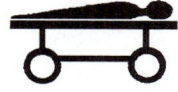

**Patient Transport**
Limit transport of patient from room to essential purposes only. Use **surgical mask** on patient during transport.

**FIGURE 7-5C** Airborne Precautions, one category of Transmission-Based Precautions (Courtesy of Brevis Corp.)

## Other Categories of Precautions

The former isolation classifications contained a category called reverse or **protective isolation** intended to protect immunosuppressed or otherwise susceptible patients. Current standards do not address protective isolation in a direct way. Individual hospitals are continuing to make it an unofficial category; signs are placed on the room doors of immunosuppressed patients. The signs direct health care workers and visitors to wear masks when entering the room if they have a cold or other contagious condition. The laboratory worker should always clarify any questions by going to the floor nurses' desk or consulting with the infection control officer.

## COMPLYING WITH THE INSTITUTION'S EXPOSURE CONTROL PLAN

Laboratory workers must observe their institution's Exposure Control Plan and CDC's safety regulations, not only in the laboratory, but also in patient rooms and all other health care situations. These procedures are discussed in depth in Lesson 1-6, Laboratory Safety: Biological Hazards. Personnel must observe Universal and Standard Precautions along with Transmission-Based Precautions. The types of Transmission-Based Precautions may be combined for diseases that have multiple modes of transmission.

## ISOLATION TECHNIQUES

Health care facilities have specific instructions and necessary supplies located outside the room of each patient requiring isolation procedures. These include handwashing and donning and removing protective barriers such as gloves, masks and gowns.

## Handwashing

Handwashing is the most important procedure in isolation techniques, just as it is in maintaining safety in the laboratory (Lesson 1-6). Proper handwashing should be the first and last step of all procedures.

Handwashing does not sterilize the hands, but removes surface contaminants, dead skin, and surface organisms. Hands and wrists should be lathered in warm water and scrubbed front and back and between fingers, rubbing thoroughly. The scrubbing process should last at least 1-2 minutes. Fingernails may be cleaned using a fingernail brush or an orange stick. The hands are then rinsed from the arm or wrist toward the tips of the fingers while holding hands in a downward position (Figure 7-6). The faucet should be turned on and off using a clean towel or tissue to avoid contaminating hands with organisms or substances that may be present on the faucet handles.

## Masks

Masks should be put on after hands are washed, avoiding touching the skin with hands. Most masks have two

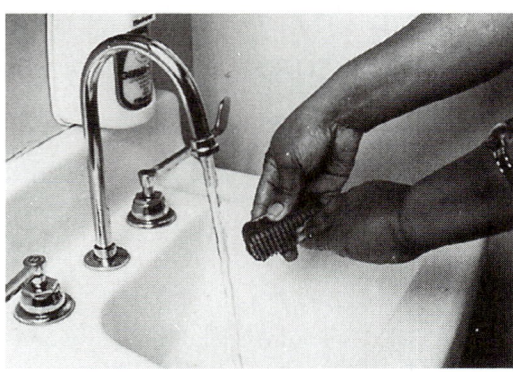

(A)

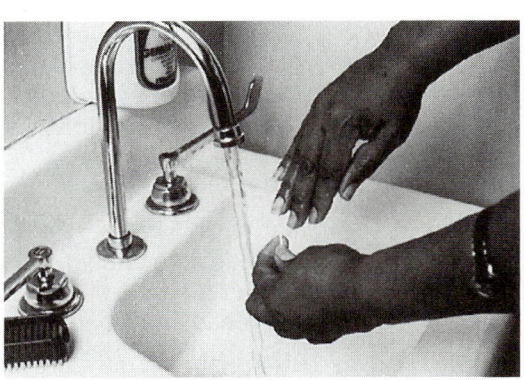

(B)

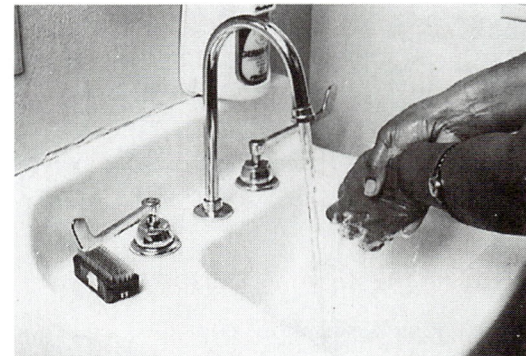

(C)

(D)

**FIGURE 7-6** Handwashing technique. (A) Interlace the fingers to clean between them. (B) Use the blunt edges of an orange stick to clean under the fingernails. (C) Use a hand brush to clean under the fingernails. (D) Rinse hands thoroughly, with the fingertips down.

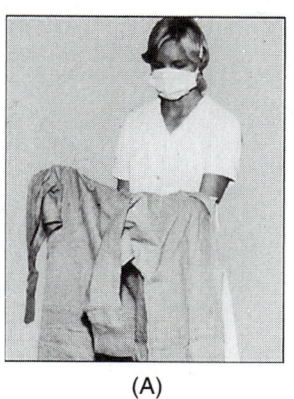 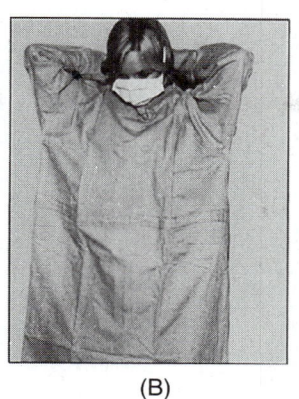 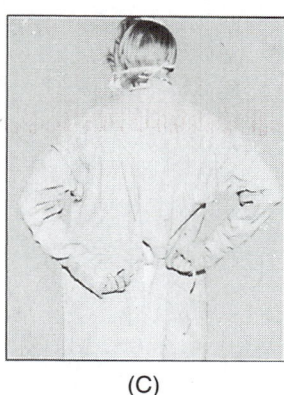

(A)                    (B)                    (C)

**FIGURE 7-7**  Putting on a clean mask and cover gown. (A) After tying on the mask, put on the gown outside the patient's room/unit. (B) Slip fingers inside the neck-band and tie gown. (C) Reach behind, overlap the ends of the gown so the uniform is covered, and secure the waist ties.

ties, one for the upper neck and one for the head (Figure 7-7). Masks should only be worn for fifteen to twenty minutes before changing into a clean one. They should not be allowed to dangle around the neck.

## Gowns

Laboratory coats should be removed before donning gowns. The gown should be touched only on the inside surface and should cover all clothing when tied (Figure 7-7). Gowns are removed by turning the inside of the gown to the outside and folding the contaminated outer side inward (Figure 7-8).

## Gloves

A clean pair of gloves must be used for each patient. The gloves are put on by pulling the cuff or wrist area over sleeve ends of the gown so all skin or clothing is covered. It is best to avoid wearing sharp rings or jewelry,

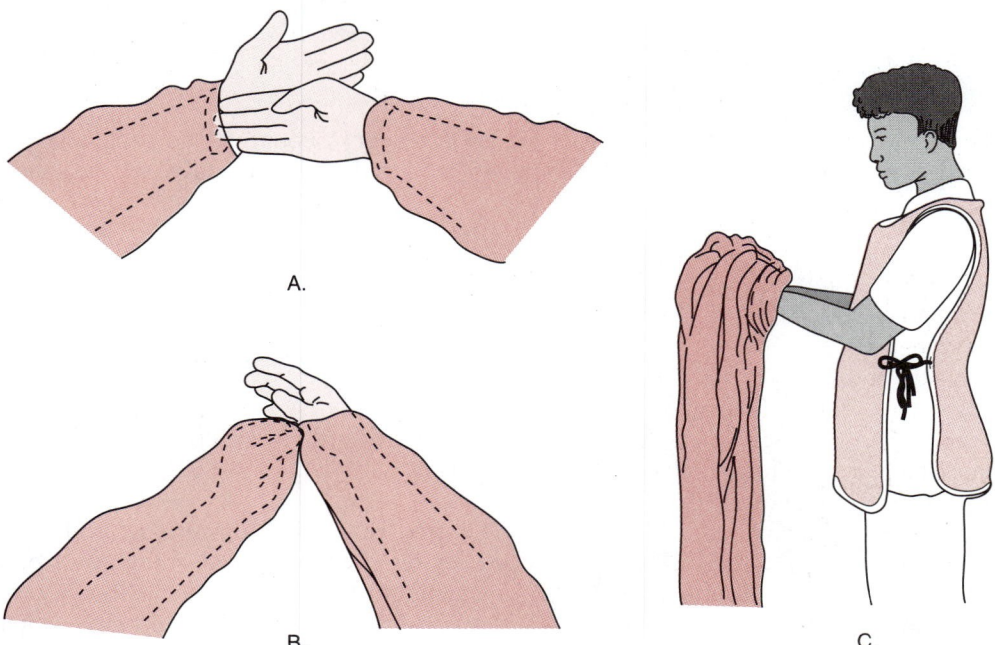

A.

B.

C.

**FIGURE 7-8**  Removing a contaminated gown. (A) Slip fingers of the right hand inside the left cuff of the gown and pull the gown as shown, over the left hand. Do not touch the outside of the gown with the right hand. (B) Using the gown-covered left hand, pull the gown down over the right hand. (C) As the gown is removed, fold with the contaminated side inward and then roll.

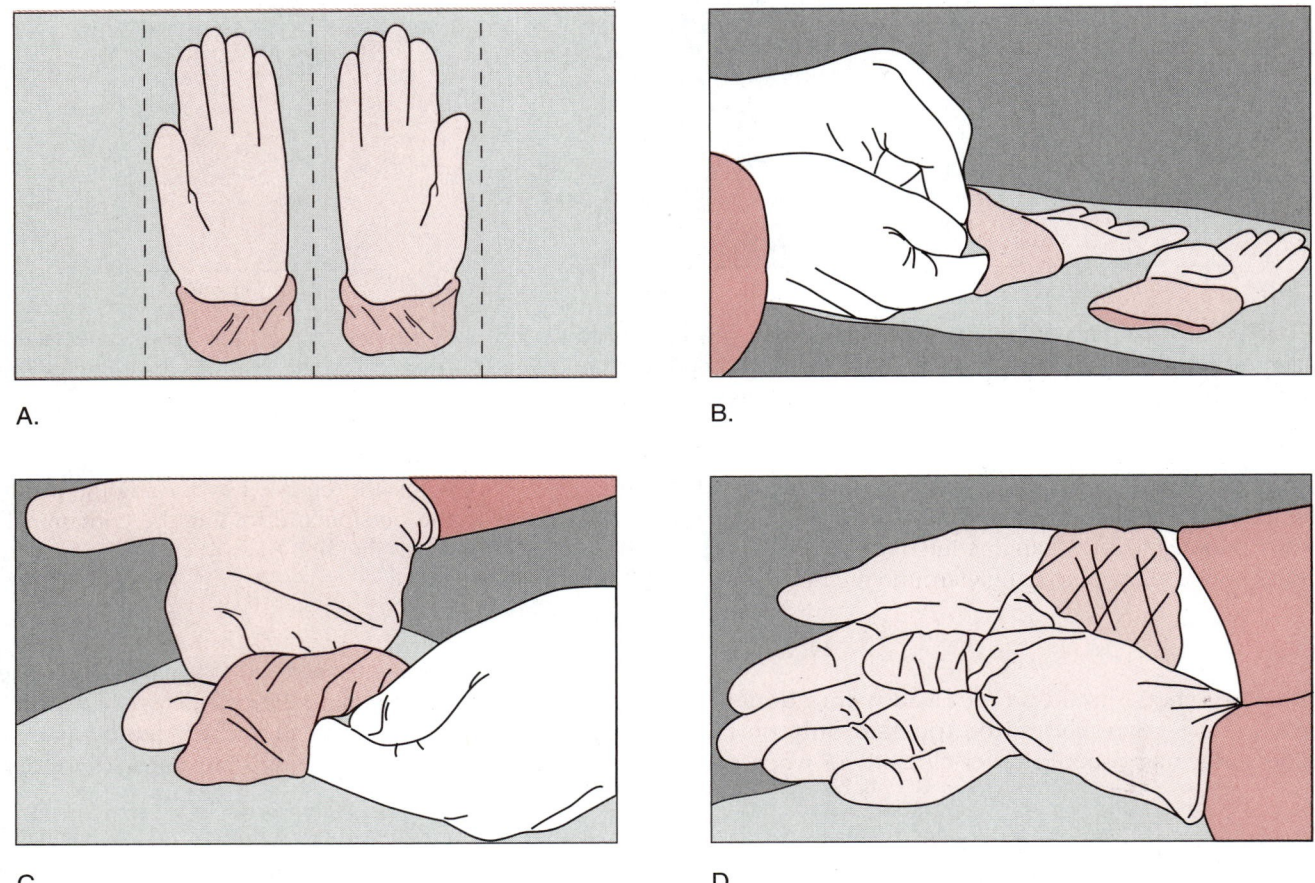

A.

B.

C.

D.

**FIGURE 7-9** Donning sterile gloves. (A) Illustration of gloves in a newly opened sterile pack. (B) Picking up first glove by the cuff to insert first hand. (C) Using the sterile-gloved hand to don second glove. (D) Adjusting gloves.

that may puncture gloves. Some types of isolation, such as reverse isolation, may require sterile gloves.

If sterile gloves are required, the worker must avoid touching the outside of the gloves with his or her hands when donning them. This is accomplished by carefully opening the sterile package, picking up a glove by the cuff, and carefully inserting the hand into the glove (Figure 7-9). The second glove is then picked up by placing the gloved fingers under the cuff and holding the glove while the hand is inserted. The cuffs are then unfolded by sliding the gloved fingers under the cuff. Sterile gloves should always be used to handle sterile equipment or instruments.

Contaminated gloves are removed by grasping the cuff of one glove with the other gloved hand and pulling the glove off over itself. The removed glove is placed into the palm of the other glove and the second glove is removed, enclosing the first glove in the sec-

ond. Used gloves are discarded in biohazard containers. Hands should always be washed with hand disinfectant after glove removal.

## Entering and Exiting an Isolation Room

The procedure used for entering and exiting isolation rooms differs according to the type of precaution. In general, most supplies are located on a cart outside the patient's room and are put on before entering (Figure 7-10).

Only items that will be used for the patient should be taken into the isolation room. Phlebotomists should leave trays and requisition slips outside the room to avoid them being contaminated. Tourniquets and pens should be left in the room for future use.

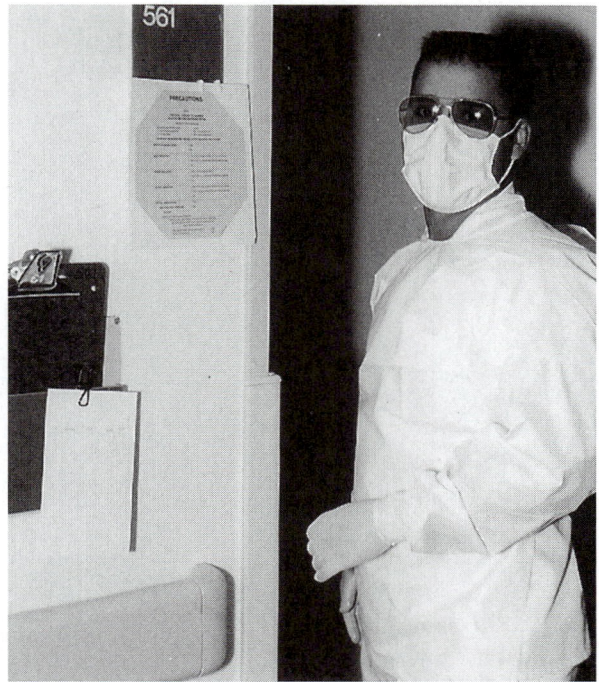

**FIGURE 7-10** Laboratory professional entering a precaution isolation room wearing gown, gloves, and mask.

When exiting the room, the used supplies should be left in a special disposal container usually located inside the room. Exceptions to this procedure include protective isolation, where disposables are usually left in a container outside the room for disposal.

## SUMMARY

Laboratory workers must observe their institution's exposure control plan, not only in the laboratory, but also in patients' rooms and all other health care situations. These procedures are discussed in depth in Lesson 1-6, Laboratory Safety: Biological Hazards.

Personnel must use Standard Precautions to prevent exposure to all blood and body fluids, whether known to be infectious or not. These precautions include:

- using proper handwashing techniques
- wearing gloves and fluid-resistant laboratory coat when handling all biological specimens, containers, or any other contaminated articles

- wearing eye protection if aerosols or splashes are likely or reasonably anticipated
- properly handling all sharps and disposing of contaminated sharps in puncture-resistant containers
- immediately cleaning up spills with an appropriate disinfectant, such as a 10% bleach solution.

## LESSON REVIEW

1. What is the function of the hospital's infection control department?
2. Explain why Transmission-Based Precautions are used.
3. Name three categories of Transmission-Based Precautions. Give an example of a condition requiring each type of precaution.
4. Explain the proper handwashing method. When is handwashing performed?
5. Explain the proper technique for putting on and removing a gown.
6. Explain how to put on gloves.
7. State five exposure-control methods for preventing exposure to blood and body fluids.
8. Explain the difference between Standard Precautions and Transmission-Based Precautions. When are Standard Precautions used?
9. What are the exposure-control methods used in each of the three categories of Transmission-Based Precautions.
10. Define Airborne Precautions, carrier, Contact Precautions, Droplet Precautions, fomites, infection, isolation, microorganism, nonpathogenic, nosocomial infection, pathogen, protective isolation, and Standard Precautions.

## STUDENT ACTIVITIES

1. Reread the information on infection control and Transmission-Based Precautions.
2. Review the glossary terms.
3. Practice the procedures for proper handwashing and donning and removal of mask, gown, and gloves, as outlined on the Student Performance Guide.

# *Student Performance Guide*

## LESSON 7-2　Infection Control and Transmission-Based Precautions

Name _____　Date _____

### ☣ INSTRUCTIONS

1. Practice the procedures for handwashing and donning mask, gown, and gloves following the step-by-step procedure.
2. Demonstrate your understanding of this lesson by:
   a. Completing a written examination successfully, and
   b. Performing the procedures for handwashing and donning mask, gown, and gloves satisfactorily for the instructor. All steps must be completed as listed on the instructor's Performance Check Sheet.

*Note:* The following procedures are intended as general guidelines for laboratory workers who must have contact with patients in isolation. The appropriate institutional policy manual must be consulted for specific instructions.

### MATERIALS AND EQUIPMENT

- sink for handwashing
- hand disinfectant
- clean paper towels
- disposable masks
- disposable gowns
- disposable gloves (sterile gloves optional)
- disposal receptacle for used items
- biohazard bags or other plastic bags with materials for labeling

### PROCEDURE

Record in the comment section any problems encountered while practicing the procedure (or have a fellow student or the instructor evaluate your performance).

S = Satisfactory
U = Unsatisfactory

| You must: | S | U | Comments |
|---|---|---|---|
| 1. Assemble equipment and materials | | | |
| 2. Wash hands:<br>a. Turn on warm water using a paper towel to turn the faucet handle, and discard the towel<br>b. Dispense soap onto hands and rub fronts and backs of hands and between fingers vigorously for one to two minutes. (If using bar soap, keep the bar in your hands during the entire lathering process)<br>c. Rinse hands, holding them fingertips downward under warm running water<br>d. Use clean towel to dry hands and turn off faucet. Dispose of towel, touching only the clean side | | | |

| You must: | S | U | Comments |
|---|---|---|---|
| 3. Don mask:<br>    a. Pick up a mask and place it over your mouth and nose, being careful not to touch your face with your fingers<br>    b. Tie the ends of the mask around your head and neck | | | |
| 4. Don gown:<br>    a. Slip arms into the sleeves of a gown, being careful to touch only the inside of gown<br>    b. Secure gown at neck and back of waist with ties, being careful to cover your clothing completely | | | |
| 5. Don gloves:<br>    a. Put on gloves, avoiding touching the outside of the gloves with your hands<br>    b. Pull the glove cuffs over the sleeves of your gown.<br>    *Note:* If using sterile gloves, open the package, being careful not to touch the outside of the gloves. Pick up the right glove by the cuff and insert your right hand. Pick up and hold the left glove by inserting the fingertips of your gloved right hand into the cuff of the left glove. Insert your left hand into glove. Position glove cuffs over your wrists by using your fingertips to push cuff toward your elbow. | | | |
| 6. Remove the gloves by folding them down and turning them inside out | | | |
| 7. Discard gloves in receptacle for contaminated materials. | | | |
| 8. Untie neck and waist ties of gown | | | |
| 9. Wash your hands following step 2 | | | |
| 10. Untie mask, touching only the ties | | | |
| 11. Hold the mask by the ties only and discard in proper receptacle | | | |
| 12. Remove gown by slipping your hands back into gown sleeve, touching only the inside of the gown | | | |
| 13. Fold the gown down over your arms inside-out and discard in appropriate receptacle | | | |
| 14. Wash your hands following step 2 | | | |
| 15. Leave the room using a clean paper towel to turn the door knob | | | |

*Evaluator Comments:*

Evaluator _____  Date _____

# Culture Techniques for Bacteria

## LESSON OBJECTIVES

**After studying this lesson, you should be able to:**

- *Explain the use of aseptic technique in bacteriology.*
- *Explain the differences between antiseptics and disinfectants and explain how they are used.*
- *Describe the different types of biological safety cabinets.*
- *Explain the differences in primary, selective, and indicator media.*
- *Describe how to inoculate different forms of media.*
- *Inoculate an agar plate using a swab and an inoculating loop.*
- *Explain the use of transport media.*
- *Define the glossary terms.*

## GLOSSARY

**agar** / seaweed derivative used to solidify microbiological media

**antiseptic** / chemical used to control the growth of microorganisms on living tissues

**aseptic technique** / measures used to prevent contamination when working with microorganisms

**disinfectant** / chemical used to kill or control microorganism growth

**HEPA filter** / high-efficiency particulate air filter used in biological safety cabinets

**indicator medium** / bacteriological medium that detects certain chemical reactions of organisms growing on it; differential medium

**inoculating loop** / instrument used to pick up and transfer bacteria

**inoculation** / process of transferring a population of microorganisms to a growth medium

**inoculum** / mass of bacteria being transferred from one medium to another

**mycoplasma** / tiny microorganism lacking a rigid cell wall

**primary medium** / medium that provides nutritional requirements for an organism and is used to recover the organism from infectious material

**quadrant** / one-fourth of a circle; one-fourth of an agar plate

**selective medium** / bacteriological medium that allows growth of some organisms while inhibiting growth of others

**sterilization** / act of eliminating all living microorganisms from an article or area

**transport medium** / medium that provides the proper environment for organisms during transport to the laboratory

## INTRODUCTION

Certain basic techniques must be mastered to work effectively in the bacteriology laboratory. Information about growth media, equipment, and reagents must be learned before beginning to work with bacteria. Safety is an important consideration; **aseptic technique** must be followed when working with bacterial cultures. Aseptic technique includes all measures used to limit exposing the worker and the environment to the bacteria; in addition, it includes preventing contamination of the bacterial culture by other unwanted organisms. The choice of medium (plural, media), a substance that provides nutrients for microorganism growth, is important. Technicians must be proficient in certain laboratory techniques, such as proper use of the **inoculating loop**, specimen preparation for reference laboratories, and bacterial transfer from the patient specimen to proper media to produce isolated colonies.

## ASEPTIC TECHNIQUE

Aseptic technique is usually thought of as a set of procedures used to prevent spread of infection during surgery. However, in the bacteriology laboratory, these are measures taken to prevent bacteria from infecting humans or contaminating surfaces, and, in some cases, to prevent contaminating the bacterial culture. Recent research has shown that the majority of laboratory-acquired infections occur by the respiratory route. Therefore, it is very important to avoid situations in which aerosols of infectious microorganisms might be formed. Aseptic technique includes physical and chemical means. Lesson 1-6 should be reviewed before before beginning this lesson.

## Physical Means of Preventing Contamination

There are several ways to incorporate aseptic technique into laboratory procedures. A fluid-resistant lab coat protects the worker's clothes from contamination, with the long sleeves protecting the culture from being contaminated by bacteria and skin cells shed from the worker's arms. The laboratory coat should be laundered at the hospital or laboratory and should never be worn home.

Handling materials and equipment is another important aspect of safety. The inoculating loop, used to transfer bacteria, must be sterilized and cooled before and after each use. It must be placed in the loop rack and never laid on the countertop (Figure 7-11). When the loop is sterilized in a flame or electric incinerator, the formation of aerosols must be avoided (Figure

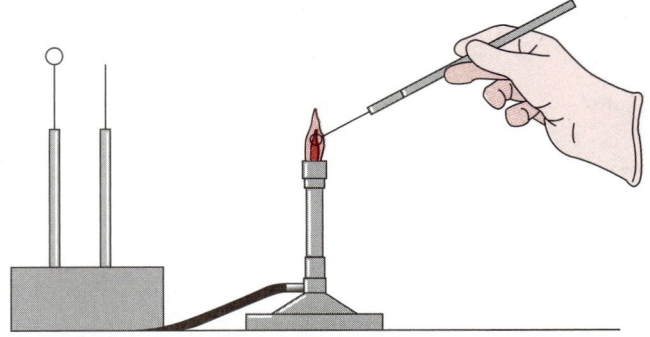

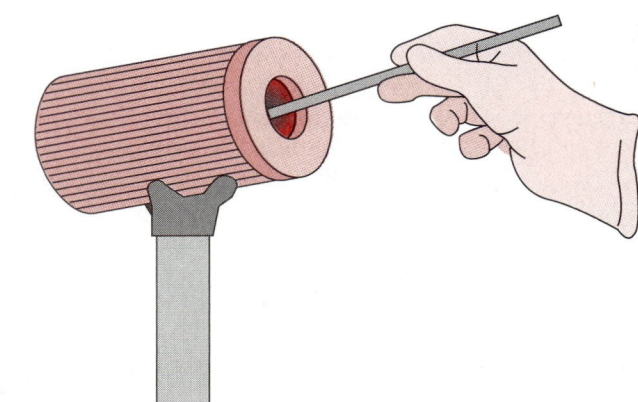

**FIGURE 7-11** Top, the proper way to sterilize the inoculating loop using a flame. A loop holder is in the background. Bottom, using an electric incinerator to sterilize the inoculating loop

7-11). Whenever possible, sterile disposable loops should be used. The lids of Petri dishes containing media should be open just enough to perform the necessary procedure (Figure 7-12).

### Microbiological Safety Cabinets.

Microbiological safety cabinets are specially designed laminar flow hoods that protect the worker from airborne infections (Figure 7-13). All work with fungi, *Mycobacterium*, and other infectious agents must be performed using a safety cabinet. These safety cabinets take in air from the room, pass it over the work area, where it picks up any airborne organisms, and then direct the air through a special high-efficiency particulate air filter, called a **HEPA filter**. The HEPA filter removes most of the contaminants from the air. This clean air is then exhausted outside.

Two classes of cabinets, Class I and Class II are found in most laboratories. Class I cabinets protect the worker, but provide little protection for the culture. The

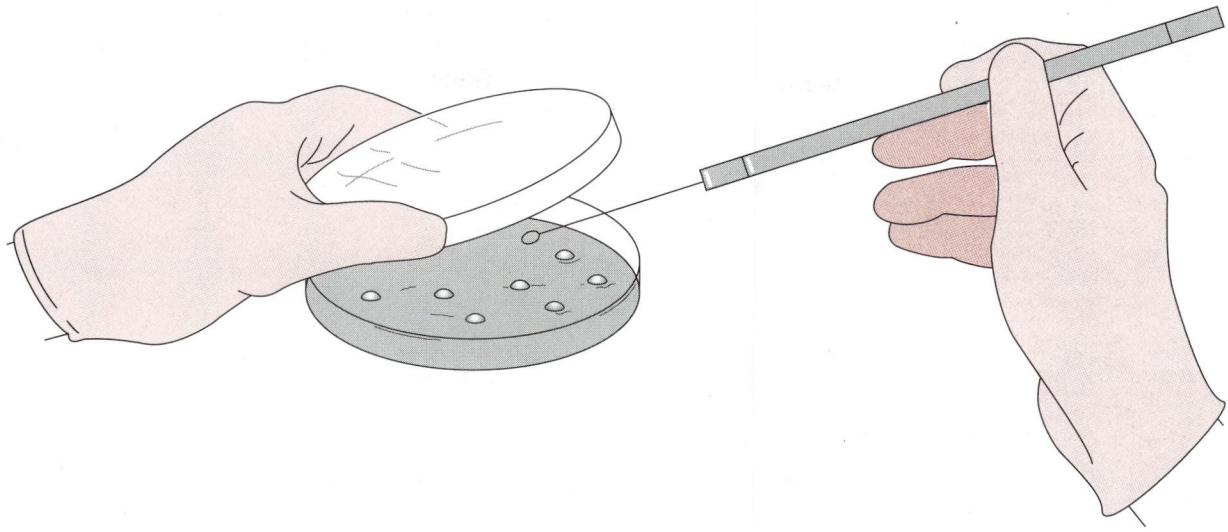

**FIGURE 7-12** Using proper technique to select colonies from an agar plate

Class II cabinet protects both the worker and the culture. Therefore, a Class II cabinet is preferred if only one can be purchased. More vigorous safety measures are used for very virulent organisms and will not be discussed here. Workers must still use aseptic technique even though the work is performed in a safety cabinet.

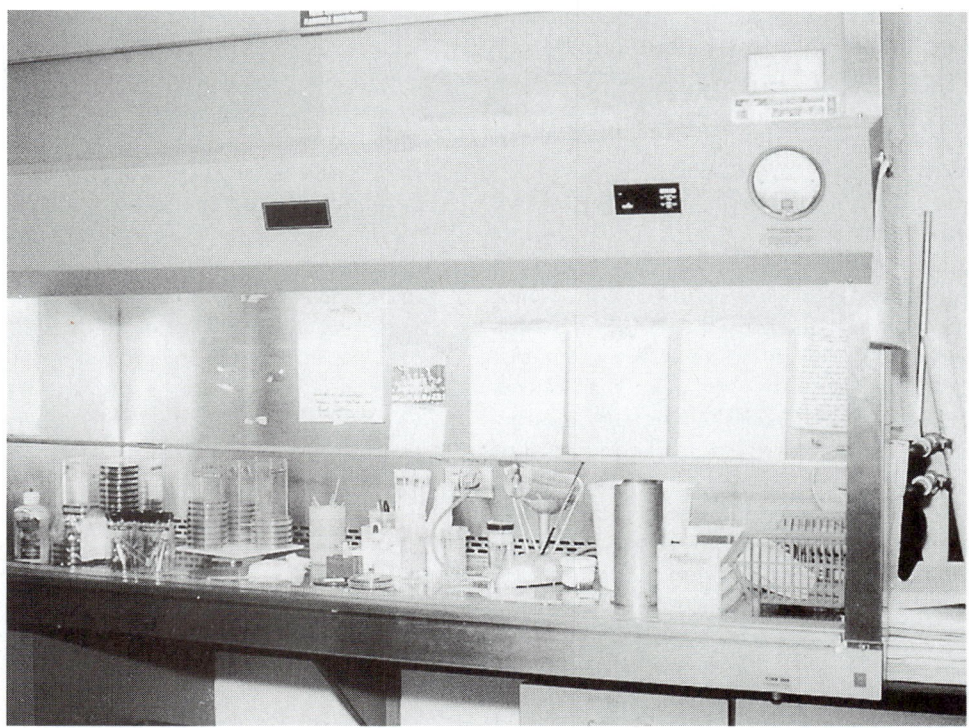

**FIGURE 7-13** Microbiological safety cabinet

**Table 7-13.** Chemicals commonly used as disinfectants

| CHEMICAL NAME OR COMMON NAME | ORGANISMS EFFECTIVE AGAINST | USE |
|---|---|---|
| Alcohols, 70-90% (isopropanol, ethanol) | Bacteria, *Mycobacterium*, and some viruses | Skin and surfaces |
| Halogens (chlorine bleach, iodine) | Especially good for viruses (protein in large amounts, such as blood spills, require increased concentration) | Surfaces |
| Aldehydes (formaldehyde and glutaraldehyde) | Bacteria, viruses, fungal and bacterial spores; *Mycobacterium* | Surfaces |
| Phenolics (Amphyl®) | Most bacteria and viruses; *Mycobacterium* | Surfaces |
| Quaternary ammonium salts | Bacteria, some fungi | Surfaces |

## Chemical Means of Preventing Contamination

Various chemicals are used as disinfectants and antiseptics. **Disinfectants** are chemicals used to kill or control the growth of microorganisms. They kill microorganisms in their active, vegetative stages, but usually not in their resting stages, such as bacterial and fungal spores. However, there are disinfectants that will kill spores (Table 7-13). Disinfection usually does not kill all microorganisms present, but reduces the number to a level that is no longer a threat to health. Bactericidal agents kill bacteria; bacteriostatic agents only slow the growth of bacteria.

**Antiseptics** are chemicals used to control the growth of microorganisms on living tissue. **Sterilization** refers to methods used to free an article or area from all living organisms. Sterilization, when performed properly, can kill spores. Table 7-13 contains a list of disinfectants, including some effective against spores and *Mycobacterium*, the organism that causes tuberculosis. Labels on the disinfectant provide information concerning the product's effectiveness on various microorganisms.

Surface disinfectants must be used liberally and often to be effective. The effectiveness of a disinfectant is influenced by its concentration, the number and type of microorganisms, the pH, the contact time, and the temperature. Also important is the microorganisms' location and the presence of interfering substances, such as protein or other organic material (Table 7-14).

Work surfaces should be wiped with a disinfectant solution before and after work is done. In addition, the area should be wiped any time a spill or splash occurs.

## GROWTH MEDIA FOR CLINICAL BACTERIOLOGY

A bacteriological medium is a substance used to grow bacteria in the laboratory. The medium may be liquid, such as a broth, or solid, such as tubes or plates of medium containing agar (Figure 7-14). **Agar** is a derivative of seaweed used to solidify liquid media.

In a clinical laboratory, the function of media is to help recover, grow, isolate, and identify microorganism(s) causing infection. A good, all-purpose medium for bacteria must support the growth of a wide variety of microorganisms and be economical. One medium that fulfills these requirements is sheep's blood agar, commonly called blood agar. Blood agar will support the growth of most microorganisms, from the tiny **mycoplasma** to most of the yeasts. Blood agar is also an indicator of bacterial *hemolysis*, the ability of certain bacteria to lyse RBCs (Color Plate 36). In general, hemolytic bacteria are more pathogenic than non-hemolytic bacteria.

**Table 7-14.** Factors affecting the action of disinfectants and antiseptics

Contact time
Temperature
pH
Concentration of chemical
Number of organisms present
Presence of organic matter, such as protein and blood

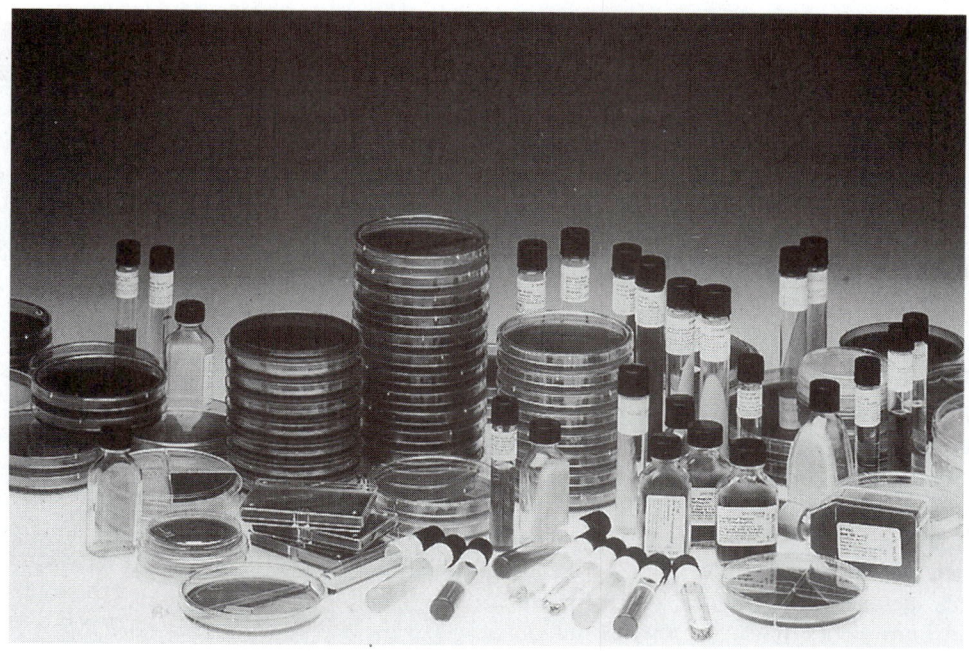

**FIGURE 7-14** Various types of media (Photo courtesy of Becton Dickinson)

## Primary Media

Choosing media to grow microorganisms is important and may determine the success of recovering the infection-causing agent (Table 7-15). The **primary medium** is the one on which the material collected from the patient is first inoculated. The primary medium is chosen based on the site of the infection; for example, the primary medium used for a wound culture would be different from that used for a urethral culture.

**Table 7-15.** Examples of primary, selective and indicator media

| TYPE | USE | ACTIVE INGREDIENT(S) | PURPOSE |
|------|-----|----------------------|---------|
| BA | Primary | Sheep or rabbit blood | Supports wide range of organisms |
| CA, MTM | Primary | Heated blood | Provides growth factors for fastidious organisms |
| EMB | Selective | Eosin y, methylene blue | Inhibits gram positive organisms |
| | Indicator | Eosin-methylene blue complex | Indicates fermentation of lactose, sucrose |
| MAC | Selective | Bile salts, crystal violet | Inhibits gram positive organisms |
| | Indicator | Neutral red | Indicates fermentation of lactose |

BA    =    blood agar
CA    =    chocolate agar
MTM   =    modified Thayer-Martin medium
EMB   =    eosin-methylene blue medium
MAC   =    MacConkey's medium

These are just a few examples of the most common media used in small laboratories or POLs; there are many other types with specialized uses.

## Selective Media

A **selective medium** contains ingredients that inhibit the growth of certain microorganisms, while allowing the growth of others. Two examples of selective media are EMB and MacConkey's (MAC), shown in Color Plates 37 and 38. Using a selective medium increases the chances of recovering a certain organism from a mixed bacterial population (Table 7-15).

## Indicator Media

An **indicator medium** (differential medium) contains substances that visibly change as a result of the metabolic activity of particular microorganisms. Indicator media can show chemical reactions of bacteria, such as fermentation of sugars. One example of an indicator medium is MAC, which produces a purple color when an organism ferments lactose. Some media, such as EMB and MAC, contain ingredients that make them function as both indicator and selective media. The results of growth on primary, selective, and indicator media can be valuable clues to a microorganism's identity. Table 7–15 gives examples of primary, selective, and indicator media, their principal ingredients, and reactions.

## PERFORMING CULTURE TECHNIQUES

In the bacteriology laboratory, the worker often must transfer culture material from one type of medium to another. The process of transferring a population of microorganisms to a growth medium is called **inoculation**. The group of microorganisms being transferred is called the **inoculum**. The first transfer of inoculum is from the site of infection to the primary medium. For example, a throat swab would be transferred to sheep's blood agar. Successfully recovering and identifying the disease-causing agent depends on properly collecting and transferring the inoculum, using aseptic technique.

## Safety

Technicians in the bacteriology laboratory must observe Standard Precautions, remembering that the specimens they handle may contain bacteria and OPIM. Handwashing and glove wearing are important when handling specimens. Other PPE should be used as required. Aseptic technique, physical methods of preventing contamination, and chemical disinfection methods must be combined to ensure the bacteriology laboratory is a safe working environment.

### *Quality Assurance*

Quality assurance or quality control is an important aspect of bacteriology. A good quality program ensures that media are not contaminated, that they will support growth of organisms, and that indicator and selective media are reacting properly. A good program will also help ensure that unknown isolates are correctly identified. The QA program may consist of internal and external components.

### Internal Program of Quality Assurance

The internal program can include specimen collection, media checks, reagent quality, equipment performance, and staff proficiency. Commercial quality control microorganism sets can be purchased that meet NCCLS requirements for testing commercially prepared media, antibiotic susceptibility testing, and help document a personal assessment program. A quality assurance program should also include monitoring and recording temperatures of all incubators and refrigerators.

### External Quality Assurance Program

Laboratories may subscribe to one of several external QA or proficiency programs. These programs can be expensive, but are a good way to ensure that staff is proficient in identifying organisms. Bacterial specimens are sent to the laboratory to be identified at specified times during the year. Regulatory agencies responsible for laboratory inspection also offer microbiology proficiency programs.

## Collecting and Transporting Specimens

Specimens must be collected with the correct type of swab. Almost all microbiological work requires use of sterile polyester or rayon swabs, since cotton contains ingredients that are harmful to some microorganisms. If the material is to be transported to another laboratory, the correct type of **transport medium** must be available (Figure 7-15). Reference laboratories usually provide transport materials and instructions for their use. The transport materials must be sterile and include ingredients that will protect the microorganisms from drying for several hours. Once the specimen arrives in the laboratory, it should be placed on the growth medium as soon as possible.

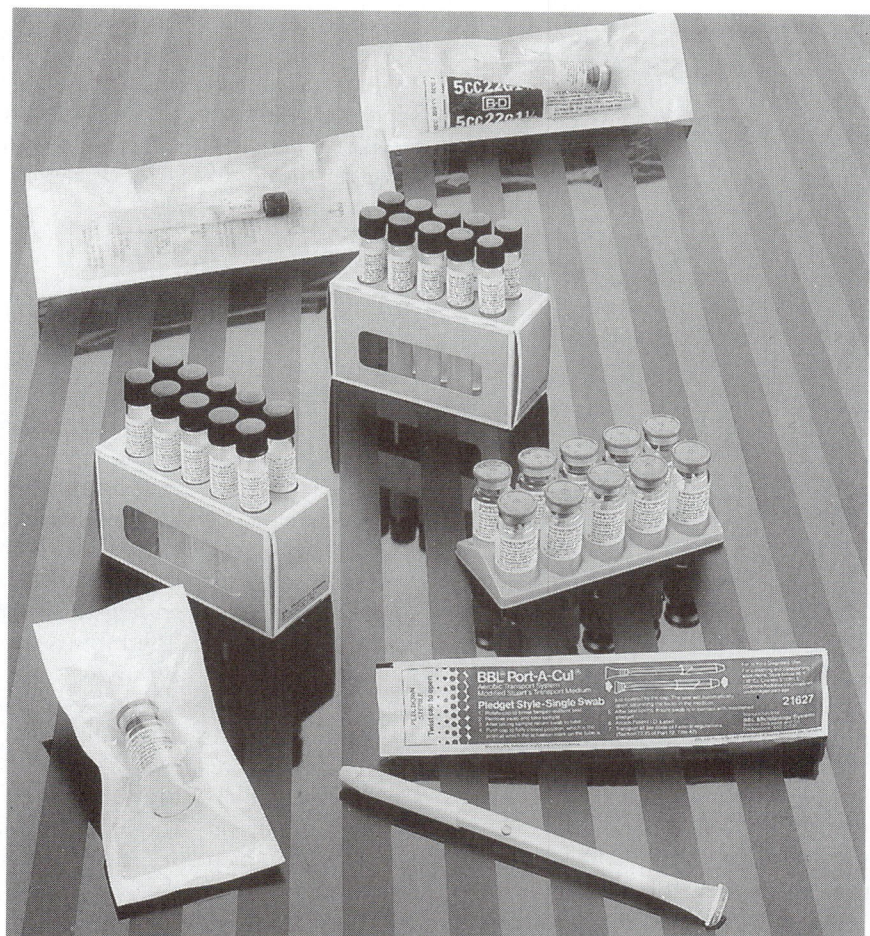

**FIGURE 7-15** Transport media (Photo courtesy of Becton Dickinson)

## Media Inoculation

### Agar Plate

The first step in inoculating a plate is labeling it with the patient's name and identification number. The Petri dish is always labeled on the *bottom*, not the lid, since the lid could get switched from one dish to another. Also, agar plates are always incubated upside down to prevent condensate that would form in the lid from dripping onto the agar.

The medium is inoculated by gently rolling the specimen swab onto one **quadrant** of the blood agar plate (Figure 7-16). When only one swab is sent, a smear can be prepared from the same swab. After the swab has been used to inoculate the plate, it is rolled across a glass microscope slide to produce a smear about 0.5-1 inch long (Figure 7-17). The swab is then discarded in a biohazard waste container.

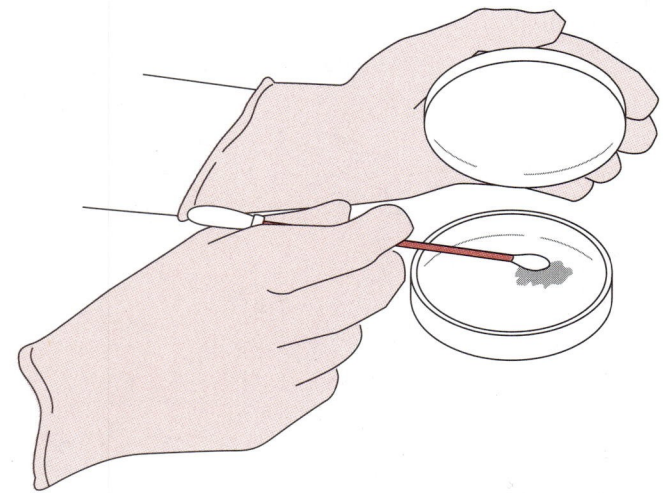

**FIGURE 7-16** Inoculating one quadrant of an agar plate using a swab

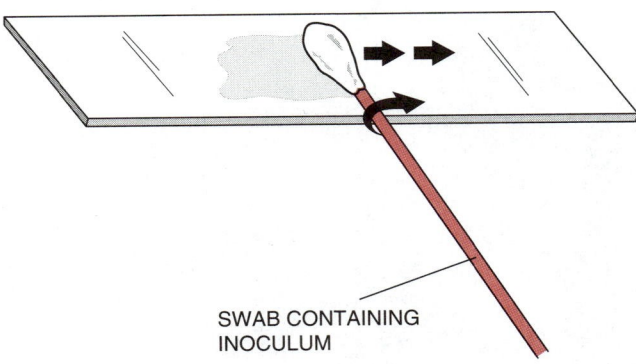

SWAB CONTAINING
INOCULUM

**FIGURE 7-17** Preparing a bacterial smear using a swab

## Streaking a Plate for Isolated Colonies

A bacterial inoculating loop is used to spread the inoculated material over the agar plate in a manner that will produce isolated colonies. This is accomplished by transferring less culture material into each successive quadrant. Gentle pressure should be used to avoid tearing the agar's surface.

The loop is sterilized, cooled, and then used to spread the material from the first quadrant into the second quadrant (Figure 7-18). After the loop is sterilized again, it is used to spread material from the second quadrant into the third quadrant, and then from the third into the fourth. In the fourth quadrant, the procedure is done carefully to produce isolated colonies of the bacteria (Figure 7-18). Some workers choose to make the streaks in the fourth quadrant in the shape of a "tornado" to increase the distance between the developing colonies. Sterile, disposable loops are available and eliminate the need for flaming when used as directed by the manufacturer. The lid of the petri dish should be raised just enough to allow room to manipulate the loop. The lid of the petri dish should never be removed completely, to avoid exposing the medium to contamination. In addition, the lid should never be laid on the countertop.

## Agar Slant

An agar slant tube should be labeled with date and patient information. Colonies are picked up from an agar plate with a sterile loop. The slant tube is held in the other hand while the fourth and fifth fingers of the hand holding the loop are used to remove the tube's cap (Figure 7-19). (The cap is not laid down, but is held in this way until the tube is recapped when the procedure has been completed.)

The loop is inserted into the tube and used to make a zig-zag pattern on the slant, starting on the slant's far end and ending at the top (Figure 7-20). The loop is withdrawn, the tube is capped, and the loop is sterilized. If the loop or culture material touched the tube's rim, the rim should be sterilized before recapping (Figure 7-19). An agar slant can also be inoculated in a similar manner using a swab.

Aseptic technique must be maintained during these operations. The loop must be sterilized in a way that reduces aerosol formation and it must not be laid down on the work surface.

## Inoculation of Indicator or Selective Medium

Additional types of media may be required to confirm an organism's identity. They are inoculated with the inoculating loop using the isolated colonies growing on the primary plate. The primary plate lid is raised just enough to insert the sterilized and cooled loop and pick

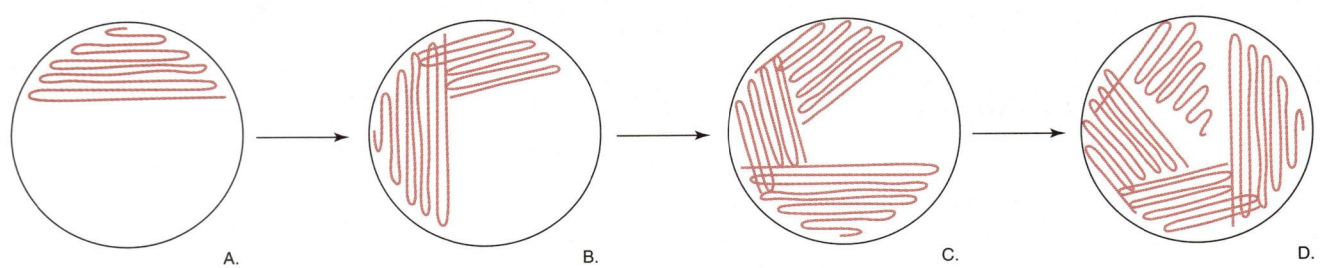

A.          B.          C.          D.

**FIGURE 7-18** Streaking an agar plate in four quadrants to produce isolated colonies: (A) inoculate first quadrant; (B) turn plate 90° and use sterile loop to streak into second quadrant; (C) turn plate another 90°, sterilize loop, and streak into third quadrant; (D) turn plate another 90°, use sterile loop to make one streak out of third quadrant in a "tornado" pattern

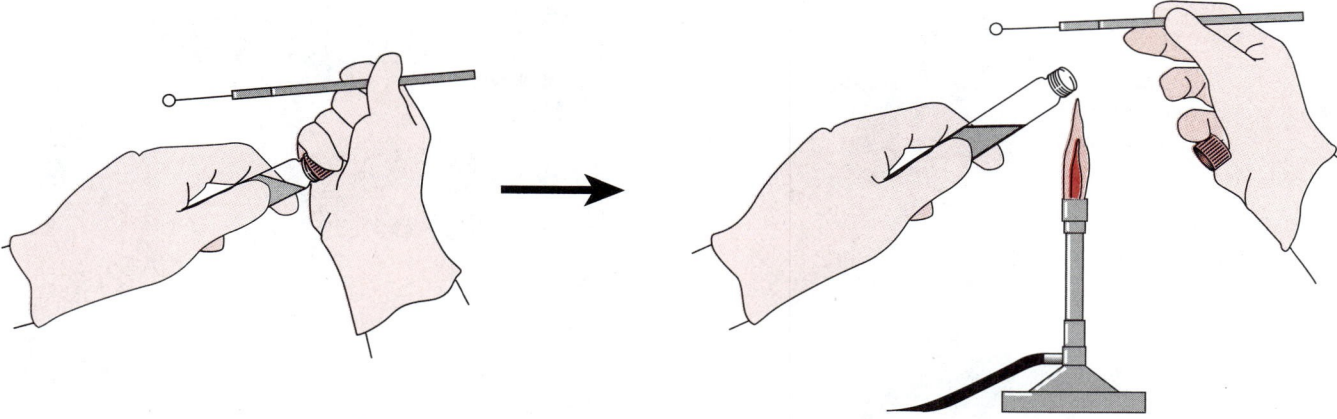

**FIGURE 7-19** Preparing to inoculate an agar slant

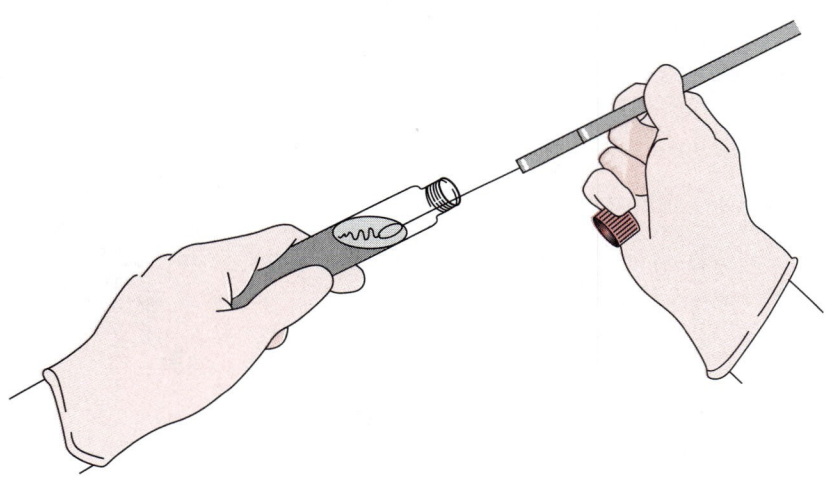

**FIGURE 7-20** Inoculating an agar slant

up one or two isolated colonies. The loop is withdrawn and the other plate's lid is raised enough to streak the plate for isolated colonies. Split plates containing two kinds of media such as blood and EMB or MAC are economical, but the streaking method must be modified (Figure 7-21).

## OBSERVING THE CULTURE AFTER TWENTY-FOUR HOURS

Most human pathogens grow best at 35–37°C. Inoculated plates are usually kept in a 35–37°C incubator overnight; if growth is not evident or is insufficient, the plate is kept an additional twenty-four hours (Figure 7-22).

When the plate is removed from the incubator, any growth can be observed through the lid, unless it is necessary to perform other tests. The plate should be inspected for the presence of isolated colonies (those not touched by others) (Figure 7-23 and Color Plate 31).

Growth on blood agar should be observed for hemolysis. Some bacteria can completely lyse RBCs so the area around the bacterial growth is almost transparent. This is called beta (β) hemolysis (Color Plate 36). Other bacteria incompletely lyse the blood cells and produce green discoloration around the colonies. This is called alpha (α) hemolysis. Absence of hemolysis is called gamma hemolysis. Observation of hemolysis is especially important in diagnosing strep throat, since

**FIGURE 7-21** Illustration of a split plate used for urine culture with blood agar on one side and EMB or MAC on the other side

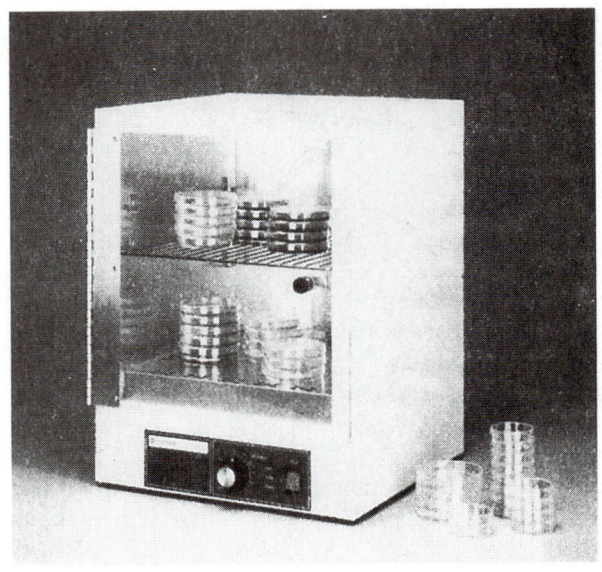

**FIGURE 7-22** A bacteriological incubator (Photo courtesy of Fisher Scientific)

*Streptococcus pyogenes*, which causes strep throat, is beta hemolytic.

Other bacterial colony characteristics that help with identification are size, color, shape, and even odor. Bacterial colonies may be white, gray, yellow, or even red. Their size may range from almost too tiny to be seen to very large. Their shape is usually round, but may also be flattened or raised like a dome. Some have distinctive odors, such as one *Pseudomonas* species that smells like grapes, and *Neisseria gonorrhoeae*, which smells to some like sweaty tennis shoes. *However, never place bacterial culture near your face or risk inhaling bacteria.*

## TRANSPORT TO ANOTHER LABORATORY

Material sent to a reference laboratory for microbiological procedures must be transported in special transport media (Figure 7-15). The Culturette® is one type of self-contained system that has a sterile swab and a medium to keep the organism alive during transport. Different systems are available for transporting aerobic and anaerobic organisms. Amies is a type of semi-solid transport medium into which the inoculated swab is inserted and the stick broken off so the tube can be capped.

Reference laboratories provide several types of transport media with which physicians and laboratory

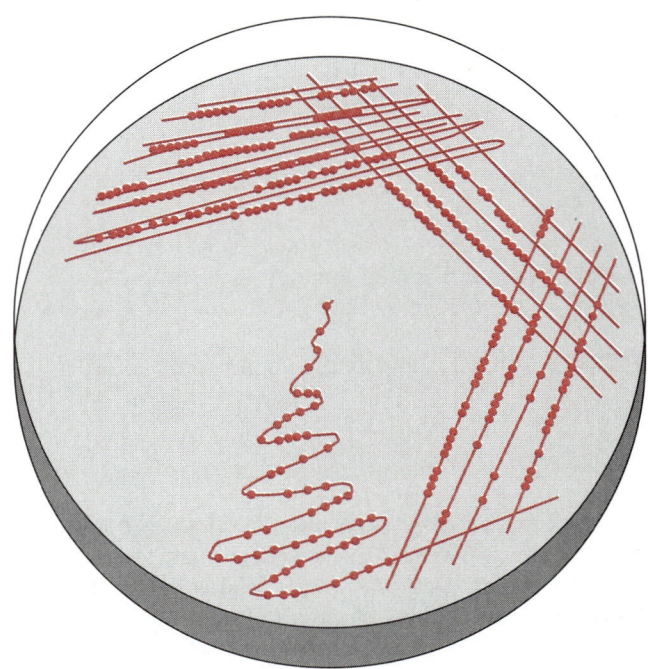

**FIGURE 7-23** Isolated colonies on an agar plate

workers must be familiar. For the transported organism(s) to survive, the transport medium must be used according to the manufacturer's instructions.

## Procedural Notes

- Always sterilize the loop before and after using it to prevent culture contamination.
- Keep agar slants or Petri dishes open only long enough to transfer the culture.
- Use aseptic technique to avoid contaminating specimens or cultures.
- Perform quality assurance checks on media and equipment to ensure proper function.
- Transfer specimens to primary media as soon possible after collection

## Safety Precautions

- Always observe Universal and Standard Precautions when handling specimens and cultures.
- Avoid formation of aerosols when sterilizing the inoculating loop.
- Always sterilize the loop after use and return it to its holder.
- Use a disposable inoculating loop whenever possible.
- Wipe work surfaces frequently with surface disinfectant.
- Wear a fluid-resistant, buttoned laboratory coat to prevent clothing contamination.
- Never wear or take the laboratory coat home.
- Never place a bacterial culture near your face or try to smell it.

## SUMMARY

Bacteriological laboratory work provides important information used in diagnosing and treating infections. Workers must be familiar with different types of media and techniques used to culture and identify organisms involved in infections. Clinical Bacteriology methods are changing from manual to automated. However, there will always be a need for technologists who understand and use good bacteriological technique.

## LESSON REVIEW

1. Discuss aseptic technique in the bacteriology laboratory.
2. Explain the differences between disinfectants and antiseptics.
3. Discuss the types of bacteriological safety cabinets and their uses.
4. Discuss the purposes of primary, selective, and indicator media.
5. Describe how to inoculate an agar plate using a swab.
6. Describe how to streak a plate for isolation.
7. Describe how to transfer an inoculum from an agar plate to an agar slant.
8. Discuss important colony characteristics that may be observed.
9. Explain how hemolytic reactions of bacteria may be used to identify the organism.
10. Explain why transport media are used.
11. Discuss quality assurance in the bacteriology laboratory.
12. Define agar, antiseptic, aseptic technique, disinfectant, HEPA filter, indicator medium, inoculating loop, inoculation, inoculum, mycoplasma, primary medium, quadrant, selective medium, sterilization, and transport medium.

## STUDENT ACTIVITIES

1. Reread the information on culture techniques for bacteriology.
2. Practice inoculating an agar plate using a swab and an inoculating loop, as outlined in the Student Performance Guide.
3. Determine the types of disinfectants used in local POLs.
4. Examine the labels of household disinfectants and compare their active ingredients with those of disinfectants used in health care settings.

# Student Performance Guide

## LESSON 7-3 Culture Techniques for Bacteria

Name _____  Date _____

## ☣ INSTRUCTIONS

1. Practice inoculating an agar plate using a swab and an inoculating loop, following the step-by-step procedure.
2. Demonstrate your understanding of this lesson by:
   a. Completing a written examination successfully, and
   b. Performing the procedure for inoculating an agar plate with a swab and inoculating loop satisfactorily for the instructor. All steps must be completed as listed on the instructor's Performance Check Sheet.

## MATERIALS AND EQUIPMENT

- gloves
- hand disinfectant
- surface disinfectant (10% chlorine bleach)
- Dacron or rayon sterile swabs, or, alternatively, the instructor may provide swabs with bacteria already applied, stored in capped culture tubes
- blood agar plates (or trypticase soy agar)
- inoculating loops, (sterile disposable preferred)
- Bunsen burner, alcohol burner, or electric incinerator
- incubator set at 35°–37°C
- educational strain of *Escherichia coli* or *Staphylococcus aureus* (less pathogenic strain used specifically for teaching purposes, available through biological supply houses), growing in tubes
- waterproof marker for writing on plastic
- matches or flint-type lighter
- test tube rack
- loop holder
- biohazard container
- paper towels

## PROCEDURE

Record in the comment section any problems encountered while practicing the procedure (or have a fellow student or the instructor evaluate your performance).

S = Satisfactory
U = Unsatisfactory

| You must: | S | U | Comments |
|---|---|---|---|
| 1. Wash hands | | | |
| 2. Assemble materials and equipment | | | |
| 3. Prepare the work area: place one or two paper towels on the counter and pour a small amount of surface disinfectant over them | | | |
| 4. Light the Bunsen burner or turn on the electric incinerator | | | |
| 5. Select an agar plate to be inoculated and label the bottom with the marker | | | |

| You must: | S | U | Comments |
|---|---|---|---|
| 6.  Select an inoculated swab or sterile swab and appropriate culture | | | |
| 7.  Set inoculating loop in holder within reach (if using disposable loop place unopened package nearby) **Note:** Put on gloves; use special care around the Bunsen burner flame | | | |
| 8.  Remove sterile swab from package by the handle | | | |
| 9.  Pick up tube of culture to be transferred in one hand; use fourth and fifth fingers of the hand holding the swab to remove the cap from the tube. (Hold cap with fingers for entire procedure; do not lay cap down) | | | |
| 10.  Insert tip of swab into culture and pick up a small amount | | | |
| 11.  Replace cap on culture tube and set tube in test tube rack. (Be careful not to touch anything with the swab tip) | | | |
| 12.  Lift the agar plate lid just enough to insert the swab and spread the inoculum over the surface of one quadrant of the agar plate | | | |
| 13.  Replace the lid on the Petri dish | | | |
| 14.  Dispose of swab in biohazard container or as directed by instructor | | | |
| 15.  Pick up inoculating loop and sterilize it by inserting loop into the middle of the flame and then moving the loop into the upper part of the flame, or sterilize the loop by placing it in an electric incinerator until the loop glows red | | | |
| 16.  Cool the loop briefly | | | |
| 17.  Streak the second quadrant of the plate by touching the loop in the first quadrant and streaking all the way across the second quadrant | | | |
| 18.  Repeat step 17 six to eight times | | | |
| 19.  Sterilize and cool the loop | | | |
| 20.  Streak the third quadrant by touching the loop to the second quadrant and streaking into the third quadrant, making six to eight strokes | | | |
| 21.  Sterilize and cool the loop | | | |
| 22.  Lift the lid of the Petri dish just enough to be able to insert the loop | | | |
| 23.  Streak the fourth quadrant in a way that produces isolated colonies: Touch the loop to the third quadrant and spread the organisms into the fourth quadrant using a continuous streak in a "tornado" pattern. Decrease the width of the streaks horizontally and increase the distance between the streaks vertically | | | |

| You must: | S | U | Comments |
|---|---|---|---|
| 24. Replace the lid on the Petri dish | | | |
| 25. Sterilize the loop and replace it in the holder | | | |
| 26. Turn off the Bunsen burner or electric incinerator | | | |
| 27. Place the agar plate upside down in the 35–37°C incubator to incubate overnight (eighteen to twenty-four hours) | | | |
| 28. Clean reusable equipment and return to proper storage; put disposables in biohazard containers | | | |
| 29. Clean work area with surface disinfectant | | | |
| 30. Remove gloves | | | |
| 31. Wash hands with hand disinfectant | | | |
| 32. The next day: Put on gloves and wipe work area with surface disinfectant or prepare as in step 3. Remove the plate from the incubator and examine the growth | | | |
| 33. Look at the colonies. Are they colored? What is the shape? Are they flat or raised? Record observations | | | |
| 34. Look for hemolysis if blood agar was used. Record as no hemolysis (gamma), alpha (α), or beta (β) | | | |
| 35. Dispose of used agar plate in biohazard container | | | |
| 36. Wipe counter with surface disinfectant | | | |
| 37. Remove and discard gloves in biohazard container and wash hands with hand disinfectant | | | |

*Evaluator Comments:*

Evaluator _____ Date _____

# Preparing a Bacteriological Smear and Performing a Gram Stain

## LESSON OBJECTIVES

**After studying this lesson, you should be able to:**

- *Discuss the use of Standard Precautions and aseptic technique.*
- *Prepare smears from a swab.*
- *Prepare smears from cultures growing on media.*
- *Heat-fix a bacteriological smear.*
- *Explain the theory of the Gram stain.*
- *Perform the Gram stain procedure.*
- *Identify gram-positive organisms on a smear.*
- *Identify gram-negative organisms on a smear.*
- *Use aseptic techniques during procedures.*
- *List the safety precautions to be observed when performing the Gram stain.*
- *Define the glossary terms.*

## GLOSSARY

**bibulous paper** / special absorbent paper used to dry slides

**counterstain** / dye that adds a contrasting color

**mordant** / substance that fixes a dye or stain to an object

## INTRODUCTION

Preparing and staining a bacteriological smear is a relatively quick and simple, yet important, process. The Gram stain reaction and morphology of an organism are significant clues to its identity and to appropriate antibiotic selection.

A smear can be prepared directly from bacteria growing on media or from a swab containing organisms from such sites as a wound or genital discharge. Since either source contains potentially infectious organisms, Standard Precautions and aseptic technique must be followed, to avoid contaminating the worker, co-workers, surroundings, and the specimen.

  **Safety**

Following the guidelines for Standard Precautions and aseptic technique is an essential part of the overall safety plan for the entire laboratory. Aseptic technique includes (1) sterilizing the loop before and after each use (or using a sterile disposable loop), (2) sterilizing the mouths of culture tubes after opening and before closing them, (3) raising the lids of Petri dishes just enough to perform a procedure and never placing them on the countertop, (4) disposing of all contaminated materials in the proper biohazard containers, and (5)

wiping the work surface area with an approved disinfectant before beginning and after finishing a procedure (Lesson 7-3).

One method of dealing with potential bacterial culture spills, especially in student laboratories, is to prepare a small work space for each person. This can be done by placing one or two paper towels on the surface and pouring on a small amount of disinfectant. If a spill occurs, the paper towels can simply be rolled up and discarded in a biohazard container. Additional rules include:

- wearing gloves when transferring patient specimens to media or slides and working with OPIM

- wearing a fluid-resistant, buttoned laboratory coat to protect clothing from contamination

- keeping the work area free of clutter

- wiping up all spills promptly with surface disinfectant

- washing hands with hand disinfectant after every procedure and any other time they may have become contaminated

- disposing of all specimens and culture materials by autoclaving (being sure to follow all applicable local, state, and federal regulations)

### *Quality Assurance*

Observing bacterial morphology on a stained smear is an important part of bacteriology. The amount of culture material applied to the slide should be such that it is barely visible when dry. Heat-fixing must also be done carefully to avoid cracking the slide or damaging the organisms with extreme heat. Gram stain reagents should not be used after the expiration date. Slides for checking the reliability of Gram stain reagents and staff technique should be used. Microscopes used to observe stained smears should be serviced on a regular basis. All lenses must be kept clean to allow for accurate observations of the stained organisms.

## PREPARING THE SMEAR

A smear can be prepared from the swab used to collect material from the patient. Such a swab could be from an infected wound or from a suspected gonorrheal discharge. *Media should be inoculated before the smear is made*. Preparing the smear first could contaminate the culture if the glass slide is not sterile. The best solution is to obtain two swabs, but that is not always practical.

## Preparing a Smear from the Swab

To prepare a smear of the organisms on the swab, a clean microscope slide is labeled with the patient's name and identification number. The swab is gently *rolled* across the surface of the slide (Figure 7-24). This action should leave just a thin film of material on the slide. When dry, a properly made smear should be barely visible on the slide before being stained. Replace the swab in its transport medium or discard in a biohazard container.

## Preparing a Smear from a Culture

Preparing a smear from bacteria growing on media is also an easy procedure. The culture may be growing on tubed media, such as an agar slant in a screw-top culture tube, or on agar in a Petri dish.

### Using a Culture on an Agar Slant

To prepare a smear using bacteria growing on a slant, a drop of water is first placed on a glass slide. The culture tube is held in one hand and the inoculating loop in the other. The fourth and fifth fingers of the hand holding the loop are used to unscrew the cap of the tube. The loop and the mouth of the tube are sterilized and allowed to cool briefly (Figure 7-25). Since several inches of the loop wire will enter the tube, the loop and about 2–2.5 inches of the wire above should be sterilized. The loop is then used to pick up a very small

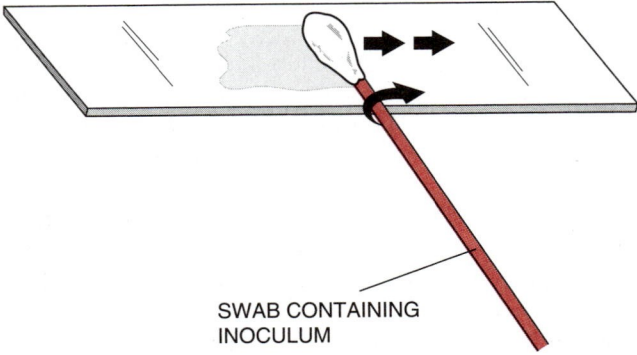

SWAB CONTAINING INOCULUM

**FIGURE 7-24** Preparing a bacterial smear using a swab

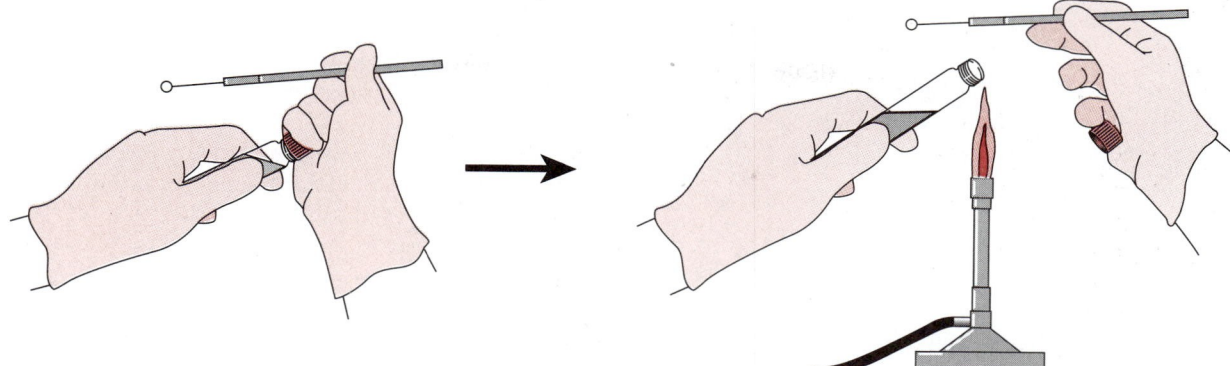

**FIGURE 7-25** Flaming a culture tube

amount of bacteria from the edge of the streak. These bacteria are mixed with a drop of water on a glass slide to make a smear about the size of a nickel (Figure 7-26). The mouth of the tube is sterilized again, the lid replaced, and the tube set in a test tube rack. The loop is then sterilized and replaced in its holder. The slide is allowed to air-dry and is then heat-fixed.

### Using a Culture in a Petri Dish

Most bacterial cultures in medical laboratories are grown on an agar medium in a Petri dish. The Petri dish lid should be raised just enough to insert the sterilized loop and touch it to a colony. The bacteria obtained are mixed with a drop of water on a clean glass slide and spread into a circle about the size of a nickel (Figure 7-27). The smear is then air-dried and heat-fixed. The dry unstained smear should be almost invisible.

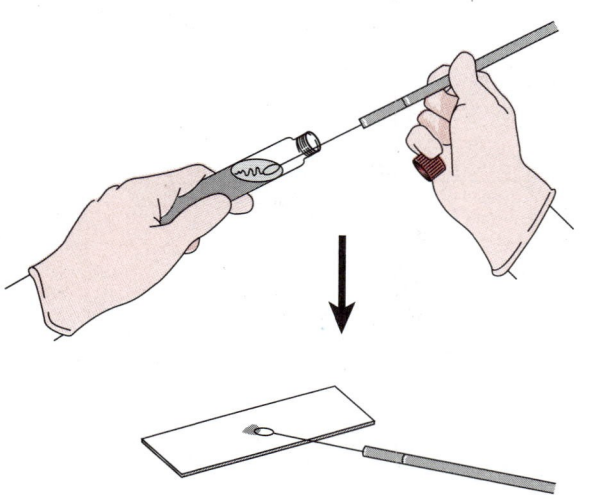

**FIGURE 7-26** Transferring bacteria from a culture tube to a slide

### Heat-Fixing the Smear

When the film on the slide is completely dry, the smear is ready to be heat-fixed. This can be done using an electric incinerator such as the Bacti-Cinerator®, an electric slide warmer, or a Bunsen burner flame (Figures 7-28 and 7-29). When using a flame, the slide is held with a spring-type clothespin or forceps and the smear is passed through the flame *briefly* two or three times (Figure 7-29). When a smear has been heat-fixed correctly, the slide should not feel hot if touched to the back of the hand.

Heat-fixing is necessary to cause the organisms to adhere to the glass slide during the staining. Excessive heating will alter or destroy the microorganism's morphology and can break the glass slide. Under-heating will cause the organisms to wash off the slide during staining and will require that the specimen be recollected if the swab has already been discarded.

## THE GRAM STAIN

The most frequently performed stain in the bacteriology laboratory is the Gram stain. Most bacterial cells are so small and possess so little color they are difficult to observe microscopically unless they are stained. The Gram stain is performed on a thin smear of bacteria that has been air-dried and heat-fixed.

Gram stain reactions are based on the chemical differences in the structures of bacterial cell walls. The staining procedure consists of applying a sequence of dye, **mordant**, decolorizer, and **counterstain**. A counterstain is a dye that adds contrasting color to the object being stained.

### Performing the Gram Stain

The air-dried and heat-fixed smear must be supported over a container to catch the staining reagents. This con-

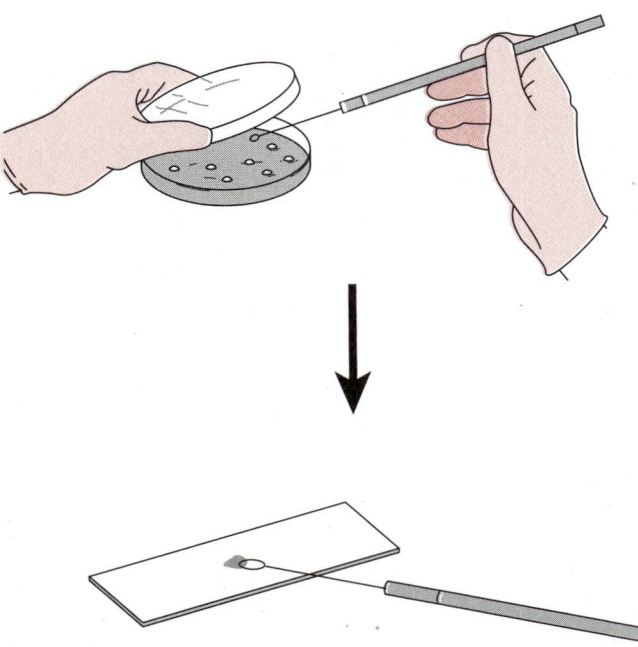

**FIGURE 7-27** Top, removing bacteria from an agar plate using the inoculating loop; bottom, making a bacterial smear using the inoculating loop

tainer can be a beaker, a glass or stainless steel pan, or a laboratory sink. A rack to fit across the top of the container can be fashioned out of glass rods and rubber tubing (Figure 7-30), or ready-made staining racks can be purchased if desired. In addition, laboratories that have large volumes of work can use automated stainers.

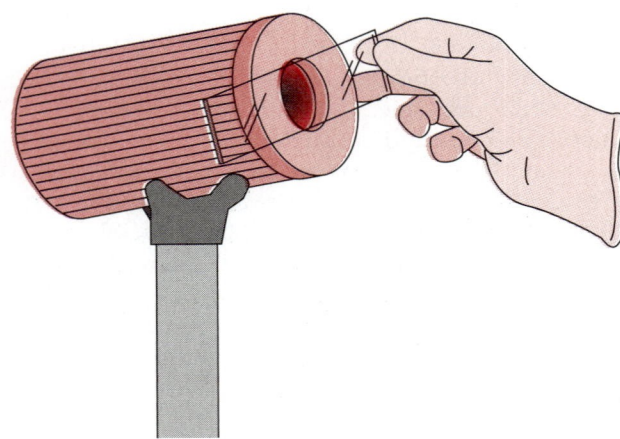

**FIGURE 7-28** Heat-fixing a bacterial smear using the BactiCinerator®

### Primary Stain

To perform the Gram stain, the heat-fixed smear is placed on the staining rack and the primary stain, a dye called crystal violet, is poured on the slide (Figure 7-31). The staining time is usually one minute, but the manufacturer's instructions must be followed. After one minute, the slide is rinsed by gently pouring tap water on it, or by holding the slide with forceps under a gentle stream of tap water.

### Gram's Iodine (Mordant)

Gram's iodine, a mordant, is then poured on the slide. A **mordant** is a substance that causes a dye or stain to adhere to the object being stained.

### Decolorizer

After one minute the slide is again rinsed with tap water. A decolorizer, such as alcohol or an alcohol-acetone mixture, is briefly added to the slide. This is best done while the slide is held with forceps and tilted downward at about a 30° angle. It is important that this not be done too long; three to five seconds, or until no more purple runs off, is long enough.

The decolorization step is an important one. At this point in the staining process, the gram-positive organisms will be dark purple-blue because their cell wall composition allows penetration and retention of the crystal violet. The gram-negative organisms will appear rather colorless because their cell walls do not retain the crystal violet in the decolorization procedure. However, prolonged decolorization can eventually remove the primary stain from the gram-positive organisms as well. This could cause incorrect identification of an organism (Figure 7-31).

### Counterstain

After the decolorizing procedure is finished, the slide is again rinsed with water to remove all decolorizer and stop the decolorization process. The slide is then flooded with the counterstain, safranin. The safranin has no

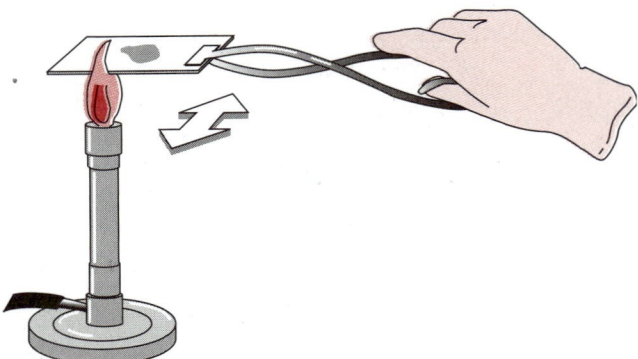

**FIGURE 7-29** Heat-fixing a bacteriological smear using a bunsen burner

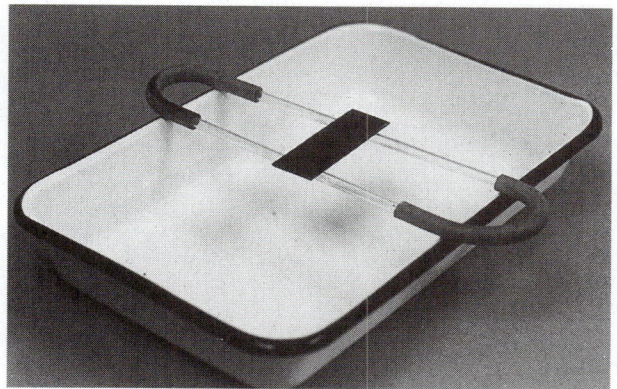

**FIGURE 7-30** Slide staining rack (Photo courtesy of John Estridge)

effect on the gram-positive cells, which retained the crystal violet, but the colorless gram-negative cells will be stained red-pink (Figure 7-31).

At the end of the counterstaining time, the slides are washed again and the excess water shaken off. The slides are then either placed standing on end to air-dry or dried by blotting between sheets of **bibulous paper** to remove the excess moisture. After the slides are completely dry, they are ready to be viewed microscopically.

## OBSERVING THE STAINED BACTERIOLOGICAL SMEAR

The stained smear should be observed using the oil-immersion objective (100X) after the stained area has been located using the low-power (10X) objective. The gram-negative organisms will appear pink-red and the gram-positive ones will appear dark blue-purple (Color Plates 32 and 33). *Staphylococcus aureus* is a common gram-positive organism that is round (coccus). Although they are not bacteria, yeasts such as *Candida albicans* stain dark purple in the Gram stain (Color Plate 35). *Escherichia coli*, an inhabitant of the intestines, is a gram-negative rod.

If the smear was prepared correctly, the bacteria should be spread out so the morphology is easy to distinguish and the color is crisp and distinct. All bacteria of the same type may not look identical, but the majority will be representative. Gram-negative rods can be slender and long, fat and long, or fat and short. Sometimes rods may be so short that they begin to appear round, like the cocci, so they are called coccobacilli. The round bacteria may appear singly or in pairs, grape-like clusters (staph), or chains similar to strings of beads (strep). Figure 7-32 illustrates some of these variations in morphology.

| Step | Time | Procedure | Result |
|------|------|-----------|--------|
| 1 | one minute | Primary stain: Apply crystal violet stain (purple) ↓ Rinse slide | All bacteria stain purple |
| 2 | one minute | Mordant: Apply Gram's iodine ↓ Rinse slide | All bacteria remain purple |
| 3 | three to five seconds | Decolorize: Apply alcohol ↓ Rinse slide | Purple stain is removed from gram-negative cells |
| 4 | one minute | Counterstain: Apply safranin stain (red) ↓ Rinse slide | Gram-negative cells appear pink-red; gram positive cells appear purple |

**FIGURE 7-31** Steps in the Gram stain procedure

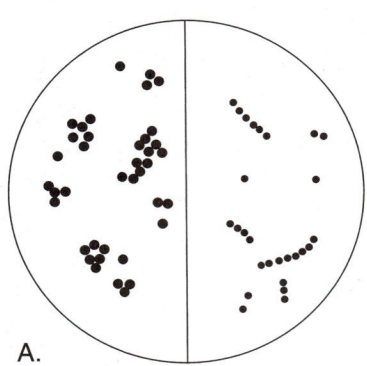
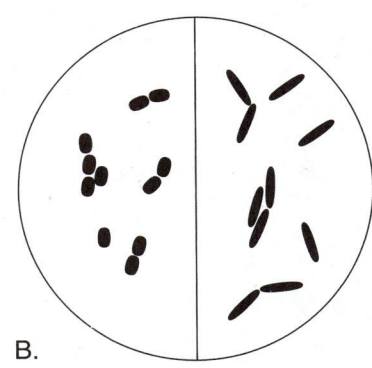
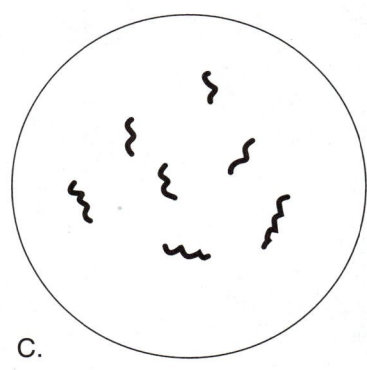

A.     B.     C.

**FIGURE 7-32** Variations in bacterial morphology: (A) cocci: left, grape-like clusters; right, bead-like chains; (B) bacilli: left, short and fat; right, long and slender; (C) spirochetes

## Procedural Notes

■ Make the smear thin enough to be just barely visible when unstained.

■ Use gentle heat to fix the slide; too much heat will distort bacterial morphology or may cause the slide to break.

■ Follow instructions carefully for the Gram stain reagents being used.

■ Ensure that the microscope objectives and eyepieces are clean.

## Safety Precautions

■ Observe Universal and Standard Precautions when handling cultures and patient specimens.

■ Wipe work surfaces with a surface disinfectant before and after procedures and anytime a spill occurs.

■ Sterilize the loop before and after use and replace it in the holder. Use sterile disposal loops when possible.

■ Avoid aerosol formation of bacterial cultures when preparing smears, heat-fixing slides, or sterilizing the loop.

■ Use care to avoid burns while heat-fixing the slide or sterilizing the loop.

■ Dispose of used slides in biohazard sharps container.

■ Discard all contaminated materials in biohazard containers, as directed by the instructor.

## LESSON REVIEW

1. Discuss the use of Standard Precautions and aseptic technique in the bacteriology laboratory.
2. Explain why it is necessary to wear a laboratory coat when working with bacteria.
3. Why is it important to gently roll the swab across the slide when preparing a smear?
4. Why is the medium inoculated with a swab before the swab is used to make a smear?
5. Explain the differences in procedures for preparing a smear from cultures growing in a tube and a Petri dish.
6. Why must the smear for Gram stain be heat-fixed before it is stained?
7. Explain how to perform a Gram stain.
8. Explain why some bacteria stain gram-positive and others stain gram-negative.
9. Describe the appearance of the gram-positive cocci and the gram-negative rods.
10. Why is it necessary to wipe countertops often with surface disinfectant?
11. Define bibulous paper, counterstain, and mordant.

## STUDENT ACTIVITIES

1. Reread the information on preparing the bacteriological smear and performing the Gram stain.
2. Review the glossary terms.
3. Practice preparing smears, performing the Gram stain, and identifying gram-negative and gram-positive organisms as outlined on the Student Performance Guide.

# Student Performance Guide

## LESSON 7-4 Preparing a Bacteriological Smear and Performing a Gram Stain

Name _____  Date _____

### INSTRUCTIONS

1. Practice preparing and staining a bacteriological smear following the step-by-step procedure.
2. Demonstrate your understanding of this lesson by:
   a. Completing a written examination successfully, and
   b. Preparing and staining bacteriological smears satisfactorily for the instructor. All steps must be completed as listed on the instructor's Performance Check Sheet.

### MATERIALS AND EQUIPMENT

- gloves
- hand disinfectant
- surface disinfectant
- educational strains (less pathogenic strains, specifically for teaching, available through catalogs) of *Escherichia coli* and *Staphylococcus aureus* growing on agar slants or in Petri dishes
- microscope with 10X, 40X, and 100X (oil-immersion) objectives

- immersion oil
- Bunsen burner, alcohol lamp, or electric incinerator
- glass microscope slides
- inoculating needle or loop (disposable preferred)
- commercially prepared slides of gram-negative and gram-positive organisms
- diamond- or carbide-tip etching pencil
- holder for inoculating loops
- sterile distilled $H_2O$
- matches or flint-type lighter
- test tube rack
- forceps or spring-type clothespins
- Gram stain kit or individual Gram stain reagents
- staining rack
- sterile Dacron swabs
- paper towels or soft laboratory tissues
- bibulous paper
- lens paper
- biohazard containers
- biohazard containers for sharps

### PROCEDURE

Record in the comment section any problems encountered while practicing the procedure (or have a fellow student or the instructor evaluate your performance).

S = Satisfactory
U = Unsatisfactory

| You must: | S | U | Comments |
|---|---|---|---|
| 1. Assemble equipment and materials | | | |
| 2. Prepare a work area: place one or two paper towels on the counter; pour surface disinfectant on them until just wet | | | |
| 3. Light the Bunsen burner or turn on the electric incinerator | | | |

| You must: | S | U | Comments |
|---|---|---|---|
| 4. Wash hands and put on gloves (use caution around flames) | | | |
| 5. Prepare one smear from each source listed below:<br>　a. Swab: prepare one smear from gram-positive organism (*S. aureus*) and one from gram-negative organism (*E. coli*), if available<br>　　(1) Obtain a microscope slide and etch the I.D. (+) onto one end with etching pencil<br>　　(2) Obtain a swab that has been inoculated with gram-positive (+) organisms<br>　　(3) Gently roll the swab across the surface of the slide to make a smear about the size of a nickel<br>　　(4) Return the swab to its container or dispose of in biohazard waste<br>　　(5) Allow the smear to air-dry completely<br>　　(6) Repeat steps a1–a5, using a gram-negative (-) organism; label slide with (-) sign<br>　　(7) Hold the gram–positive (+) slide by the edge using forceps or spring clothespin and pass it through the flame two to three times to heat-fix. If using an electric incinerator, hold slide flat against opening for a few seconds. (Do not heat excessively)<br>　　(8) Heat fix the gram-negative slide following steps in #7<br>　　(9) Allow the slides to cool before staining | | | |
| 　b. Tubed media<br>　　(1) Obtain a microscope slide and a culture of a gram-positive organism and a gram-negative organism growing on agar slants in tubes<br>　　(2) Sterilize and cool the loop and transfer one drop of sterile water to the center of the microscope slide<br>　　(3) Hold the tube of gram-positive culture in one hand and the inoculating loop in the other<br>　　(4) Use the fourth and fifth fingers of the hand holding the loop to twist the cap off the tube<br>　　(5) Sterilize 2–2.5 inches of the loop and cool the loop again<br>　　(6) Sterilize the mouth of the culture tube and use the cooled loop to pick up a small amount of bacteria from the edge of the growth on the slant<br>　　(7) Sterilize the mouth of the tube, replace the cap, and set the tube in a test tube rack<br>　　(8) Mix the bacteria on the loop with the water on the slide and spread the mixture to make a smear about the size of a nickel. Do not make the smear too thick<br>　　(9) Repeat steps b1–8 using the gram negative culture<br>　　(10) Allow smears to air-dry completely<br>　　(11) Heat-fix the smears (as in 5a7)<br>　　(12) Allow the slides to cool | | | |
| 　c. Petri dish<br>　　(1) Obtain microscope slides and a gram-negative and a gram-positive culture growing in Petri dishes | | | |

| You must: | S | U | Comments |
|---|---|---|---|
| (2) Sterilize and cool the inoculating loop and transfer one drop of water to the microscope slides <br> (3) Sterilize and cool the loop again <br> (4) Lift the lid of the first Petri dish just enough so the inoculating loop can fit into it <br> (5) Touch the sterile loop to a bacterial colony and transfer a small amount to the drop of water on the slide <br> (6) Replace the lid on the Petri dish <br> (7) Use the loop to mix the bacteria and water together and spread the mixture into a nickel-sized area <br> (8) Repeat steps c1–c7 using the second Petri dish culture <br> (9) Allow smears to air-dry completely <br> (10) Heat-fix the smears (as in 5a7) <br> (11) Allow the slides to cool | | | |
| 6. Turn off the burner or electric incinerator | | | |
| 7. Assemble staining rack and reagents | | | |
| 8. Place smears from all three sources on the staining rack, if space allows | | | |
| 9. Flood the slides with crystal violet for the manufacturer's recommended time, usually one minute | | | |
| 10. Rinse the stain off the slides with a gentle stream of water from a beaker, faucet, or plastic squeeze bottle | | | |
| 11. Tilt the slides to remove excess water | | | |
| 12. Flood the slides with Gram's iodine for the recommended time | | | |
| 13. Rinse the slides as in step 10 and 11 | | | |
| 14. Hold the slides, one by one, by the short edge using forceps or clothespin. Add the decolorizer by squeeze bottle or Pasteur pipet until no more purple color runs off the slide <br> *Note:* It is important to decolorize no longer than a few seconds to prevent over-decolorization | | | |
| 15. Rinse the slides immediately to remove the decolorizer; tilt the slides to remove excess water | | | |
| 16. Counterstain the smears by flooding the slides with safranin for the recommended time | | | |
| 17. Rinse the slides, tilt to remove excess water; wipe the back of the slide with paper towel to remove stain; stand slides on end or blot between sheets of bibulous paper to dry | | | |
| 18. Place the completely dry slide of the gram-positive cocci on the microscope stage | | | |
| 19. Use the low-power (10X) objective to locate the stained smear | | | |
| 20. Place a drop of immersion oil on the stained area | | | |

| You must: | S | U | Comments |
|---|---|---|---|
| 21. Carefully rotate the oil-immersion objective into place | | | |
| 22. Observe that the *Staphylococcus* organisms are gram-positive cocci, with the majority being arranged in grape-like clusters | | | |
| 23. Rotate the low-power objective into position and remove the slide | | | |
| 24. Repeat steps 18–21, using the slide of gram-negative rods | | | |
| 25. Observe that the *E. coli* are gram-negative rods | | | |
| 26. Rotate the low-power objective into place and remove the slide | | | |
| 27. Observe the third slide, repeating steps 18–21; observe the morphology and Gram stain reaction of the organisms present | | | |
| 28. Rotate the low-power objective into place and remove the slide | | | |
| 29. Clean the oil-immersion objective and the top of the microscope condenser with lens paper | | | |
| 30. Return equipment to proper storage; wipe oil off slides gently and store slides, or discard in sharps container | | | |
| 31. Return cultures to storage or discard in proper biohazard container to be autoclaved or picked up for disposal | | | |
| 32. Clean work surfaces with disinfectant | | | |
| 33. Remove and discard gloves in biohazard container and wash hands with hand disinfectant | | | |

*Evaluator Comments:*




Evaluator _____  Date _____

# Throat Culture and Rapid Tests for Group A Streptococcus

## LESSON OBJECTIVES

**After studying this lesson, you should be able to:**

- *Discuss the importance of identifying Group A Streptococcus.*
- *Collect a throat swab and transfer it to blood agar.*
- *Interpret the results of a throat culture.*
- *Use a bacitracin disk to identify Group A Streptococcus.*
- *List the two main types of technology used in rapid tests for Group A Streptococcus.*
- *Define the glossary terms.*
- *Perform a rapid test for Group A Streptococcus.*

## GLOSSARY

**fossae** / in the throat, shallow depressions where the tonsils were located before surgical removal

**hemolysis** / destruction of RBCs, resulting in the release of hemoglobin from the cells

**pharyngeal** / having to do with the back of the throat or pharynx

## INTRODUCTION

The throat culture is one of the most frequently performed microbiology laboratory tests, especially in children and young adults. The test is performed anytime the patient reports clinical symptoms of "strep throat." Strep tonsillitis is an infection by *Streptococcus pyogenes*, a gram-positive coccus, which belongs to Lancefield Group A. Therefore, it is often referred to as Group A *Streptococcus* (GAS). Only 5-10% of patients with sore throats test positive for Group A strep. However, because the complications of untreated strep infection are serious, all patients who report symptoms should be tested. An untreated Group A *Streptococcus* infection can result in scarlet fever, rheumatic fever, rheumatic endocarditis, or glomerulonephritis. These complications are most common in patients under twenty-five.

Group A *Streptococcus* is just one of several Lancefield groups of streptococci. There are additional groups that cause tonsillitis and other infections in humans. The two most common of these are Lancefield Group C and Group G. These two groups may cause illness in some patients, leaving others asymptomatic. *Streptococcus* grouping kits are now available to test for the other groups if a symptomatic patient tests negative for Group A.

## DETECTION OF GROUP A *STREPTOCOCCUS*

Confirmation of the preliminary diagnosis of Group A *Streptococcus* can be made either by identifying the organism in culture or by performing a rapid immuno-assay test.

 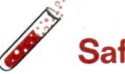 **Safety**

Personnel in the small laboratory may collect the specimen from the throat and also culture the organism or perform the rapid test for Group A *Streptococcus*. Appropriate PPE must be worn. A buttoned, fluid-resistant laboratory coat will protect the technician from clothing contamination by organisms or test reagents. Gloves and protective eyewear should also be worn. Hands must be washed before gloving, after glove removal, and any other time there is a possibility of contamination.

Eating, drinking, applying cosmetics, or putting any objects (such as pencils) in the mouth are not allowed while working with specimens or while in the laboratory. Contact lenses must not be touched.

Work surfaces must be wiped with a bactericidal agent before and after use. The area on which specimens are placed when brought to the lab should also be cleaned. Clutter should be removed to help prevent accidental spills. Bunsen burners and electric incinerators must be used with caution to avoid burns. All waste must be placed in the appropriate biohazard containers.

## Performing the Throat Culture

### Collecting the Specimen

A throat culture is performed by swabbing the **pharyngeal** surfaces to pick up any organisms present. The swab should be gently passed across the surface of both tonsils or the **fossae** (if tonsils have been removed), and the back of the throat (Figure 7-33). Touching the tongue or the inside of the mouth with the swab should be avoided. These surfaces are covered with normal flora of the mouth, which may grow on the medium and contaminate the culture.

### Inoculating the Media

This throat swab is immediately used to inoculate one quadrant of a blood agar plate. A sterile loop is then used to streak for isolated colonies. The loop can also be used to make two or three stabs into the blood agar. This is done by touching the inoculated area in the first quadrant with the sterile loop and then "stabbing" the loop into the agar two or three times in the fourth quadrant.

Blood agar supplies the required nutrients for growth of throat isolates and also demonstrates bacterial **hemolysis**, the lysis of the RBCs by the organisms (Color Plate 36). Hemolysis is indicated by clear areas around colonies on the blood plate and in the stabs. The hemolysis can be complete (beta, β) or incomplete (alpha, α). Absence of hemolysis is referred to as

---

*Quality Assurance*

The quality of the results from bacteriology laboratory procedures is only as good as the quality of the work performed. Quality assurance programs must be in place to ensure reliability of media and the performance of staining reagents and test kits. Many commercial check systems are available for use with these programs. (See Lesson 7-3 for a review.)

New media shipments must be checked for reliability. Blood agar should be inoculated with a known culture of Group A *Streptococcus* to check for growth support and hemolysis. Rapid tests for Group A *Streptococcus* contain internal controls. The worker must be certain the control is reacting properly before reporting the patient's results. The reliability of Gram stain reagents must be checked by using one of the commercially available sets of known gram-negative and gram-positive organisms.

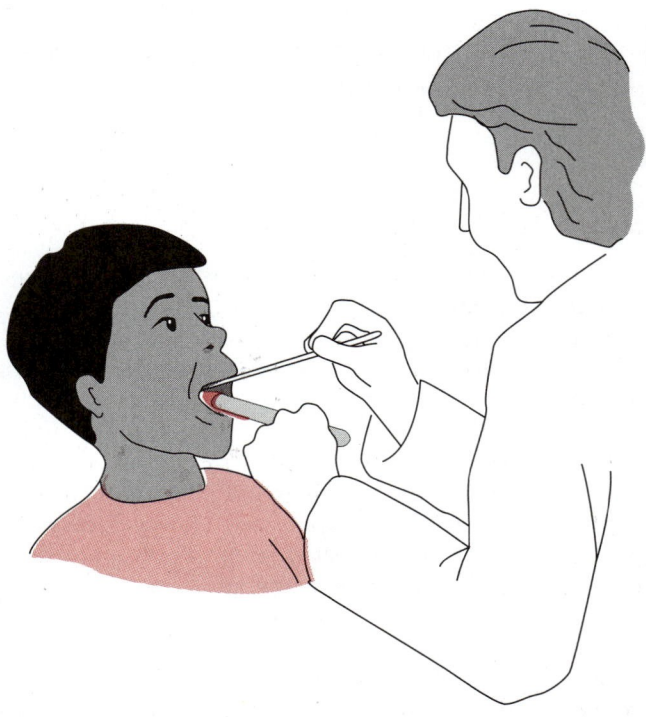

**FIGURE 7-33** Swabbing the throat for culture

gamma hemolysis. A paper disk containing the antibiotic bacitracin can be placed on the concentrated streak in the first quadrant of the newly streaked plate before it is placed in the incubator.

## Incubating the Culture

Growth of most streptococci is enhanced by incubation in an increased $CO_2$ environment. A $CO_2$ concentration of 10% increases the growth of hemolytic streptococci and inhibits the growth of other throat flora. This can be accomplished with a special $CO_2$ incubator, or, more simply for the smaller laboratory, by using candle jars. These are made by placing the culture plate in a large wide-mouth (restaurant condiment) jar, setting a short lighted white candle on top of the plate, and closing the lid. The candle uses up most of the oxygen and extinguishes itself, leaving 5-10% $CO_2$ inside the jar. Commercial gas-generating systems are also available that accomplish this by chemical means.

If there is a delay in getting the specimen to the laboratory, a transport medium suitable for streptococci must be used to maintain viability of the organism until it is placed on growth media. Laboratory personnel must know which of the several types of transport media provided by reference laboratories should be used for throat cultures.

## Interpreting the Throat Culture

After overnight incubation, the initial blood plate is examined for growth, which is noted as scant, moderate, or heavy. The agar is then examined for signs of hemolysis and for growth around the bacitracin disk. The stabs in the agar are closely examined because beta hemolysis will show up in the stabs even if it is difficult to see on the plate surface. If there are beta-hemolytic colonies on the medium and a zone of inhibition around the disk, Group A *Streptococcus* is indicated. Many laboratories select an isolated beta-hemolytic colony, streak it to another plate for confluent growth, and place a bacitracin disk to be interpreted the next day.

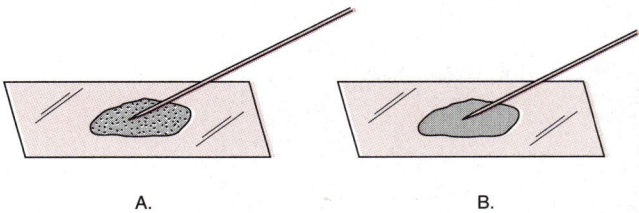

A.             B.

**FIGURE 7-34** Latex slide agglutination tests: (A) positive, (B) negative

If there is need to confirm Group A, isolated beta-hemolytic colonies are tested with a panel of antibodies against the various groups of *Streptococcus*. These antibodies are available in kits. Alternatively, isolated beta-hemolytic colonies can be tested with some of the rapid Group A strep kits.

## Performing a Rapid Test for Group A *Streptococcus*

Although the throat culture is still used, many rapid tests for detecting Group A *Streptococcus* are used by small and large laboratories to quickly identify the organism. Most of the kits give test results in about five minutes. Two basic technologies used are latex agglutination and immunoassay.

### Latex Agglutination Tests

The latex agglutination kits use the organism from the specimen as the *antigen* and provide the *antibodies* to Group A *Streptococcus* coated on microscopic latex beads. A throat swab is performed as usual and the swab is placed into an acid solution to extract the antigen. This extract is mixed with the antibody-coated latex beads for a certain length of time on a test slide. After the incubation time, the slide is examined for agglutination, visible aggregates of antigen-antibody latex. A positive test should have strong agglutination. Absence of agglutination indicates a negative test (Figure 7-34). Reusable slides must be cleaned thoroughly before use to avoid false-positive results. Occasionally, a shipment of swabs will produce false positives. New shipments of swabs should be tested with the kit reagents before being used for patient tests.

### Immunoassay for Group A *Streptococcus*

Several Strep A test kits using enzyme immunoassay (EIA) technology are on the market. This test method is very sensitive and specific for the organism. The EIA tests also use an extract of the organisms from the throat swab. Some are two-step tests, an acid extraction, and the addition of the extract to the test system. Others have additional steps, such as adding a conjugate or wash solution.

Results are displayed in different ways, based on the patterns the manufacturers used to apply the antibody to the test membrane. Some test systems produce a plus (+) sign for positive and a minus (-) sign for negative (Figure 7-35). If no Group A antigen is present, the horizontal bar serves as a control to prove that the test is working. Any Group A antigen present will bind and cause the vertical line to be visible, making a (+) sign.

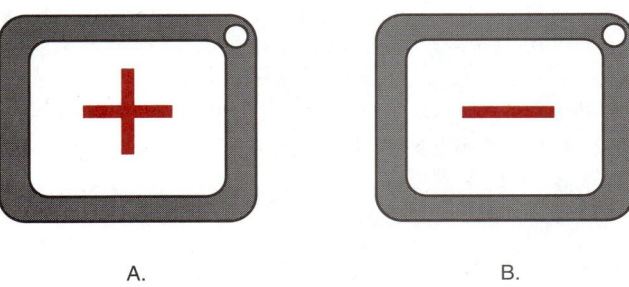

A.                              B.

**FIGURE 7-35** Examples of strep test kits that use the positive (+) and the negative (−) signs for indicating results

Other test kits use a colored dot or parallel colored lines on the test membrane to indicate results.

The ICON® Fx Strep A test, marketed by Beckman Coulter, is another type of immunochemical assay for Group A *Streptococcus* (Figure 7-36). The test device membrane contains two colorless stripes of absorbed antibodies conjugated to visualizing particles that form a color in the presence of the Strep A antigen. If Strep A antigen is detected in the patient sample, a colored line will appear in the patient area and another will appear in the control area if the procedure and reagents are correct. The procedure for this test is described in the Student Performance Guide.

To perform the test, the patient's throat is swabbed, the swab is inserted into the test device, and two extraction reagents are added. After one minute the device is closed and sealed. Five minutes later the results are visible in the window on the device front. A negative result is indicated by a single colored line in the control area, meaning that no Strep A antigen was detected but the test procedure was correct. A positive result is indicated by colored lines in both the patient and control areas. No lines, or a line in the patient area only, indicates a invalid test and the test must be repeated by collecting another sample and using a new test device (Figure 7-37).

## Considerations in Using Rapid Tests for Group A *Streptococcus*

Many of the rapid strep kits on the market have high sensitivity and specificity when the number of bacteria in the throat (colony count) is high. However, the results of these tests are not as accurate if the patient has few colonies or the swabbing is not thorough. In addition, it is best if the patient has not eaten, drunk, or gargled in the thirty minutes before the swab is taken. It is generally recommended that any negative rapid strep test be confirmed by a throat culture, which does not significantly add to the cost of patient care. A false-negative test for Group A *Streptococcus* infection could have serious consequences for children and young adults if an infection goes untreated.

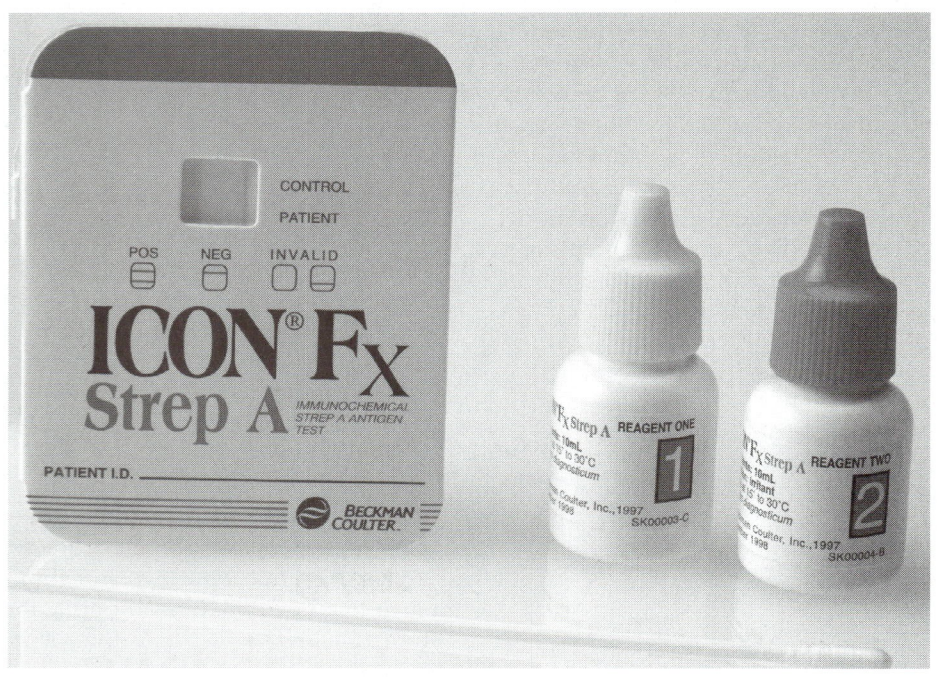

**FIGURE 7-36** ICON® Fx Strep A test kit. (Photo courtesy of Beckman Coulter, Fullerton, CA)

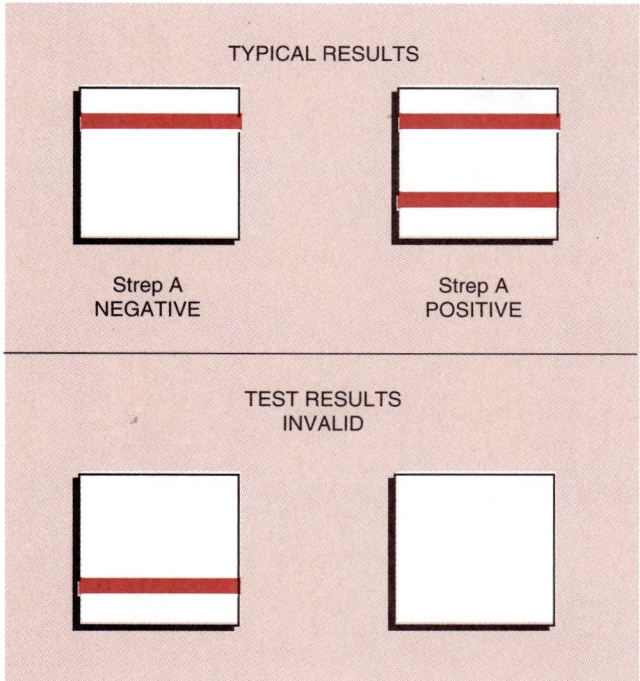

TYPICAL RESULTS

Strep A
NEGATIVE

Strep A
POSITIVE

TEST RESULTS
INVALID

**FIGURE 7-37** Results of a rapid strep test. Illustration of typical results obtained with the ICON® Fx Strep A test. When patient is negative for Group A *Streptococcus*, only the top line of color appears. Two lines of color indicate a positive test. Any other combination or no lines are an invalid result and the test must be repeated.

## Procedural Notes

- Touch only the tonsils and back of the throat with the swab to avoid contamination with mouth and tongue flora.
- Check the expiration date on media, disks, and kits.
- Always follow the manufacturers' directions for the material used.
- Incubate the culture in a 5–10% $CO_2$ atmosphere.
- Use caution when interpreting any hemolysis present.

## Safety Precautions

- Follow Universal and Standard Precautions.
- Wear appropriate protective clothing.
- Treat used swabs as if infectious.
- Wipe the work area frequently with surface disinfectant.
- Wear a mask and safety glasses when collecting the throat swab if the patient is coughing excessively.

## LESSON REVIEW

1. Discuss the importance of early diagnosis of Group A *Streptococcus* infection.
2. Explain why the tongue and mouth should not be swabbed when testing for strep throat.
3. Explain why a throat culture is inoculated to blood agar.
4. Explain the purpose of the bacitracin disk.
5. Explain the reason for making stabs in the agar.
6. Discuss the different types of hemolysis.
7. Discuss agglutination tests and rapid EIA tests for Group A *Streptococcus*.
8. Explain the danger of a false negative rapid strep test.
9. List four safety procedures that must be observed when collecting or processing throat culture swabs.
10. Define fossae, hemolysis, and pharyngeal.

## STUDENT ACTIVITIES

1. Reread the information on throat culture and rapid tests for Group A *Streptococcus*.
2. Review the glossary terms.
3. Practice the procedure for performing a throat culture, as outlined in the Student Performance Guide.
4. Practice performing the procedure for rapid tests for Group A *Streptococcus*, as outlined in the Student Performance Guide.
5. Survey local POLs to find out which rapid tests for Group A *Streptococcus* are used and what procedure is followed when a rapid test is negative.

## *Student Performance Guide*

## **LESSON 7-5** Throat Culture and Rapid Tests for Group A *Streptococcus*

Name _____ Date _____

  ### INSTRUCTIONS

1. Practice performing a throat culture and rapid test for Group A *Streptococcus*, following the step-by-step procedure.
2. Demonstrate your understanding of this lesson by:
   a. Completing a written examination successfully, and
   b. Performing the throat culture and the rapid test for Group A *Streptococcus* satisfactorily for the instructor. All steps must be completed as listed on the instructor's Performance Check Sheet.

*Note:* The instructions given are for the ICON® Fx Strep A test (Beckman Coulter). Manufacturer's instructions must be followed for whichever test kit is used. Inclusion of this method does not constitute endorsement by the authors.

### MATERIALS AND EQUIPMENT

- gloves
- sterile Dacron or rayon swabs
- blood agar plate
- inoculating loop
- Bunsen burner or electric incinerator
- incubator set at 35–37°C
- $CO_2$ incubator or candle jars
- bacitracin disks
- commercial rapid EIA test kit for Group A *Streptococcus*
- biohazard container
- surface disinfectant
- hand disinfectant

### PROCEDURE

Record in the comment section any problems encountered while practicing the procedure (or have a fellow student or the instructor evaluate your performance).

S = Satisfactory
U = Unsatisfactory

| You must: | S | U | Comments |
|---|---|---|---|
| 1. Assemble equipment and materials | | | |
| 2. Wash hands and put on gloves | | | |
| 3. Collect throat specimen<br>*Note:* Often the same swab can be used for the culture plate and the rapid test. However, some test kits recommend collecting two swabs | | | |
| 4. Transfer the bacteria to the properly labeled blood agar plate:<br>a. Roll the swab gently on the surface of one quadrant of the blood agar plate. Save the swab for the rapid test or discard in biohazard container, if two were collected | | | |

| You must: | S | U | Comments |
|---|---|---|---|
| b. Sterilize a loop for streaking the plate or use a sterile disposable plastic loop <br> c. Streak the plate for isolated colonies as described in Lesson 7-2. Make two to three stabs in agar. Place bacitracin disk on quadrant one <br> d. Place the plate upside down in the 37°C incubator (with increased $CO_2$) overnight (or use candle jar in incubator) | | | |
| 5. Perform ICON® Fx Strep A rapid test for Group A *Streptococcus.* (Follow manufacturer's instructions on package insert) <br> a. Open the test device just prior to use; lay it so it stays flat <br> b. Insert the patient or control swab into the green triangle; gently push until the tip of the swab is visible in the hole above the triangle <br> c. Hold Reagent One bottle vertical and add four drops to the triangle <br> d. Hold Reagent two bottle vertical and add four drops to the triangle <br> e. Rotate the swab to the right (clockwise) three times by twirling the shaft between the thumb and index finger <br> f. Wait one minute <br> g. Peel off the adhesive lines from the right edge of the test device and close and securely seal it. <br> h. Wait five minutes before reading the result <br> i. Interpret the results: <br> (1) A negative sample will give a single, colored control line in the top half of the window. This indicates that the procedure and reagents were correct, but no Strep A antigen was detected <br> (2) A positive sample will give two colored lines <br> (3) If no lines are present or only the patient area contains a colored line, the test is invalid and must be repeated | | | |
| 6. Dispose of all contaminated materials in biohazard container | | | |
| 7. Return all equipment to proper storage | | | |
| 8. Wipe work area with surface disinfectant | | | |
| 9. Remove and discard gloves in biohazard container | | | |
| 10. Wash hands with hand disinfectant | | | |
| 11. Observe the throat culture plate after overnight incubation. Quantitate the growth: No growth, scant, moderate, or heavy growth | | | |
| 12. Observe for hemolysis and record the type: alpha, beta, or gamma (Be certain to examine the agar stabs) | | | |
| 13. Observe for zone of inhibition around the bacitracin disk if beta (β) hemolysis is present. If none is seen, record "no β-hemolytic strep isolated" | | | |
| 14. Wash hands and put on gloves | | | |

| You must: | S | U | Comments |
|---|---|---|---|
| 15. Inoculate another blood plate using beta-hemolytic isolated colonies, streaking the whole plate for continuous growth (if required for identification). Place a Bacitracin disk in the center of the plate. Incubate overnight at 35–37°C | | | |
| 16. Clean equipment and return to storage | | | |
| 17. Wipe work area with surface disinfectant | | | |
| 18. Remove and discard gloves in biohazard container | | | |
| 19. Wash hands with hand disinfectant | | | |
| 20. Examine the plate from step 15 after overnight incubation. If there are beta-hemolytic colonies on the medium and a zone of inhibition (no growth) around the bacitracin disk, report as "β-hemolytic streptococci present" | | | |
| 21. Dispose of all contaminated materials in the biohazard container | | | |
| 22. Wipe the counter with surface disinfectant | | | |
| 23. Wash hands with hand disinfectant | | | |

*Evaluator Comments:*

Evaluator _____ Date _____

# Urine Culture, Colony Count, and Antibiotic Susceptibility Testing

## LESSON OBJECTIVES

**After studying this lesson, you should be able to:**

- *Use the proper technique to inoculate a urine culture.*
- *Select a calibrated inoculating loop to inoculate a urine culture.*
- *Select the correct primary medium and indicator medium for a urine culture.*
- *Streak a urine culture for colony count.*
- *Perform a colony count on a urine culture.*
- *Explain the purposes of the catalase and coagulase tests.*
- *Perform an antibiotic susceptibility test.*
- *Describe the safety precautions to observe when performing urine culture, colony count, and antibiotic susceptibility testing.*
- *Define the glossary terms.*

## GLOSSARY

**coliform** / certain gram-negative intestinal bacteria including *Escherichia coli*

**colony count** / method of estimating the number of organisms in urine by counting the colonies on a urine culture plate

## INTRODUCTION

The urine culture is one of the most frequently requested tests in the bacteriology laboratory. Urinary tract infection (UTI) occurs when bacteria migrate up the urethra into the bladder, or even further into the kidneys. Although females are prone to UTIs because of their anatomy, UTIs also occur in males. The microorganism most commonly responsible is *Escherichia coli* (*E. coli*), a gram-negative rod that is part of the normal flora of the intestinal tract. Other gram-negative bacilli, such as *Pseudomonas, Proteus,* and *Klebsiella,* can also cause UTI. A gram-positive organism frequently found as the causative agent in urinary tract infections is *Staphylococcus saprophyticus.*

## PERFORMING THE URINE CULTURE

The physician orders a urine culture when a patient has UTI symptoms, including frequent urination, pain and burning during urination, blood in the urine, and sometimes fever and backache (Table 7-16). In asymptomatic patients, a culture may be requested because bacteria were noted in a routine urinalysis.

###  Safety

The procedures performed in urine culture, **colony count**, and antibiotic susceptibility testing expose the technician to potentially infectious body fluids and to

**Table 7-16.** Symptoms associated with urinary tract infections

Frequent urination
Blood in urine
Pain or burning sensation when urinating
Fever
Backache

cultures of unknown bacteria (if educational strains are not used). Standard Precautions must be observed, in addition to laboratory chemical safety guidelines. Gloves must be worn when handling the urine and when handling the plates containing bacterial growth. The Petri dish lid must be opened only as wide as required to pick up colonies for further testing. Aerosol formation must be avoided when sterilizing the inoculating loop. All contaminated materials must be discarded in biohazard waste containers, as directed by the instructor. All work surfaces must be wiped with a surface disinfectant. Hands must be washed with antibacterial hand soap after gloves have been removed.

*Quality Assurance*

Results from the urine culture are used to guide the physician in confirming and treating UTIs. The specimen for urine culture and sensitivity must be collected before antibiotic therapy is begun. The patient must be instructed in the proper method of urine collection to avoid contamination of the urine. A UTI usually has only one causative agent; the presence of three or more colony types on the primary culture plate suggests the urine was not clean-catch. Quality assurance programs to assure reliability of growth media, stain reagents, and other chemicals must be in place.

## Collecting the Specimen

The specimen to be cultured must be collected by clean-catch, as described in Lesson 5-2. Females should be careful to avoid contaminating the specimen with vaginal material, which may contain microorganisms. If vaginal flora grow on the culture, they can interfere with the process of identifying the organism causing the

infection. The urine container should be labeled on the side (not on the lid) with the patient's name and identification number and time of collection. The urine should be cultured within one hour of collection if not refrigerated. If the specimen is to be sent to a reference laboratory, the instructions and transport supplies of that laboratory must be used.

## Streaking the Plate for Colony Count

Urine specimens are streaked onto the primary medium, usually blood agar, and onto an indicator/selective medium such as EMB or MAC. Most urinary tract pathogens will grow on blood agar. Both EMB and MAC inhibit the growth of gram-positive organisms and indicate fermentation reactions of gram-negative organisms (Color Plates 37 and 38). Split plates, which have blood agar on one side and EMB or MAC on the other, are cost-effective and save space (Lesson 7-3, Figure 7-21).

A calibrated platinum or sterile plastic loop with a capacity of either 0.01 mL or 0.001 mL is used to inoculate the blood agar plate. The loop is sterilized and cooled, then dipped into a well-mixed urine sample. The loop is observed to be sure it is full of urine and then is used to make a vertical streak down the center of the blood agar plate. Fifteen to twenty horizontal cross streaks are then made all the way across the plate, crossing the vertical streak each time. In some laboratories, a third set of streaks is made at right angles to the second set (Figure 7-38). The EMB or MAC is inoculated in the same manner. The loop is sterilized after use and placed in its rack. The culture plates are placed in the 35–37°C incubator overnight.

## COLONY COUNT AND INTERPRETATION

After eighteen to twenty-four hours or overnight incubation, the plates are removed from the incubator and observed for growth. Any distinguishing characteristics of the growth, such as colony color and morphology, and hemolysis on the blood agar plate, should be noted. Both gram-positive and gram-negative organisms can grow on the blood plate. Only gram-negative organisms should grow on EMB or MAC.

## The Colony Count

Colonies are counted on the blood agar plate (Figure 7-39). If a 0.001 mL loop was used, the number of colonies counted is multiplied by 1000 to calculate the

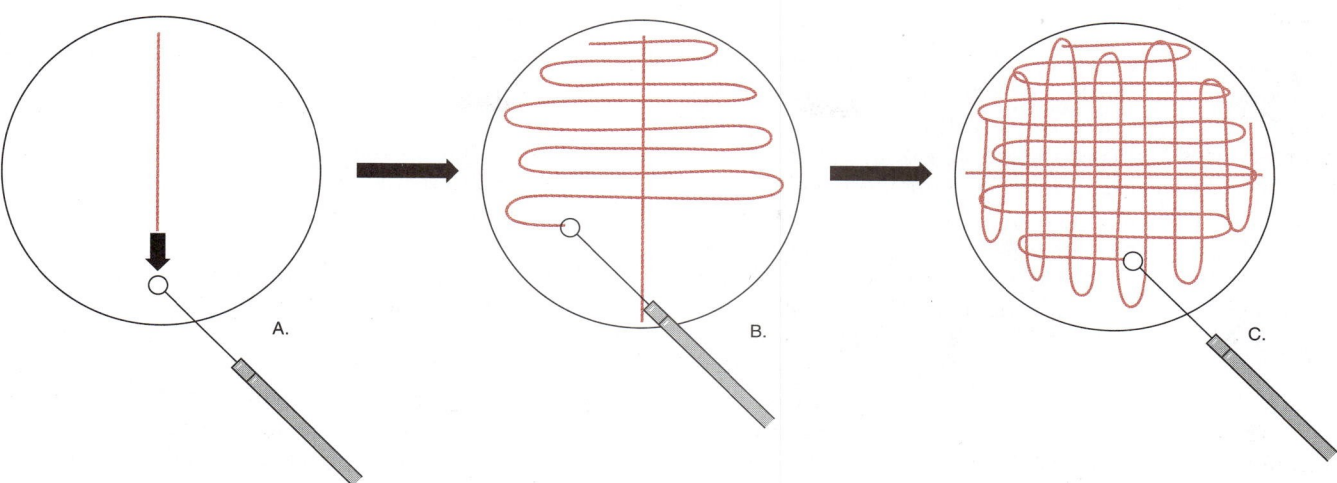

**FIGURE 7-38** Streaking a urine culture plate: (A) make one streak down the center of the plate using a calibrated loop; (B) make several streaks at right angles to the initial streak, crossing over the original streak several times; (C) optional: make several streaks at right angles to the second set of streaks so the plate is almost solidly streaked

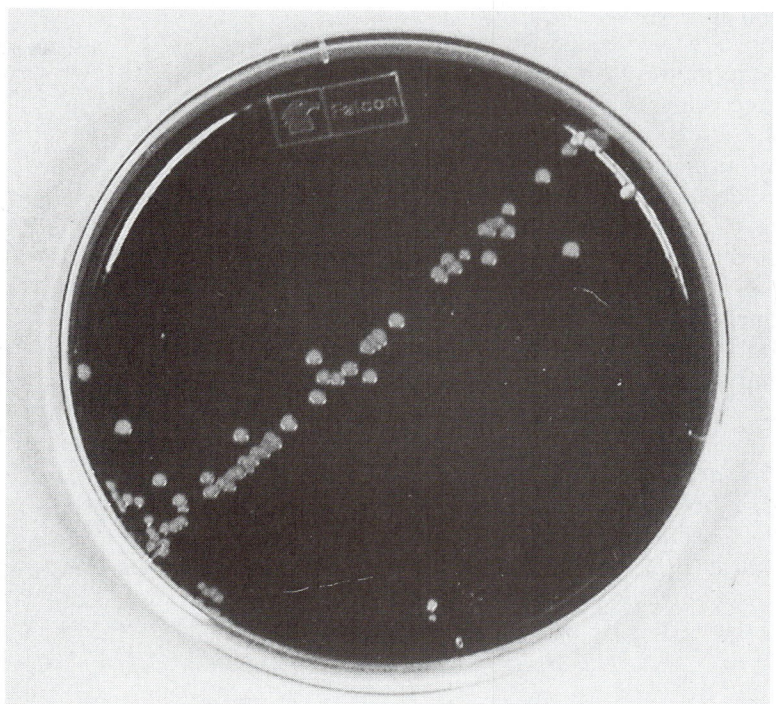

**FIGURE 7-39** Isolated colonies from a urine culture (Photo courtesy of John Estridge)

colony count per mL of urine. If a 0.01 mL loop was used, the number of colonies is multiplied by 100. A count of 100,000/mL or greater is evidence of UTI, whether or not the patient has symptoms. However, in patients who have symptoms or have frequent UTIs, colony counts as low as 1000/mL may be significant.

## Gram-Positive Organisms

A Gram stain should be made of organisms on the blood agar plate. If gram-positive cocci are present, a catalase test must be performed to differentiate between *Streptococcus* and *Staphylococcus*.

## Catalase Test

To perform the catalase test, a tiny portion of colony is picked up with a sterile applicator stick and placed in a drop of 3% hydrogen peroxide ($H_2O_2$) on a clean microscope slide. (Picking up any blood agar on the loop must be avoided, since the hemoglobin will cause a false-positive catalase test.)

If bubbles develop within ten seconds, the organism is catalase-positive and can be presumptively identified as *Staphylococcus* species (Figure 7-40). The report might read "gram-positive cocci, morphologically resembling *Staphylococcus*; catalase-positive." A positive catalase test should be followed by a coagulase test.

The absence of bubbles is a negative catalase test and indicates *Streptococcus* species. It could be reported as "gram-positive cocci, morphologically resembling *Streptococcus* species, catalase-negative."

## Coagulase Test

If the bacteria are catalase-positive, gram-positive cocci arranged in grape-like clusters, a coagulase test should be performed to differentiate between *Staphylococcus aureus* and other staphylococci. The coagulase test can be performed by the slide method or tube method. However, the tube test is recommended as more reliable.

A small amount of culture is mixed with a commercially available coagulase plasma (rabbit plasma) on a slide or in a tube. The slide is read for the presence of clumping, which is a positive result. The inoculated tube of plasma is incubated for four hours and checked at one-hour intervals to see if the plasma has formed a fibrin clot (solidified or thickened) (Figure 7-41).

A positive result could be reported as "gram-positive cocci, morphologically resembling *Staphylococcus*; coagulase-positive." This would be a presumptive identification of *S. aureus*.

An organism with a negative coagulase result would be reported as "gram-positive cocci, morphologically resembling *Staphylococcus* species; coagulase-negative." The result indicates the organism is not *S. aureus* and could be *S. saprophyticus*, a common gram-positive organism involved in UTI.

## Gram-Negative Organisms

The growth on EMB or MAC should be observed after overnight incubation to presumptively identify any gram-negative rods that have grown. A Gram stain of bacteria growing on EMB or MAC should confirm the gram-negative bacteria, since both media inhibit growth of gram-positive organisms.

Many gram-negative microorganisms have distinctive colony morphologies on selective and indicator media. *Klebsiella* species has distinctive, bubblegum pink, mucoid colonies. *E. coli* forms a green metallic sheen on EMB (Color Plate 38) and can be reported as "gram-negative rods, **coliform** by EMB." Coliform refers to certain gram-negative intestinal bacteria.

The physician may treat the patient on the basis of these reports and then check the results of antibiotic susceptibility tests to see if the prescribed antibiotic will be effective. However, the physician may also request a definitive identification of the isolated organism.

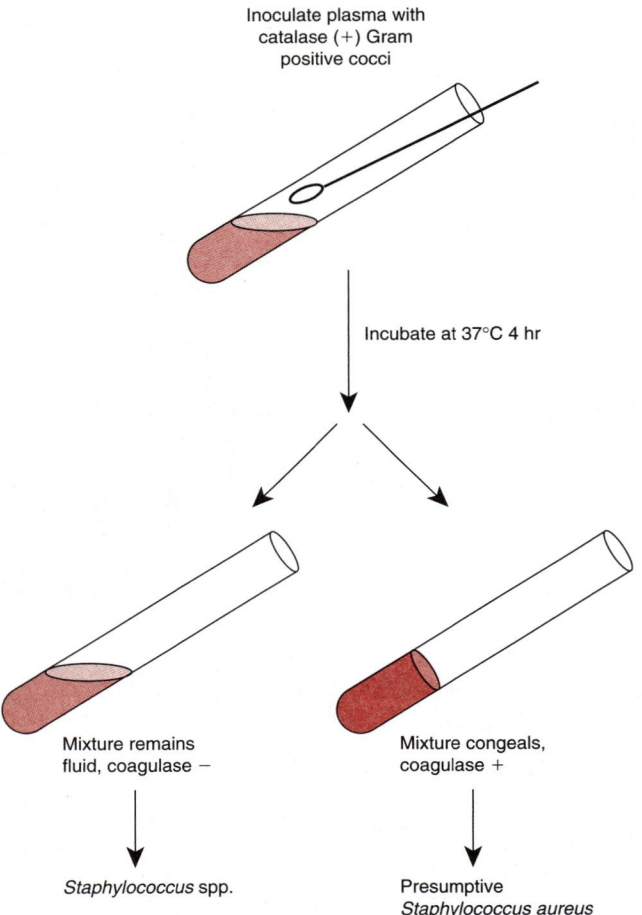

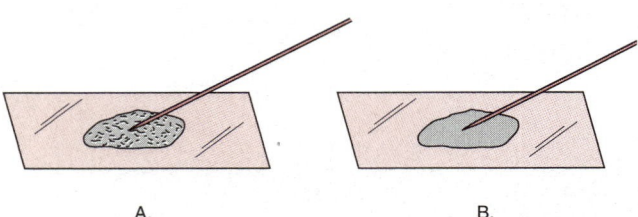

A.   B.

**FIGURE 7-40** The catalase test: (A) bubbles, indicating a positive test; (B) absence of bubbles, indicating a negative test

**FIGURE 7-41** The coagulase test

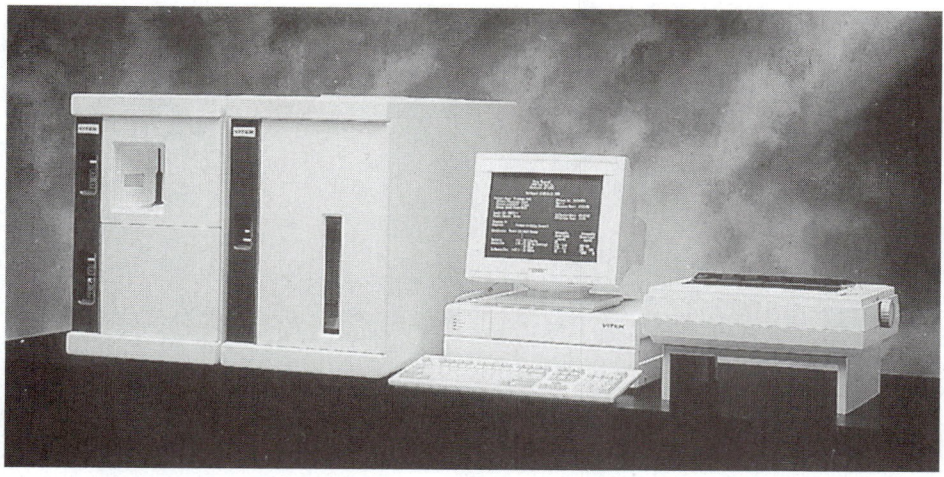

**FIGURE 7-42** The VITEK® fully automated microbiology identification system (Photo courtesy of bioMerieux, Inc.)

## Bacterial Identification Systems

Many bacterial identification systems are available, some automated and some manual. The automated systems are used at most larger institutions and reference laboratories, where the volume of cultures performed per month is several thousand. Two automated systems now on the market are the WALKAWAY® by Microscan and the ITEK® by bioMerieux, Inc. (Figure 7-42). These instruments can identify the organism and also determine its antibiotic susceptibility.

Manual identification systems are used in small, low-volume laboratories or as back-ups to automated systems in larger laboratories. These manual systems, such as the API strip shown, are inoculated with a suspension of the organism and incubated (Figure 7-43 and Color Plate 39). The results of various biochemical reactions, such as fermentation of certain sugars, are used to make identifications. Other manual systems are the Enterotube® II® by Roche Diagnostics Corp.and the Mini-Tek® by BBL.

## ANTIBIOTIC SUSCEPTIBILITY TESTING

When a culture and sensitivity (C & S) is ordered, the susceptibility of an organism to antibiotics is assessed by either the MIC (minimum inhibitory concentration) method or the disk method of Bauer and Kirby. The MIC, performed in special welled plates, tests the organism against antibiotic dilutions to determine the minimum antibiotic concentration that inhibits its growth. The procedure requires a special instrument to read the results (Figure 7-44).

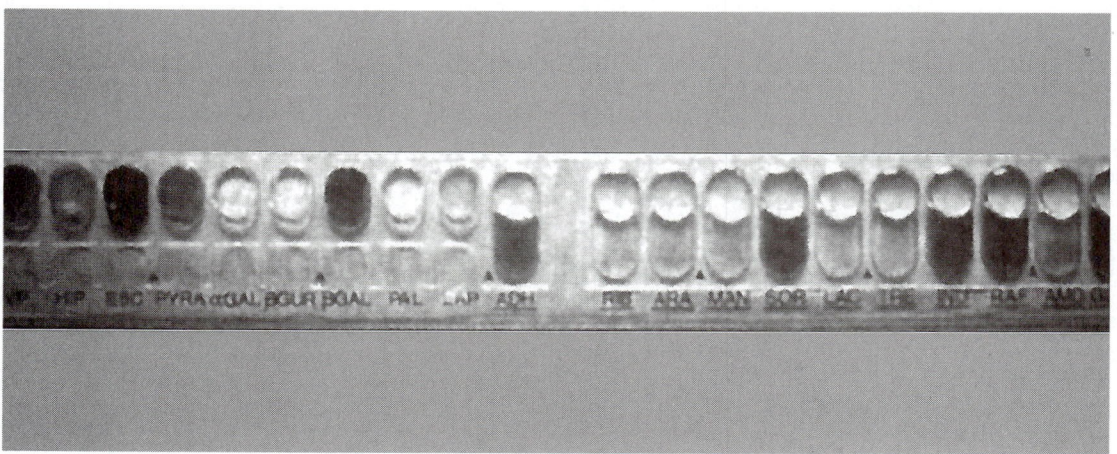

**FIGURE 7-43** A manual bacterial identification system

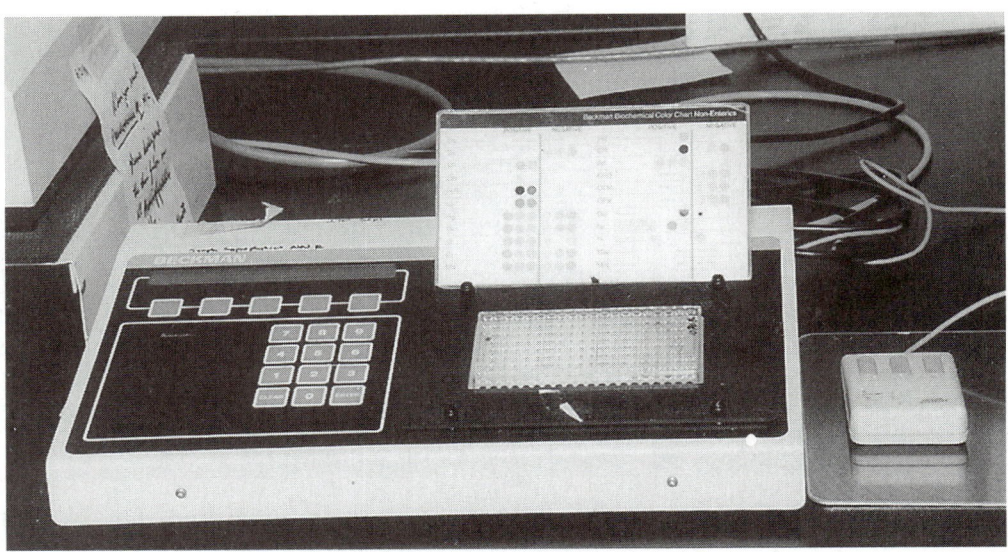

**FIGURE 7-44** MIC system showing the welled plate and reading instrument

## Performing the Disk Antibiotic Susceptibility Test

To perform the Bauer-Kirby antibiotic susceptibility test, a standardized suspension is made of the organism to be tested. This can be prepared in soy broth and the turbidity compared to a standard suspension, such as a McFarland's standard, available in sets of varying concentrations. Alternatively, commercial kits such as the Prompt™ by BBL can be used to standardize the procedure.

The suspension is thoroughly mixed just before use. A sterile swab is wet in the suspension, pressed against the inside of the tube to express any excess fluid, and then used to streak the surface of a Mueller-Hinton plate.

The entire plate is streaked by beginning at the top edge and making continuous streaks all the way across the agar to the bottom edge. The plate is then turned 90° and streaked from the top edge all the way to the bottom edge, resulting in an almost continuous mat of growth after incubation. This is called a "lawn" (Figure 7-45).

The antibiotic disks, which are paper disks impregnated with antibiotics, are placed on the surface of the Mueller-Hinton agar while the surface of the plate is still wet from the inoculum. If only a small number of tests are being performed, sterile forceps are used to place the selected antibiotic disks. Disks should be evenly spaced in a circular pattern around the outer edge of the agar (Figure 7-46). Disk dispensers that dispense a set of twelve or more disks at a time are available from Difco and BBL. The disks must be well-tamped down onto the surface of the agar, so they will not fall off when the plate is turned upside down to incubate overnight.

## Interpreting the Antibiotic Susceptibility Test

After overnight incubation at 35–37°C, the plates are read for inhibition of growth around the antibiotic disks (Figure 7-47 and Color Plate 41). The zones of inhibition can be measured using transparent templates such as the Zone Interpretation Overlay Set by BBL, calipers, or a ruler (Figure 7-48).

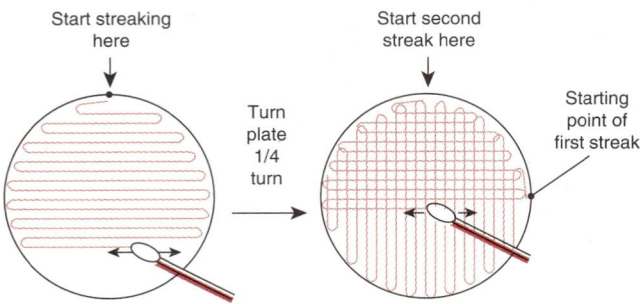

**FIGURE 7-45** Streaking the Mueller-Hinton plate

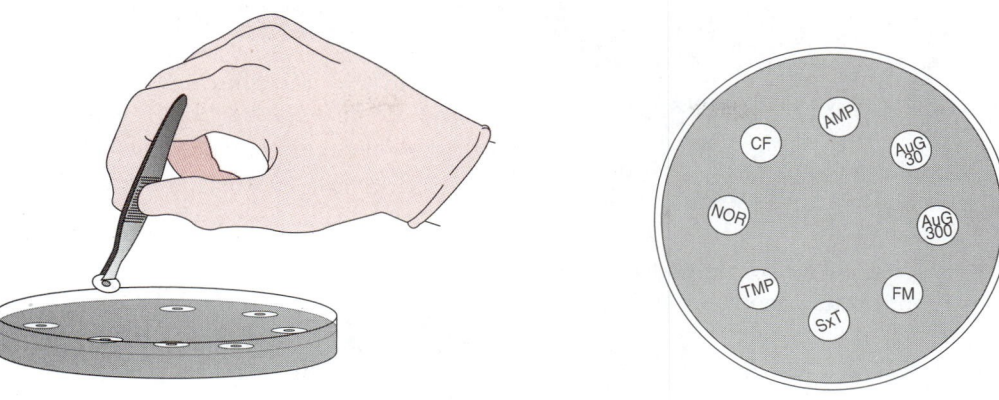

**FIGURE 7-46** Using forceps to place the antibiotic disks on the Mueller-Hinton agar

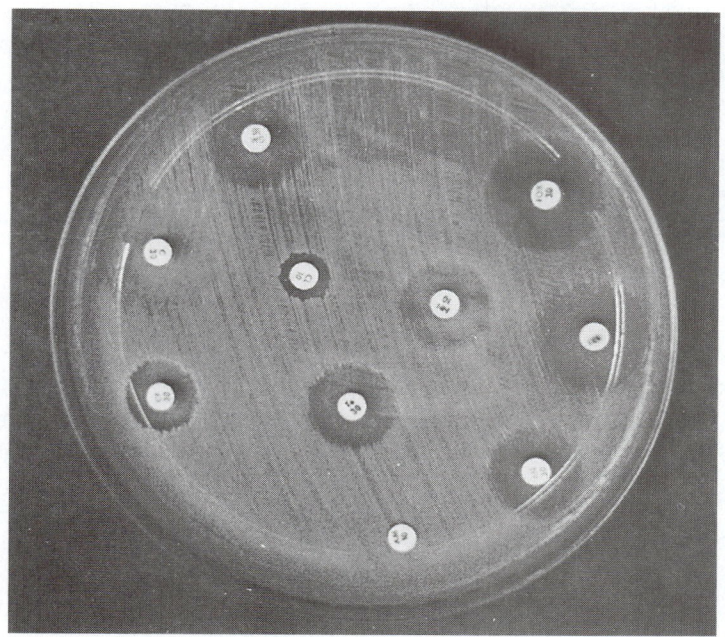

**FIGURE 7-47** Antibiotic susceptibility test plate showing zones of inhibition after eighteen- to twenty-four-hour incubation (Photo courtesy of John Estridge)

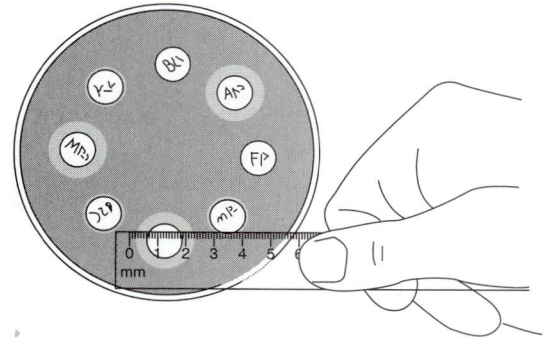

**FIGURE 7-48** Measuring the zones of inhibition using a ruler

Each antibiotic produces a specific zone size for each organism. The zone size is used to classify the organism as sensitive (S), resistant (R), or intermediate (I), based on information in the package insert provided with each cartridge of antibiotic disks. The organism is said to be intermediate (I) if the zone size is between sensitive and resistant. An antibiotic that produces a "sensitive" zone should be prescribed for the infection. The physician may prescribe an "intermediate" antibiotic, but in more frequent or larger-than-usual doses.

## Procedural Notes

- Instruct patient in proper method of clean-catch urine collection.
- Perform colony count from the blood agar plate to include both gram-positive and gram-negative organisms.
- Consult your facility's manual for the procedure to follow if three or more colony types are present.
- Incubate the culture plates upside down.
- Ensure that the Bauer-Kirby suspension is standardized when performing the antibiotic susceptibility test.

## Safety Precautions

- Observe Universal and Standard Precautions.
- Wear a fluid-resistant, buttoned laboratory coat.
- Observe chemical safety guidelines.
- Avoid aerosol formation.
- Wipe work surfaces with disinfectant before beginning work, when finished, and every time a spill occurs.

## LESSON REVIEW

1. Explain why a clean-catch urine sample must be used for urine culture.
2. Discuss the types of media used for urine culture.
3. Describe how to streak the blood agar plate and EMB or MAC.
4. Discuss estimating the bacterial colony count in urine; how does the loop used for streaking affect it?
5. Discuss how to presumptively identify bacteria.
6. Explain the catalase test.
7. Explain the coagulase test.
8. List two automated methods used to identify bacteria.
9. Give an example of a manual method of identifying bacteria by biochemical reactions.
10. Explain how to set up a disk antibiotic susceptibility test.
11. Describe how the zones of inhibition around the disks are measured.
12. Define coliform and colony count.

## STUDENT ACTIVITIES

1. Reread the information on performing a urine culture, colony count, and antibiotic susceptibility test.
2. Review the glossary terms.
3. Practice performing the urine culture and colony count and the antibiotic susceptibility test, as outlined in the Student Performance Guide.

*Student Performance Guide*

## LESSON 7-6 Urine Culture and Colony Count

Name _____ Date _____

### ☣ THE URINE CULTURE AND COLONY COUNT

### INSTRUCTIONS

1. Practice performing the urine culture and colony count following the step-by-step procedure.
2. Demonstrate your understanding of this lesson by:
   a. Completing a written examination successfully, and
   b. Performing the procedure for urine culture and colony count satisfactorily for the instructor. All steps must be completed as listed on the instructor's Performance Check Sheet.

### MATERIALS AND EQUIPMENT

- gloves
- clean-catch urine specimen (the instructor may desire to "seed" a urine specimen with inoculum of an educational strain of *Escherichia coli*)
- culture of *E. coli*, educational strain (optional)
- blood agar plates
- EMB or MAC agar plates
- calibrated loop (0.01 mL or 0.001 mL)
- Bunsen burner, alcohol burner, or electric incinerator
- matches or flint-type lighter
- wax pencil or marking pen
- surface disinfectant
- hand disinfectant
- biohazard container

### PROCEDURE

Record in the comment section any problems encountered while practicing the procedure (or have a fellow student or the instructor evaluate your performance).

S = Satisfactory
U = Unsatisfactory

| You must: | S | U | Comments |
|---|---|---|---|
| 1. Assemble equipment and materials | | | |
| 2. Light the Bunsen burner or turn on the electric incinerator | | | |
| 3. Wash your hands and put on gloves | | | |
| 4. Obtain a clean-catch urine specimen (Lesson 5-2) | | | |
| 5. Label the bottom of a blood agar plate and an EMB or MAC plate | | | |
| 6. Mix the urine by swirling, and remove the lid from the urine container carefully, to avoid forming splashes or aerosols | | | |
| 7. Sterilize and cool the calibrated loop | | | |

| You must: | S | U | Comments |
|---|---|---|---|
| 8. Insert the loop into the well-mixed urine sample. Remove the loop and check to see that the loop is filled with urine | | | |
| 9. Transfer the loopful of urine to the surface of the blood agar plate by making a streak down the center of the plate | | | |
| 10. Spread the urine over the plate by making twenty to twenty-five cross-streaks at right angles to the center streak, crossing it each time | | | |
| 11. Turn the Petri dish one-quarter turn (90°) and streak twenty to twenty-five times at right angles to the first set, crossing all of them each time (follow facility policy for streaking) | | | |
| 12. Replace the lid on the Petri dish | | | |
| 13. Repeat steps 7–12, using an EMB or MAC plate | | | |
| 14. Sterilize the loop and return it to the holder | | | |
| 15. Turn off the Bunsen burner or electric incinerator | | | |
| 16. Return equipment to proper storage | | | |
| 17. Place agar plates upside down in 35–37°C incubator for eighteen to twenty-four hours (overnight) | | | |
| 18. Dispose of contaminated materials in biohazard container | | | |
| 19. Wipe counter with surface disinfectant | | | |
| 20. Remove and discard gloves in biohazard container | | | |
| 21. Wash hands with hand disinfectant | | | |
| 22. The next day: Wash hands and put on gloves. Examine the plates | | | |
| 23. Count the number of colonies on the blood agar plate | | | |
| 24. Calculate the number of organisms by multiplying the number of colonies from step 23 by 1000 if the 0.001 mL loop was used, or 100 if the 0.01 mL loop was used | | | |
| 25. Record the results | | | |
| 26. *Keep the plates to perform the antibiotic susceptibility test* or discard the plates in the biohazard container | | | |
| 27. Wipe the counter with surface disinfectant | | | |
| 28. Remove gloves and discard in biohazard container | | | |
| 29. Wash your hands with hand disinfectant | | | |

*Evaluator Comments:*

Evaluator _____ Date _____

# Student Performance Guide

## LESSON 7-6 Antibiotic Susceptibility Test

Name _____  Date _____

## ☣ ANTIBIOTIC SUSCEPTIBILITY TEST

### INSTRUCTIONS

1. Practice performing the antibiotic susceptibility test following the step-by-step procedure.
2. Demonstrate your understanding of this lesson by:
   a. Completing a written examination successfully, and
   b. Performing the procedure for the antibiotic susceptibility test satisfactorily for the instructor. All steps must be completed as listed on the instructor's Performance Check Sheet.

### MATERIALS AND EQUIPMENT

- gloves
- Mueller-Hinton plates
- Trypticase soy broth, 5 mL per tube, or a commercial kit such as Prompt™ by BBL
- McFarland's standard #2 (not necessary if using a commercial system to produce a standard suspension)
- wax pencil or marking pen
- Bunsen burner, alcohol burner, or electric incinerator
- matches or flint-type lighter
- surface disinfectant
- hand disinfectant
- biohazard container
- antibiotic disks (Sensi-Discs™ from BBL: ampicillin, Augmentin®, norfloxacin, nitrofurantoin, trimethoprim, Bactrim™, and cephalothin are often used for urines)
- forceps
- calipers, ruler, or special transparent template to measure zones of inhibition
- culture of *E. coli*, educational strain, growing on agar
- sterile swabs

## PROCEDURE

Record in the comment section any problems encountered while practicing the procedure (or have a fellow student or the instructor evaluate your performance).

S = Satisfactory
U = Unsatisfactory

| You must: | S | U | Comments |
|---|---|---|---|
| 1. Assemble materials and equipment: Mueller-Hinton plate, culture plate with bacterial colonies (or colony count plate from urine culture procedure), sterile swab, forceps, broth, antibiotic disks, and marker | | | |
| 2. Light the burner or electric incinerator. Wash hands and put on gloves (use care around flame) | | | |

| You must: | S | U | Comments |
|---|---|---|---|
| 3. Write the identification on the bottom of Mueller–Hinton plate | | | |
| 4. Prepare bacterial suspension using broth and McFarland's standard #2 (or following the manufacturer's instructions if using a commercial system):<br>a. Use sterile swab to pick up a few colonies from the culture plate<br>b. Remove cap from broth and insert swab into broth, gently swishing the swab around to make a slightly turbid suspension of bacteria<br>c. Compare with McFarland's #2 standard<br>d. Press the swab against the side of the tube to express excess liquid. Replace cap on broth tube and set tube in rack | | | |
| 5. Use the swab to streak the Mueller-Hinton agar: Starting at the top edge of the agar, make horizontal streaks the whole width of the plate, from top to bottom | | | |
| 6. Turn the plate 90° and streak from top to bottom, using the same swab; the agar surface should be almost completely covered with the broth inoculum (Figure 7-45) | | | |
| 7. Dispose of swab in biohazard container | | | |
| 8. Sterilize the forceps, pick up one disk out of the cartridge, and place it on the surface of the still-wet agar (Sterilize forceps before picking up each disk) | | | |
| 9. Continue to place disks until all to be used are in place (they should form a circle along the outer edge of the agar, if several are used). A disk dispenser may be used if available | | | |
| 10. Sterilize the forceps and return them to storage. Turn off burner or electric incinerator | | | |
| 11. Replace the Petri dish lid and incubate the plate upside down at 35–37°C overnight (eighteen to twenty-four hours) | | | |
| 12. Remove gloves and wash your hands with hand disinfectant | | | |
| 13. The next day: Wash your hands and put on gloves | | | |
| 14. Remove Mueller-Hinton plate from incubator and observe for zones of inhibition; some disks may not be inhibitory, depending on which organism is present | | | |
| 15. Measure zones, using a metric ruler, calipers, or a special transparent template, which has many sizes of zones printed on it | | | |
| 16. Record the susceptibility of the organism to each antibiotic disk as sensitive (S), resistant (R), or intermediate (I), following the guidelines included on the package insert for each disk cartridge | | | |
| 17. Discard agar plate in biohazard container | | | |

| You must: | S | U | Comments |
|---|---|---|---|
| 18. Clean equipment and return to storage | | | |
| 19. Wipe counter with surface disinfectant | | | |
| 20. Remove gloves and discard in biohazard container | | | |
| 21. Wash your hands with hand disinfectant | | | |

*Evaluator Comments:*

Evaluator _____ Date _____

# Laboratory Detection of Sexually Transmitted Diseases

## LESSON OBJECTIVES

**After studying this lesson, you should be able to:**

- *Explain the importance of early detection of sexually transmitted diseases (STDs).*
- *Discuss the steady increase in incidence of STDs.*
- *Explain why it is important for POLs and other small laboratories to be knowledgeable about STD testing.*
- *Discuss four basic types of tests used to detect STDs.*
- *List five STDs prevalent in the United States.*
- *Name one method of detection for each of the five prevalent STDs.*
- *Discuss the need for confirmatory tests for certain STDs.*
- *Define the glossary terms.*

## GLOSSARY

***Candida albicans*** / fungus that causes vaginitis in females, especially following antibiotic therapy for bacterial infections

***Chlamydia*** / gram-negative intracellular bacteria; *Chlamydia trachomatis* is a cause of STDs

**gonorrhea** / contagious infection spread by sexual contact and caused by *Neisseria gonorrhoeae*

**HIV** / human immunodeficiency virus, a retrovirus that has been identified as the cause of AIDS

**HSV-1** / Herpes simplex virus, type 1; the cause of oral herpes

**HSV-2** / Herpes simplex virus, type 2; the cause of genital herpes

**nongonococcal urethritis** / gonorrhea-like STD caused by organisms other than gonococci

**oxidase test** / enzyme test used to identify certain bacteria such as *Neisseria*

**spirochetes** / motile bacteria with a helical or spiral shape

**STD** / sexually transmitted disease

**syphilis** / infectious, chronic, sexually transmitted disease caused by a spirochete, *Treponema pallidum*

**trichomoniasis** / sexually transmitted infection of the genitourinary tract caused by the parasitic protozoan, *Trichomonas vaginalis*

**urethritis** / inflammation of the urethra

**vaginitis** / inflammation of the vagina

**venereal** / having to do with, or transmitted by, sexual contact

## INTRODUCTION

Sexually transmitted diseases (**STDs**) are transmitted primarily through sexual intercourse or other sexual contact. This lesson introduces basic laboratory methods used to detect STDs in males and females. The causative agents of STDs may be bacteria, protozoa, fungi, or viruses. The infections usually occur in the genitourinary tract, but may be found in other areas. As sexual practices change, many microorganisms once limited to the genitourinary tract are found in other sites in the body. Tests for STDs should not be limited to specimens from the genitourinary tract. For example, in suspected cases of **gonorrhea**, urethral, rectal, and pharyngeal swabs may be collected.

The most common STDs detected in the United States are **Chlamydial** infections, gonorrhea, herpes, hepatitis B and C, **trichomoniasis**, **syphilis**, and candidiasis (Table 7-17). In the United States, the incidence of STD cases rose dramatically until the appearance of AIDS in the 1980s. STDs then began to decline, and have continued to decline except for certain diseases, such as chlamydial infection.

Formerly, most STD testing was performed in hospital laboratories or state public health laboratories because of complex testing methods. However, due to the increasing incidence of STDs, more private practitioners are seeing patients who require testing for STDs. Many diagnostic methods for STD detection can be used in POLs. Physicians and laboratory technicians need to know how to collect specimens to send to a reference laboratory for testing and also which tests are suitable for smaller laboratories. Several manufacturers market kits that produce reliable results for detecting the various STD agents. However, a number of procedures are still performed only in larger laboratories.

## SYMPTOMS OF SEXUALLY TRANSMITTED DISEASES

**Venereal** disease, or sexually transmitted disease, can have long-lasting effects in both males and females. In males, STDs usually produce symptoms such as a penile discharge or burning upon urination. However, evidence indicates that more males than previously thought may be positive for STDs, although asymptomatic. Any male whose sex partner is positive for an STD must be tested or treated. Females may be asymptomatic and untreated for some STDs, a factor important in disease transmission and in infertility for many women.

## DETECTION OF STDS IN FEMALES

Female patients may be tested for STDs because of findings during a routine examination, reporting of symptoms, or because a partner has tested positive for STDs. Many STDs cause **vaginitis**, an inflammation of the vagina. Vaginitis may be caused by bacteria, fungi, or protozoa. Some of the most common organisms are *Gardnerella vaginalis* (formerly *Hemophilus vaginalis*), *Mobiluncus* species, *Streptococcus* Group B, *Chlamydia trachomatis*, *Neisseria gonorrhoeae*, and ***Candida albicans***. Infection by bacteria may occur because of changes in the vaginal pH or alteration in normal flora. Detection methods include Gram stain, culture, wet mounts, serum antibody tests, immunoassays, and DNA probes. Table 7-18 gives examples of STD detection methods.

### The Three-Slide Test

The three-slide test is an important part of discovering the cause of vaginitis. A relatively simple procedure, most of its results can be available in about thirty minutes, while the patient is still in the office. It is a CLIA-waived physician-performed microscopy test. Components of the three-slide test include:

- Saline wet mount preparation of vaginal secretions for *Trichomonas* and "clue cells".

- KOH (potassium hydroxide) preparation of vaginal secretions for yeasts and fungi.

- Gram stain of endocervical secretions for bacteria and yeasts.

**Table 7-17.** Common STDs detected in the United States and their causative agents

| DISEASE | AGENT |
| --- | --- |
| Chlamydial infection | *Chlamydia trachomatis* |
| Gonorrhea | *Neisseria gonorrhoeae* |
| Herpes, type 1 | Herpes simplex virus, type 1 (HSV-1) |
| Herpes, type 2 | Herpes simplex virus, type 2 (HSV-2) |
| Hepatitis B | Hepatitis B virus (HBV) |
| Hepatitis C | Hepatitis C virus (HCV) |
| AIDS | Human immunodeficiency virus (HIV) |
| Trichomoniasis | *Trichomonas vaginalis* |
| Candidiasis | *Candida albicans* |
| Syphilis | *Treponema pallidum* |

**Table 7-18.** Sexually transmitted diseases and examples of tests available for their detection

| DISEASE | TEST METHODS |
| --- | --- |
| Chlamydial infection | EIA, ELISA, DNA probe, cell culture |
| Gonorrhea | Culture, Gram stain, DNA probe, monoclonal antibody agglutination test |
| Herpes | Cell culture, EIA, serology for IgG and IgM |
| Candidiasis | KOH wet prep, culture, Gram stain, rapid chemical confirmation test |
| Trichomoniasis | Saline wet prep |
| Syphilis | |
|   Screen | VDRL, RPR |
|   Confirmatory | FTA-ABS, MHA-TP, direct smear |
| AIDS | |
|   Screen | EIA for anti-HIV-1 |
|   Confirmatory | Western blot, culture, p24 antigen |
| Hepatitis B | Anti-HBcAg (acute), anti-HBsAg (chronic), or hepatitis panel |

Specimens for other tests may be collected at the same time, such as a swab for *N. gonorrhoeae* culture, or a swab for *C. trachomatis* or *N. gonorrhoeae* DNA probe tests. If suspected herpes lesions are present, a specimen can be collected from the lesions and sent to the reference laboratory in viral transport medium.

## Saline Wet Preparation

The saline wet prep is prepared by mixing a drop of vaginal specimen with a drop of 0.85% saline on a microscope slide and adding a coverslip. A depression slide can also be used. The physician may examine the slide microscopically in the examination room or send it to the laboratory. It must be examined within thirty minutes of collection to detect *Trichomonas vaginalis*, a parasitic protozoan, which causes trichomoniasis. If *Gardnerella vaginalis* is present, "clue cells," which are vaginal epithelial cells covered with the bacteria, may also be seen (Figure 7-49 and Color Plate 44).

## The KOH Preparation

A drop of vaginal material is mixed with one to two drops of 10% KOH solution on a microscope slide or in a depression slide to look for fungi, such as *C. albicans*. The KOH destroys structures such as epithelial cells and WBCs; any fungi present will appear as tangled masses resembling hairs or threads (Figure 7-50).

## *Neisseria gonorrhoeae* Culture

A sterile rayon or Dacron swab is used to collect the specimen for culture of *N. gonorrhoeae*, the organism that causes gonorrhea. The swab is used to streak the modified Thayer-Martin (MTM) agar in the shape of a "Z" or a "W." The culture must be transported to the laboratory and the plate cross-streaked using a sterile loop (Figure 7-51). The culture plate is immediately placed in an increased $CO_2$ environment and incubated at 35–37°C to prevent loss of viability of any organisms present.

## The Smear for Gram Stain

The same swab used to inoculate the media for Neisseria culture can be used to prepare the smear, as described in

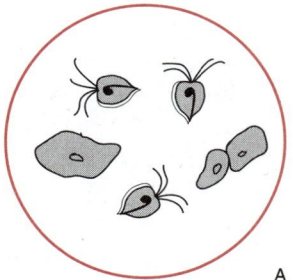
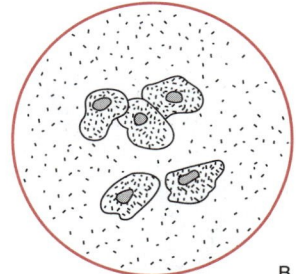

A        B

**FIGURE 7-49** Saline wet preparation: (A) trichomonads, (B) "clue" cells

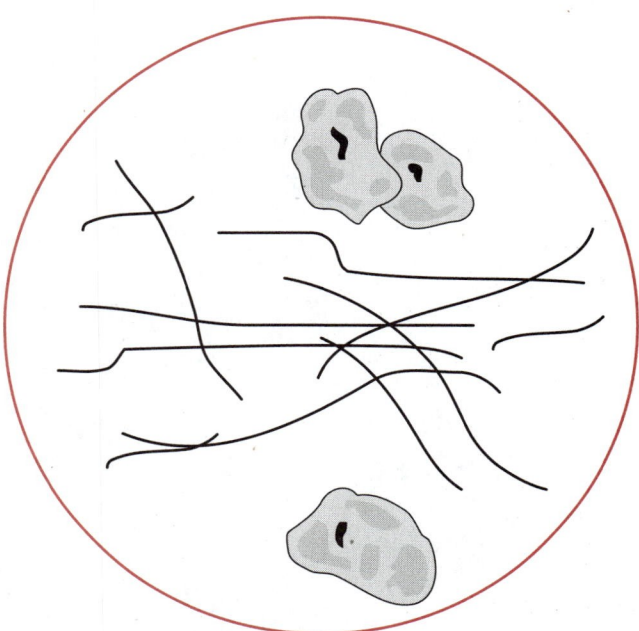

**FIGURE 7-50** KOH preparation showing presence of fungal elements

Lesson 7-4. The smear is Gram-stained and examined for the presence of bacteria and pus cells (WBCs) using the oil-immersion objective of the microscope. Smears from uninfected females should have a moderate amount of *Lactobacillus* (gram-positive rods), few or no WBCs, and few epithelial cells (Color Plate 43).

G. vaginalis is a gram-variable microorganism, which means it may stain either gram-negative or gram-positive. If present on the smear, the tiny organisms will be scattered over the other constituents on the smear, especially the vaginal epithelial cells (Color Plate 44). If yeast cells are present, they will stain dark purple (Color Plate 35).

The smear is also examined for the presence of *N. gonorrhoeae*, a gram-negative kidney-bean-shaped diplococcus. The organism can be found both inside neutrophilic leukocytes (intracellular) and also extracellular on smears from infected patients (Figure 7-51 and Color Plate 42).

## DETECTION OF STDS IN MALES

Male STD patients usually have symptoms of **urethritis**, an inflammation of the urethra. The major symptoms are a burning sensation on urination, or the presence of a penile discharge. Tests may include a urinalysis and culture, a Gram stain, a culture or DNA probe test for *N. gonorrhoeae*, immunoassay or DNA probe for *C. trachomatis*, and serology tests for herpes simplex virus (HSV), HIV, and syphilis.

Males also sometimes develop a "nonspecific" or **"nongonococcal" urethritis** in which the organisms causing the condition cannot be identified. In these cases, the physician tries treatments for the standard microorganisms usually implicated in urethritis.

## Urinalysis and Culture

If there are strong indications of STDs in a male patient, the specimens for those tests should be collected before the patient collects the urine sample.

The results of the urinalysis can help determine if the symptoms are due to UTI or STD. If the midstream urine specimen contains RBCs, bacteria, WBCs, or protein, the patient may have a UTI instead of an STD. The results of urine culture can be used to confirm the urine microscopic findings. If the urine results are negative, the problems may be due to an STD.

## The Urethral Gram Stain

A smear is made of the urethral discharge using a sterile Dacron or rayon swab. The smear is Gram-stained in the laboratory and examined microscopically. The entire smear is searched for evidence of bacteria, especially *N. gonorrhoeae*, other microorganisms, and WBCs. The presence of many WBCs is a strong indicator of gonorrhea (Color Plate 42).

## The Urethral Culture

The urethral discharge is collected on a urogenital swab and cultured for *N. gonorrhoeae*. It is inoculated onto a modified Thayer–Martin (MTM) plate by touching the urogenital swab to the plate five or six times. The plate is transported to the laboratory immediately, where it is cross-streaked using a sterile loop, and placed into a 35–37°C incubator in an increased $CO_2$ environment (Figure 7-53).

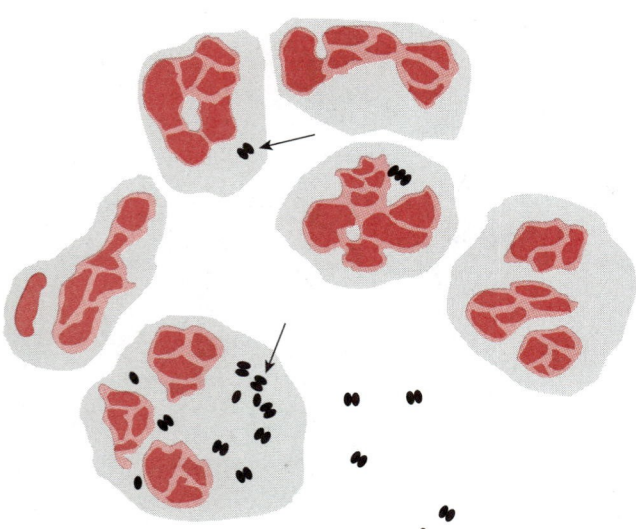

**FIGURE 7-51** The Gram stain showing WBCs and intracellular (arrows) and extracellular diplococci

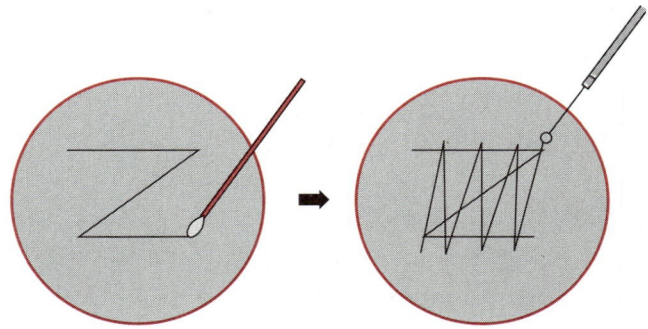

**FIGURE 7-52** Cross-streaking the Thayer-Martin plate for vaginal culture

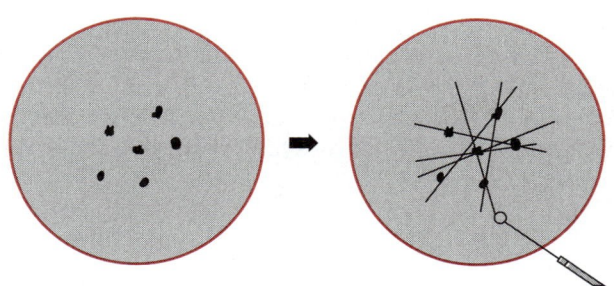

**FIGURE 7-53** Cross-streaking the Thayer-Martin plate for urethral culture

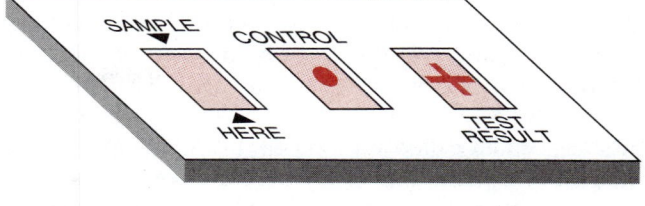

**FIGURE 7-54** Illustration of one EIA test design

## EXAMINATION OF CULTURES FOR *NEISSERIA*

After overnight incubation, the Thayer-Martin plate is examined for growth. *N. gonorrhoeae* appear as tiny, shiny, grayish colonies growing along the streak pattern. If scant or no growth is present, the plate is incubated for an additional twenty-four hours. Other bacteria and yeasts may also grow on Thayer-Martin.

### Confirmatory Tests for *Neisseria*

The **oxidase test** can be used to help identify colonies of *N. gonorrhoeae*, an oxidase-positive organism. Suspected *Neisseria* colonies should be tested with oxidase reagent. Oxidase-positive organisms turn purple-black on exposure to the reagent. If the reaction is positive, a smear should be made and a Gram stain performed on one of the oxidase-positive colonies. The presence of gram-negative diplococci on the smear is presumptive for *N. gonorrhoeae* and a test must be done to confirm identification. Dupont's Gonochek® II identifies *N. gonorrhoeae, N. lactima, N. meningitidis,* and gives presumptive identification for *Branhamella catarrhalis*. GonoGen® from Becton Dickinson Microbiology Systems is a fifteen-minute agglutination test. Other identification kits are available from Microbiologics and Pharmacia Diagnostics.

## TESTS FOR OTHER STDS

Many types of tests are available for detecting other STDs such as AIDS, herpes, hepatitis, syphilis, and chlamydial infection. Methods include negative staining, electron microscopy, fluorescent antibody techniques, enzyme immunoassays (EIAs), serological tests, monoclonal antibody agglutination, and nucleic acid (DNA and RNA) probes (Table 7-18). The physician may order tests for one or more of these other diseases, depending on the sexual history of the patient or the patient's symptoms.

An increasing number of easy-to-use test systems are becoming available, so that more testing can be performed in the smaller laboratory and the POL. Figure 7-54 illustrates an example of an EIA test. However, other tests are still used that are more time-consuming, technically advanced, or infrequently performed; specimens for these tests must be sent to a reference laboratory.

### Tests for Herpes Infection

Herpes simplex virus (HSV) infections have chronic, painful, recurring episodes. If herpes lesions are present, a vesicle can be broken with a sterile swab or needle and the vesicle fluid collected using another sterile swab. The swab is then inserted into viral transport medium and sent to a reference laboratory for culture.

Two common types of tests for herpes infection are cell culture and serum antibody levels of anti-HSV. Cell-culture results are available in twenty-four to forty-eight hours. A sample of the patient's blood can also be sent to a reference laboratory for serum titers of IgG and IgM to herpes simplex virus, type 1 (**HSV-1**) and type 2 (**HSV-2**). The titers indicate whether the patient has active herpes or has ever had herpes type 1 or type 2 in the past.

### Tests for *Chlamydia* Infection

*Chlamydia* infection can be detected by EIA, cell culture, and DNA probes. In the female patient, *C. trachomatis* infection may cause the cervix to bleed easily just from the touch of a swab during examination. The cervix is said to be "friable."

*C. trachomatis* infection is a common cause of urethritis in males, especially in young adults. Since urination temporarily flushes out any microorganisms inhabiting the urethra, for best chances of detection, the patient should not have urinated in the last one to two hours before the specimen collection.

There are several tests for *C. trachomatis*. The same specimen swab can be used to test for both *Chlamydia* and *N. gonorrhoeae* in some of the DNA probe kits. DNA probe tests have high sensitivity and specificity. A piece of DNA with a specific sequence of nucleic acids, called the "probe DNA," is added to a mixture containing the DNA from any organisms in the patient specimen. If the probe DNA and the organism's DNA match and combine, they will produce a signal such as a color or luminescence that can be measured by a special instrument.

Immunoassay tests are also available for *C. trachomatis*. Two of these are the Premier® *Chlamydia* by Meridian and CLEARVIEW™ *Chlamydia* from Wampole Laboratories. These tests have built-in positive and negative controls. The tests can be used to screen urines for *Chlamydia* in male patients, but their lower urine test sensitivity means negative results should be confirmed by another method.

Each of the various tests has its own instructions and supplies. For example, procedures and supplies will be different for a DNA probe and an immunoassay. The technologist and the clinician must be sure to follow instructions for the method being used.

## Tests for Syphilis

**Syphilis** is another venereal disease spread by sexual contact. Syphilis is caused by *Treponema pallidum*, a spiral bacterium (**spirochete**). Early (primary) syphilis is characterized by skin lesions. Organ or tissue damage occurs in the secondary stage. Late-stage (tertiary) syphilis can affect the cardiovascular and central nervous systems.

Because of the difficulty in growing *Treponema* in culture, the diagnostic method of choice has been serum antibody titers. The *Venereal Disease Research Laboratory (VDRL)* test and the *rapid plasma reagin (RPR)* test are serological screening tests for syphilis. The VDRL test can only be performed by laboratories certified in its use. The RPR is a simpler procedure.

### The VDRL Test

Patients infected with *T. pallidum* produce a nonspecific antibody-like substance called reagin. When the VDRL antigen mixture, made of cardiolipin, cholesterol, and lecithin, is reacted with serum containing reagin, a visible reaction, flocculation, occurs. The test is "reactive" in 70–99% of primary and secondary syphilis cases, but is usually nonreactive in tertiary cases.

### The RPR Test

The RPR test has a carbon-containing cardiolipin antigen that reacts with the antibody-like substance (reagin) produced in response to syphilis and other conditions.

This is also a flocculation test, with the carbon causing black clumps on a white background in a reactive test. Test results are reported as "reactive" or "nonreactive." A reactive result *does not* mean the patient definitely has syphilis; it only indicates the presence of these nonspecific antibodies.

### Confirmation of a Reactive Syphilis Screening Test

A "reactive" result in a serum syphilis screening test must be confirmed by a more specific test method, since "biologic false positives" (BFPs) can occur. Many nonsyphilitic conditions can cause BFPs, including tuberculosis, hepatitis, pneumonia, pregnancy, and rheumatoid arthritis.

The fluorescent treponemal antibody-absorption (FTA-ABS) test is specific for *Treponema* antibodies. The *Treponema* antigen is used to detect patient serum antibodies. The *T. pallidum* microhemagglutination assay (MHA-TP) also detects antibodies to the syphilis organism. Both the FTA-ABS and the MHA-TP are specific treponemal antigen tests that may be used to confirm a reactive RPR or VDRL test. The newest test methods available use enzyme-linked immunosorbent assays (ELISAs). (An illustration of a fluorescently stained spirochete is shown in Color Plate 34.)

## Tests for HIV

Human immunodeficiency virus (**HIV**) is transmitted sexually and by contact with infectious body fluids. The main approach to HIV testing is to assay for anti-HIV in the patient's serum. Since this antibody usually does not appear until several months to a year after exposure, a negative test must be followed by another test in about six months. These tests are usually performed in reference laboratories and state public health laboratories.

Murex Corporation has marketed the SUDS® Test for HIV-1 antibodies, which gives results in ten minutes. According to the manufacturer, negative results can be reported immediately, but reactive specimens must be confirmed by a more specific test method, such as Western blot. The test could be useful in emergency care situations, physicians' offices, and "stat labs." However, the implications of a positive HIV test require patient counseling before testing.

Since saliva and urine from HIV-infected patients contain HIV antibodies, tests have been developed to detect these. As HIV infections progress, the virus multiplies and can be cultured and isolated. Other tests detect viral components such as the p24 antigen. The p24 antigen can be detected very early after HIV infection, then disappears, and cannot be detected again until the late stages of the disease.

## Tests for Hepatitis B Infections

The hepatitis B virus (HBV) can cause serious illness and even be fatal because of its effects on the liver. A patient may remain chronically infected with HBV after seeming to have recovered. This chronic infection can cause liver cancer (hepatocarcinoma). HBV transmission can be through sexual contact, or contact with infectious body fluids, or contaminated surfaces. An HBV vaccine is available that is effective up to five to seven years. At-risk health care workers must be immunized or must sign a refusal statement waiving employer liability.

A wide range of tests are available for detecting HBV antigens and antibodies. Test methods include radioimmunoassays, EIA, and ELISA. The most common screening test is the test for HBV surface antigen (HBsAg). A positive result indicates the patient now has, or recently has had, an acute HBV infection. The finding of HBsAg several months after infection indicates the person is a chronic HBV carrier. The anti-HBsAg titer is used to check for immunity after receiving the HBV vaccine. Detecting anti-HBcAg (antibody to the HBV core antigen) is another test for HBV infection.

## SUMMARY

This lesson presents only basic information about the microorganisms involved in STDs and the test methods used to detect them. There is a great need for laboratory personnel who are familiar with the epidemiology and test methods for common STDs. The incidence of some of these diseases has been rising in recent years and is still on the increase. Some of the diseases, including AIDS, hepatitis B, and syphilis, are life-threatening. Early detection with laboratory tests may mean earlier treatment, increased survival chances or life span for the patient, and a decrease in transmission of the diseases.

## LESSON REVIEW

1. Explain the importance of early detection of STDs.
2. Discuss the correlation between STD incidence and the number of HIV infections.
3. Discuss why personnel in POLs and other small laboratories should be knowledgeable about STDs and the methods used to detect them.
4. List five STDs prevalent in the United States.
5. Name one method of detection for each of five STDs.
6. Explain what the presence of HBsAg indicates about a patient.
7. Discuss the danger of chronic HBV infection.
8. Explain why patients should be tested for both herpes simplex virus type 1 and type 2.
9. Define *Candida albicans, chlamydia*, gonorrhea, HIV, HSV-1, HSV-2, non-gonococcal urethritis, oxidase test, spirochetes, STD, syphilis, trichomoniasis, urethritis, vaginitis, and venereal.

## STUDENT ACTIVITIES

1. Reread the information on laboratory detection of STDs.
2. Review the glossary terms.
3. Survey POLs in your community to find out the extent of STD testing performed.
4. Determine how a nearby reference laboratory confirms positive HIV tests and reactive RPR tests.

# LESSON 7-8

# Fecal Occult Blood Test

## LESSON OBJECTIVES

**After studying this lesson, you should be able to:**

- *State the purpose of the fecal occult blood test.*
- *State the principle of the guaiac reaction.*
- *List two causes of false-positive tests.*
- *List one cause of a false-negative test.*
- *Instruct a patient on how to collect a specimen for the fecal occult blood test.*
- *Perform a slide test for fecal occult blood.*
- *List safety precautions to be observed in performing the fecal occult blood test.*
- *Define the glossary terms.*

## GLOSSARY

**guaiac** / chemical derived from the resin of the *Guaiacum* tree

**malignant** / cancerous; not benign

**occult** / concealed or hidden

## INTRODUCTION

The fecal **occult** blood test is a simple, inexpensive screening test for colon cancer, a leading cause of death in the United States. The test aids in early detection of colon cancer, during the period when a patient has no or few symptoms. As **malignant** cells grow, they cause microscopic bleeding in the intestine that cannot be detected by the naked eye. The fecal occult blood test detects this hidden, or **occult**, bleeding in the colon through a chemical test for blood on a small portion of stool specimen. Early detection of intestinal bleeding helps the physician find and treat a malignancy before it becomes widespread.

## PRINCIPLE OF THE FECAL OCCULT BLOOD TEST

The fecal occult blood test is a good screening procedure, since it can detect amounts of blood too small to be visible. The test is performed on a slide that contains paper squares coated with **guaiac**, a chemical derived from tree resin. A small portion of stool (fecal) specimen is applied to the paper in the slide. A developer solution containing hydrogen peroxide ($H_2O_2$) is added to the paper. If blood is present in the specimen, the iron (Fe) in the hemoglobin catalyses the reaction between the guaiac in the paper and the ($H_2O_2$). The completed reaction forms a blue color. A simplified reaction equation is shown as:

$$\text{Alpha guaiaconic acid} + H_2O_2 \xrightarrow{\text{hemoglobin (Fe)}} \text{Blue quinone compound}$$

The guaiac reaction is not specific for blood. Certain foods and drugs can cause either a false-negative or false-positive reaction (Table 7-19). The peroxidase enzyme, found in horseradish and turnips, will produce a false-positive result; in addition, the blood in red meat will react positively. Cimetidine, a medication for ulcers, contains a blue pigment that can cause confusion in reading the test result. Excess dietary vitamin C can inhibit the reaction and cause a false-negative result.

Several manufacturers offer card tests for occult blood. Beckman Coulter offers Hemoccult® and Hemoccult® SENSA® test kits (figure 7-55). Another test, Coloscreen®, is manufactured by Helena Laboratories.

 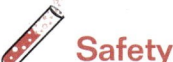 **Safety**

Universal and Standard Precautions must be observed when handling fecal specimens or slides that have had specimens applied to them. Slides mailed to the laboratory for testing must be in an approved safety pouch or container.

## Quality Assurance

Patients should be instructed in the proper diet and drug restrictions to follow before collecting the fecal specimen. If the slides are prepared by the patient at home, they must be delivered to the laboratory and tested within two days, since a further delay has been shown to cause a false-negative result. Control areas (performance monitors) on the slides must always be developed. The test must be considered invalid if the performance monitor areas fail to react properly.

**Table 7-19.** Dietary factors causing false-negative and false-positive fecal occult blood tests

| FALSE POSITIVES | FALSE NEGATIVES |
|---|---|
| Turnips | Excess vitamin C |
| Horseradish | |
| Excess red meat | |
| Any food containing peroxidase enzyme | |
| The ulcer medication cimetidine contains a blue pigment that can interfere with test interpretation | |

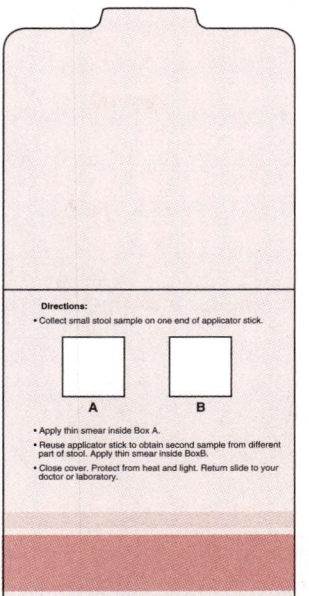 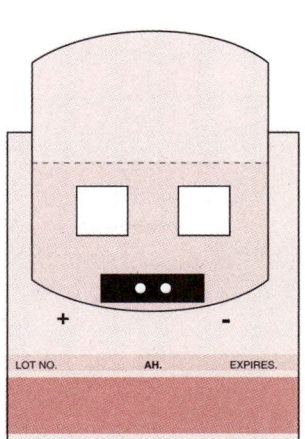

**FIGURE 7-55** Hemoccult® slide: left Hemoccult® slide with front flap open, revealing boxes A and B; and (right) with back flap open, showing the test area (reverse sides of boxes A and B), and the Performance Monitor areas

## Collecting the Specimen for Fecal Occult Blood

The fecal sample can be collected by the physician during a rectal examination or sigmoidoscopy. Alternatively, the patient can collect specimens at home, apply the samples to the test slides, and bring them to the laboratory to be analyzed.

### Patient Instructions

The patient should be given a list of instructions concerning dietary and drug restrictions. Detailed instructions can be found in manufacturers' product inserts.

Collection containers such as urine cups may be provided to the patient for home use. After the sample has been obtained, the patient should use an applicator stick (usually provided in the kits) to apply a thin feces smear to one of the specimen areas (boxes) (Figure 7-56). The applicator should be reused to obtain a second sample from another specimen area and apply it to the remaining box. To increase the likelihood of detecting occult blood, specimens should be collected from bowel movements on three successive days and applied to three different test slides.

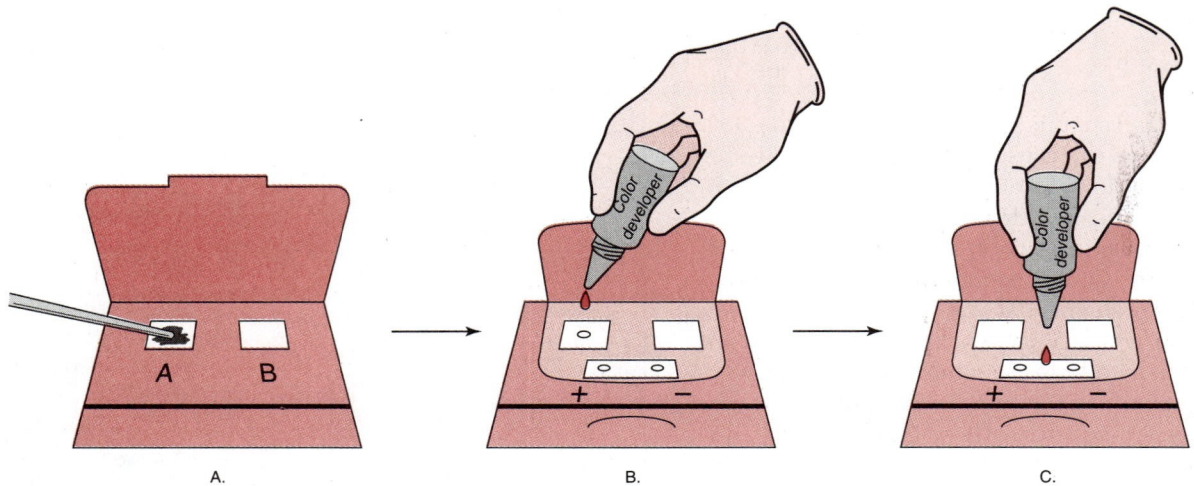

**FIGURE 7-56** (A) Apply a thin smear of fecal sample to a slide test; (B) apply two drops of color developer to test area after opening the back flap of slide; (C) apply one drop of color developer between the positive and negative Performance Monitor areas

## Performing the Fecal Occult Blood Test

If the screening test was done at home, the patient information on the front side of the slides should be confirmed when the slides arrive in the laboratory. Standard Precautions must be used when handling these slides, since they contain biological specimens and are potentially infectious. The flap on the back of the slide is opened and two drops of developer are applied to each sample area (Figure 7-56). Any blue color developing around the fecal smears within sixty seconds is a positive test. Color photos of positive and negative smears are included with every test kit for comparison.

## Quality Control

Quality control is provided by developing the performance monitor built into each card. One negative and one positive control spot are included near the test areas. One drop of developer is applied between the positive and negative spots (Figure 7-56). If the slide and developer are functioning properly, within ten seconds, a blue color will appear in the positive spot; the negative spot will have no blue color.

If a patient who has not been on the restricted diet tests positive on one or more of the three specimens submitted, the tests should be repeated, using the restrictions. However, even if the results of the second series are negative, more diagnostic procedures should be ordered, since the bleeding may be sporadic.

### *Procedural Notes*

- Be sure slides are tested within two days of preparation.
- Protect the slides from heat and light.
- Interpret test results before applying developer to the performance monitors.
- Wait three to five minutes after applying the fecal sample to the paper before adding developer.
- Do not use slides after expiration date.

### *Safety Precautions*

- Observe Universal and Standard Precautions.
- Treat patient samples and all materials that come in contact with them as potentially infectious.
- Avoid contacting eyes and skin with developer.

## LESSON REVIEW

1. What is the purpose of the fecal occult blood test?
2. What is the principle of the guaiac reaction?
3. List two causes of false-positive tests and tell why they occur.
4. List one cause of a false-negative test result.
5. Explain how to instruct a patient in collecting the fecal specimen and preparing the slides.
6. Why should patient samples be regarded as potentially infectious?
7. Why is colon cancer a leading cause of death?
8. Why should the fecal occult blood test be performed in a series of three?
9. Define guaiac, malignant, and occult.

## STUDENT ACTIVITIES

1. Reread the information on the fecal occult blood test.
2. Review the glossary terms.
3. Practice instructing a patient in collecting the specimen and applying it to the slides.
4. Practice performing a test for detecting fecal occult blood as outlined in the Student Performance Guide.

## *Student Performance Guide*

### **LESSON 7-8** Fecal Occult Blood Test

Name _____ Date _____

 **INSTRUCTIONS**

1. Practice performing a test for fecal occult blood following the step-by-step procedure.
2. Demonstrate your understanding of this lesson by:
   a. Completing a written examination successfully, and
   b. Performing the test for fecal occult blood satisfactorily for the instructor. All steps must be completed as listed on the instructor's Performance Check Sheet.

*Note:* Procedure given is general. Package insert for test kit used should be consulted for specific instructions before performing the test.

## MATERIALS AND EQUIPMENT

- gloves
- surface disinfectant (10%) chlorine bleach solution)
- timer
- test kit for fecal occult blood (Hemoccult®, Coloscreen® or other)
- applicator sticks
- cups for collecting fecal specimens
- fecal specimens
- biohazard container
- laboratory tissues and paper towels
- aerosol air deodorizer

## PROCEDURE

Record in the comment section any problems encountered while practicing the procedure (or have a fellow student or the instructor evaluate the performance).

S = Satisfactory
U = Unsatisfactory

| You must: | S | U | Comments |
|---|---|---|---|
| 1. Wash your hands and put on gloves | | | |
| 2. Assemble materials and equipment | | | |
| 3. If the specimen has already been applied to the slide, proceed to step 5. If slides are to be taken home, practice instructing a patient in collecting the specimen and preparing the slides. Show the patient the instructions on the slide cover and ask if there are any questions | | | |
| 4. If the specimen is available, but not applied to the slide, proceed as follows:<br>a. Fill out the patient information on the front of the slide package | | | |

| You must: | S | U | Comments |
|---|---|---|---|
| b. Open the flap on the front to expose the two paper guaiac squares.  Follow the directions and obtain a small portion of the stool sample on the applicator stick.  Apply a thin smear to box A<br>c. Reuse the applicator stick to obtain a second sample from a different part of the specimen.  Apply a thin smear to box B<br>d. Close the cover and wait three to five minutes for the smears to dry | | | |
| 5.  Turn the slide over and open the perforated flap to expose the backs of boxes A and B, and the Performance Monitor (control) area | | | |
| 6.  Apply two drops of the developer onto each smear (boxes A and B) and start the timer | | | |
| 7.  Read the results after the appropriate time interval | | | |
| 8.  Compare the colors on the slide to the color guide in the package insert. Any blue color is a positive test | | | |
| 9.  Apply *one* drop of developer between the positive (+) and the negative (-) Performance Monitor areas.  Read the results after the appropriate time interval.  If the Performance Monitors do not react properly, repeat the test, using a new slide | | | |
| 10.  Record the results | | | |
| 11.  Dispose of all potentially infectious materials in a biohazard container | | | |
| 12.  Wipe the counter with surface disinfectant | | | |
| 13.  Return equipment to proper storage | | | |
| 14.  Remove gloves and discard in biohazard container | | | |
| 15.  Wash your hands with hand disinfectant | | | |

*Evaluator Comments:*

Evaluator _____ Date _____

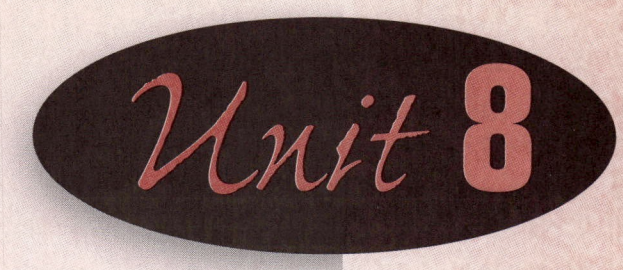

# Basic Parasitology

## UNIT OBJECTIVES

**After studying this unit, you should be able to:**
- *Discuss the functions of the parasitology section of the medical laboratory.*
- *Discuss mechanisms of parasitic infection.*
- *Describe parasite control methods.*
- *Describe appropriate diagnostic techniques for blood, tissue, and intestinal parasites.*
- *Explain the procedures for properly collecting and processing specimens for parasite examination.*
- *Prepare and perform a cellophane tape test for pinworms.*
- *Prepare fecal specimens for microscopic parasite examination.*
- *Prepare smears for examining blood parasites.*

## UNIT OVERVIEW

Many types of parasitic organisms cause human disease. Most parasitic diseases in the United States have been brought under control with education, improved sanitation techniques, and insect control measures. However, worldwide, millions of people are infected with parasites, and in many parts of the world parasites remain a major cause of disease and death.

As world travel has become commonplace, parasitic infections are detected more frequently in U.S. medical laboratories. Additionally, organisms such as *Pneumocystis, Toxoplasma,* and *Cryptosporidium* are becoming an increasing problem because they can cause severe disease in immunocompromised transplant, AIDS, and chemotherapy patients.

Parasitology is usually a part of the microbiology department. Only in large reference or research laboratories is parasitology a stand-alone department. Because of the large variety of parasites and the infrequency with which they are found, most laboratory workers do not gain much experience in parasite identi-

fication. Therefore, many laboratories routinely send specimens for parasite examination to a reference or state health laboratory.

The stool, or fecal, specimen is the one most frequently examined for parasites. However, parasites may be present in and on all parts of the body, so specimens vary with the patient's symptoms. Since the malarial parasite infects RBCs, the hematology technician may be the first to detect that organism. *Trichomonas,* a flagellated parasite, may inhabit the genitourinary tract and may be detected during the microscopic part of a routine urinalysis. Organisms such as lice can infest body hair. Tapeworms, roundworms, amoebae, and *Cryptosporidium* infect the intestinal tract. Organisms such as *Toxoplasma* may be found in tissue.

Unit 8 provides information about basic parasitology concepts and laboratory procedures. Lesson 8-1 is a brief introduction to the field of parasitology. Groups of the more common human parasites, modes of transmission, life cycles, and diagnostic methods are outlined.

Lesson 8-2 describes specimen collection and processing for parasite examination and describes the procedure for the cellophane tape test for detecting pinworm. Methods of preparing fecal specimens for microscopic examination for parasites are presented in Lesson 8-3. Lesson 8-4 describes the procedure for preparing, staining, and examining blood smears for parasites.

This unit represents only an introduction to the field of clinical parasitology. Becoming expert in parasite identification requires much practice and study. Specimens must be collected and processed correctly to increase the likelihood of detecting any parasite(s) present. Personnel should also have a basic knowledge of parasites and be able to recognize parasitic forms. Technicians in laboratories that do not perform frequent parasitology examinations may not be able to identify all parasites, but they must be alert enough and sufficiently trained to recognize something unusual in the specimen that requires expert evaluation.

## SUGGESTED READINGS AND REFERENCES

Ash, L. R. & Orihel, T. C. (1987). *Parasites: A guide to laboratory procedures and identification.* Chicago: ASCP Press.

Ash, L. R., Orihel, T. C. & Savioli, L. (1994). *Bench aids for the diagnosis of intestinal parasites.* World Health Organization.

Ash, L. R. & Orihel, T. C. (4th ed.). (1997). *Atlas of human parasitology.* Chicago: ASCP Press.

Ash, L. R. (4th ed.). (1997). *Human parasitology: Teaching slide set.* Chicago: ASCP Press.

Bogitsh, B. & Cheng, T. C. (2nd ed.). (1998) *Human parasitology.* San Diego: Academic Press.

Brooke, M. M. & Melvin, D. M. (1984). *Morphology of diagnostic stages of intestinal parasites of man.* HHS Publication No. (CDC) 84-8116.

Despommier, D. D., Gwadz, R. W., & Hotez, P. J. (3rd ed.). (1995). *Parasitic diseases.* New York: Springer-Verlag.

Diggs, L. W., Sturm, D., & Bell, A. (5th ed.). (1988). *The morphology of human blood cells.* Abbott Park IL: Abbott Laboratories.

Fleck, S. L. & Moody, A. H. (1988). *Diagnostic techniques in medical parasitology.* London: John Wright.

Forbes, B. A., Sahm, D. F., Trevino, E., & Weissfeld, A. (10th ed.). (1998). *Scott's diagnostic microbiology.* St. Louis: Mosby Year Book.

Garcia, L. S. & Bruckner, D. A. (3rd ed.). (1996). *Diagnostic medical parasitology.* Washington, DC: American Society for Microbiology.

Gillespie, S. H. & Hawkey, P. M. (Eds.) (1995). *Medical parasitology: A practical approach.* Oxford: Oxford University Press.

Henry, J. B. (Ed.). (19th ed.). (1997). *Clinical diagnosis and management by laboratory methods.* Philadelphia: W. B. Saunders.

Koneman, E. W., Allen, S. D., & Janda, W. M. (5th ed.). (1997). *Color atlas and textbook of diagnostic microbiology.* Philadelphia: Lippincott-Raven.

Leventhal, R., & Cheadle, R. F. (4th ed.). (1995). *Medical parasitology: A self-instructional text.* Philadelphia: F. A. Davis Company.

Marshall, J. R. (1993). *Fundamental skills for the clinical laboratory professional.* Albany, NY: Delmar Publishers, Inc.

Melvin, D. M. & Brooke, M. M. (3rd ed.). (1985). *Laboratory procedures for the diagnosis of intestinal parasites.* Atlanta: U.S. Dept. of Health and Human Services, Public Health Service, CDC.

Ravel, R. (6th ed.). (1995). *Clinical laboratory medicine: Clinical application of laboratory data.* Chicago: Mosby Year Book.

Schmidt, G. D., Roberts, L. S., & Janovy, J. (5th ed.). (1995). *Foundations of parasitology.* St. Louis: WCB/McGraw-Hill.

Schmidt, G. D. (5th ed.). (1992). *Essentials of parasitology.* William C. Brown/McGraw-Hill Publishers.

Wentworth, B. B. (Ed.) (7th ed.). (1988). *Diagnostic procedures for mycotic and parasitic infections.* Washington, DC: American Public Health Association, Inc.

# Introduction to Parasitology

**After studying this lesson, you should be able to:**

- *Name the three major morphological parasite groups.*
- *List three ways in which parasite infections are transmitted.*
- *List three methods used in diagnosing parasitic infections.*
- *List four specimens that may be examined for parasites.*
- *List four ways to control or prevent parasitic infections.*
- *Name three blood parasites.*
- *Name three intestinal protozoan parasites.*
- *Name three types of parasitic helminths.*
- *Explain how immunological tests are useful in the parasitology laboratory.*
- *Define the glossary terms.*

## GLOSSARY

**arthropod** / member of the phylum Arthropoda, which includes crustaceans, insects, and arachnids

**cestode** / tapeworm; member of the class Cestoda

**commensal** / organism that lives with, on, or in another, without causing injury to either

**congenital** / acquired during fetal development, and present at the time of birth, but not inherited

**definitive host** / host in which the sexual or adult form of the parasite is found

**ectoparasite** / parasite that lives on the outer surface of a host

**endemic** / recurring in a specific location or population

**helminth** / worm, especially a parasitic worm; in parasitology, the group comprising the roundworms and flatworms

**host** / organism from which a parasite obtains nutrients and in which some or part of the parasite's life cycle is carried out

**immunocompromised** / having reduced or absent ability to produce a normal immune response

**intermediate host** / host in which the asexual, immature, or larval form of the parasite is found

**nematode** / roundworm; any unsegmented worm of the class Nematoda

**opportunistic parasite** / organism that causes disease only in immunocompromised hosts

**ova** / eggs

**parasite** / organism that lives in or on another species and at the expense of that species

**pathogenic** / capable of causing damage or injury to the host

**proglottid (pl. proglottides)** / segment of a tapeworm that contains male and female reproductive systems

**protozoa** / unicellular eukaryotic organisms, both free-living and parasitic

**reservoir host** / host, other than the usual host, in which the parasite lives and is infectious

**tremadode** / fluke; any parasitic flatworm of the class Trematoda

**vector** / agent that transports a pathogen from an infected host to a noninfected host

## INTRODUCTION

Clinical parasitology is the study of parasites, parasitic diseases, methods of diagnosing and identifying parasites, and treating and controlling parasitic diseases. Parasites may be classified in several ways. They may be grouped according to the site in which they normally are found; for example, intestinal parasites, blood parasites, or **ectoparasite**s (parasites on the exterior of the host). Or they may be grouped according to morphological characteristics; for example, worms (tapeworms, roundworms, and flukes), protozoa, and arthropods (insects and arachnids).

Parasitic infections are usually diagnosed by finding and identifying the parasite, either macroscopically or microscopically, or by immunological tests. Occasionally, the organism may be cultured. This lesson presents an overview of the field of clinical parasitology as it relates to medical laboratory procedures. Clinical parasitology textbooks and atlases should be consulted for more comprehensive information.

## WHAT ARE PARASITES?

**Parasites** are organisms that live in or on another organism, the **host**, and live at the expense of the host organism. In other words, the parasite depends on the host for nutrients, which results in injury to the host.

Many parasites cause little obvious harm to the host, for example head lice. Others, such as the malarial parasite, may cause severe disease and even death if left untreated. These are called **pathogenic** parasites. **Opportunistic parasite**s are those that cause few or no symptoms in healthy hosts, but may cause severe disease in **immunocompromised** hosts.

## CHARACTERISTICS OF PARASITES AND PARASITIC INFECTIONS

### Classifying Parasites

Parasites, like other living organisms, are grouped according to international rules of zoological classification based on morphology and other characteristics. Although organisms may be called by various common names, such as "hookworm" or "beef tapeworm," they have two-part latinized scientific names that are recognized internationally. Scientific names of organisms are always italicized, with genus names also capitalized.

### Types of Hosts

To complete their life cycles, most parasites have specific requirements. Although essentially all animal species have parasites, these parasites are often very host-specific. However, if conditions are right, parasites normally found in one host may survive or even thrive in an unnatural host. An example of this is the dog heartworm, *Dirofilaria immitis*. This parasite is considered to be host-specific, with dogs being the natural host. However, the dog heartworm can infect other animals, such as cats. These infections are not usually as serious as infections in dogs.

The **definitive host**, or main host, is the organism in which the sexually mature (adult) form of a parasite is found. Some parasites require two or more different host species to complete their life cycle.

The **intermediate host** is an organism required to complete a parasite's life cycle in addition to the definitive host. The intermediate host usually harbors an asexual or larval form of the parasite. For example, *Plasmodium*, which causes malaria, lives in both humans and mosquitoes. In humans, *Plasmodium*'s intermediate host, the parasite reproduces asexually. Sexual reproduction of *Plasmodium* occurs in the mosquito, the definitive host.

A **reservoir host** is an organism other than the main host that can harbor a parasite and serve as a source of infection.

A **vector** is a living carrier that transmits the parasite to an uninfected host. A *biologic vector* is a host essential to the life cycle, for example the mosquito is a biologic vector for *Plasmodium*. *Mechanical vectors* transmit the parasite mechanically. For example, flies that land on infected feces and then land on food may carry infective parasite stages from one site to another.

## Geographical Distribution of Parasites

Parasites are only found where the appropriate hosts are available to allow the organism's life cycle to develop. Environmental factors, such as humidity and temperature, are important to the survival of most parasites, especially those that require arthropod vectors. Temperature extremes and dry conditions may be detrimental to parasitic forms. Therefore, the majority of parasites are found in temperate to tropical climates. Some parasites also depend on arthropod vectors or animal reservoirs to perpetuate their life cycle.

## Life Cycles of Parasites

A parasitic life cycle is the complete process of a parasite infecting (or infesting) a host, growing, developing, reproducing, and being transmitted to a new host. Parasite life cycles may be simple or complex. Some parasites spend their whole life in one host. Others require different types of hosts during different parts of their life cycles. Still others may only be parasitic for a portion of their life and free-living at other times. Knowledge of the specific life-cycle requirements of each type of parasite is valuable in preventing parasitic infections and in determining the appropriate specimen to examine when parasitic infection is suspected.

The "infective stage" of the parasite is the stage of the life cycle during which the parasite is capable of infecting a host. The "diagnostic stage" is the life cycle stage that can be detected in a specimen and helps in diagnosis. Knowledge of the diagnostic stage is required to select the proper diagnostic method.

Sometimes the diagnostic and infective stages are the same, particularly for intestinal parasites. For example, in the life-cycle diagram of *Giardia* shown in Fugure 8-1, the cyst is the infective stage, as well as a diagnostic stage.

Parasites that live on external body surfaces, such as lice, cause infestations. Parasites that live within the host cause infections. Parasites may infect (or infest) external body surfaces, external body cavities, the intestinal tract, blood, and organs such as the liver, bone marrow, and other tissues. Many parasites have specific tissue requirements and will migrate through the body to a specific organ.

## Diagnosing Parasitic Infections

Most parasitic diseases have generalized symptoms such as fever, pain, chills, diarrhea, or fatigue and loss of vitality, symptoms that could be caused by a variety of conditions or diseases. Therefore, a definitive diagnosis usually depends on finding and identifying the parasite's diagnostic stage.

Specimens that may be examined for evidence of parasites include feces, urine, sputum, aspirations, and blood and other tissues. For some parasites, immunological tests are available. Patient history is also very important in diagnosing parasitic infections, particularly if the patient has any history of travel to **endemic** areas, areas where the organism occurs naturally.

### Transmitting Parasitic Infections

There are only a few ways to transmit parasitic infections. Most parasitic infections are acquired through ingestion of an infective form in food or water, insect bites, or contact with an infected person. A few organisms can be acquired through **congenital** infection and some organisms, such as hookworm, can penetrate intact skin. Table 8-1 lists some parasitic diseases, their usual routes of transmission, and their infective stages.

### Infection Sites

The site infected by a parasite is determined by how the parasite enters the body, the parasite's tissue specificity, and the host's immunity.

## How Parasites Cause Disease

Parasitic disease occurs when the damage caused by the parasite to the host becomes severe enough to cause pathologic changes in the host. Parasitic infec-

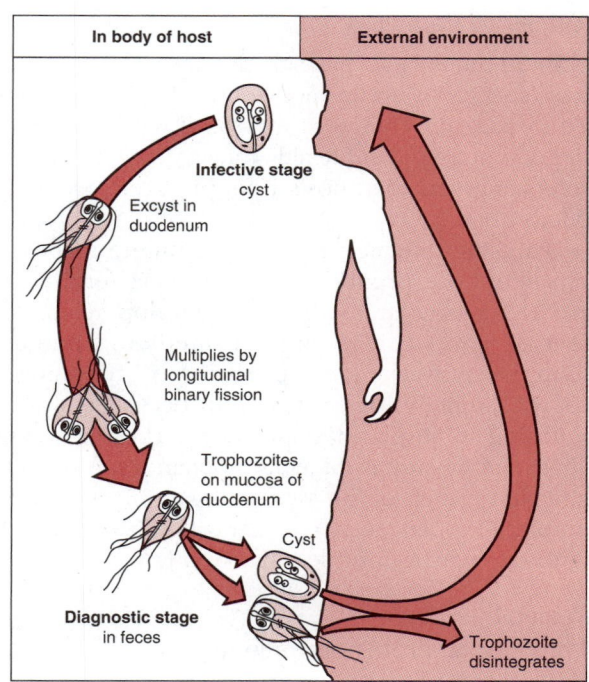

**FIGURE 8-1** Diagram of life cycle for *Giardia lamblia*

**Table 8-1.** Examples of parasitic diseases, their transmission routes, and their infective stages

| DISEASE | CAUSATIVE ORGANISM | TRANSMISSION ROUTE | INFECTIVE STAGE |
|---|---|---|---|
| Amebiasis | *Entamoeba histolytica* | Ingestion | Cyst |
| Giardiasis | *Giardia lamblia* | Ingestion | Cyst |
| Malaria | *Plasmodium* | Mosquito bite | Sporozoite |
| Toxoplasmosis | *Toxoplasma gondii* | Ingestion or congenital | Oocysts or zoite |
| Trichomoniasis | *Trichomonas vaginalis* | Sexual contact | Trophozoite |
| Babesiosis | *Babesia bigemina* | Tick bite | Sporozoite |
| Cryptosporidiosis | *Cryptosporidium* | Ingestion | Oocyst |
| Trichinosis | *Trichinella spiralis* | Ingestion | Larva |
| Enterobiasis | *Enterobius vermicularis* | Ingestion | Ova |
| Hookworm | *Necator, Ancylostoma* | Skin penetration | Larva |
| Ascariasis | *Ascaris lumbricoides* | Ingestion | Ova |

tions can result in no symptoms, mild or moderate symptoms, or even death.

Many factors determine the effect a parasite will have on the host, including the parasite's number, size, location, and toxicity, as well as the host's condition. Damage may be mechanical, such as obstructing an organ or vessel; irritative; toxic, due to substances produced or released by the parasite; or an allergic reaction. Some infections are self-limiting. Common problems seen with parasitic infections include anemia, jaundice, secondary bacterial infections, organ dysfunction, and interference with normal physiological processes.

## Immunity to Parasites

Absolute immunity to parasites is rare unless the individual (species) is an unsuitable host. In general, resistance to parasitic infection increases with age. Hosts with good nutrition and health are less likely to develop severe symptoms than hosts from impoverished socioeconomic conditions.

Parasitic infection produces immune responses much like those produced in viral or bacterial infections. This means antibodies may develop against the infecting parasite and the cell-mediated immune response may be stimulated. Because of the immune response, immunological tests can be used to aid in diagnosing some parasitic infections. These are especially useful when it is difficult to obtain a specimen for examination, such as in tissue or organ infections. For example, toxoplasmosis is a parasitic disease usually diagnosed by measuring serum antibody.

## Parasitic Infections
## in Immunocompromised Patients

A large part of the recent increase in reported parasitic infections is due to parasitic diseases occurring in immunocompromised patients, such as AIDS, organ transplants, or chemotherapy or radiation patients. Infections with organisms such as *Toxoplasma* and *Cryptosporidium* can be life-threatening to these patients, and must be treated with vigorous drug therapy. Immunodiagnosis in these patients may be difficult because antibody levels may be below detection limits.

## Treating Parasitic Infections

Several drugs are effective against parasites, but most have some level of toxicity. The degree of treatment success depends on the infecting parasite, the extent of infection, the host's health, and the infection site. Surgery may be required in some cases.

## PREVENTING PARASITIC INFECTIONS

The key to preventing parasitic infections is to understand the transmission methods and the location of the parasite's infective stages. Parasite-control methods include:

- blocking transmission of the infective form
- providing health education
- improving sanitation
- identifying and treating infected individuals to prevent the spread of infection

## Blocking Transmission of the Infective Form

One of the most important ways of preventing parasite infections is to block transmission of the parasite's infective stage by breaking a link in the organism's life cycle. For this reason, it is important to understand the life history of the parasite, where it is found, what host is required for its reproduction, and how transmission occurs. When the infective stage of the parasite is known, it is possible to plan effective control and prevention methods. For example, in the 1800s in North America, malaria was found as far north as southern Canada. When it was discovered that the malarial parasite was transmitted to man through the bite of infected mosquitoes, mosquito control measures were implemented in the United States. This rapidly and drastically reduced the malaria infection rate, so that by the 1950s, the U.S. was no longer considered endemic for malaria.

## Health Education and Improved Sanitation

Health education about proper personal hygiene and food handling has contributed to a drop in parasitic diseases. Improved sanitation techniques and standards (water quality, sewage treatment, and waste disposal) reduce the incidence of infection with waterborne parasites.

## Recent Outbreaks of Parasitic Infections

It only takes a small lapse for parasitic infections to emerge. Natural disasters, such as the 1993 flooding seen in the midwestern U.S., increase the risk of water being contaminated with untreated sewage, resulting in increased parasitic infections. A 1993 water treatment plant failure in Milwaukee, WI, caused more than 400,000 people to become ill due to *Cryptosporidium*, an intestinal parasite. *Cryptosporidium* causes diarrhea of one to two weeks' duration in healthy immunocompetent individuals, but can cause life-threatening illness in immunocompromised individuals. Several fatalities occurred as a result of the Milwaukee cryptosporidiosis outbreak.

Since 1995, several foodborne outbreaks of cyclosporiasis have been reported in the U.S. and Canada. Cyclosporiasis is caused by infection with *Cyclospora*, a coccidian parasite causing symptoms similar to those caused by *Cryptosporidium*. Most of the outbreaks were traced to ingesting contaminated produce, primarily raspberries. Although the food contamination's source has still not been agreed on, improved sanitation techniques in food harvesting and processing likely could have prevented most of these outbreaks.

## ORGANISMS PARASITIC FOR HUMANS

The parasites that infect humans can be grouped into three large groups: **protozoa**, **helminths**, and **arthropods** (Figure 8-2).

## Protozoa

Protozoa are single-celled eukaryotic organisms that are larger than most bacteria. Parasitic protozoa include amoebae, flagellates, ciliates, and apicomplexans (formerly sporozoa) (Table 8-2). All four of these groups contain organisms parasitic to man and animals. Protozoa can infect most body sites, including blood, tissues, the intestinal and genitourinary tracts, and the oral cavity.

## Helminths

Helminth is the common name used for parasitic worms. These include flatworms, such as flukes and tapeworms, and roundworms, such as whipworms and hookworms (Table 8-3). Most helminth infections occur in the intestinal tract. However, other tissues are sometimes infected by certain helminths.

## Arthropods

Arthropods include arachnids, such as spiders, ticks, and mites, and insects, such as lice, bugs, fleas, flies, and mosquitoes. Some arthropods, such as lice, fleas, and mosquitos, are parasitic to humans, while others, such as flies, are important in transmitting the infective stage of parasites to humans (Table 8-4).

## IDENTIFYING PARASITES IN THE LABORATORY

A useful parasite classification for the medical laboratory is based on the organ system in which the parasites are found. The ectoparasites are usually easily seen and identified. However, endoparasites present more of a problem and require special specimen preparation. Two broad categories of endoparasites are:

- intestinal and atrial parasites
- blood and tissue parasites.

## Intestinal and Atrial Parasites

Of the several types of organisms that can infect the intestinal tract (Table 8-5), some are pathogenic, whereas others are **commensal**, that is, not harmful.

Intestinal parasites are usually identified by the morphology seen during microscopic examination of fecal specimens. Atlases of parasite morphology are indispensable in the parasitology laboratory.

### Atrial Protozoa

Atrial parasites infect body cavities. *Entamoeba gingivalis* is an amoeba that may be present in the mouth,

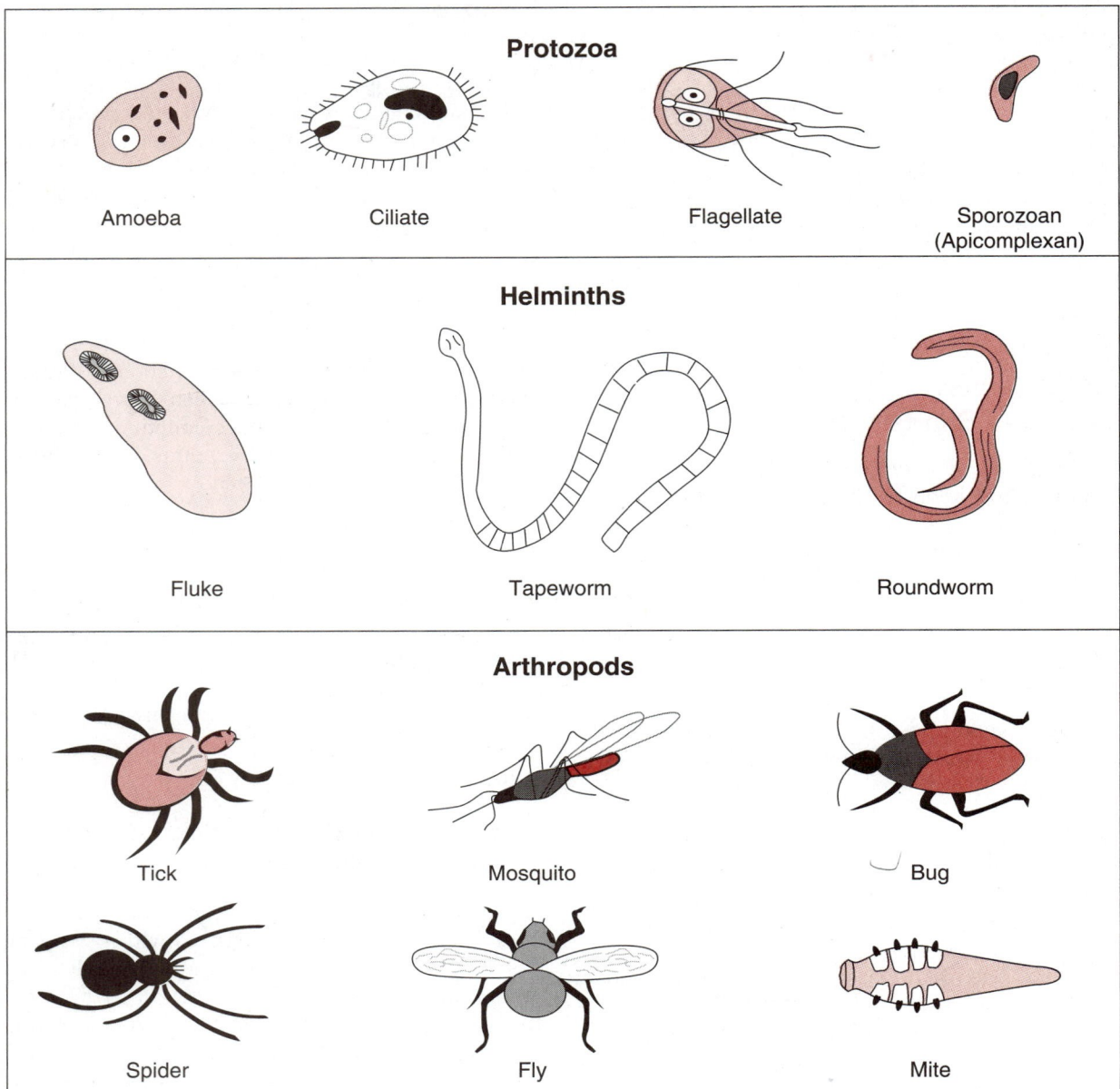

**FIGURE 8-2** Three groups of parasites: protozoa, helminths, and arthropods

**Table 8-2.** Medically important protozoa

| PROTOZOAN GROUP | EXAMPLES |
|---|---|
| Amoebae | *Entamoeba, Naegleria* |
| Flagellates | *Trichomonas, Giardia* |
| Ciliates | *Balantidium* |
| Apicomplexans | *Plasmodium, Toxoplasma, Cryptosporidium* |

**Table 8-3.** Medically important helminths

| HELMINTH GROUP | EXAMPLES |
|---|---|
| Trematodes (flukes) | Liver fluke, lung fluke |
| Cestodes (tapeworms) | Beef tapeworm, pork tapeworm |
| Nematodes (roundworms) | Pinworm, hookworm, whipworm, filarial worms |

**Table 8-4.** Medically important arthropods

| ARTHROPOD GROUP | EXAMPLES |
| --- | --- |
| Arachnids | Spiders, ticks, mites |
| Insects | Lice, bugs, fleas, flies, mosquitoes |

**Table 8-5.** Examples of intestinal parasites

| PROTOZOA | |
| --- | --- |
| Amoebae | Entamoeba |
| Ciliates | Balantidium |
| Flagellates | Giardia |
| Apicomplexans | Cryptosporidium, Isospora Cyclospora |
| **HELMINTHS** | |
| Trematodes | Fasciolopsis |
| Cestodes | Taenia, Dipylidium |
| Nematodes | Enterobius, Ascaris |

but is usually considered commensal. *Trichomonas vaginalis* is a flagellate that may occur in the urogenital tract.

## Intestinal Protozoa

Intestinal protozoa that may be pathogenic include *Entamoeba histolytica, Giardia lamblia, Cyclospora, Isospora belli*, and *Cryptosporidium. Giardia* is the most common intestinal protozoan pathogen in the United States and is a frequent cause of diarrhea in children in day care centers. It is estimated that over 7% of the U.S. population is infected with *Giardia*. Nonpathogenic protozoa common to the intestinal tract include other *Entamoeba* sp., *Endolimax, Chilomastix,* and *Iodamoeba*.

## Intestinal Helminths

The three groups of helminths that can infect the human intestinal tract are **nematode**s (roundworms), **tremat̄odes**, (flukes), and **cestode**s (tapeworms) (Table 8-5). The most common helminths are nematodes. These include *Enterobius vermicularis* (pinworm), *Trichuris trichiura* (whipworm), *Ascaris lumbricoides* (roundworm), and hookworms (*Necator* and *Ancylostoma*). Trematodes found in the intestinal tract include *Fasciolopsis, Fasciola, Heterophyes, Metagonimus,* and *Clonorchis*. The most common tapeworm infection in the U.S. is caused by the dwarf tapeworm, *Hymenolepis nana*. Other tapeworms that may infect humans include the beef tapeworm (*Taenia saginata*), the pork tapeworm (*Taenia solium*), the fish tapeworm (*Diphyllobothrium latum*), and the dog tapeworm (*Dipylidium caninum*).

## Laboratory Detection of Intestinal and Atrial Parasites

Intestinal protozoa are identified by the morphology of cysts, trophozoites, or oocysts in fecal specimens. Because protozoa are so small, identification of genus and species may be difficult. However, it is very important to distinguish pathogens from commensals.

Roundworm infections are diagnosed by identifying **ova** (eggs), larvae, or adults in fecal or perianal specimens. Trematode infections may also be diag-

nosed by identifying eggs in fecal specimens. *Paragonimus* and *Schistosoma* worms inhabit the lungs and blood vessels, respectively, but their eggs are often found in feces or urine (*Schistosoma*). Tapeworms are identified by finding ova or **proglottides** (tapeworm segments) in feces.

Immunological tests are being developed to detect a few intestinal protozoa. These tests are coming into wider use because they have some advantages over traditional microscopic methods of identifying parasites. The technician does not need to have morphological expertise to interpret the results of immunoassays with color endpoint reactions. The assays often have high sensitivity, that is, they can detect low levels of antigen, levels that might require microscopic examination of several specimens before the parasite could be detected.

Antigen capture immunoassays (modified enzyme immunoassays) are available for detecting some parasite antigens in fecal specimens. An example is the Triage® Parasite Panel by Biosite® Diagnostics. *Entamoeba histolytica, Giardia,* and *Cryptosporidium* antigens can be detected in fifteen minutes using a single self-contained test cassette that also includes controls for the three organisms.

Other immunological tests available include kits that detect serum antibody to *E. histolytica* and fluorescent antibody kits to detect *Giardia* and *Cryptosporidium* in fecal specimens as well as in water supplies.

## Blood and Tissue Parasites

Worldwide, the blood and tissue parasites are a diverse group (Table 8-6). However, in the United States only a few organisms infect the blood and tissue.

**Table 8-6.** Examples of blood and tissue parasites

| PARASITES FOUND IN BLOOD | PARASITES FOUND IN TISSUE |
|---|---|
| Plasmodium | Toxoplasma |
| Babesia | Trichinella |
| Trypanosoma | Leishmania |
| Filarial worms | Trypanosoma |
| | Amoebae |
| | Schistosoma |
| | Filarial worms |

## Blood Parasites

The most common blood parasite is the malarial parasite (*Plasmodium* sp.). Other blood parasites include the trypanosomes, *Babesia*, and the filarial worms.

## Tissue Parasites

Tissue parasites include *Toxoplasma*, parasitic and free-living amoebae (*Naegleria* and *Acanthamoeba*), *Leishmania, Schistosoma,* some filarial worms, microsporidia, trypanosomes, and *Trichinella*.

## Laboratory Detection of Blood and Tissue Parasites

The specimen required for detecting blood and tissue parasites is determined by the location or site of infection and the organism suspected. Blood parasites are identified by microscopic examination of stained blood smears, described in Lesson 8-4.

Tissue parasites may be identified by microscopic examination of stained biopsy material, aspirates, sputum, skin snips, or by immunological tests, such as serum antibody tests for *Toxoplasma*.

*Pneumocystis carinii* is an opportunistic pathogen found in the lungs. It causes pneumonia in immunocompromised individuals and has been responsible for many AIDS deaths. In the past, *Pneumocystis* has been grouped with protozoa because it can be identified with stains typically used for protozoan parasites. Although recent research provides evidence that *Pneumocystis* should be grouped with the fungi, most parasitology laboratories continue to provide diagnostic testing for *Pneumocystis*.

## SUMMARY

Organisms capable of parasitizing humans are quite diverse. In the United States, parasites are not frequently observed in clinical specimens. Because of this, most laboratory personnel do not have much experience in parasite identification. Specimens for parasite examination are often sent to reference or state public health laboratories, where more expert staff can perform the examinations.

Medical laboratory personnel should be familiar with characteristics of common parasitic infections so the appropriate specimens are collected and correctly processed for examination. This greatly increases the chances of discovering parasites in the laboratory examination. Lesson 8-2 gives the procedures for processing specimens to examine for parasites.

## LESSON REVIEW

1. How are parasitic infections usually diagnosed?
2. What are the three major groups of organisms that contain human parasites?
3. How does geography or climate affect the incidence of parasites?
4. What body sites can be infected by parasites?
5. Name three factors that affect the severity of parasitic infections.
6. Name three ways parasitic diseases can be transmitted.
7. Name four methods used to prevent or control parasite infections.
8. Name four groups of protozoan parasites.
9. Name three groups of parasitic helminths.
10. How are intestinal parasitic infections usually diagnosed?
11. How are infections with blood or tissue parasites usually diagnosed?
12. Define arthropod, cestode, commensal, congenital, definitive host, ectoparasite, endemic, helminth, host, immunocompromised, intermediate host, nematode, opportunistic parasite, ova, parasite, pathogenic, protozoa, reservoir host, trematode, and vector.

## STUDENT ACTIVITIES

1. Reread the introduction to parasitology.
2. Review the glossary terms.
3. Research a parasitic disease. Report on the life cycle, transmission, symptoms, diagnostic methods, and treatment course.

# Collecting and Processing Specimens for Parasite Examination

## LESSON OBJECTIVES

**After studying this lesson, you should be able to:**

- *Explain the procedure for collecting fecal specimens for parasite examination.*
- *Name two preservatives commonly used for fecal specimens.*
- *Describe safety precautions to observe when handling fecal specimens.*
- *Describe the proper transport procedure for fecal specimens.*
- *Demonstrate preparing and using a cellophane tape swab for perianal specimens.*
- *Name two nonfecal specimens that may be examined for parasites.*
- *Define the glossary terms.*

## GLOSSARY

**cyst** / nonmotile, nonfeeding stage of a protozoan parasite; usually an infective stage

**PVA** / polyvinyl alcohol, a preservative used for fecal specimens

**trophozoite** / motile, feeding stage of protozoan parasites

## INTRODUCTION

The two most common parasitology laboratory requests are for blood examination for malarial parasites and fecal examination for ova and parasites (O & P). The O & P test requires a fecal specimen, and the malarial smear requires a fresh blood specimen.

Although small laboratories do not usually perform the actual microscopic examination for parasites, laboratory personnel must provide instructions for specimen collection, and must process the specimen before it is sent to a reference laboratory. A basic understanding of parasite life cycles is required to be sure the most appropriate specimen is obtained, thus increasing the chances of finding and identifying any parasites present.

This lesson describes routine specimen collection and processing to detect intestinal parasites. Lesson 8-3 describes the procedures for preparing fecal wet mounts and smears for staining, as well as fecal-concen-tration techniques. The procedure for preparing and staining blood smears for detection of blood parasites is described in Lesson 8-4.

## TYPES OF SPECIMENS FOR PARASITE EXAMINATION

### Fecal (Stool) Specimens

The fecal specimen is the specimen most commonly examined when infection with intestinal parasites is suspected. Helminths, amoebae, and other intestinal protozoa can be identified during microscopic examination performed on unstained, stained, and concentrated fecal specimens. Fecal specimens are also used for immunological tests that detect *Giardia*, *Cryptosporidium*, and *Entamoeba histolytica* antigens in the specimens.

## Blood Specimens

Blood is the specimen examined when infection with blood parasites such as the malarial parasite, filiarial worms, or certain trypanosomes is suspected. Specially prepared and stained blood smears or wet mounts of blood are examined. Collecting blood specimens at timed intervals may be required, as when testing for malaria.

## Specimens for Serological or Immunological Tests

Although immunological tests are being developed for many parasites, only a few have widespread use. Tests available for *Toxoplasma, Giardia,* and *Entamoeba histolytica* have fairly reliable results. Tests may be designed to detect parasite antigen in fecal specimens, as for *Giardia* (see "Fecal Specimens" above), or to detect anti-parasite antibody in serum, as for *Toxoplasma*. In the case of suspected acute infections, such as toxoplasmosis, paired serum samples (samples collected two to three weeks apart) are tested for the presence of IgM and IgG, or for a rising antibody titer.

## Other Specimens

Specimens other than blood or stool can be tested or examined for parasites. The type of specimen required depends on what organism(s) is suspected, based on the patient's symptoms and medical history. For example, sputum specimens may be examined for *Pneumocystis* or *Paragonimus*. Vaginal secretions may be examined for *Trichomonas*. Tissue specimens, usually processed and stained by the histology laboratory, may be examined when *Trichinella, Pneumocystis, Toxoplasma,* or other tissue parasites are suspected. Examples of organisms that may be found in non-fecal specimens are listed in Table 8-7.

## COLLECTING AND PROCESSING FECAL SPECIMENS

 ### Safety

Several risks are present when collecting and processing specimens for parasite examination. These risks include exposure to infective parasite cysts, oocysts, eggs, or larvae in stool specimens and to non-parasitic pathogens that may be present in stool and biological fluids. Workers must use Universal and Standard Precautions, as well as standard microbiology safety practices. Precautions must be observed even with pre-

**Table 8-7.** Examples of organisms found in nonfecal specimens

| TYPE OF SPECIMEN | POSSIBLE ORGANISMS |
| --- | --- |
| Sputum | *Paragonimus, Ascaris* |
| Blood | *Plasmodium, Babesia, Trypanosoma* |
| CSF | Amoebae, *Toxoplasma, Trypanosoma* |
| Liver | Amoebae, *Leishmania, Schistosoma* |
| Urine | *Trichomonas, Schistosoma* |
| Muscle | *Trichinella* |
| Bronchial washes | *Pneumocystis** |
| Duodenal aspirates | *Giardia, Isospora* |
| Vaginal secretions | *Trichomonas* |

\* recently grouped with fungi

served (fixed) specimens, since some parasite forms remain viable for weeks even after formalin fixation.

Good safety practices include, but are not limited to, wearing fluid-resistant protective clothing and gloves, using biological safety cabinets, decontaminating work surfaces frequently, washing hands before donning gloves and after removing gloves, and disposing of all sharp objects in a sharps container for biohazards.

Specimens may be processed in a fume hood to avoid inhaling preservative fumes and minimize unpleasant odors. All specimens and processing materials should be disposed of in the same manner as bacterial or biohazardous specimens.

### Quality Assurance

Specimens must be collected and processed according to established procedure. Specimen collection timing is critical for some tests, such as blood smears for malaria and the scotch tape test for pinworm. Specimens must be collected from a patient before anti-parasite drugs are administered and should not be collected within seven days after administration of antacids, mineral oil, barium, bismuth, or certain antidiarrheal medications, or within three weeks after certain antimicrobial agents and dyes.

To maintain the morphology of some parasites, specimens must be processed as quickly as possible after collection. If looking for motile forms in unfixed stool specimens, microscopic examination must be performed within thirty minutes to one hour of collection.

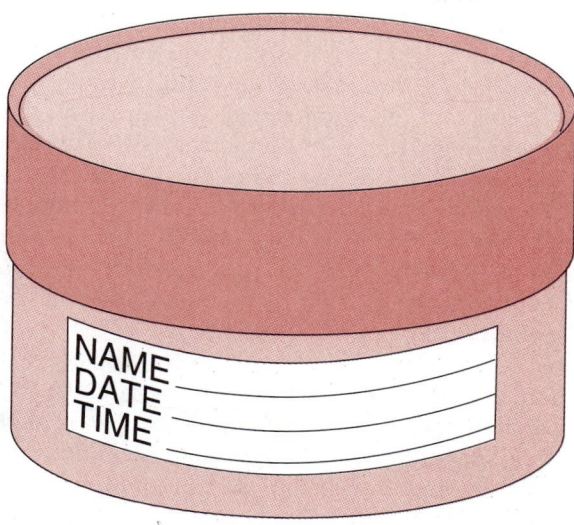

FIGURE 8-3 Container for collecting fecal specimens

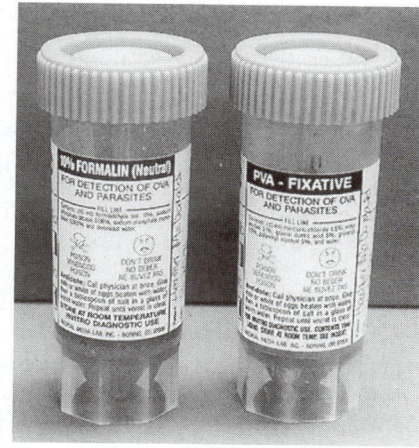

FIGURE 8-4 Fixative vials for preserving fecal specimens

## FECAL SPECIMEN COLLECTION

Fecal samples should be collected in a clean, dry, wide-mouth, leakproof container that has a tight-fitting lid (Figure 8-3). Specimens may be collected in a bedpan and transferred to the container, but the sample *must not* be contaminated with urine or water. Patients should wait one week after ingesting antidiarrheal medication, radiopaque compounds (barium), or oily laxatives before collecting fecal specimens for parasite examination.

The specimen container must be labeled with the patient's name and the date and time of collection. It is recommended that at least three separate specimens be collected over a period of three to five days. Specimens should be delivered to the laboratory as soon as possible (within two hours of collection). If specimen transport must be delayed, kits containing vials with preservatives and containers for mailing are available (Figures 8-4 and 8-5).

## FECAL SPECIMEN PROCESSING

Specimens should be processed and examined as soon as possible after arrival at the laboratory. It is especially important to process watery specimens quickly (within thirty minutes to one hour), because parasites such as protozoan **trophozoites** will deteriorate rapidly.

Fecal specimens should be visually examined, microscopically examined, and concentrated for additional microscopic examination (see also Lesson 8-3). Portions of the specimen should be preserved for further examination and for staining.

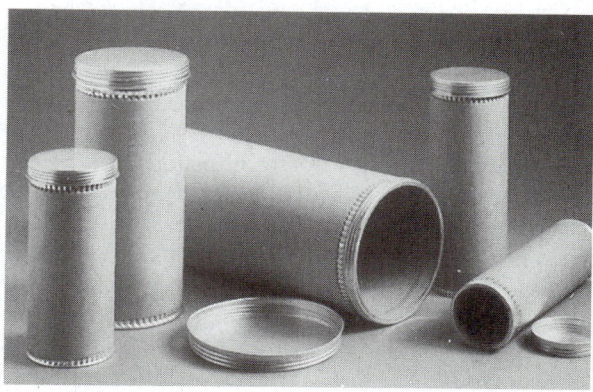

FIGURE 8-5 Containers for transporting or mailing biological specimens (Photo courtesy of Fisher Scientific)

### Visual Examination of Fecal Specimens

The specimen should be visually examined. The consistency of the specimen should be recorded (watery, loose, soft, or formed). Adult worms or tapeworm proglottids may sometimes be seen. Portions of blood or mucus, if present in the fecal sample, should be selected for examination. In protozoan parasitic infections, trophozoite forms are more likely to be found in the more fluid specimens and cyst forms in the more formed specimens.

### Preservation of Fecal Specimens

Portions of the specimen should be preserved for future examination and for staining. Most laboratories use a two-vial technique (Figure 8-4). A portion of the specimen is placed in a vial of 10% formalin to preserve eggs, **cysts**, and larvae. Formalinized specimens can be used for wet mounts, immunoassays, stains, and concentration techniques.

Another portion of the specimen is placed in a fixative such as polyvinyl alcohol (**PVA**), which preserves cysts and trophozoites and permits the specimen to be stained. Other preservatives sometimes used in place of PVA are sodium acetate-acetic acid-formalin (SAF) and merthiolate-iodine formalin (MIF).

### Specimen Transport

Fecal specimens to be mailed or otherwise transported should be placed in fixative vials and appropriately labeled. The vials should be enclosed in leakproof containers or bags and placed in labeled mailing/transport cartons (Figure 8-5). Specimens to be mailed must be in containers approved for biological materials by the United States Postal Service.

## PROCEDURE: CELLOPHANE TAPE TEST FOR PINWORMS

### Enterobiasis

The most common roundworm infection in the United States is enterobiasis, infection with the human pinworm or seatworm, *Enterobius vermicularis*. This organism is frequently found in young children in day care centers and elementary schools. It is estimated that, in the United States, approximately 40 million people are infected at any one time.

Pinworm infections are acquired by ingesting the pinworm ova. The ova hatch in the small intestine, releasing larvae that mature into adult worms within about thirty days. The adult female pinworm lives in the colon and migrates out of the anus to deposit eggs in the perianal region during the night. This leads to the characteristic symptom, anal itching, and contributes to reinfection when children scratch and their hands become contaminated with eggs. Pinworm infections are easily spread when eggs become airborne from contaminated clothing and bedding.

A simple diagnostic technique for pinworms is to prepare a cellophane tape swab or perianal swab for the parent to take home (Figure 8-6). The parent should collect a specimen from the perianal region between 9 p.m. and midnight or in the early morning before the child has bathed. It may be necessary to collect several specimens over a period of days, because the female worm does not migrate every night.

### Preparing Cellophane Tape Swab

To prepare the swab, a piece of clear cellophane tape four to five inches long is attached to the underside of a microscope slide, wrapped around the end of the slide, and smoothed into place on the top of the slide. For labeling and easy lifting, a paper tab is attached to the tape's free end (Figure 8-6). Unused slides may be stored in a cool place for weeks. Commercially prepared swabs are also available.

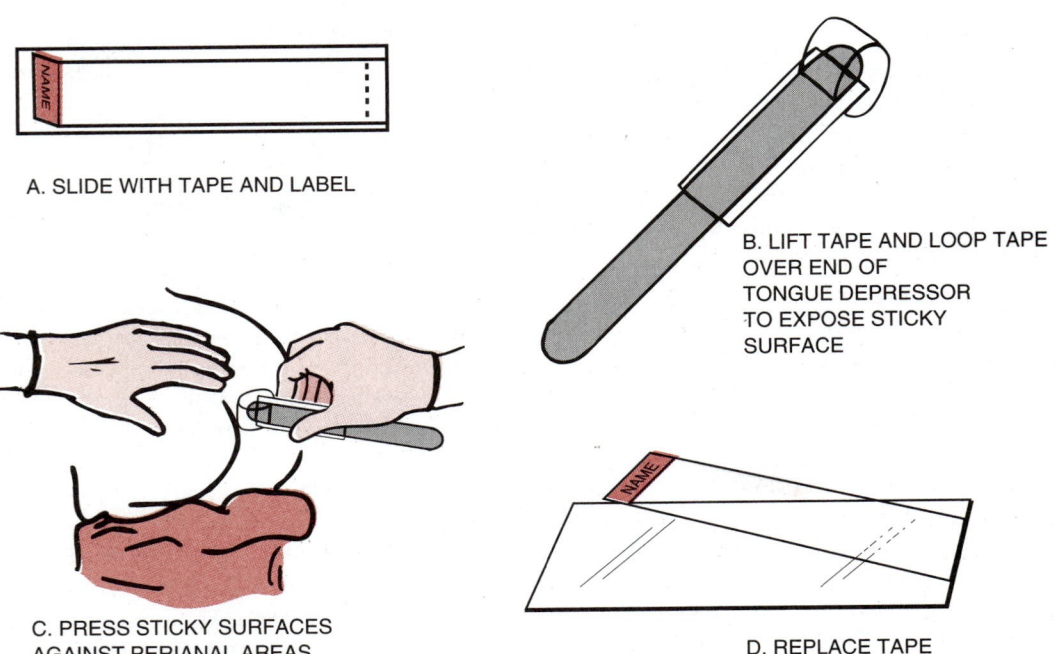

A. SLIDE WITH TAPE AND LABEL

B. LIFT TAPE AND LOOP TAPE OVER END OF TONGUE DEPRESSOR TO EXPOSE STICKY SURFACE

C. PRESS STICKY SURFACES AGAINST PERIANAL AREAS

D. REPLACE TAPE

**FIGURE 8-6** Technique for preparing and using a cellophane tape swab

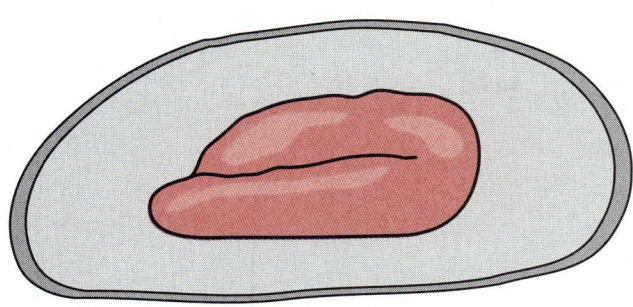

**FIGURE 8-7** Microscopic appearance of *Enterobius* ovum (approximately 55 μm x 25 μm)

## Collecting the Specimen with a Cellophane Tape Swab

To collect the specimen, the slide is placed on a tongue depressor, and the tape is lifted and looped over the end of the depressor, sticky side out (Figure 8-6B). The sticky center surface of the tape is pressed against several areas of the perianal region while spreading the buttocks apart. The tape is then smoothed back onto the slide, sticky side down, and the slide is delivered to the laboratory for examination.

## Microscopic Examination of Cellophane Tape Swab

The slide is examined for eggs using the low-power (10X) objective (Figure 8-7). A drop of toluene or xylene can be placed under the tape to clear the glue and allow for easier egg identification. Since these eggs remain viable (infective) for weeks, the specimen should be handled with care. *Enterobius* eggs have a characteristic appearance (Figure 8-7). They are approximately 55 μm x 25 μm, colorless, and flattened on one side. The eggs have a thick-walled shell, and contain a developing larva.

### Procedural Notes

■ Collect specimens according to established procedures.

■ Collect specimens at proper time intervals.

■ Process specimens within two hours of collection.

### Safety Precautions

■ Observe Standard and Universal Precautions when handling specimens.

■ Avoid contacting skin with preservatives and inhaling fumes.

■ Handle preserved specimens as if infectious.

■ Wear appropriate PPE when handling specimens.

## SUMMARY

Examining blood, stool, tissues, and other biological specimens helps diagnose parasitic infections. Established procedures for proper specimen collection and processing must be carefully followed to ensure the specimen is suitable for testing. Success in detecting parasites depends on having a proper specimen to examine.

## LESSON REVIEW

1. Explain the proper method for collecting fecal specimens.
2. Which type of fecal specimen must be processed quickly? Why?
3. What terms are used to describe the consistency of fecal specimens?
4. Name two preservatives used for fecal specimens.
5. What safety precautions must be observed when handling and processing fecal specimens? Why?
6. What parasite is best detected using a cellophane tape swab (perianal swab)?
7. Explain how to prepare a cellophane tape swab. How is the specimen collected?
8. What specimens other than feces are examined for parasites? Blood, Urine
9. Name three parasites found in nonfecal specimens. ring worm
10. Define cyst, PVA, and trophozoite.

## STUDENT ACTIVITIES

1. Reread the information on collecting and processing specimens for parasite examination.
2. Review the glossary terms.
3. Practice instructing a patient in properly collecting a fecal specimen for parasite examination as outlined on the Student Performance Guide.
4. Practice preparing a perianal swab (cellophane tape swab) as outlined on the Student Performance Guide.
5. Practice processing fecal specimens for parasite examination as outlined in the Student Performance Guide.

# *Student Performance Guide*

## LESSON 8-2 Collecting and Processing Specimens for Parasite Examination

Name _____ Date _____

### INSTRUCTIONS

1. Practice the procedures for collecting and processing specimens for parasite examination, following the step-by-step procedure.
2. Demonstrate your understanding of this lesson by:
   a. Completing a written examination successfully, and
   b. Performing the procedures for collecting and processing specimens for parasite examination satisfactorily for the instructor. All steps must be completed as listed on the instructor's Performance Check Sheet.

### MATERIALS AND EQUIPMENT

- gloves
- hand disinfectant
- 10% chlorine bleach solution
- wooden tongue depressors
- wooden applicator sticks
- microscope slides
- clear cellophane tape
- xylene or toluene
- microscope
- biohazard disposal container
- sharps disposal container
- leakproof vials for transporting specimens
- 10% formalin
- PVA (or other appropriate) fixative
- fecal specimens (students may bring pet specimens for practice)
- fecal specimen containers
- atlas of parasitic morphology containing illustrations of *Enterobius* ova (optional)

### PROCEDURE

Record in the comment section any problems encountered while practicing the procedure (or have a fellow student or the instructor evaluate your performance).

S = Satisfactory
U = Unsatisfactory

| You must: | S | U | Comments |
|---|---|---|---|
| 1. Instruct a patient in the proper procedure for collecting a fecal specimen (steps 1a–c): <br> a. Give patient a fecal specimen container with lid and label <br> b. Explain the fecal collection procedure to the patient, emphasizing the following precautions: <br>   (1) Specimen must not be contaminated with urine or water <br>   (2) Outer surface of specimen container must not be contaminated <br>   (3) Container must be labeled with the patient's name, date, and time of specimen collection | | | |

| You must: | S | U | Comments |
|---|---|---|---|
| (4) Unpreserved specimens must be transported to a laboratory immediately following collection (within two hours)<br>(5) Specimens should not be collected until at least a week after ingesting interfering substances such as oily laxatives, barium or radiopaque contrast media, or antidiarrheal medications<br>c. If immediate transport to a laboratory is not possible, instruct the patient in the proper way to preserve the specimen, following the instructions in step 2. | | | |
| 2. Prepare a fecal specimen for transport (steps 2a–i)<br>  a. Wash your hands and put on gloves<br>  b. Obtain a fecal specimen, fixative vials, and transport containers. Check label to be sure required patient information is present (name, date, time of collection)<br>  c. Open container and observe consistency of specimen. Record as watery, loose, soft, or formed<br>  d. Obtain a vial of 10% formalin and one of PVA fixative<br>  e. Use disposable applicators to obtain a portion of specimen approximately one-third the volume of the fixative<br>  f. Place specimen in vial and mix thoroughly using applicator. Discard applicator(s) into biohazard container. Label vial with patient information<br>  g. Repeat procedure (steps 2e–f) with the second vial of fixative, using clean applicators<br>  h. Disinfect work area with surface disinfectant<br>  i. Remove and discard gloves in biohazard container and wash your hands with hand disinfectant | | | |
| 3. Prepare a cellophane tape perianal swab (steps 3a–e)<br>  a. Obtain tape, clean microscope slide, and paper tab<br>  b. Attach a four-to-five-inch section of tape to one end of the microscope slide's back<br>  c. Fold the tape around the end of the slide and smooth down over the slide top, so the tape adheres to the slide, leaving a small portion free at the end<br>  d. Attach a small paper tab to the free end of the tape to use as a label and lifting tab<br>  e. Store the prepared slide in a cool, dust-free location | | | |
| 4. Demonstrate the use of the cellophane tape swab (steps 4a–k)<br>  a. Wash your hands and put on gloves<br>  b. Obtain a clean wooden tongue depressor<br>  c. Obtain previously prepared cellophane tape slide (step 3) and label the tab<br>  d. Place the cellophane tape swab near one end of the depressor, tape side up<br>  e. Lift the cellophane tape and form a loop around the end of the tongue depressor, sticky side of tape to the outside<br>  f. Explain how to obtain the pinworm specimen by touching sticky surface of the tape to perianal region | | | |

| You must: | S | U | Comments |
|---|---|---|---|
|    g. Remove the tape from the tongue depressor and smooth back into place on the microscope slide, being careful not to touch the sticky surface | | | |
|    h. Discard the tongue depressor in biohazard container (if actually used for specimen collection) | | | |
|    i. Place the slide on a microscope stage and demonstrate how to observe for eggs using the low-power (10X) objective | | | |
|    j. Clear glue from tape by placing a drop of xylene or toluene under the tape if desired (follow proper precautions in handling these chemicals) | | | |
|    k. Remove the slide from the microscope stage and discard in bio-hazard sharps container | | | |
| 5. Discard specimen in appropriate biohazard container, as directed by instructor | | | |
| 6. Discard used materials appropriately | | | |
| 7. Return supplies to storage | | | |
| 8. Disinfect work area with surface disinfectant | | | |
| 9. Remove and discard gloves in biohazard container and wash your hands with hand disinfectant | | | |

*Evaluator Comments:*

Evaluator _____    Date _____

# Microscopic Methods of Detecting Intestinal Parasites

## LESSON OBJECTIVES

**After studying this lesson, you should be able to:**

- *Name three types of preparations used for the microscopic examination of fecal specimens.*
- *Explain how to prepare saline and iodine wet mounts for microscopic examination.*
- *Name two types of concentration procedures for fecal specimens.*
- *Explain fecal flotation and sedimentation procedures.*
- *Prepare fecal smears from fresh or fixed fecal specimens.*
- *Define the glossary terms.*
- *List safety precautions to be observed when preparing fecal specimens for microscopic examinations.*
- *Define the glossary terms.*

## GLOSSARY

**micrometer** / ruled device for measuring small objects

**trichrome stain** / stain commonly used for fecal specimens

## INTRODUCTION

The majority of parasitic infections are diagnosed by the microscopic identification of the parasite in blood, tissue, or fecal specimens. Much experience is required to become expert in parasite identification.

The procedures for examining blood for parasites are described in Lesson 8-4. The procedures for examining tissues for parasites are usually performed in the histology laboratory, where tissues are fixed, sectioned, and stained with special stains for parasite detection. This lesson describes the methods of preparing fecal specimens for microscopic parasite examination.

## MICROSCOPIC EXAMINATION OF FECAL SPECIMENS

The routine fecal specimen examination for parasites includes microscopic examination of wet mounts from fresh or fixed specimens, wet mounts of concentrated specimens, and stained smears (Figure 8-8).

 **Safety**

Preparing fecal specimens for microscopy presents biological and chemical hazards. Standard and Universal Precautions must be followed when handling fecal specimens. Even though a specimen may have had fixative added, it is still potentially infectious, since some parasites (particularly helminth eggs and protozoan cysts) are not immediaterly killed by fixatives.

Procedures such as concentration techniques, that use fixatives and volatile chemicals, should be performed in a fume hood to eliminate the possibility of inhaling fumes. Appropriate PPE, including chemical resistant gloves, must be worn to prevent exposing skin to the fixatives.

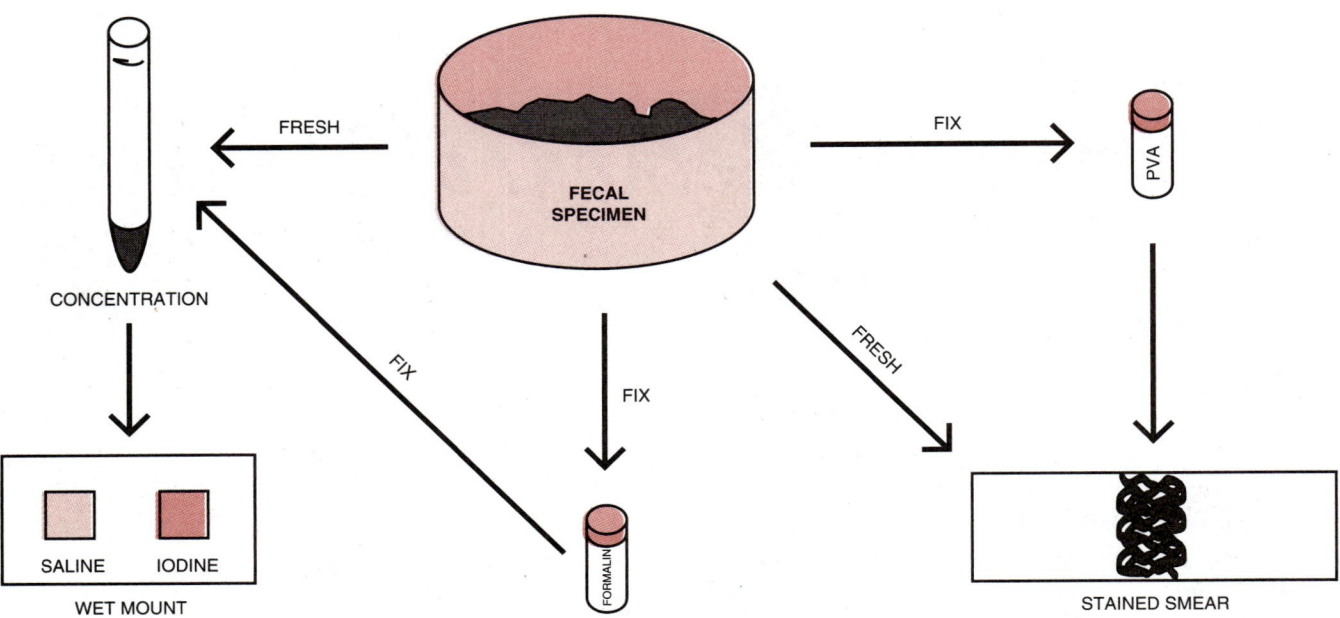

**FIGURE 8-8** Flowchart for preparing fecal specimens for microscopic examination

### Quality Assurance

Procedures must be carefully followed when performing concentration techniques. Centrifuge speed should be checked and recorded at designated intervals using a tachometer. The specific gravity of reagents used in concentration methods must be verified. Reagent containers must remain tightly capped when not in use to prevent evaporation and changes in specific gravity.

## Wet Mounts

Wet mounts are prepared from fresh or fixed (preserved) fecal specimens. Motile trophozoites (trophs) can be observed in wet mounts of *fresh* specimens. Observing motility (movement) is helpful, because preserved trophozoites are very small, lack many distinguishing characteristics, and may be easily overlooked by the microscopist. Wet mounts from fixed specimens are used to detect cysts, ova, and larva.

### Preparing Wet Mounts

Wet mounts are prepared by mixing a small amount of fresh or fixed specimen with a drop of saline on one end of a microscope slide (Figure 8-8). A similar portion of specimen is mixed with a drop of iodine solution on the other end of the slide and coverglasses are placed over the specimens. If desired, the coverglass edges may be sealed with petroleum jelly to retard drying. The preparations should be thin enough so newsprint can just be read through the specimen when the slide is placed on newspaper (Figure 8-9).

### Examining Wet Mounts

The entire wet mount preparation should be examined using the 10X or 20X objective. Most ova and larvae can be seen at this magnification. The 40X (high-power) objective should be used to examine the preparation for protozoa. Helminth eggs retain better morphology in the saline mount; iodine provides good morphology of protozoan cysts. An ocular **micrometer** (rule) should be used to measure any organisms seen.

## Concentration Techniques for Fecal Specimens

Concentration techniques increase the likelihood of detecting the parasite and decrease the amount of fecal debris. Fresh or formalin-fixed specimens may be concentrated by sedimentation or flotation techniques. Commercial systems for fecal concentration are available,

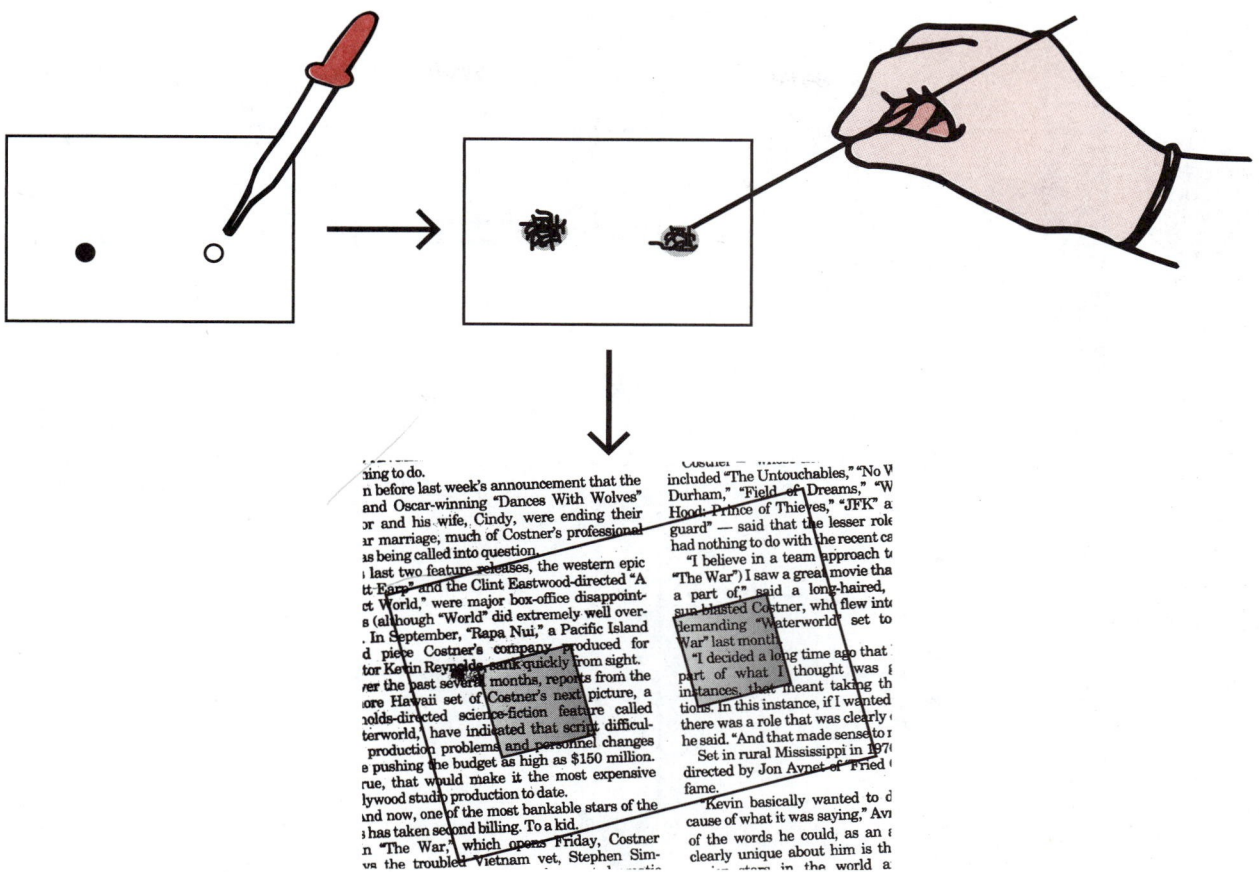

**FIGURE 8-9** Preparing wet mounts of fecal material for microscopic examination: top left, drops of iodine and saline are placed on slide; top right, portions of feces are mixed with drops; and (bottom) density of mounts is checked after coverslips are added

such as CON-Trate® by Meridian Diagnostics, and Parasep®, by Intersep Filtration Systems.

Sedimentation techniques use solutions of lower specific gravity than that of the parasites, causing the parasites to collect in the sediment when the specimen is centrifuged. Sedimentation methods detect parasites such as helminth ova and larvae and protozoan oocysts. One common sedimentation technique is the formalin-ethyl acetate method.

Flotation techniques use solutions of high specific gravity to cause the less dense parasitic forms to float to the solution's top while fecal debris settles to the tube's bottom. These methods yield a cleaner sample than sedimentation techniques, and recover most organisms and ova, although the morphology of some cysts and ova may be distorted. Using formalin-fixed specimens prevents distortion of ova and larvae. Two flotation techniques are the zinc sulfate and Sheather's sugar methods.

## Formalin-Ethyl Acetate Sedimentation Procedure

To perform a formalin-ethyl acetate sedimentation, a well-mixed formalin-treated specimen is strained through gauze into a 15 mL conical tube. The tube is filled with saline or 10% formalin and centrifuged, and the supernatant is decanted into a container of disinfectant. Formalin is mixed with the sediment remaining in the tube and ethyl acetate is added to the mixture. The tube is capped, shaken, and centrifuged again. The tube contents will separate into four layers: ethyl acetate, fecal debris, formalin, and sediment (Figure 8-10). The top three layers are removed and the sediment is used to make saline and iodine wet mounts for microscopic examination.

## Formalin-Zinc Sulfate Flotation Procedure

To perform a formalin-zinc sulfate flotation, a well-mixed formalin-treated specimen is strained through

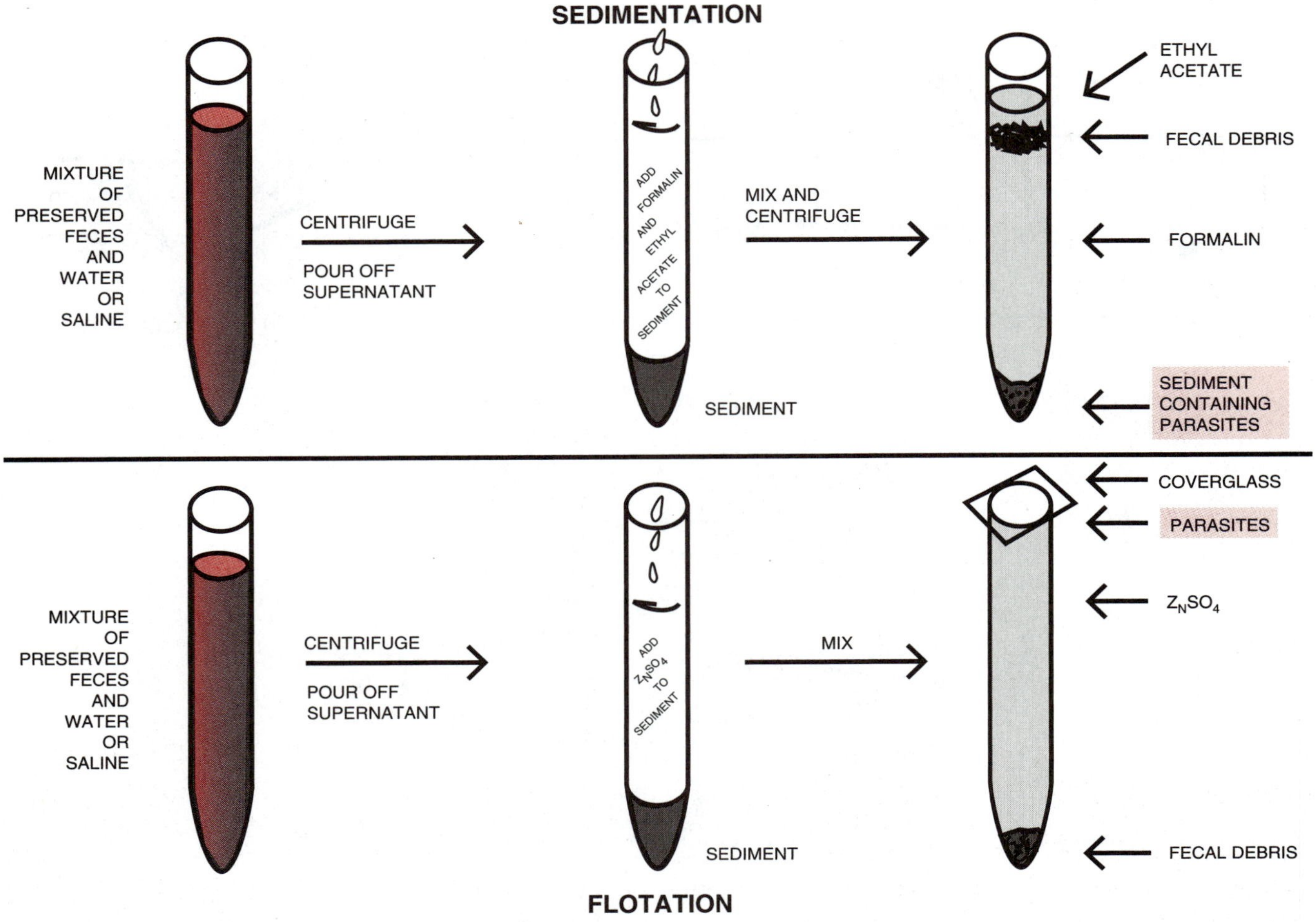

**SEDIMENTATION**

**FLOTATION**

**FIGURE 8-10** Sedimentation (top) and flotation (bottom) techniques

gauze into a tube and centrifuged (Figure 8-10). The supernatant is discarded in disinfectant. Zinc sulfate solution (specific gravity 1.190–1.200) is mixed with the sediment and the tube is filled to the top with zinc-sulfate with the tube in a vertical position. A clean coverglass is placed over the tube's top so the underside touches the fluid and the tube is left undisturbed for ten minutes. The coverglass is then carefully lifted in a straight, upward motion and lowered onto a drop of iodine or saline on a microscope slide.

Alternatively, the tube may be centrifuged for one minute at 1500 rpm after it is filled with zinc sulfate. A loop or capillary pipet is then used to remove a drop of the top film and prepare the wet mounts.

### Sucrose Flotation Procedure

Sheather's sugar solution, a sucrose solution with a specific gravity of 1.18, can be used to concentrate protozoan oocysts and cysts. A portion of fecal specimen is mixed with the sucrose solution in a conical centrifuge tube and centrifuged. Parasite cysts and oocysts, as well as some ova, float to the top of the solution. Wet mounts are prepared from the top layer of sucrose and examined microscopically. This method is useful for recovering *Cryptosporidium* oocysts.

## Stains for Fecal Specimens

Stained smears should be prepared for all fecal specimens examined. The smears can be made from fresh or fixed specimens. Stained smears are particularly important for positive identification of protozoan parasites.

Several stains are useful for parasite identification. Most laboratories use a modification of the **trichrome stain**, which seems to be the easiest to perform and gives the most consistent results. Trichrome-stained protozoa are blue-green to purple with red nuclei; helminths are purple. Immunofluorescent stains or modified acid-fast stains are used to identify *Cryptosporidium*.

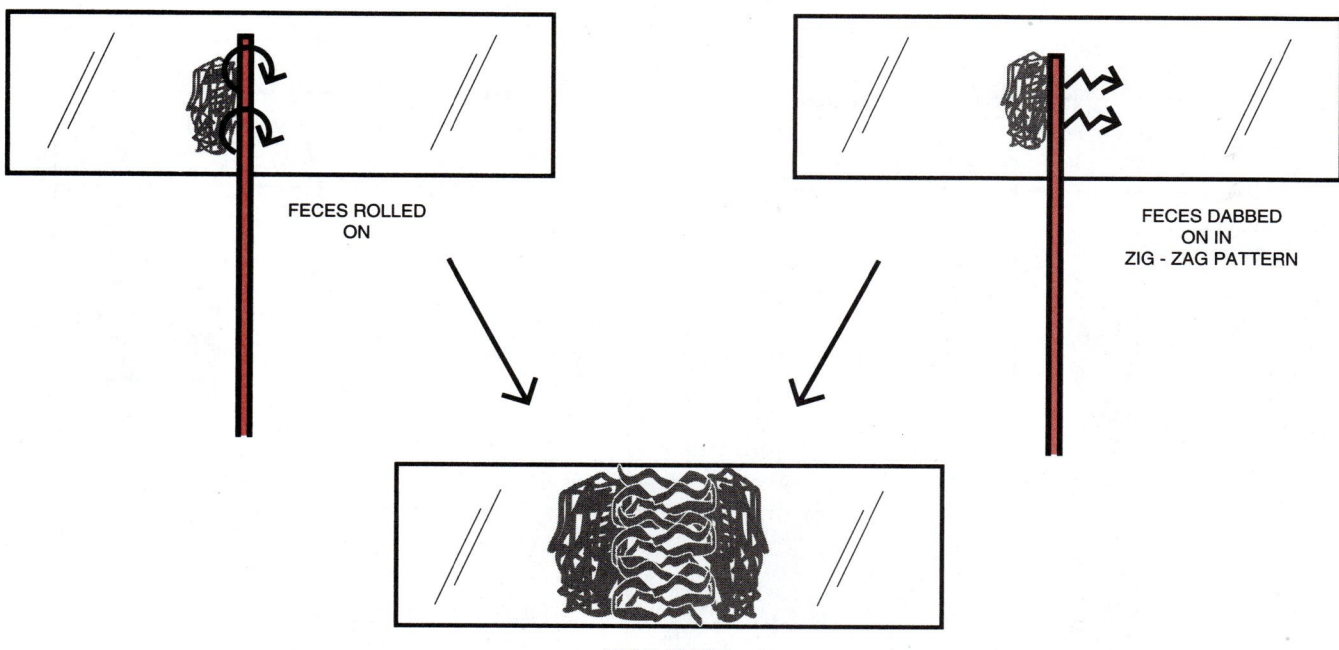

FECES ROLLED ON

FECES DABBED ON IN ZIG - ZAG PATTERN

FECAL SMEAR

**FIGURE 8-11** Preparing fecal smears

## Preparing Fecal Smears

Smears from polyvinyl alcohol (PVA)-fixed specimens are prepared by removing a portion of well-mixed specimen and spreading over a large area extending from the top to the bottom of the slide (Figure 8-11). The smear should dry for at least four hours (or overnight) at 35°C before staining.

Smears from fresh specimens are prepared similarly. A portion of specimen is removed with an applicator stick and spread over a large area of the slide. Smears of fresh specimens must be placed in fixative *before* they are allowed to dry. Smears can remain in fixative several days. After fixation, the smears may be stained.

## Staining Fecal Smears

Staining techniques for fecal specimens are complex and time-consuming. Most laboratories prepare the smears when processing the specimens and save the smears to stain in a batch. For this reason, final laboratory O & P reports may not be available until several days after the specimen is received.

## Organisms Seen in Fecal Specimens

Intestinal protozoa are identified by the morphology of cysts, trophozoites, or oocysts in fecal specimens. Helminths are identified by ova, larvae, or adults in fecal specimens.

Pathogenic intestinal protozoa include *Entamoeba histolytica, Dientamoeba fragilis, Giardia lamblia, Balantidium coli, Isospora belli, Cryptosporidium, Cyclospora,* and possibly *Blastocystis hominis.* Nonpathogenic intestinal protozoa include other *Entamoeba* sp., *Endolimax, Chilomastix,* and *Iodamoeba.* Any helminth found in a fecal specimen is considered of clinical importance.

Figures 8-12, 8-13, and 8-14 contain diagrams of amoebic, flagellate, ciliate, apicomplexan, and helminth forms of the more common human parasites. More information on these parasites can be found in Lesson 8-1 and textbooks of clinical parasitology.

### *Procedural Notes*

- Follow laboratory procedure manual for concentration technique(s).
- Observe proper centrifugation times and speeds.
- Check specific gravity of solutions regularly.
- Do not use reagents after expiration dates
- Allow fecal smears to dry several hours or overnight before staining.
- Place smears made from fresh specimens in fixative before the smears dry.

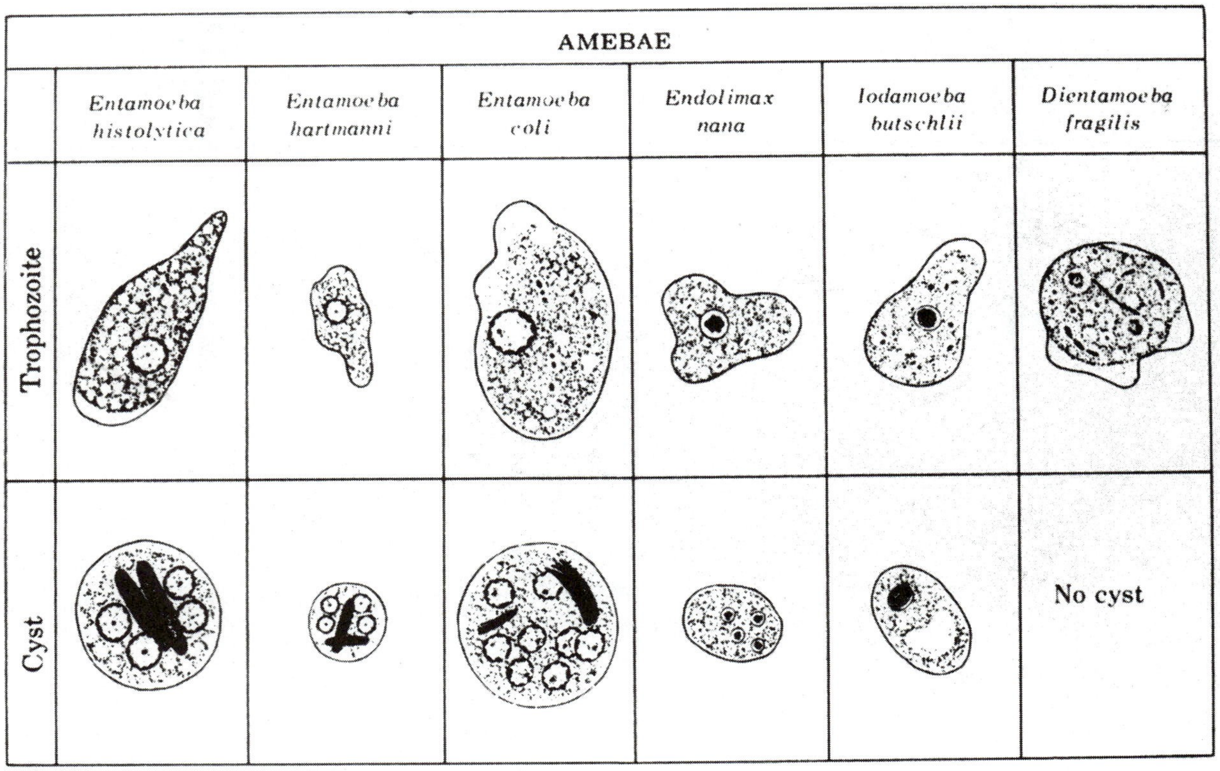

| AMEBAE | | | | | |
|---|---|---|---|---|---|
| *Entamoeba histolytica* | *Entamoeba hartmanni* | *Entamoeba coli* | *Endolimax nana* | *Iodamoeba butschlii* | *Dientamoeba fragilis* |

(rows labeled **Trophozoite** and **Cyst**; Dientamoeba fragilis Cyst cell reads "No cyst")

**FIGURE 8-12** Intestinal amoebae (*Dientamoeba* is a flagellate) (Adapted from Centers for Disease Control Publication No. 84-8116, U.S. Department of Health and Human Services)

## Safety Precautions

- Follow Universal and Standard Precautions when handling fresh and preserved fecal specimens.
- Dispose of specimens in biohazard containers.
- Balance load before turning centrifuge on.
- Do not open centrifuge lid until rotor has completely stopped.
- Avoid exposure to fixatives and other chemicals by working in a fume hood and wearing protective clothing and gloves.

## LESSON REVIEW

1. What are three types of preparations used for microscopically examining intestinal parasites?
2. What specimens are used for wet mounts? *saline, iodine*
3. What diluents are used for wet mounts?
4. Name three methods of concentrating fecal specimens. Where are the concentrated parasites found in each method?
5. How are fecal smears prepared for staining?
6. What stain is used for fecal specimens? *Giemsa,*
7. Why must a fume hood be used when preparing fecal specimens for microscopy?
8. Why must Universal and Standard Precautions be used when handling preserved fecal specimens?
9. Define micrometer and trichrome stain.

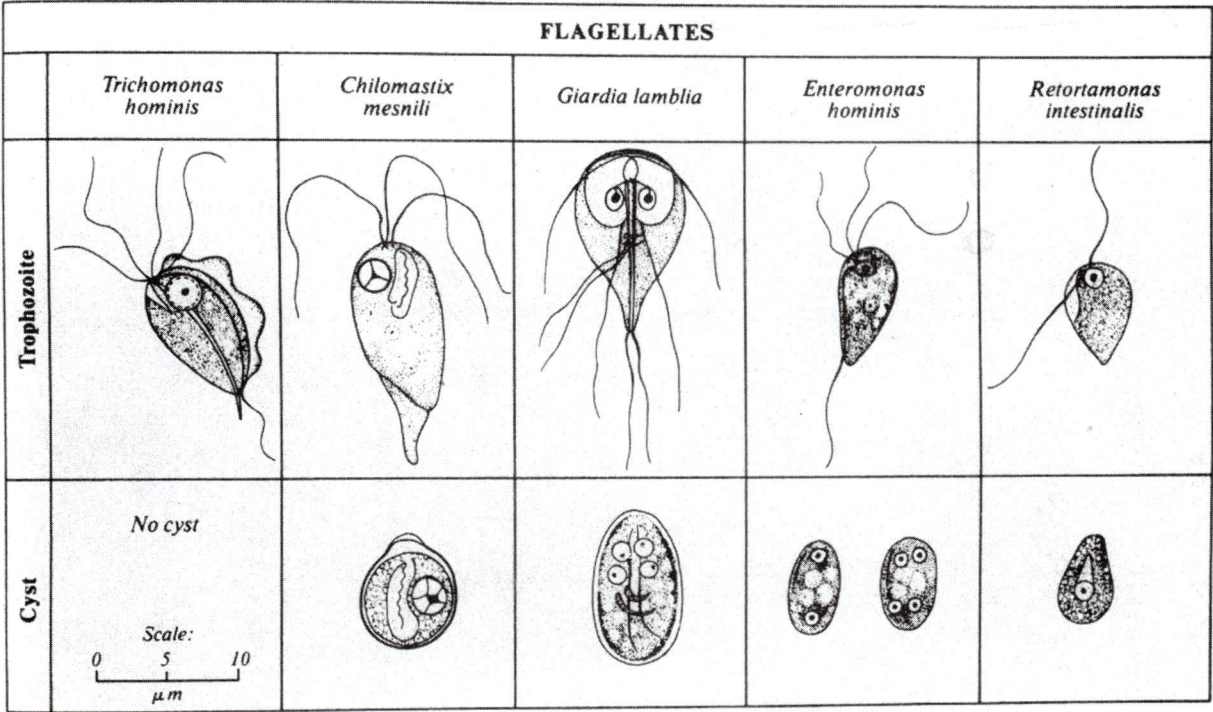

**FIGURE 8-13** Intestinal ciliates, coccidia, and flagellates (Adapted from Centers for Disease Control Publication No. 84-8116, U.S. Department of Health and Human Services)

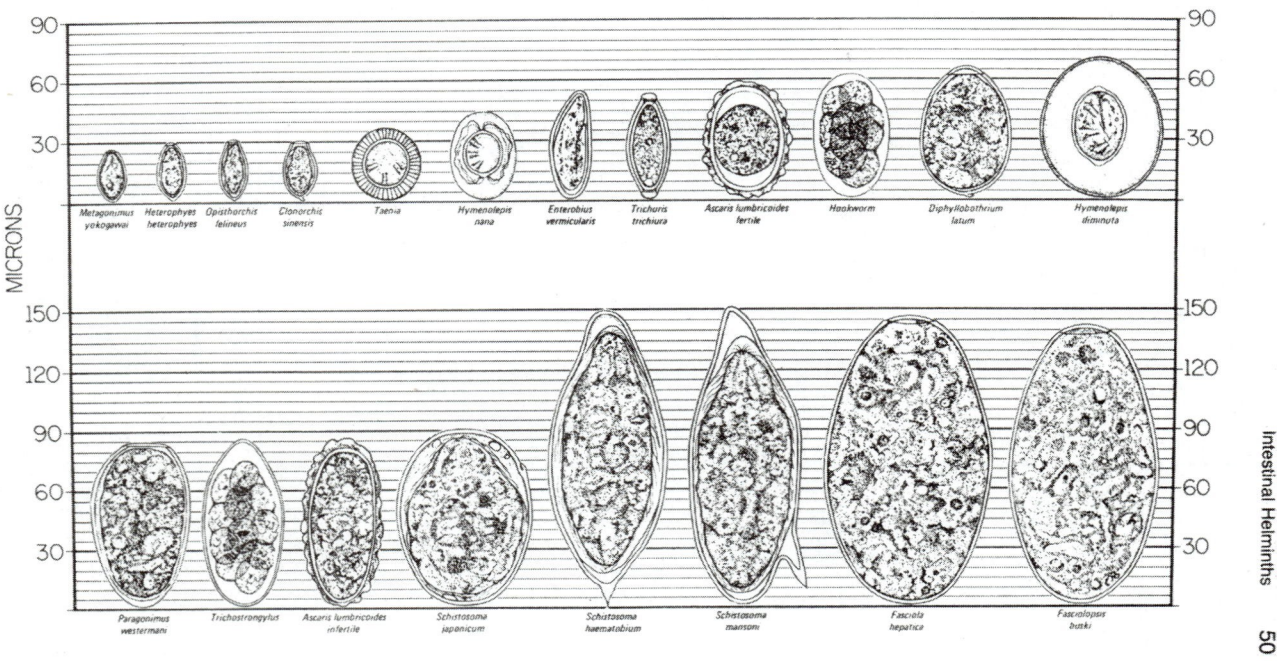

**FIGURE 8-14**   Helminth ova (Adapted from Centers for Disease Control Publication No. 84-8116, U.S. Department of Health and Human Services)

## STUDENT ACTIVITIES

1. Reread the information on microscopic methods for detecting intestinal parasites.
2. Review the glossary terms.

3. Practice preparing specimens for detecting intestinal parasites as outlined on the Student Performance Guide.

## *Student Performance Guide*

### **LESSON 8-3** Microscopic Methods for Detecting Intestinal Parasites

Name _____   Date _____

### INSTRUCTIONS

1. Practice preparing fecal specimens for microscopic examination for intestinal parasites, following the step-by-step procedure.
2. Demonstrate your understanding of this lesson by:
   a. Completing a written examination successfully, and
   b. Preparing fecal specimens for microscopic examination for intestinal parasites satisfactorily for the instructor. All steps must be completed as listed on the instructor's Performance Check Sheet.

## MATERIALS AND EQUIPMENT

- gloves
- hand disinfectant
- surface disinfectant (10% chlorine bleach solution)
- absorbent lab paper
- puncture-proof container for sharps
- biohazard containers
- wooden applicator sticks
- fecal specimens preserved in 10% formalin and in PVA (specimens from pets may be used)
- fume hood

### *Materials for Wet Mounts:*

- coverglasses, 22 mm²
- glass microscope slides, 2 x 3 inch preferable
- saline (0.85% NaCl)

- iodine solution for fecal wet mounts (Lugol's, Dobell and O'Connors, or D'Antoni's)
- dropping pipets
- D'Antoni's Iodine:

  Add 1.0 g potassium iodide (KI) and 1.5 g iodine crystals to 100 mL distilled water in a dark bottle. Shake well and filter daily before use.

### *Materials for Preparing Fecal Smear for Staining:*

- 35°C incubator or laboratory oven
- microscope slides, 1 x 3 inch
- wooden applicator sticks

### *Materials for Formalin-Ethyl Acetate Sedimentation (or a commercial stool concentration kit):*

- conical centrifuge tubes, 15 mL capacity (preferably disposable)
- 10% formalin
- ethyl acetate
- cotton swabs
- gauze or cheesecloth
- plastic funnel
- clinical centrifuge capable of spinning 15 mL conical tubes at 500 xg
- wooden applicator sticks

***Optional:*** Preserved fecal specimens containing parasites, atlases, diagrams, stained microscope slides, photographs, or videos of intestinal parasites

# PROCEDURE

Record in the comment section any problems encountered while practicing the procedure (or have a fellow student or the instructor evaluate your performance).

S = Satisfactory
U = Unsatisfactory

| You must: | S | U | Comments |
|---|---|---|---|
| 1. Assemble equipment and materials | | | |
| 2. Wash your hands and put on gloves | | | |
| 3. Prepare a work area by placing absorbent lab paper on counter or in fume hood | | | |
| 4. Demonstrate the procedure for preparing a fecal smear for staining, following steps 4a–d<br>a. Obtain PVA-fixed fecal specimen and two 1 x 3 inch microscope slides<br>b. Use applicator stick to mix specimen and remove a portion<br>c. Spread specimen evenly on slide by rolling stick across slide or smearing in a zig-zag fashion (see Figure 8-11). Smear should cover one-third to one-half the length of the slide and should extend from the slide's top to bottom edges. Prepare a second slide from the same specimen<br>d. Label slides and place them in 35°C incubator to dry for at least four hours, preferably overnight | | | |
| 5. Demonstrate the procedure for preparing saline and iodine wet mounts from a formalin-fixed fecal specimen, following steps 5a–i<br>a. Obtain a formalin-fixed specimen<br>b. Place a 2 x 3 inch glass slide on work area<br>c. Place one drop of saline on left half of slide and one drop of iodine solution on right half of slide<br>d. Use applicator stick to mix specimen<br>e. Remove a small portion of specimen with applicator stick and mix in with saline drop. Place a coverglass over the drop<br>f. Remove another small portion of fecal specimen and mix in with iodine drop. Place a coverglass over the drop. Discard applicator in biohazard container<br>g. Place slide over newsprint and check thickness of wet mounts (letters should be readable through the specimen)<br>h. **Optional:** Place slide on microscope stage and scan specimens with the low-power and high-power objectives. Use visual aids such as atlases, diagrams, or photographs to help recognize parasitic forms<br>i. Discard slide in biohazard sharps container | | | |

| You must: | S | U | Comments |
|---|---|---|---|
| 6. Demonstrate the procedure for formalin-ethyl acetate sedimentation, following steps 6a-k, or skip to step 7<br>  a. Obtain a formalin-fixed fecal specimen<br>  b. Mix the specimen and strain 5mL through wet gauze into a conical centrifuge tube<br>  c. Add saline or formalin to a volume of 15 mL and centrifuge the tube at 500 xg for 10 min<br>  d. Decant supernatant into a container of disinfectant, leaving approximately 1mL in tube<br>  e. Add 9 mL of 10% formalin to tube and mix using applicator stick<br>  f. Add 4 mL ethyl acetate, cap tube securely, and shake it vigorously by inversion for one-half minute<br>  g. Centrifuge tube for ten minutes at 500 xg<br>  h. Use a wooden applicator to ring the debris plug<br>  i. Pour off the top layers of ethyl acetate, debris, and formalin (see Figure 8-10), leaving 0.5–1.0 mL of sediment in tube<br>  j. Use a cotton swab to remove debris from the inside of tube. Add a few drops of 10% formalin to resuspend sediment<br>  k. Mix sediment with applicator stick and prepare saline and iodine wet mounts from portions of sediment, as in step 5b–i | | | |
| 7. Discard all contaminated materials in appropriate biohazard containers | | | |
| 8. Discard or store preserved specimens, as directed by instructor. | | | |
| 9. Disinfect work area and reusable supplies with 10% chlorine bleach solution | | | |
| 10. Remove and discard gloves in biohazard container and wash your hands with hand disinfectant | | | |

*Evaluator Comments:*




Evaluator _____ Date _____

# Preparing and Staining Smears for Blood Parasites

## LESSON OBJECTIVES

**After studying this lesson, you should be able to:**

- *Describe how to properly collect a blood specimen for parasite examination.*
- *Explain the purpose of preparing thin and thick blood smears for detecting blood parasites.*
- *Prepare thin and thick blood smears.*
- *Stain thin and thick blood smears with Giemsa stain.*
- *List safety precautions to be observed when preparing and staining blood smears for parasites.*
- *Define the glossary terms.*

## GLOSSARY

**Anopheles** / genus of mosquito that is the definitive host for the human malaria parasites (genus *Plasmodium*) and is capable of transmitting the organism to humans

**Giemsa stain** / polychromatic stain used for staining blood cells and blood parasites

**malaria** / in humans, a disease caused by infection with protozoan parasites of the genus *Plasmodium*

**microfilariae** / immature forms of filarial worms

**parasitemia** / parasites in the blood

**paroxysm(s)** / cycle(s) of chills and fever associated with malaria that occur thirty-six to seventy-two hours apart, depending on the *Plasmodium* species

**Plasmodium** / protozoan genus that includes the organisms causing human malaria

## INTRODUCTION

Several parasites have forms or stages that are present in the blood of infected individuals during part of the parasite's life cycle. Examples of these are the parasites that cause malaria, African sleeping sickness (trypanosomiasis), babesiosis, and dog heartworm disease.

The most common method for detecting the blood parasites is microscopic blood examination. This lesson explains the proper techniques of preparing and staining blood smears for detecting and identifying blood parasites. Much experience is required to recognize and identify the various species of blood parasites. Identifying specific blood parasites is beyond the scope of this lesson.

# HUMAN BLOOD PARASITES
## Human Malaria

Human **malaria** is caused by any one of four species of protozoan parasites belonging to the genus *Plasmodium* (Table 8-8). The parasites are transmitted to humans bitten by infected *Anopheles* mosquitoes or, rarely, through transfusion of infected blood. Mosquitoes become infected when they ingest blood from an infected person. Figure 8-15 shows a malarial parasite's life cycle.

**Table 8-8.** *Plasmodium* species that cause human malaria

| SPECIES | DISEASE CAUSED | PAROXYSMS |
|---|---|---|
| P. vivax | Benign tertian malaria | Every 48 hr |
| P. ovale | Ovale malaria | Every 48 hr |
| P. malariae | Quartan malaria | Every 72 hr |
| P. falciparum | Malignant malaria | Every 36–38 hr |

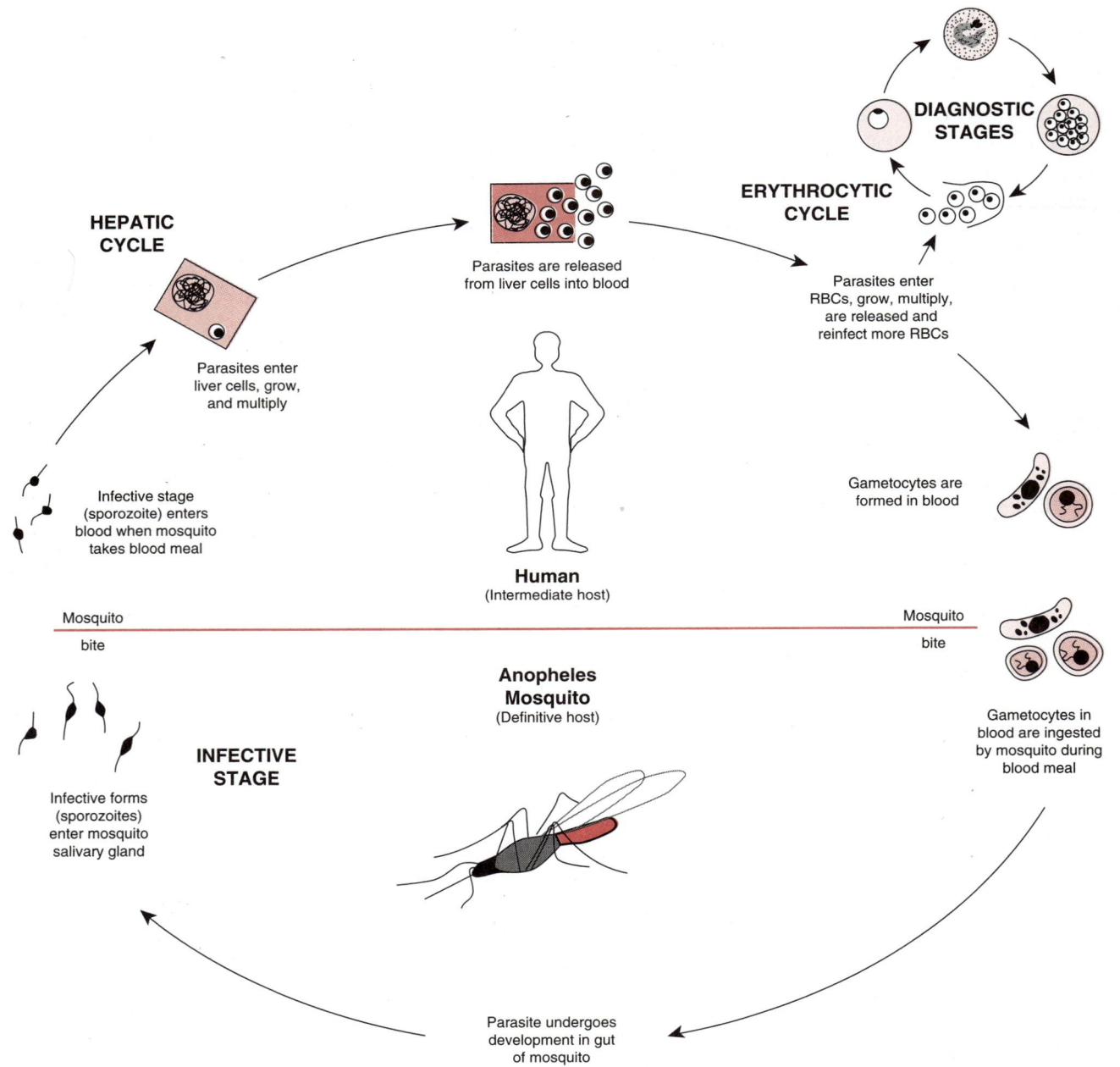

**FIGURE 8-15**  Life cycle of *Plasmodium*, the organism causing malaria

## Symptoms Associated with Malarial Infection

*Plasmodium* infection causes anemia, an enlarged spleen, and cycles of chills, fever, and sweats called **paroxysms**. The parasites infect liver cells and also RBCs. As the parasites develop in RBCs, they eventually cause the infected cells to rupture, releasing toxins and parasites, and initiating the cycle of chills, fever, and sweats.

Malaria cases may range from mild to fatal, depending on which species of *Plasmodium* causes the infection. Therefore, rapid identification of the infecting species is important.

## Epidemiology

Malaria has essentially been eliminated in the United States, but remains a major problem in the tropics of Asia, Africa, and Central and South America. Because of increased world travel, however, it is not uncommon to find patients with malaria in the United States. Malaria should be considered a possible cause of unexplained fever even for patients in so-called malaria-free countries, and these patients' recent travel history should be obtained. Recently, drug-resistant strains of *Plasmodium* and insecticide-resistant mosquitoes have become a problem in successfully treating and controlling the disease.

## Other Blood Parasites

Among the several other blood parasites that can cause infections are the protozoans *Babesia* and *Trypanosoma* and the filarial worms. These organisms are seen infrequently in humans in the U.S. Table 8-9 lists some of the bloodborne parasites, their transmission methods, and the diseases they cause.

The dog heartworm, *Dirofilaria immitis*, is a filarial parasite transmitted by mosquitoes and common in the U.S. Heartworm infection is diagnosed by examining dog blood for **microfilariae**, immature forms (larvae) of the heartworm.

## LABORATORY DETECTION OF BLOOD PARASITES

 **Safety**

Universal and Standard Precautions must be used to protect health care workers and patients. Appropriate PPE must be worn when collecting blood specimens and handling any biological specimen. Needles and lancets must be discarded in biohazard containers for sharps. Hands should be washed before donning and after removing gloves.

**Table 8-9.** Examples of parasites found in blood, their modes of transmission, and the diseases they cause

| ORGANISM | TRANSMISSION | DISEASE CAUSED |
|---|---|---|
| *Plasmodium spp.* | mosquito bite | malaria |
| *Babesia microti* | tick bite | babesiosis |
| *Trypanosoma brucei* | tsetse fly bite | African sleeping sickness, trypanosomiasis |
| *Trypanosoma cruzi* | Reduviid bug bite contaminated with bug's infected feces | Chagas' disease, American trypanosomiasis |
| *Wuchereria bancrofti* | mosquito bite | filariasis, elephantiasis |
| *Brugia spp.* | mosquito bite | filariasis, elephantiasis |
| *Leishmania donovani* | sand fly bite | visceral leishmaniasis, Kala azar, dumdum fever |
| *Toxoplasma gondii* | ingestion of oocysts, eating undercooked infected meat, congenital | toxoplasmosis |

### Quality Assurance

Established procedures for preparing blood smears for parasite examination must be followed. Since some parasitemias exhibit periodicity, collection timing is critical. Specimens may need to be collected at several intervals over two to three days to ensure a specimen containing the parasites.

Since anticoagulants can alter parasite morphology and staining characteristics, capillary specimens are preferred, especially for malaria. Blood specimens should be collected before treatment is initiated.

Blood should be examined as soon as possible after collection. Positive control slides should be stained with each fresh dilution of Giemsa stain.

## COLLECTING THE BLOOD SPECIMEN

Blood for parasite examination may be obtained by capillary puncture or venipuncture. However, blood to be examined for parasites should *not* be anticoagulated.

Anticoagulants distort parasite morphology and interfere with staining of parasitic stages.

Blood collection timing in suspected malaria cases is important. Blood should be collected between paroxysms, which may occur from thirty-six to seventy-two hours apart depending on the infecting species (Table 8-8).

*[handwritten note: Thick Smear is for present of Para and Thin is to Identify Para. morpholgy]*

## Preparing the Blood Smears

Two types of blood smears are prepared: thin and thick. The thick smear is used for screening; it contains ten to thirty times as much blood per microscopic field as a thin smear. Therefore, examining thick smears increases the chance of detecting parasites in a "light infection" because of the greater volume of blood screened. The thin film or smear is used to identify the parasite because the morphology is better in thin than in thick smears.

### Preparing a Thin Smear

A thin smear is prepared from freshly collected *anticoagulant-free* blood in the manner described in Lesson 2-8. A drop of blood is spread on a clean glass slide in the same way as for a differential count (Figure 8-16). The smear is allowed to air-dry in a slide rack. It is then immersed in absolute methanol for thirty to sixty seconds to fix the smear and is again allowed to air-dry. A

minimum of two thin smears should be prepared from each blood collection.

### Preparing a Thick Smear

There are two methods of preparing thick blood smears (Figure 8-17). A few small drops of blood can be placed in the center of a slide and spread into a dime-sized (approximately 2 cm) circle with the corner of another glass slide; or a drop of capillary blood can be touched from a fingerstick to a slide, and spread in a circular motion using slight pressure against the finger (Figure 8-17). A *minimum* of two thick smears should be prepared from each blood collection.

Thick smears should be allowed to dry flat at room temperature several hours or overnight before staining. A properly prepared thick film should be thin enough to read through when the slide is laid on a newspaper. Too-thick smears may peel off the slide during staining. Thick smears are *not* fixed before staining and should be stained within twenty-four hours of preparation.

## Staining Blood Smears for Parasites

The preferred stain for identifying parasites in blood is **Giemsa stain**. This polychromatic stain is similar to Wright's, but does not have fixative incorporated into it. Wright stain, which is routinely used for hematological studies, may be used for thin smears if rapid results are required. However, parasites do not stain as well with Wright's as with Giemsa stain and results from Wright-stained smears should be confirmed by examination of a Giemsa-stained smear.

Giemsa stain may be purchased as a stock solution to be diluted before use. Optimal dilutions and staining times should be determined for the brand and stain lot used. Staining times range from twenty minutes to two hours, depending on the stain dilution. "Quick"

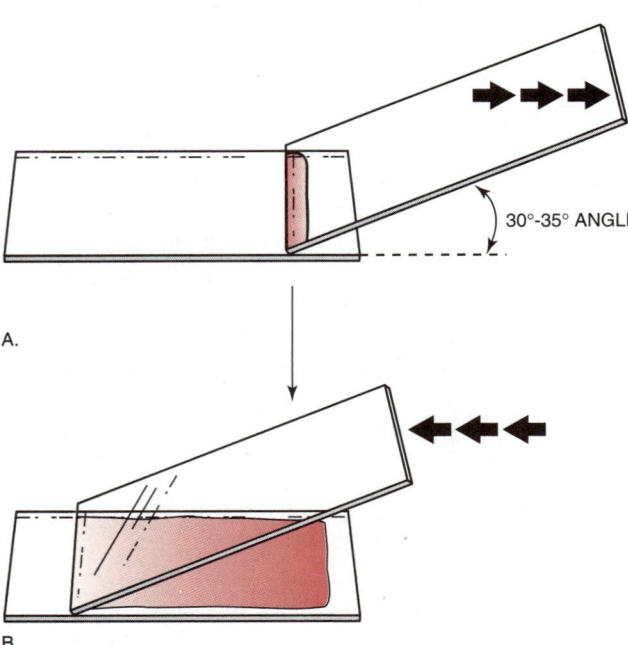

30°-35° ANGLE

A.

B.

**FIGURE 8-16** Preparing a thin blood smear

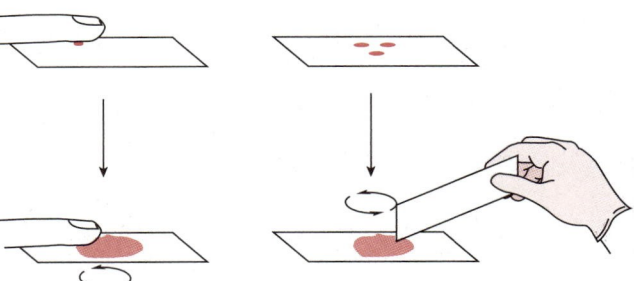

**FIGURE 8-17** Two methods of preparing thick blood smears: (Left) make smear directly from finger puncture; (right) use slide to spread the blood

Giemsa stains are available that do not require the long staining times, but staining results are usually not as good as with traditional Giemsa stain.

### Preparing Stain

A fresh dilution of Giemsa stain should be made daily. The stock Giemsa solution should be diluted with phosphate-buffered water, pH 7.0–7.2. Commonly used dilutions are 1:20, 1:50, or 1:100, with 1:50 being the most common (Table 8-10).

### Staining the Smears

Only one set of smears should be stained initially. This leaves a backup set in case a problem occurs during staining or smears need to be sent to a reference laboratory.

***Staining Thin Smears.*** A thin smear previously fixed in absolute methanol should be immersed in freshly diluted Giemsa stain for the appropriate time (see Table 8-10). After staining, the slide should be rinsed briefly in phosphate-buffered water and air-dried in a slide rack. Stained slides should be stored in covered slide boxes protected from light.

***Staining Thick Smears.*** Thick films should not be fixed before staining. During staining, the RBCs will be laked or lysed (destroyed) and only WBCs, platelets, and parasites (if present) will be visible. This makes it possible to scan the thick areas without the RBCs obscuring the field of view.

The dry slide should be immersed in Giemsa stain diluted 1:40 or 1:50 for fifty minutes (for other staining options see Table 8-10). The smear is then rinsed for three to five minutes in buffered water and allowed to air-dry in a slide rack. The dry, stained smears should be stored in slide boxes as mentioned above.

## Microscopically Examining Smears for *Plasmodium*

To examine smears for malarial parasites, the oil-immersion objective is used. The thin smear should be examined for thirty minutes using a back-and-forth serpentine motion to screen adjacent fields as in the differential count (Figure 8-18). RBCs are examined for parasitic inclusions.

To screen the thick film, 100–200 microscopic fields should be examined using the oil-immersion objective. WBCs, platelets, and parasites (if present) will be stained.

Although species identification is beyond the scope of this lesson, Figure 8-19 and Color Plates 47 and 48 depict some stages of *Plasmodium* that may be seen in infected RBCs. The typical appearance of malarial stages in stained thick smears is shown in a composite photograph, Color Plate 46.

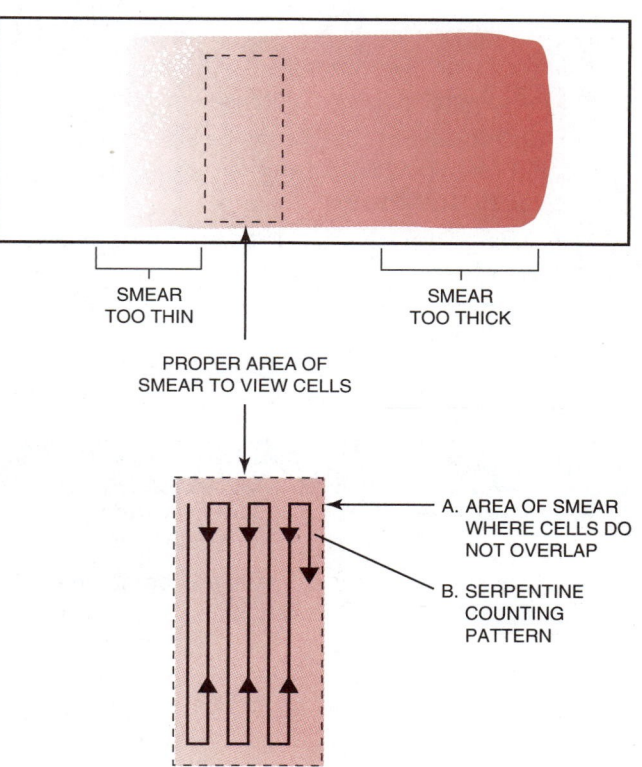

**FIGURE 8-18** Method of scanning adjacent microscopic fields in a thin blood smear

| Table 8-10. Dilutions and staining times for blood smears using commercial Giemsa stain | | |
|---|---|---|
| **DILUTION** | **STAINING TIME** | **DIRECTIONS FOR MAKING DILUTION** |
| 1:20 | 20 minutes | 2 mL Giemsa* + 38 ml bH$_2$O** |
| 1:50 | 50 minutes | 1 mL Giemsa + 49 ml bH$_2$O |
| 1:100 | 2 hours | 1 mL Giemsa + 99 ml bH$_2$O |

\* stock Giemsa stain, available commercially
\*\* phosphate-buffered water, pH 7.0–7.2

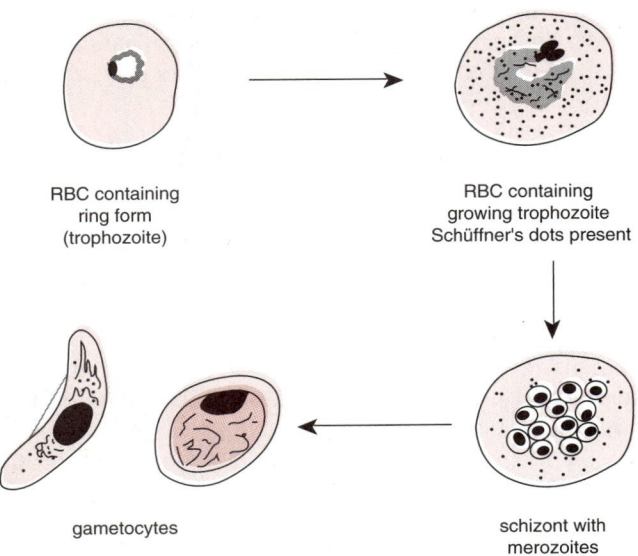

RBC containing
ring form
(trophozoite)

RBC containing
growing trophozoite
Schüffner's dots present

gametocytes

schizont with
merozoites

**FIGURE 8-19** Examples of erythrocytic stages that may be seen in *Plasmodium* infections

## Procedural Notes

- Use only fresh anticoagulant-free blood to make the smears.
- Do not make thick smears too thick.
- Make fresh dilutions of Giemsa stain daily.
- Blood smears should always be screened and interpreted by qualified workers experienced in parasite identification.
- Include positive control slides each time a new batch of stain is used.

## Safety Precautions

- Follow Universal and Standard Precautions when collecting and handling blood.
- Use caution in handling methanol; do not inhale fumes or allow it to contact skin.

## LESSON REVIEW

1. What is the proper blood specimen for making smears for parasite examination? *Capillary, Venipunct.*
2. Why are both thin and thick smears prepared? *thick present / thin br. ? dont*
3. Explain the procedure for making the thin blood smear. *drop of bld & spread*
4. Explain the procedure for making the thick blood smear. *drop Bld, or finger drop & spread.*
5. What is the preferred stain for blood smears for parasite examination? *Giemsa stain*
6. What safety precautions must be observed when preparing malarial smears? *expose, glove, caution*
7. Why is the blood-collection time important when malaria is suspected? *avoid coagulation mosquitoes infected by (orasm)*
8. Define *Anopheles*, Giemsa stain, malaria, paroxysm, and *Plasmodium*. *stain br. smear.*

## STUDENT ACTIVITIES

1. Reread the information on preparing and staining smears for blood parasites.
2. Review the glossary terms.
3. Practice the procedure for preparing and staining smears for blood parasites as outlined on the Student Performance Guide.
4. Optional: To observe another type of blood parasite, obtain freshly collected canine blood (less than one day old) from a local veterinary practice. Prepare and stain thin and thick smears from the blood. If the dog is infected with heartworm (*Dirofilaria* sp.) the stained microfilaria can be seen with the low-power objective. (Microfilaria will stain even in anticoagulated blood.) Stained microfilaria will appear as long, purple worms. Wet preps may also be performed: Place a small drop of blood on a glass slide and place a coverslip over it. Observe the specimen using the low-power objective. If the blood specimen is fresh and contains microfilaria, they will be seen moving under the coverslip.

## Student Performance Guide

## LESSON 8-4 Preparing and Staining Smears for Blood Parasites

Name _____    Date _____

### INSTRUCTIONS

1. Practice preparing and staining smears for blood parasites, following the step-by-step procedure.
2. Demonstrate your understanding of this lesson by:
   a. Completing a written examination successfully, and
   b. Performing the procedure for preparing and staining smears for blood parasites satisfactorily for the instructor. All steps must be completed as listed on the instructor's Performance Check Sheet.

### MATERIALS AND EQUIPMENT

- gloves
- hand disinfectant
- surface disinfectant
- biohazard container
- puncture-proof container for sharp objects
- acrylic safety shield or face protection

- Materials for capillary puncture
- clean glass slides
- absolute methanol
- stock Giemsa stain
- staining jars (Coplin jars)
- phosphate-buffered water, pH 7.2
  Recipe for Giemsa buffer (phosphate-buffered water):
  39 mL 0.067 M $NaH_2PO_4$
  61 mL 0.067 M $Na_2HPO_4$
  900 mL distilled water
  check pH. Should be 7.0–7.2
- microscope
- immersion oil
- lens paper
- slide box

***Optional visual aids:*** commercially prepared stained slides of *Plasmodium* and *Babesia*; commercially prepared stained slides of filarial worms, such as dog heartworm (*Dirofilaria* sp.); charts, Kodachrome slides, and figures showing morphology of blood parasites

***Note:*** Consult manufacturer's instructions accompanying Giemsa stain for recommended optimal dilution and staining time.

### PROCEDURE

Record in the comment section any problems encountered while practicing the procedure (or have a fellow student or the instructor evaluate the performance).

S = Satisfactory
U = Unsatisfactory

| You must: | S | U | Comments |
|---|---|---|---|
| 1. Wash your hands and put on gloves | | | |
| 2. Assemble equipment and materials for capillary puncture | | | |
| 3. Perform a capillary puncture (as described in Lesson 2-2) | | | |
| 4. Wipe away the first drop of blood | | | |

| You must: | S | U | Comments |
|---|---|---|---|
| 5. Apply a small drop of blood to a clean glass slide and use a clean spreader slide to form a thin blood film (as in Lesson 2-8). Make duplicate smears and set slides aside to air-dry | | | |
| 6. Immerse dried thin smears in absolute methanol for thirty to sixty seconds and air-dry. | | | |
| 7. Make a thick smear by holding a clean slide under the patient's finger and allowing one or two large drops of blood to fall on the center of the slide | | | |
| 8. Spread the blood evenly into a dime-sized circle to form the thick smear, using *slight* pressure against the fingertip (or use the corner of a clean glass slide to spread the blood). Make duplicate smears | | | |
| 9. Check the thickness of the thick smears by laying the slides on printed material. The print should be readable through the blood film | | | |
| 10. Place the slides on a flat surface in a dust-free place and allow them to air-dry at room temperature for several hours or overnight. DO NOT FIX. | | | |
| 11. Have patient apply pressure to puncture site with sterile gauze when satisfactory smears have been obtained. (At this point, if staining is to be done another day, work area may be cleaned, gloves removed, and hands washed, steps 20-25. Reglove before handling smears for staining procedure) | | | |
| 12. Stain smears by immersing slides in a freshly prepared 1:50 dilution of Giemsa stain for fifty minutes. (Be sure thin smear has been fixed and thick smear has dried for several hours) | | | |
| 13. Rinse stained smears in buffered water: rinse thin smear one to two minutes; rinse thick smear three to five minutes | | | |
| 14. Place rinsed slides in slide rack and allow to air-dry | | | |
| 15. Place thin smear on microscope stage and observe cells using oil-immersion objective. Observe quality of stain: RBCs should be pinkish, WBC nuclei should be blue-purple. Examine RBCs for stained intracellular parasitic inclusions. (Refer to charts, figures, or commercially prepared slides, if available) | | | |
| 16. Remove thin smear from microscope stage and place thick smear in position | | | |
| 17. Examine thick smear using oil-immersion objective. WBCs and platelets should be visible, but RBCs should have been destroyed in the staining process. If parasites were present in the blood specimen, they will be stained. (Refer to charts, figures, or commercially prepared slides, if available) | | | |
| 18. Remove slide from microscope stage | | | |
| 19. Clean oil from microscope objective with lens paper | | | |
| | | | |

| You must: | S | U | Comments |
|---|---|---|---|
| 20. Place slides in covered slide box | | | |
| 21. Discard capillary puncture materials in appropriate biohazard containers | | | |
| 22. Clean equipment and return to proper storage | | | |
| 23. Clean work area with surface disinfectant | | | |
| 24. Remove and discard gloves in biohazard container | | | |
| 25. Wash your hands with hand disinfectant | | | |

*Evaluator Comments:*




Evaluator _____ Date _____

# Glossary

**AABB** / American Association of Blood Banks

**AAMA** / American Association of Medical Assistants

**absorbance (A)** / a logarithmic expression of the amount of light absorbed by a substance containing colored molecules; optical density (O.D.)

**accessioning** / the process by which a specimens are logged in, labeled, and assigned a specimen number

**accreditation** / a voluntary process in which a private, independent agency grants recognition to institutions or programs that meet or exceed established standards of quality

**accuracy** / a measure of how close a determined value is to the true value

**acidosis** / abnormal condition in which blood pH falls below 7.35

**acquired immunodeficiency syndrome (AIDS)** (ah-KWEYE-ird im-YOU-no-deh-FISH-en-see SIHN-drohm) / a form of immune deficiency induced by infection with human immunodeficiency virus (HIV)

**acute phase proteins** / proteins that increase rapidly in serum during acute infection, inflammation, or following tissue injury

**adhesion** / the act of two parts or surfaces sticking together

**aerobic** / requiring oxygen

**aerosol** (EHR-oh-sol) / liquid in the form of a very fine mist

**agar** / a derivative of seaweed used to solidify microbiological media

**agglutination** (ah-gloo-tih-NAY-shun) / the clumping or aggregation of particulate antigens due to reaction with a specific antibody

**agglutination inhibition** / interference with or prevention of agglutination

**aggregate** / the total substances making up a mass; a cluster or clump of particles

**aggregation** / the collecting of separate objects into one mass

**Airborne Precautions** / a CDC category of isolation designed to prevent the transmission of infectious diseases such as pulmonary tuberculosis, rubeola (measles), and varicella (chickenpox)

**alanine aminotransferase (ALT)** (AL-ah-neen am-MEEN-oh-TRANS-fer-aze) / enzyme that is present in high concentration in liver tissue and that is measured to assess liver function; SGPT

**albumins** (al-BYOU-mihns) / a homogeneous group of serum proteins that are made in the liver and help maintain osmotic balance

**alimentary tract** / (al-ih-MEN-tah-ree tract) the digestive tube from the mouth to the anus

**alkaline phosphatase (ALP or AP)** / enzyme widely distributed in the body, especially in the liver and bone

**alkalosis** / abnormal condition in which blood pH rises above 7.45

**allergy** / a condition resulting from an exaggerated immune response; hypersensitivity

**amorphous** / without definite shape

**AMT** / American Medical Technologists

**anaerobic** / growing only in the absence of oxygen

**anamnestic response** (an-am-NES-tik ree-SPANS) / rapid increase in blood immunoglobulins following a second exposure to an antigen; booster response or secondary response

**anemia** / decrease below normal in the RBC count or in the blood hemoglobin level

**angioplasty** (AN-jee-oh-plast-ee) / surgical repair of a vessel

**anisocytosis** (an-IH-soh-seye-TOH-sis) / marked variation in the sizes of erythrocytes when observed on a peripheral blood smear

***Anopheles*** (an-AH-fehl-eez) / the genus of mosquito that is the definitive host for the human malaria parasites (genus *Plasmodium*) and is capable of transmitting the organism to humans

**antibiotic susceptibility testing** / determining of the susceptibility of microorganisms to specific antibiotics

**antibody (Ab)** / serum protein that is induced by and reacts specifically with a foreign substance (antigen); immunoglobulin

**anticoagulant** (an-tee-koh-AG-you-lant) / a chemical that prevents blood coagulation

**antigen (Ag)** (AN-tih-jen) / "foreign" substance that induces an immune response by causing production of antibodies and/or sensitized lymphocytes that react specifically with that substance; immunogen

**antiseptic** / a chemical used to control the growth of microorganisms on living tissues

**antiserum** / serum that contains antibodies

**anuria** (an-YOUR-ee-ah) / complete failure of kidney function and suppression of urine formation; absence of urine production

**aperture** / an opening

**artery** / a blood vessel that carries oxygenated blood from the heart to the tissues

**arthropod** / a member of the phylum Arthropoda, which includes crustaceans, insects, and arachnids

**ASCLS** / American Society for Clinical Laboratory Science (formerly American Society for Medical Technology, ASMT)

**ASCP** / American Society of Clinical Pathologists

**ASPT** / American Society of Phlebotomy Technicians

**aseptic technique** / measures used to prevent contamination when working with microorganisms

**aspartate aminotransferase (AST)** (ASS-par-tate ah-MEEN-oh-TRANS-fer-aze) / enzyme that is present in many tissues, including cardiac, muscle, and liver, and that is measured to assess liver function; SGOT

**atherosclerosis** (ath-er-oh-skleh-ROH-sis) / a condition in which lipids, calcium, and other substances deposit on the inner surface of the arteries

**autoantibody** / an antibody that is directed against the self (one's own tissues)

**autoclave** (AW-toh-klayv) / an instrument that uses pressurized steam for sterilization

**autoimmune disease** / disease resulting when the immune response is directed at one's own tissues (self-antigens)

**average** / the sum of a set of values divided by the number of values; the mean

**B lymphocyte, B cell** / a type of lymphocyte primarily responsible for the humoral immune response

**bacillus** (ba-SIHL-uhs)/ a rod-shaped bacterium

**band cell** / an immature granulocyte with a nonsegmented nucleus; a "stab cell"

**basophil** (BAY soh-fil)/ a leukocyte containing basophilic-staining granules in the cytoplasm

**basophilic** (BAY-soh-FIL-ik)/ blue in color; having affinity for the basic stain

**basophilic stippling** (BAY-soh-fil-ik STIP-ling)/ fine granular remnants of RNA and other basophilic nuclear material remaining inside the erythrocyte after the nucleus is lost from the cell

**Beer's Law** / a mathematical relationship that demonstrates the linear relationship of concentration to absorbance and forms the basis for spectrophotometric analysis

**bibulous paper** / a special absorbent paper used to dry slides

**bilirubin** (BIHL-ee-roo-bihn)/ a product formed in the liver from the breakdown of hemoglobin

**binocular** / having two oculars or eyepieces

**biological safety cabinet** / a special cabinet that provides protection while working with infectious microbiological agents

**blast cell** / an immature blood cell normally found only in the bone marrow

**blood bank** / department in the medical laboratory where blood components are tested and stored until needed for transfusion; refrigerated unit used for the storage of blood components

**blood group antibody** / a serum protein (immunoglobulin) that reacts specifically with a blood group antigen

**blood group antigen** / a substance or structure on the red blood cell membrane that causes antibody formation and reacts with that antibody

**bloodborne pathogens (BBP)** / pathogens that may be present in human blood (and blood-contaminated body fluids) and that cause disease in humans

**Bloodborne Pathogens (BBP) Standard** / OSHA guidelines for preventing occupational exposure to pathogenic microorganisms present in human blood and body fluids, including, but not limited to, human immunodeficiency virus (HIV) and hepatitis B virus (HBV); final OSHA standard of December 6, 1991, effective March 6, 1992

**Bowman's capsule** / the portion of the nephron that receives the glomerular filtrate

**buffer** / a substance that lessens change in pH of a solution when acid or base (alkali) is added

**buffy coat** / a light-colored layer of leukocytes and platelets that forms on top of the RBC layer when a sample of blood is centrifuged or allowed to stand undisturbed

**BUN** / blood urea nitrogen; a test measuring urea in blood

**CAAHEP** / Commission on Accreditation of Allied Health Education Programs (formerly CAHEA)

*Candida albicans* / a fungus that causes vaginitis in females, especially following antibiotic therapy for bacterial infections

**CAP** / College of American Pathologists

**capillary** / a minute blood vessel that connects the smallest arteries to the smallest veins, and that serves as an exchange vessel

**capillary action** / the action by which a fluid enters a tube because of the attraction between the fluid and the tube

**capillary tube** / a glass or plastic tube of very small diameter used for laboratory procedures

**carcinogen** (kar-SIHN-o-jen) / a substance with the potential to produce cancer

**cardiopulmonary circulation** (kar-dee-oh-PUHL-muh-nair-ree sir-kyou-LAY-shun)/ the system of blood vessels that circulates blood from the heart to the lungs and back to the heart

**carrier** / a person who harbors an organism and has no symptoms or signs of disease, but is capable of spreading the organism to others

**cast** / in urinalysis, a protein matrix formed in the kidney tubules and washed out in the urine

**caustic** (KAW-stihk)/ a substance that burns or destroys skin and flesh; capable of destroying tissue

**CBC** / complete blood count; a commonly performed group of hematological tests

**CDC** / Centers for Disease Control and Prevention

**cell diluting fluid** / a solution used to dilute blood for cell counts

**Celsius scale** / temperature scale where the freezing point of water is zero (0°) and the boiling point is 100°; indicated by "C"; also called centigrade

**centi** / prefix used to indicate one-hundredth of a unit; $10^{-2}$

**centrifugal analysis** / a type of discrete chemical analysis in which the reagents and sample are mixed together by centrifugal action

**centrifuge** (SEHN-trih-fewj)/ an instrument that spins tubes at high speeds, forcing heavy particles in samples to the bottom of the tubes

**cephalic vein** / a superficial vein of the arm commonly used for venipuncture

**cephaloplastin** (SEF-al-oh-plast-in) / a commercial preparation of partial thromboplastin

**cestode** / tapeworm; member of the class *Cestoda*

*Chlamydia* (klah-MIHD-ee-a) / gram-negative intracellular bacteria; *Chlamydia trachomatis* is a cause of STD

**chromogen** / a substance that becomes colored when it undergoes a chemical change

**clean-catch urine** / a midstream urine sample collected after the urethral opening and surrounding tissues have been cleansed

**CLIA '88** / Clinical Laboratory Improvement Amendments of 1988

**clinical laboratory science** / the field of medical technology

**clinical laboratory scientist (CLS)** / medical technologist

**clinical laboratory technician (CLT)** / medical laboratory technician

**coagulation** / the process of forming a fibrin clot

**coagulation factors** / a group of plasma proteins involved in blood clotting

**coarse adjustment** / control that adjusts position of microscope objectives; used to initially bring objects into focus

**coccus** (KAH-kuhs)/ a spherical bacterium

**coefficient of variation** / a calculated value that compares the relative variability between different sets of data

**COLA** / Commission on Office Laboratory Accreditation

**coliform** / certain gram-negative intestinal bacteria, including *Escherichia coli*

**collagen** / a protein connective tissue found in skin, bone, ligaments, and cartilage

**colony** / a defined mass of bacteria assumed to have grown from a single organism

**colony count** / a method of estimating the number of organisms in urine by counting the colonies on a urine culture plate

**commensal** / an organism that lives with, on or in another, without causing injury to either

**communicable** / able to be transmitted directly or indirectly from one individual to another

**complement** / a group of plasma proteins that participates in immune reactions to cause cell lysis and the inflammatory response

**condenser** / apparatus located below the microscope stage that directs light into the objective

**congenital** (cahn-JEHN-ih-tahl)/ acquired during fetal development, and present at the time of birth, but not inherited

**Contact Precautions** / CDC category of isolation designed to prevent transmission of diseases spread by close or direct contact

**control serum** / a serum with a known concentration of the same constituents as those being measured in the patient sample

**corrosive** / a chemical agent, such as an acid, that has the ability to gradually destroy a material

**cortex** / the outer layer or portion of an organ

**coumarin** / an anticoagulant administered orally to prevent or slow clotting

**counterstain** / a dye that adds a contrasting color

**creatine kinase (CK)** / enzyme that is present in large amounts in brain tissue and in heart and skeletal muscle and is measured to aid in the diagnosis of heart attack

**creatinine** / a breakdown product of creatine that is normally excreted in the urine

**critical measurements** / measurements made when the accuracy of a solution's concentration is important; measurements made using glassware manufactured to strict standards

**culture** / growth of microorganisms in a special medium; the process of growing microorganisms in the laboratory

**cyanmethemoglobin** (seye-an-met-HEE-moh-gloh-bin)/ a stable colored compound formed when hemoglobin is reacted with Drabkin's reagent; hemiglobincyanide (HiCN)

**cyst** / the nonmotile, nonfeeding stage of a protozoan parasite; usually an infective stage

**cystitis** (sis-TEYE-tis)/ inflammation of the urinary bladder

**cytoplasm** (SEYE-to-plaz-m)/ the fluid portion of the cell surrounding the nucleus

**D-dimer** / a small molecule cleaved by plasmin from the cross-linked fibrin in a clot during fibrinolysis

**definitive host** / the host in which the sexual or adult form of the parasite is found

**deionized water** (dee-EYE-oh-neyezd wah-ter)/ water that has had most of the mineral salts removed

**deoxyhemoglobin** (dee-AHK-see HEE-moh-gloh-bin)/ the hemoglobin formed when oxyhemoglobin releases oxygen to tissues

**DHHS** / Department of Health and Human Services

**diabetes mellitus** / a disorder of carbohydrate metabolism characterized by a state of hyperglycemia due to insulin deficiency

**differential count** / a determination of the relative numbers of each type of leukocyte in a stained blood smear

**discrete analysis** / a method of analysis in which the assay procedure for each sample is performed in its own separate container within the instrument

**disinfectant** / a chemical used to kill or control the growth of microorganisms

**disseminated intravascular coagulation** / a bleeding disorder characterized by widespread thrombotic and secondary fibrinolytic reactions

**distal convoluted tubule** / the portion of a renal tubule that empties into the collecting tubule

**distilled water** / the condensate collected from steam after water has been boiled

**diuresis** (deye-yer-EE-sis)/ output of abnormally large urine volume

**diurnal** / having a daily cycle

**DNA** / a nucleic acid that is found primarily in the nucleus of all living cells and carries genetic information; deoxyribonucleic acid

**Drabkin's reagent** / a hemoglobin diluting reagent that contains iron, potassium, cyanide, and sodium bicarbonate

**Droplet Precautions** / a CDC isolation category designed to prevent the transmission of diseases spread through the air over short distances

**dysfunction** / impaired or abnormal function

**ectoparasite** / a parasite that lives on the outer surface of a host

**EDTA** / ethylenediaminetetra-acetic acid; an anticoagulant commonly used in hematology

**EIA** / enzyme immunoassay

**electrolyte** / a solution that conducts electricity

**electrolytes** / the cations and anions important in maintaining fluid and acid-base balance

**embolus (pl. emboli)** / a mass (clot) of blood or foreign matter carried in the circulation

**endemic** / recurring in a specific location or population

**endogenous** (ehn-DAH-jen-uhs) / produced within; growing from within

**endothelium** (en-doh-THEEL-ee-um) / the layer of epithelial cells that lines the cavities of blood vessels and the serous cavities of the body

**engineering control** / using available technology and equipment to isolate the worker from hazards

**enzyme** (EN zeye-m) / a protein that causes or accelerates changes in other substances without being changed itself

**enzyme immunoassay (EIA)** (EN-zeye-m ihm-you-noh-ASS-ay) / a serological test that uses an enzyme-labeled antibody as a reactant

**eosin** / a red-orange stain or dye

**eosinophil** (EE-oh-SIHN-oh-fil)/ a leukocyte containing eosinophilic granules in the cytoplasm

**epidemiology** / the study of the factors that cause disease and determine disease frequency and distribution

**epitope** / the portion of an antigen that reacts specifically with an antibody; antigenic determinant

**Epstein-Barr virus (EBV)** / a virus that infects lymphocytes and causes infectious mononucleosis

**erythrocyte** (eh-RITH-roh-seye-t) / blood cell that transports $O_2$ to the tissues and carbon dioxide ($CO_2$) to the lungs; red blood cell (RBC)

**erythrocytosis** (eh-RITH-roh-seye-TOH-sis)/ an excess of RBCs in the peripheral blood; sometimes called polycythemia

**ethics** / a system of conduct or behavior; rules of professional conduct

**exogenous** (eks-AH-jen-uhs)/ originating from the outside

**exposure incident** / an accident, such as a needlestick, in which an individual has been exposed to possible infection through contact with body substances from another individual; especially refers to bloodborne pathogens

**eyepiece** / ocular

**Fahrenheit scale** / temperature scale where the freezing point of water is 32° and the boiling point is 212°; indicated by "F"

**fastidious organism** / an organism that requires special nutritional factors to survive

**FDP** / fibrinogen-degradation products formed when plasmin cleaves fibrinogen

**fecal** / pertaining to waste matter discharged from the intestines

**femtoliter (fL)** / a unit of volume; $10^{-15}$L

**fibrin** (FEYE-brin) / a protein formed from fibrinogen by the action of thrombin

**fibrinogen** (Feye-BRIN-oh-jehn) / a plasma protein produced in the liver and converted to fibrin through the action of thrombin

**fibrinolysis** (feye-brin-oh-LEYE-sis)/ enzymatic breakdown of a blood clot

**fine adjustment** / control that adjusts position of microscope objectives; used to sharpen focus

**fission** / asexual reproduction of a microorganism

**fixative** / preservative; a chemical that prevents deterioration of cells or tissues

**fluorescent** / having the property of emitting light of one wavelength when exposed to light of another wavelength

**folic acid** / a member of the B vitamin complex

**fomites** / inanimate objects, such as bed rails, linens, or eating utensils, that may be contaminated with infectious organisms and serve as a means of their transmission

**formalin** / a solution of formaldehyde used as a fixative or preservative

**fossae** (FAH-see) / in the throat, shallow depressions where the tonsils were located before surgical removal

**fume hood** / a device that draws contaminated air out of an area and either cleanses and recirculates it, or discharges it to the outside

**gamma glutamyl transferase (GGT)** / enzyme that is present in liver, kidney, pancreas, and prostate, and that is measured to assess liver function

**gauge** / a measure of the diameter of a needle

**Gaussian curve** / a graph plotting the distribution of values around the mean; normal frequency curve

**Giemsa stain** (GEEM-sah stayn) / a polychromatic stain used for staining blood cells and blood parasites

**globin** / the protein portion of the hemoglobin molecule

**globulins** / a heterogeneous group of serum proteins with varied functions

**glomerular filtrate** (gloh-MER-you-ler FIHL-trayt) / the fluid that passes from the blood into the nephron and from which urine is formed

**glomerulonephritis** (gloh-mer-you-loh-neh-FREYE-tis) / inflammation of the glomeruli

**glomerulus (pl. glomeruli)** (gloh-MER-you-lus) / a small bundle of capillaries that is the filtering portion of the nephron

**glucagon** / a pancreatic hormone that increases blood glucose concentration by promoting the conversion of glycogen to glucose

**glucose dehydrogenase** / enzyme used in glucose analytical methods that converts glucose to gluconolactone

**glucose oxidase** / an enzyme that converts glucose to gluconic acid and that is used in many glucose analytical methods

**glucose tolerance test (GTT)** / a test analyzing blood glucose at timed intervals following ingestion of a standard glucose dose; oral glucose tolerance test

**glycogen** (GLEYE-koh-jen) / the storage form of glucose found in high concentration in the liver

**glycolysis** / energy production as a result of the metabolic breakdown of glucose

**glycosuria** (gleye-koh-SYOUR-ree-ah) / glucose in the urine; glucosuria

**gonorrhea** (gahn-oh-REE-ah) / a contagious infection spread by sexual contact and caused by *Neisseria gonorrhoeae*

**gout** / a painful condition in which blood uric acid is elevated and urates precipitate in joints

**gram (g)** / basic metric unit of weight or mass

**gram-equivalent weight** / the gram formula weight divided by the total positive charge (valence) of a molecule

**gram-formula weight** / the weight in grams of the entity represented by a chemical formula

**gram negative** / designation for bacteria that lose the crystal violet (purple stain) and retain the safranin (red stain) in the Gram stain procedure

**gram positive** / designation for bacteria that retain the crystal violet (purple stain) in the Gram stain procedure

**Gram stain** / a differential stain used to classify bacteria

**granulocyte** (GRAN-you-loh-seye-t) / a leukocyte containing granules in the cytoplasm; any of the neutrophilic, eosinophilic, or basophilic leukocytes

**guaiac** (GWEYE-ak) / a chemical derived from the resin of the *Guaiacum* tree

**HCFA** / Health Care Financing Administration

**hCG** / human chorionic gonadotropin, a hormone present in pregnancy; uterine chorionic gonadotropin (uCG)

**HDL cholesterol** / high-density lipoprotein fraction of total blood cholesterol

**helminth** / a worm, especially a parasitic worm; in parasitology, the group comprising the roundworms and flatworms

**hemacytometer** (hee-mah-seye-t-OH-mee-ter) / a heavy glass slide made to precise specifications and used to count cells microscopically; a counting chamber

**hemacytometer coverglass** / a special coverglass of uniform thickness used with a hemacytometer

**hematocrit** (heh-MAT-oh-crit) / the volume of erythrocytes packed by centrifugation in a given volume of blood and expressed as a percentage; abbreviated "crit" or Hct

**hematology** / the study of blood and the blood-forming tissues

**hematoma** / the swelling of tissue around a vessel due to leakage of the blood into the tissue

**hematuria** (hee-ma-TYOUR-ee-ah) / the presence of blood in the urine

**heme** / the iron-containing portion of the hemoglobin molecule

**hemiglobincyanide (HiCN)** (HEE-meg-gloh-bin-SEYE-ah-nide) / cyanmethemoglobin

**hemoglobin (Hb, Hgb)** (HEE-moh-gloh-bin) / the major functional component of red blood cells that serves as the oxygen-carrying protein

**hemolysis** (hee-MAHL-ih-sihs) / the destruction of red blood cells resulting in the release of hemoglobin from the cells

**hemolytic disease of the newborn (HDN)** / a condition in which antibody from the mother destroys the red blood cells of the fetus

**hemophilia** (hee-moh-FIHL-ee-ah) / a bleeding disorder resulting from a hereditary coagulation factor deficiency or dysfunction

**hemopoiesis** (hee-moh-poy-EE-sis) / the process of blood cell formation and development; hematopoiesis

**hemorrhage** (HEM-or-ihj) / excessive or uncontrolled bleeding

**hemostasis** (hee-moh-STAY-sis) / the process of stopping bleeding

**HEPA filter** / *h*igh-*e*fficiency *p*articulate *a*ir filter used in biological safety cabinets

**heparin** / an anticoagulant used in certain laboratory procedures

**hepatitis B virus (HBV)** / a virus that causes hepatitis and is transmitted by contact with infected blood or other body fluids

**hepatitis C virus (HCV)** / a virus that causes hepatitis and is transmitted by contact with infected blood or other body fluids

**heterophile antibodies** / antibodies that are increased in infectious mononucleosis

**hexokinase** (hex-oh-KEYE-naze) / an enzyme that is used in glucose analytical methods and that converts glucose to glucose-6-phosphate

**histogram** / a graph that illustrates the size and frequency of occurrence of articles being studied

**HIV** / human immunodeficiency virus, a retrovirus that has been identified as the cause of acquired immunodeficiency syndrome (AIDS)

**homeostasis** / the tendency toward steady state or equilibrium of body processes

**host** / an organism from which the parasite obtains nutrients and in which some or part of the parasite's life cycle is carried out

**Howell-Jolly body** / nuclear remnant remaining in red blood cells after the nucleus is lost; common in pernicious anemia and hemolytic anemia

**HSV-1** / Herpes simplex virus, type 1; the cause of oral herpes

**HSV-2** / Herpes simplex virus, type 2; the cause of genital herpes

**human immunodeficiency virus (HIV)** / a retrovirus that has been identified as the cause of AIDS

**hyaline** (HEYE-ah-luhn)/ transparent, pale

**hypercalcemia** (heye-per-kal-SEE-mee-ah)/ blood calcium levels above normal

**hyperglycemia** / blood glucose concentration above normal

**hyperkalemia** / blood potassium levels above normal

**hyperlipidemia** (heye-per-lip-ih-DEE-mee-ah)/ excessive amount of fat in blood

**hypernatremia** / blood sodium levels above normal

**hyperthyroidism** (heye-per-THEYE-royd-izm)/ excessive functional activity of the thyroid gland; excessive secretion of thyroid hormones

**hyphae** (HEYE-fee) / filaments of mold that make up the mycelium

**hypoalbuminemia** (heye-poh-al-byou-min-EE-mee-a)/ marked decrease in serum albumin concentration

**hypocalcemia** (heye-poh-kal-SEE-mee-ah) / blood calcium levels below normal

**hypochromic** (heye-poh-KROHM-ik) / having reduced color or hemoglobin content

**hypodermic needle** / a hollow needle used for injections or for obtaining fluid specimens

**hypoglycemia** / blood glucose concentration below normal

**hypokalemia** / blood potassium levels below normal

**hyponatremia** / blood sodium levels below normal

**hypothyroidism** (heye-poh-THEYE-royd-izm)/ deficiency of thyroid function

**immunity** / resistance to disease or infection

**immunization** / the process of producing immunity to an antigen

**immunoassay** (ihm-you-noh-ASS-ay)/ a diagnostic method using antigen-antibody reactions

**immunocompetent** (ihm-you-noh-COMP-o-tent)/ capable of producing a normal immune response

**immunocompromised** (ihm-you-noh-COMP-roh-meyez-d) / having reduced or inability to produce a normal immune response

**immunoglobulins (Ig)** (ihm-you-noh-GLOB you-lihns)/ antibodies; serum proteins that are induced by and react specifically with antigens (immunogens)

**immunohematology** (ihm-you-noh-hee-mah-TAHL-oh-jee)/ the study of blood group antigens and antibodies; blood banking

**immunology** / the branch of medicine involving the study of the immune processes and immunity

**immunosuppression** / suppression of the immune response by physical, chemical, or biological means

**impedance** / resistance in an electrical circuit

**index of refraction** / the ratio of the velocity of light in one medium, such as air, to its velocity in another medium

**indicator medium** / a bacteriological medium that detects certain chemical reactions of the organisms growing on it; differential medium

**indices** (IN-dih-sees)/ plural of index; indexes; erythrocyte indices are values that compare cells in a blood sample to standard values

**infection** / a pathological condition caused by growth of microorganisms in the host

**inflammation** / tissue reaction to injury

**inoculating loop** / an instrument used to pick up and transfer bacteria

**inoculation** / process of transferring a population of microorganisms to a growth medium

**inoculum** / mass of bacteria being transferred from one medium to another

**insulin** / a pancreatic hormone essential for proper metabolism of blood glucose and maintenance of blood glucose levels

**intermediate host** / the host in which the asexual, immature, or larval form of the parasite is found

**intravascular** / inside the blood vessels

**ion-selective electrode** / an electrode manufactured to respond to the concentration of a specific ion

**iris diaphragm** (EYE-rihs DEYE-ah-fram)/ device that regulates the amount of light striking the specimen being viewed through the microscope

**ISCLT** / International Society for Clinical Laboratory Technology

**isolation** / the practice of limiting the movement and social contact of a patient who is potentially infectious or who must be protected from exposure to infectious agents

**isotonic solution** / a solution that has the same concentration of dissolved particles as that solution or cell with which it is compared

**JCAHO** / joint Commission on Accreditation of Healthcare Organizations, an independent accrediting agency

**ketones** (KEE-tohns)/ a group of chemical substances produced during increased metabolism of fat; ketone bodies

**ketonuria** (kee-toh-NYOUR-ee-ah)/ ketones in the urine

**kidney** / the organ in which urine is formed

**kilo** / prefix used to indicate one thousand units; $10^3$

**lactate dehydrogenase (LD or LDH)** (LAK-tate dee-heye-DRO-jen-aze) /enzyme widely distributed in the body and measured to assess liver function

**lancet** / a sterile, sharp-pointed blade used to perform a capillary puncture

**laser** / a narrow and extremely intense beam of light that has only one wavelength and goes in only one direction

**lateral** / toward the side

**LDL cholesterol** / low-density lipoprotein fraction of total blood cholesterol

**lens** / a curved transparent material that spreads or focuses light

**lens paper** / a special nonabrasive material used to clean optical lenses

**leukemia** (loo-KEE-mee-ah)/ a chronic or acute disease involving unrestrained growth of leukocytes in the bone marrow and peripheral blood

**leukocyte** (LOO-koh-seye-t)/ blood cell that functions in immunity; white blood cell (WBC)

**leukocytosis** (loo-koh-seye-TOH-sis)/ increase above normal in the number of leukocytes (white blood cells) in the blood

**leukopenia** (loo-koh-PEE-nee-ah) / less than the normal in the number of leukocytes (white blood cells) in the blood;

**Levey-Jennings chart** / a quality control chart used to record daily quality control values

**lipemic** / having a cloudy appearance due to excess lipid content

**lipids** / any one of a group of fats or fat-like substances

**liter (L)** / basic metric unit of volume

**loop of Henle** / the U-shaped portion of a renal tubule between its proximal and distal portions

**lumen** / the open space within a tubular organ or tissue

**lymphocyte** (LIM-foh-seye-t)/ a small basophilic-staining leukocyte having a round or oval nucleus and playing a vital role in the immune process

**lymphocytosis** / more than the normal number of lymphocytes in the blood

**lymphokine** (LIHM-foh-keye-n)/ any of several small molecules that are produced by lymphocytes and help regulate the immune response

**lyophilize** (leye-AYF-ihl-eyez)/ to remove water from a frozen solution under vacuum; freeze-dry

**macrocytic** (mak-roh-SIH-tik)/ having a larger than normal cell size

**malaria** / in humans, a disease caused by infection with protozoan parasites of the genus *Plasmodium*

**malignant** / cancerous; not benign

**material safety data sheet (MSDS)** / safety information that must be supplied by manufacturers of hazardous materials

**mean** / the sum of a set of values divided by the number of values; the average

**mean corpuscular hemoglobin (MCH)** (mee-n kor-PUHS-kyou-lar HEE-moh-gloh-bin)/ mean cell hemoglobin; average red blood cell hemoglobin expressed in picograms (pg)

**mean corpuscular hemoglobin concentration (MCHC)** (mee-n kor-PUHS-kyou-lar HEE-moh-gloh-bin con-sehn-tray-shun)/ mean cell hemoglobin concentration; comparison of the weight of hemoglobin in a red blood cell to the size of the cell expressed in percentage or g/dL

**mean corpuscular volume (MCV)** (mee-n kor-PUHS-kyou-lar vahl-youm) / mean cell volume; average red blood cell volume; an estimate of the volume of a red blood cell in a blood sample, expressed in femtoliters (fL) or cubic microns (μ³)

**median cubital vein** / a superficial vein located in the bend of the elbow (cubital fossa) that connects the cephalic vein to the basilic vein

**medical laboratory technician (MLT)** /a professional who has completed a minimum of two years of specific training in an accredited medical laboratory technician program and has passed a national certifying examination; clinical laboratory technician

**medical technologist (MT)** / a professional who has a baccalaureate degree from an accredited college or university, has completed clinical training in an accredited medical technology program, and has passed a national certifying examination; clinical laboratory scientist

**medical technology** / the health profession concerned with performing laboratory analyses used in diagnosing and treating disease as well as in maintaining good health; clinical laboratory science

**medium** / a substance used to provide nutrients for growing microorganisms

**medulla** / the inner or central portion of an organ

**megakaryocyte** (meh-gah-KAIR-e-oh-seye-t) / a large bone marrow cell from which platelets are derived

**melanin** / a dark pigment of skin, hair, and certain tumors

**meniscus** (mehn-IS-kuhs)/ the curved upper surface of a liquid in a container

**meter (M)** / basic metric unit of length or distance

**methylene blue** (MEH-thel-een blue)/ a blue stain or dye

**micro** / prefix used to indicate one-millionth of a unit; 10⁻⁶

**microbiology** / a branch of biology dealing with microscopic forms of life

**microcytic** (mik-roh-SIH-tik)/ having a smaller than normal cell size

**microfilaria (pl. microfilariae)** (meye-kroh-fihl-A-ree-a)/ immature form of filarial worms

**microfuge** (MEYE-kroh-fewj)/ a centrifuge that spins microcentrifuge tubes at high rates of speed

**microhematocrit** / a hematocrit performed in a capillary tube using a small quantity of blood

**microhematocrit centrifuge** / an instrument that spins capillary tubes at a high speed to rapidly separate liquid from cellular components

**micrometer** / a ruled device for measuring small objects

**microorganism** / a single-celled microscopic organism

**micropipet** / a pipet that measures or holds volumes less than 1 mL

**microscope arm** / the portion of the microscope that connects the lenses to the base

**microscope base** / the portion of the microscope that rests on the table and supports it

**midstream urine** / a urine sample collected in the middle of voiding

**milli** / prefix used to indicate one-thousandth of a unit; 10⁻³

**minimum inhibitory concentration (MIC)** / the minimum concentration of an antibiotic required to inhibit growth of a microorganism

**molar solution (M)** / a solution containing one mole of solute per liter of solution

**mole** / the formula weight of a substance expressed in grams

**monochrometer** / a device that isolates a narrow portion of the light spectrum

**monoclonal antibody** / antibody derived from a single cell line or clone

**monocular** (mahn-AHK-you-lahr)/ having one ocular or eyepiece

**monocyte** (MAHN-oh-seye-t)/ a large leukocyte usually characterized by a convoluted or horseshoe-shaped nucleus

**mordant** / a substance that fixes a dye or stain to an object

**morphology** (mor-FAHL-oh-jee)/ the form and structure of cells, tissues, and organs

**mutagen** (MYOU-tah-jehn)/ a substance with the potential to make a stable change in a gene that is then passed on to offspring

**mycelium** (meye-SEEL-ee-uhm)/ a mass of hyphae that makes up the vegetative body of molds

**mycology** / the study of fungi

**mycoplasma** / a tiny microorganism lacking a rigid cell wall

**mycosis** (meye-KOH-sis)/ infection caused by fungi

**myocardial infarction (MI)** (meye-oh-KAR-dee-ahl in-FARK-shun)/ heart attack caused by obstruction of the blood supply to the heart or within the heart

**myoglobin** / a pigmented protein found in muscle tissue

**NAACLS** / National Accrediting Agency for Clinical Laboratory Sciences

**nano** / prefix used to indicate one-billionth of a unit; 10⁻⁹

**NCA** / National Credentialing Agency for Laboratory Personnel

**NCCLS** / National Committee for Clinical Laboratory Standards; a nonprofit, educational organization that establishes standards of best current practice for clinical laboratories

**nematode** / roundworm; any unsegmented worm of the class Nematoda

**nephron** (NEF-ron)/ the structural and functional unit of the kidney

**nephrotoxic** (nef-roh-TOKS-ihk)/ toxic or destructive to kidney cells

**neutrophil** (NOO-troh-fil)/ a neutral-staining leukocyte, usually the first line of defense against infection

**nocturia** (noc-TYOUR-ee-ah)/ excessive urination at night

**noncritical measurements** / measurements that are estimated; measurements made in containers that estimate volume (such as the Erlenmeyer flask)

**nongonococcal urethritis** (nahn-gahn-oh-KAHK-ahl YOU-ree-THREYE-tis)/ a gonorrhea-like STD caused by organisms other than gonococci

**nonpathogenic** / not normally causing disease in a healthy individual

**normal flora** / microorganisms that are normally present at a specific site

**normal solution (N)** / a solution containing one gram equivalent weight of a substance per liter of solution

**normochromic** (nor-moh-KROH-mik)/ having normal color

**normocytic** (nor-moh-SIH-tik)/ having a normal cell size

**nosepiece** / revolving unit to which microscope objectives are attached

**nosocomial infection** (nohz-oh-KOH-mee-ahl ihn-FEHK-shun)/ infection acquired in a hospital or health-care facility

**nucleus (pl. nuclei)** / the central structure of a cell that contains DNA and controls cell growth and function

**objective** / magnifying lens closest to the object being viewed with a microscope

**occult** / concealed or hidden

**ocular** (AHK-you-lahr)/ eyepiece of the microscope, containing a magnifying lens

**oliguria** (ahl-ee-GYOUR-ee-ah)/ decreased production of urine

**oncologist** / a physician specializing in the study and treatment of tumors or cancers

**opalescent** (oh-pah-LEHS-ent)/ having a milky iridescence

**OPIM** / Other Potentially Infectious Materials; any and all body fluids, tissues, organs, or other specimens from a human source

**opportunistic parasite** / an organism that causes disease only in immunocompromised hosts

**opportunistic pathogen** / a microorganism that causes disease in the host only when normal defense mechanisms are impaired or absent

**OSHA** / Occupational Safety and Health Administration; the federal agency that monitors the Occupational Safety and Health Act of 1971

**osmolality** (ahs-moh-LAL-iht-ee) / a measure indicating the number of dissolved solids in a fluid, usually serum or urine

**ova** / eggs

**oxidase test** / an enzyme test used to identify certain bacteria, such as *Neisseria*

**oxyhemoglobin** (ahk-see-HEE-mo-gloh-bin)/ the form of hemoglobin that binds and transports oxygen

**packed cell column** / the layers of blood cells that form when a tube of whole blood is centrifuged

**palpate** / to examine by touch

**parasite** / an organism that lives in or on another species of organism and at the expense of that organism

**parasitemia** (pair-ah-siht-EE-mee-ah)/ parasites in the blood

**parenteral** (pair-EHN-ter-al)/ any route other than alimentary canal; intravenous, subcutaneous, intramuscular, or mucosal

**parfocal** / the ability to maintain focus of an image when changing from one power of objective lens to another

**paroxysm(s)** (pair-AHKS-ihzm) / the cycle(s) of chills and fever associated with malaria that occurs from thirty-six to seventy-two hours apart, depending on the *Plasmodium* species

**partial thromboplastin** / the lipid portion of thromboplastin, available as a commercial preparation

**pathogen** / an organism or agent capable of causing disease in a host

**pathogenic** (path-oh-JEHN-ihk) / capable of causing damage or injury to the host

**pathologist** / a physician specially trained in the nature and cause of disease

**percent transmittance (%T)** / the percentage of light that passes through a solution

**peroxidase** (per-OKS-ih-daze)/ the enzyme that converts hydrogen peroxide to water and oxygen

**personal protective equipment (PPE)** / specialized clothing or equipment used by workers to protect themselves from direct exposure to blood or other potentially hazardous materials; includes, but is not limited to, gloves, laboratory apparel, eye protection, and breathing apparatus

**petechiae** (puh-TEE-kee-uh)/ small, purplish hemorrhagic spots on the skin

**Petri dish** / a shallow, covered dish made of plastic or glass

**pH** / a measurement of the hydrogen ion concentration expressing the degree of acidity or alkalinity of a solution

**pharyngeal** (fair-ihn-JEE-ahl)/ having to do with the back of the throat or pharynx

**phlebotomist** (fleh-BOT-oh-mist)/ one trained to draw blood; venipuncturist

**phlebotomy** / venipuncture; entry of a vein with a needle

**physiological saline** / a 0.85% (0.15M) sodium chloride solution

**picogram (pg)** / micromicrogram; $1 \times 10^{-12}$ gram

**plasma** / the liquid portion of blood in which blood cells are suspended; the straw-colored liquid remaining after blood cells are removed from anticoagulated blood

**plasma cell** / a cell that produces antibodies and is derived from a B lymphocyte

**plasmin** (PLAZ-min)/ an enzyme that binds to fibrin and initiates breakdown of the fibrin clot

**plasminogen** (plaz-MIN-oh-jen)/ the inactive precursor of plasmin

*Plasmodium* / the protozoan genus that includes the organisms causing human malaria

**platelet**/ a formed element in circulating blood that plays an important role in blood coagulation; a small disk-shaped fragment of cytoplasm derived from a megakaryocyte; a thrombocyte

**POCT** / point-of-care test(ing); testing outside the traditional laboratory setting; also called bedside testing, off-site testing and alternate-site testing

**poikilocytosis** (POY-kihl-oh-seye-TOH-sis)/ significant variation in the shape of erythrocytes

**POL** / physician office laboratory

**polychromatic** / having many colors

**polyclonal antibodies** / antibodies derived from more than one cell line

**polycythemia** (PAHL-ee-sih-THEE-mee-ah)/ an excess of red blood cells in the peripheral blood

**polyuria** (pahl-ee-YOUR-ee-ah)/ excessive production of urine

**population** / the entire group of items or individuals from which the samples under consideration are presumed to have come

**porphyrins** (POR-fihr-ins)/ a group of pigments that are required for in the synthesis of hemoglobin

**postprandial** (pohst-PRAN-dee ahl)/ after eating

**precipitation** / formation of an insoluble antigen-antibody complex

**precision** / reproducibility of results; the closeness of obtained values to each other

**prefix** / modifying word or syllable(s) placed at the beginning of a word

**primary lymphoid organs** / organs in which B and T lymphocytes acquire their special characteristics; in humans, the bone marrow and thymus

**primary medium** / a medium that provides nutritional requirements for an organism and is used to recover the organism from infectious material

**progeny** / offspring or descendants

**proglottid (pl. proglottides)** (pragh-LAH-tid)/ segment of a tapeworm that contains male and female reproductive systems

**proportion** / the relation in number or amount of one portion compared to another or to the whole

**protective isolation** / isolation category designed to protect highly susceptible patients from exposure to infectious agents; reverse isolation

**proteinuria** / protein in the urine, usually albumin

**prothrombin** (pro-THROM-bin) / the precursor of thrombin; factor II

**prothrombin time (PT)** / a coagulation screening test used to monitor oral anticoagulant therapy

**protozoa** / unicellular eukaryotic organisms, both free-living and parasitic

**proximal convoluted tubule** / the portion of a renal tubule that collects the filtrate from Bowman's capsule

**PVA** / polyvinyl alcohol, a preservative used for fecal specimens

**pyelitis** (peye-ih-LEYE-tihs)/ inflammation of the renal pelvis

**pyelonephritis** (peye-eh-loh-neh-FREYE-tis) / inflammation of the kidney and the renal pelvis

**quadrant** / one-fourth of a circle; one-fourth of an agar plate

**radioimmunoassay (RIA)** (ray-dee-oh-ihm-you-noh-ASS-ay) / a serological test using a test component labeled with a radioisotope

**random error** / error whose source cannot be definitely identified

**random urine specimen** / a urine specimen collected at any time, without regard to diet or time of day

**ratio** / relationship in number or degree between two things

**reactive lymphocyte** / lymphocyte that occurs in response to viral infections; common in infectious mononucleosis; atypical lymph

**reagent** / substance or solution used in laboratory analyses; substance involved in a chemical reaction

**reciprocal** / inverse; one of a pair of numbers (as 2/3 and 3/2) that has a product of one

**reference laboratory** / an independent regional laboratory that offers routine and specialized testing to hospitals and physicians

**reflectance photometer** / an instrument that measures the light reflected from a colored reaction product

**refractometer** / an instrument for measuring refraction

**renal hilus** (REE-nahl HEYE-lus)/ the concavity in the kidneys where nerves and vessels enter or exit

**renal pelvis** / the cavity in the kidney that receives urine from the renal tubules and the site where the ureter enters the kidney

**renal threshold** / the blood concentration above which a substance not normally excreted by the kidneys appears in the urine

**reservoir host** / a host, other than the usual host, in which the parasite lives and is infectious

**resolving power** / the ability of a microscope to distinguish between two separate but adjacent objects; resolution

**reticulocyte** (reh-TIK-you-loh-seyte) / an immature erythrocyte that has retained RNA in the cytoplasm

**reticulocytopenia** (reh-TIK-you-loh-seye-toh-PEE-nee-ah)/ a decrease below the normal number of reticulocytes

**reticulocytosis** / an increase above the normal number of reticulocytes in the circulating blood

**reticulum** / (reh-TIK-you-lum) a network

**Rh (D) immune globulin (RhIG)** / a concentrated, purified solution of human anti-D antibody used for injection

**rheumatoid arthritis (RA)** (ROO-mah-toyd ar-THREYE-tis)/ an inflammatory disease characterized by inflammation of the joints

**rheumatoid factors (RF)** (ROO-mah-toyd fak-tors)/ autoantibodies that are directed against human IgG that are often present in the serum of patients with rheumatoid arthritis

**RNA** / a nucleic acid found in all living cells that is important in protein synthesis; ribonucleic acid

**rotor** / the part of a centrifuge that holds the tubes and rotates during the operation of the centrifuge

**rouleau(x)** (roo-LOH) / group(s) of red blood cells arranged like a roll of coins

**sample** / in statistics, a subgroup of a population

**secondary lymphoid tissue** / tissues in which lymphocytes are concentrated, such as the spleen, lymph nodes, and tonsils

**sediment** / solids that settle to the bottom of a liquid

**sedimentation** / the process of solid particles settling to the bottom of a liquid

**selective medium** / a bacteriological medium that allows growth of some organisms while inhibiting the growth of certain others

**seroconversion** / the appearance of antibody in the serum of an individual following exposure to an antigen

**serofuge** (SEE-roh-fewj)/ a centrifuge that spins small tubes such as those used in blood banking

**serology** / the study of antibodies and antigens in serum using immunological methods

**serum** / the liquid obtained from blood that has been allowed to clot

**shift** / an abrupt change from the established mean indicated by the occurrence of all control values on one side of the mean

**shift to the left** / the appearance of an increased number of immature neutrophil forms in the peripheral blood; occurs in response to bacterial infections

**SI units** / standardized units of measure; international units

**solid-phase chemistry** / an analytical method in which the sample is added to a strip or slide containing, in dried form, all the reagents for the procedure

**solute** / a liquid, gas, or solid dissolved in a liquid to make a solution

**solvent** / the liquid in which substances are dissolved; a liquid that holds a solute in solution

**specific gravity** / the ratio of the weight of a solution to the weight of an equal volume of distilled water; a measurement of density

**spectrophotometer** / an instrument that measures intensities of light in different parts of the light spectrum

**spirochetes** (SPEYE-roh-keets)/ motile bacteria having a helical or spiral shape

**stage** / platform that holds the object to be viewed microscopically

**standard** / a chemical solution of a known concentration that can be used as a reference or calibration substance

**standard deviation** / a measure of the spread of a population of values around the mean

**Standard Precautions** / a set of CDC safety procedures designed to protect patients and healthcare workers from infectious agents

**stat test** / a test that must be performed immediately

**statistics** / the science of collecting and classifying data to show their significance

**STD** / sexually transmitted disease

**stem** / main part of a word; root word; the part of a word remaining after removing the prefix or suffix

**stem cell** / a primitive, undifferentiated bone marrow cell

**sterilization** / the act of eliminating all living microorganisms from an article or area

**suffix** / modifying word or syllable(s) placed at the end of a word

**supernatant** (SOO-per-nay-tant)/ the clear liquid remaining at the top of a solution after centrifugation or settling out of solid substances

**supravital stain** / a dye that stains living cells or tissues

**syphilis** / an infectious, chronic, sexually transmitted disease caused by a spirochete, *Treponema pallidum*

**syringe** / a hollow, tube-like container with a plunger, used for injecting or withdrawing fluids

**systematic error** / a variation that may influence results to be consistently higher or lower than the real value

**systemic circulation** / the system of blood vessels that carries blood from the heart to the tissues and back to the heart

**TC** / to contain

**TD** / to deliver

**T lymphocyte, T cell** / a type of lymphocyte responsible for the cell-mediated immune response

**terminology** / terms used in any specialized field

**thalassemia** (thal-ah-SEE-mee-ah) / a genetic condition in which abnormal hemoglobin is produced, resulting in anemia

**thrombin** / a protein formed from prothrombin by the action of thromboplastin and other factors in the presence of calcium ions; factor $II_a$

**thrombocyte** (THRAHM-boh-seye-t) / a blood platelet

**thrombocytopenia** (throm-boh-seye-toh-PEE-ne-a) / abnormal decrease in the number of platelets in the blood

**thrombocytosis** (throm-boh-seye-TOH-sis) / abnormal increase in the number of platelets in the blood

**thromboplastin** / a lipoprotein found in endothelium and other tissue; coagulation factor III, also called tissue factor

**thrombus (pl. thrombi)** / a blood clot that obstructs a blood vessel

**thymus** (THEYE-mus)/ a gland located near the thyroid that is considered a primary lymphoid tissue

**thyroxine** (theye-ROKS-en)/ a thyroid hormone, commonly called T4

**titer** (TEYE-ter)/ reciprocal of the highest dilution that gives the desired reaction; concentration of a substance determined by titration

**tourniquet** / a band used to constrict blood flow

**transport medium** / a medium that provides the proper environment for organisms during transport to the laboratory

**trematode** / fluke; any parasitic flatworm of the class *Trematoda*

**trend** / an indication of error in the analysis, detected by increasing or decreasing values in the control sample

**trichomoniasis** (trih-koh-moh-NEYE-ah-sis) / a sexually transmitted infection of the genitourinary tract caused by the parasitic protozoan, *Trichomonas vaginalis*

**trichrome stain** / a stain commonly used for fecal specimens

**triglycerides** / the major storage form of lipids

**triiodothyronine** (treye-eye-oh-doh-THEYE-roh-neen) / one of the thyroid hormones, commonly called T3

**trophozoite** / the motile, feeding stage of protozoan parasites

**tubular necrosis** (TOO-byou-lar neh-KROH-sis) / death of the tissue comprising the renal tubules

**turbid** / having a cloudy appearance

**Universal Precautions** / a method of infection control in which all human blood and other body substances are treated as if infectious

**ureter** / the tube carrying urine from the kidney to the urinary bladder

**urethra** (you-REE-thra) / a canal through which urine is discharged from the urinary bladder

**urethritis** (YOU-ree-THREYE-tis) / inflammation of the urethra

**uric acid** / breakdown product of nucleic acids

**urinary bladder** / an organ for the temporary storage of urine

**urine** / excretory fluid produced by the kidneys

**urinometer** / a float with a calibrated stem used for measuring specific gravity

**urobilinogen** (you-roh-bihl-IN-oh-jehn) / a breakdown product of bilirubin formed by the action of intestinal bacteria

**urochrome** / the yellow pigment that gives urine its color

**UTI** / urinary tract infection

**vacuole** (VAK-you-ohl) / in cell cytoplasm, a clear compartment

**vaginitis** / inflammation of the vagina

**vasoconstriction** (VAS-oh-cahn-STRIKT-shun) / a narrowing of the diameter of a blood vessel

**vector** / an agent that transports a pathogen from an infected host to a noninfected host

**vein** / a blood vessel that carries deoxygenated blood from the tissues to the heart

**venereal** / having to do with, or transmitted by, sexual contact

**venipuncture** / entry of a vein with a needle; a phlebotomy

**virology** (vir-AHL-oh-jee) / the study of viruses

**vitamin B12** / a vitamin essential to the proper maturation of blood cells and other cells in the body

**Westergren tube** / a slender pipet marked from 0-200 mm used in the Westergren erythrocyte sedimentation rate method

**Westgard's rules** / a set of rules used to determine when a method is out of control

**whole blood** / blood that contains all components

**Wintrobe tube** / a slender thick-walled tube marked from 0–100 mm; used in the Wintrobe method of macrohematocrit and Wintrobe erythrocyte sedimentation rate

**work practice controls** / methods of performing tasks that reduce the worker's exposure to blood and other potentially hazardous materials

**working distance** / distance between the microscope objective and the microscope slide when the object is in sharp focus

**XDP** / fibrin-degradation products that contain the D-dimer cross-linked region

**zone of inhibition** / in the antibiotic susceptibility test, the area around an antibiotic disk that contains no bacterial growth

# Appendix A

## SOURCES OF INFORMATION:
## HEALTH CARE ACCREDITING AND CREDENTIALING AGENCIES,
## PROFESSIONAL SOCIETIES, GOVERNMENTAL AGENCIES

### ACCREDITING AGENCIES

American Association of Blood Banks (AABB)
8101 Glenbrook Road
Bethesda, MD 20814-2749
301.907.6977
www.aabb.org

College of American Pathologists, Laboratory Accreditation
  Program
325 Waukegan Road
Northfield, IL 60093-2750
800.323.4040
www.cap.org

Commission on Accreditation of Allied Health Education
  Programs (CAAHEP)
35 E. Wacker Dr. Suite 1970
Chicago, IL 60606-2208
312.553.9355
e-mail: caahep@caahep.org
www.caahep.org

Commission on Office Laboratory Accreditation (COLA)
9881 Broken Land Pkwy, Suite 200
Columbia, MD 21046-1158
410.381.6581
800.981.9883
e-mail: info@COLA.org
www.cola.org

Council for Higher Education Accreditation
One Dupont Circle NW, Suite 510
Washington, DC 20036-1135
202.955.6126
e-mail: chea@chea.org
www.chea.org

Joint Commission on Accreditation of Healthcare
  Organizations (JCAHO)
One Renaissance Blvd.
Oakbrook Terrace, IL 60181
630.792.5000
www.jcaho.org

National Accrediting Agency for Clinical Laboratory Sciences
  (NAACLS)
8410 W. Bryn Mawr Ave., Suite 670
Chicago, IL 60631-3415
773.714.8880
e-mail: naaclsinfo@naacls.org
www.naacls.org

### CREDENTIALING AGENCIES, PROFESSIONAL SOCIETIES AND OTHER SOURCES OF INFORMATION

Advance for Medical Laboratory Professionals
2900 Horizon Drive, Box 61556
King of Prussia, PA 19406-0956
800.355.1088
www.advanceweb.com

American Association for Clinical Chemistry
2101 L. Street NW, Suite 202
Washington, DC 20037
800.892.1400 or 202.857.0717
www.aacc.org
Journal/Publications: *Clinical Laboratory News,
Clinical Chemistry*

American Association of Blood Banks (AABB)
8101 Glenbrook Road
Bethesda, MD 20814-2749
301.907.6977
www.aabb.org

American Association of Medical Assistants
20 N Wacker Dr. Suite 1575
Chicago, IL 60606-2903
312.899.1500
www.aama-ntl.org
Journal: *PMA-The AAMA Journal*

American Association of Bioanalysts (AAB)
Associate Member Section (formerly ISCLT)
917 Locust Street, Suite 1100
St. Louis, MO 63101-1413
314.241.1445
www.aab.org

American Medical Association
515 North State Street
Chicago, IL 60610
312.464.5000
www.ama-assn.org

American Medical Technologists (AMT)
710 Higgins Road
Park Ridge, IL 60058-5765
847.823.5169
www.amt1.com

American Society for Clinical Laboratory Science (ASCLS)
7910 Woodmont Avenue, Suite 530
Bethesda, MD 20814
301.657.2768
e-mail: ascls@ascls.org
www.ascls.org

American Society for Microbiology (ASM)
1325 Massachusetts Ave. NW
Washington, DC 20005-4171
202.942.9319
www.asmusa.org
Journals: *Journal of Clinical Microbiology, Clinical Microbiology Reviews, Clinical and Diagnostic Laboratory Immunology, Journal of Virology*

American Society of Hematology
1200 19th St. NW, #300
Washington, DC 20036
202.857.1118
www.hematology.org
Journal: *Blood*

American Society of Phlebotomy Technicians (ASPT)
1109 2nd Ave. S.W.
P.O. Box 1831
Hickory, NC 28602
704.322.1334
www.aspt.org

Association for Professionals in Infection Control and Epidemiology (APIC)
1275 K Street NW, Suite 1000
Washington, DC 20005-4006
202.789.1890
e-mail: APICinfo@apic.org
www.apic.org
Journal: *American Journal of Infection Control*

Association of Schools of Allied Health Professions
1730 M Street, Suite 500
Washington, DC 20036
202.293.4848
e-mail: asahp1@asahp.org
Journal: *Journal of Allied Health*

Board of Registry
American Society of Clinical Pathologists (ASCP)
P. O. Box 12277
Chicago, IL 60612-0277
312.738.1336
e-mail: info@ascp.org
www.ascp.org

Centers for Disease Control and Prevention
1600 Clifton Road
Atlanta, GA 30333
404.639.3534
404.639.3311
800.311.3435
www.cdc.gov

Clinical Laboratory Management Association
989 Old Eagle Road, Suite 815
Wayne, PA 19087-1704
610.995.9580
www.clma.org
Journals: *Clinical Laboratory Management Review, Vantage Point*

Food and Drug Administration (FDA)
5600 Fishers Lane
Rockville, MD 20857
888.INFO.FDA
www.fda.gov

Health Care Financing Administration (HCFA)
7500 Security Blvd.
Baltimore, MD 21244
410.786.3000
www.hcfa.gov

International Association of Medical Laboratory Technologists
Adolf Fredriks Kyrkogata 11
S-11137 Stockholm, Sweden
e-mail: m.haag@iamlt.se
www.iamlt.se
Journal: *Med Tec International*

National Credentialing Agency for Laboratory Personnel (NCA)
P. O. Box 15945-289
Lenexa, KS 66285
913.438.5110
www.applmeapro.com/nca/

National Institutes of Health (NIH)
Bethesda, MD 20892
e-mail: NIHInfo@OD.NIH.GOV
www.nih.gov

National Institute for Occupational Safety and Health (NIOSH)
200 Independence Ave. S.W., Room 715H
Washington, DC 20201
800.35NIOSH
www.cdc.gov/niosh

National Technical Information Service (NTIS)
U. S. Dept. of Commerce
Springfield, VA 22161
703.605.6000
800.553.6847
www.ntis.gov

NCCLS
(National Committee for Clinical Laboratory Standards)
940 West Valley Road, Suite 1400
Wayne, PA 19087-1898
610.688.0100
e-mail: info@nccls.org
www.nccls.org

Occupational Safety and Health Administration (OSHA)
U. S. Dept. of Labor
Public Affairs Office, Room 3647
200 Constitution Ave. NW
Washington, DC 20210
202.693.1999
www.osha.gov

Superintendent of Documents
U. S. Government Printing Office
Washington, DC 20402
202.512.1800
FAX 202.512.2250
www.access.gpo.gov

## PROFICIENCY TESTING

Several agencies as well as some state public health laboratories have DHHS approved proficiency testing programs. Contact individual state agencies or HCFA for additional information. A listing of approved proficiency testing programs may be obtained through CDC's Public Health Practice Program Office, Division of Laboratory Systems, www.phppo.cdc.gov/dls/

# Appendix B

## GUIDE TO STANDARD PRECAUTIONS

Standard Precautions were issued by CDC in 1996 to replace Universal Precautions and Body Substance Isolation. Shown below are icons and descriptions of the components of Standard Precautions.

 **Wash Hands** (Plain soap). Wash after touching **blood, body fluids, secretions, excretions** and **contaminated items**. Wash immediately **after gloves are removed** and **between patient contacts**. Avoid transfer of microorganisms to other patients or environments.

 **Wear Gloves.** Wear when touching **blood, body fluids, secretions, excretions** and **contaminated items**. Put on **clean** gloves just **before touching mucous membranes** and **nonintact skin**. Change gloves between tasks and procedures on the same patient after contact with material that may contain high concentrations of microorganisms. Remove gloves promptly after use, before touching noncontaminated items and environmental surfaces, and before going to another patient, and wash hands immediately to avoid transfer of microorganisms to other patients or environments.

 **Wear Mask and Eye Protection or Face Shield.** Protect mucous membranes of the eyes, nose and mouth during procedures and patient-care activities that are likely to generate **splashes** or **sprays of blood, body fluids, secretions**, or **excretions**.

 **Wear Gown.** Protect skin and prevent soiling of clothing during procedures that are likely to generate **splashes** or **sprays of blood, body fluids, secretions**, or **excretions**. Remove a soiled gown as promptly as possible and wash hands to avoid transfer of microorganisms to other patients or environments.

 **Patient-Care Equipment.** Handle used patient-care equipment soiled with **blood, body fluids, secretions**, or **excretions** in a manner that prevents skin and mucous membrane exposures, contamination of clothing, and transfer of microorganisms to other patients and environments. Ensure that reusable equipment is not used for the care of another patent until it has been appropriately cleaned and reprocessed and single use items are properly discarded.

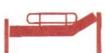 **Environmental Control.** Follow hospital procedures for routine care, cleaning, and disinfection of environmental surfaces, beds, bedrails, bedside equipment and other frequently touched surfaces.

 **Linen.** Handle, transport, and process used linen soiled with **blood, body fluids, secretions**, or **excretions** in a manner that prevents exposures and contamination of clothing, and avoids transfer of microorganisms to other patients and environments.

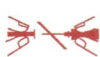 **Occupational Health and Bloodborne Pathogens.** Prevent injuries when using needles, scalpels, and other sharp instruments or devices; when handling sharp instruments after procedures; when cleaning used instruments; and when disposing of used needles.

 **Never recap used needles using both hands** or any other technique that involves directing the point of a needle toward any part of the body; rather, use either a one-handed "scoop" technique or a mechanical device designed for holding the needle sheath.

 Do not remove used needles from disposable syringes by hand, and do not bend, break, or otherwise manipulate used needles by hand. Place used disposable syringes and needles, scalpel blades and other sharp items in puncture-resistant sharps containers located as close as practical to the area in which the items were used, and place reusable syringes and needles in a puncture resistant container for transport to the reprocessing area.

Use **resuscitation devices** as an alternative to mouth-to-mouth resuscitation.

 **Patient Placement.** Use a private room for a patient who contaminates the environment or who does not (or cannot be expected to) assist in maintaining appropriate hygiene or environmental control. Consult Infection Control if a private room is not available.

# Appendix C

## ABBREVIATIONS COMMONLY USED IN MEDICAL LABORATORIES

| | | | |
|---|---|---|---|
| A | absorbance | CSF | cerebrospinal fluid |
| Ab | antibody | cu mm | cubic millimeter, $mm^3$ |
| AFB | acid-fast bacillus | diff | leukocyte differential |
| Ag | antigen | EBV | Epstein-Barr virus |
| AIDS | acquired immunodeficiency syndrome | EIA | enzyme immunoassay |
| ALL | acute lymphocytic leukemia | ESR | erythrocyte sedimentation rate |
| ALP, AP | alkaline phosphatase | E.U. | Ehrlich units |
| ALT | alanine aminotransferase (formerly SGPT) | F | Fahrenheit |
| AML | acute myelogenous leukemia | FBS | fasting blood sugar |
| APTT | activated partial thromboplastin time | FDP | fibrinogen-degradation products |
| ARC | AIDS-related complex | FUO | fever of unknown origin |
| AST | aspartate aminotransferase (formerly SGOT) | g, gm | gram |
| | | Gc | gonococcus, gonorrhea |
| bacti | bacteriology | GGT | gamma glutamyl transferase |
| BBP | blood-borne pathogen | GI | gastrointestinal |
| BP | blood pressure | GTT | glucose tolerance test |
| BT | bleeding time | GU | genitourinary |
| BUN | blood urea nitrogen | HAV | hepatitis A virus |
| C | Celsius, centigrade | Hb, Hgb | hemoglobin |
| CBC | complete blood count | HBV | hepatitis B virus |
| cc, ccm | cubic centimeter | hCG | human chorionic gonadotropin |
| CCU | coronary care unit | HCl | hydrochloric acid |
| CGL | chronic granulocytic leukemia | $HCO_3^-$ | bicarbonate |
| CK | creatine kinase | Hct | hematocrit |
| Cl | chloride | HCV | hepatitis C virus |
| CLL | chronic lymphocytic leukemia | HDL Chol | high density lipoprotein cholesterol |
| cm | centimeter | HDN | hemolytic disease of newborn |
| CNS | central nervous system | H & H | hemoglobin and hematocrit |
| C & S | culture and sensitivity | HIV | human immunodeficiency virus |
| CO | carbon monoxide | $H_2O$ | water |
| $CO_2$ | carbon dioxide | HPF | high power field |
| CPK | creatine phosphokinase | HSV | herpes simplex virus |
| crit | hematocrit | ICU | intensive care unit |

| | | | | |
|---|---|---|---|---|
| IgG | immunoglobulin G | | POL | physician office laboratory |
| IgM | immunoglobulin M | | PP | postprandial |
| IM | infectious mononucleosis | | PPE | personal protective equipment |
| i.m. | intramuscular | | PRC | packed red cells |
| ITP | idiopathic thrombocytopenic purpura | | PSA | prostate specific antigen |
| IU | international unit | | PT | prothrombin time, pro-time |
| IV, i.v. | intravenous | | qns | quantity not sufficient |
| K | potassium | | qs | quantity sufficient |
| kg | kilogram | | RA | rheumatoid arthritis |
| L | liter | | RBC | red blood cell |
| LD, LDH | lactate dehydrogenase | | RF | rheumatoid factors |
| LDL Chol | low density lipoprotein cholesterol | | RIA | radioimmunoassay |
| LPF | low power field | | RNA | ribonucleic acid |
| M | molar | | RPR | rapid plasma reagin |
| MCH | mean corpuscular hemoglobin | | sed rate | erythrocyte sedimentation rate |
| MCHC | mean corpuscular hemoglobin concentration | | SGOT | serum glutamic oxaloacetic transaminase |
| MCV | mean corpuscular volume | | SGPT | serum glutamic-pyruvic transaminase |
| μg | microgram | | S.I. | international units (Le Systéme International d'Unités) |
| μL, μl | microliter | | SICU | surgical intensive care unit |
| mEq | milliequivalent | | sp.gr. | specific gravity |
| mg | milligram | | Staph | *Staphylococcus* |
| MI | myocardial infarction | | stat | immediately |
| mL, ml | milliliter | | STD | sexually transmitted disease |
| MLT | medical laboratory technician | | STI | sexually transmitted infection |
| mm | millimeter | | Strep | *Streptococcus* |
| mmol | millimole | | STS | serological tests for syphilis |
| MRI | magnetic resonance imaging | | TIBC | total iron binding capacity |
| MT | medical technologist | | TIA | transient ischemic attack |
| N | normal, normality | | UA | urinalysis, uric acid |
| Na | sodium | | URI | upper respiratory infection |
| NaCl | sodium chloride | | UTI | urinary tract infection |
| nm | nanometer | | μmol | micromole |
| O.D. | optical density | | uv | ultraviolet |
| O & P | ova and parasites | | VD | venereal disease |
| OPIM | other potentially infectious material | | VDRL | Venereal Disease Research Laboratory |
| PCV | packed cell volume | | VLDL | very low density lipoproteins |
| pH | hydrogen ion concentration | | WBC | white blood cell |
| PMN | polymorphonuclear neutrophil | | XDP | fibrin-degradation products |
| POCT | point-of-care test | | | |

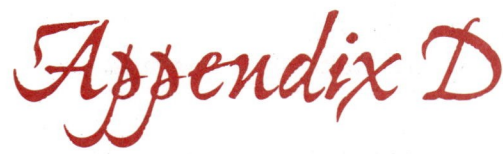

# METRIC CONVERSION TABLES

## COMMONLY USED PREFIXES IN THE METRIC SYSTEM

| ABBREVIATION | PREFIX | MEANING | MULTIPLE OF BASIC UNIT | WEIGHT GRAM (G) | LENGTH METER (M) | VOLUME LITER (L) |
|---|---|---|---|---|---|---|
| k | kilo | 1000 | $10^3$ | kg | km | kL |
| h | hecto | 100 | $10^2$ | hg* | hm* | hL* |
| da | deca | 10 | $10^1$ | dag* | dam* | daL* |
| d | deci | .1 | $10^{-1}$ | dg* | dm* | dL |
| c | centi | .01 | $10^{-2}$ | cg* | cm | cL* |
| m | milli | .001 | $10^{-3}$ | mg | mm | mL |
| μ | micro | .000001 | $10^{-6}$ | μg | μm | μL |
| n | nano | | $10^{-9}$ | ng | nm | nL* |
| p | pico | | $10^{-12}$ | pg | pm* | pL* |

*Units not commonly used in the laboratory

## COMMON METRIC EQUIVALENTS

**Mass**
$10^{-3}$ kg = 1 gram = $10^3$ mg = $10^6$ μg
$10^{-3}$ g = 1 mg = $10^3$ μg = $10^6$ ng
$10^{-9}$ g = 1 ng = $10^3$ pg

**Volume**
$10^{-3}$ kL = 1 liter = $10^3$ mL = $10^6$ μL
$10^{-3}$ L = 1 mL = $10^3$ μL = $10^6$ nL
$10^{-1}$ L = 1 dL = $10^2$ mL

**Length**
$10^{-3}$ km = 1 meter = $10^3$ mm = $10^6$ μm
$10^{-3}$ m = 1 mm = $10^3$ μm = $10^6$ nm
$10^{-2}$ m = 1 cm = 10 mm = $10^4$ μm
$10^{-3}$ mm = 1 nm = 10 Å

# CONVERSION OF ENGLISH UNITS TO METRIC UNITS

| | ENGLISH UNIT | ENGLISH ABBREVIATION | MULTIPLY BY | TO GET METRIC UNIT | METRIC ABBREVIATION |
|---|---|---|---|---|---|
| Distance | 1 mile | mi | = 1.6 | kilometers | km |
| | 1 yard | yd | = 0.9 | meters | m |
| | 1 inch | in | = 2.54 | centimeters | cm |
| Mass | 1 pound | lb | = 0.454 | kilograms | kg |
| | 1 pound | lb | = 454 | grams | g |
| | 1 ounce | oz | = 28 | grams | g |
| Volume | 1 quart | qt | = 0.95 | liters | L |
| | 1 fluid ounce | fl. oz. | = 30 | milliliters | mL |
| | 1 teaspoon | tsp | = 5 | milliliters | mL |

# CONVERSION OF METRIC TO ENGLISH UNITS

| | METRIC UNIT | METRIC ABBREVIATION | MULTIPLY BY | TO GET ENGLISH UNIT | ENGLISH ABBREVIATION |
|---|---|---|---|---|---|
| Distance | 1 kilometer | km | = 0.6 | miles | mi |
| | 1 meter | m | = 3.3 | feet | ft |
| | 1 meter | m | = 39.37 | inches | in |
| | 1 centimeter | cm | = 0.4 | inches | in |
| | 1 millimeter | mm | = .04 | inches | in |
| Mass | 1 gram | g | = .0022 | pounds | lb |
| | 1 kilogram | kg | = 2.2 | pounds | lb |
| Volume | 1 liter | L | = 1.06 | quarts | qt |
| | 1 milliliter | mL | = .03 | fluid ounces | fl. oz. |

# SI UNITS AND COMMON EQUIVALENTS

| COMMON USAGE | SI EQUIVALENT |
|---|---|
| micron ($\mu$) | micrometer ($\mu$m; $10^{-6}$ meter) |
| cubic micron ($\mu^3$) | femtoliter (fl; $10^{-15}$ liter) |
| micromicrogram ($\mu\mu$g) | picogram (pg; $10^{-12}$ gram) |
| microgram (mcg) | microgram ($\mu$g; $10^{-6}$ gram) |
| Angstrom (Å) | nm x $10^{-1}$ |
| millimicron (m$\mu$) | nanometer (nm; $10^{-9}$ meter) |
| lambda ($\lambda$) | microliter ($\mu$l; $10^{-6}$ liter) |

# EXAMPLES OF USAGE OF SI UNITS IN REPORTING LABORATORY TEST RESULTS

| Cell counts | cells/mm$^3$ or cells/cumm | cells/$\mu$L or cells/liter |
|---|---|---|
| Hematocrit | % (Ex: 41%) | Percent expressed as decimal (Ex: 0.41) |
| Hemoglobin | g/dL | g/liter |
| MCV | $\mu^3$ | fl |
| MCH | $\mu\mu$g | pg |
| MCHC | % | g/dL (or g/L) |

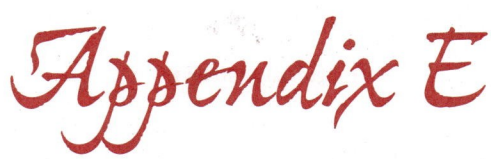

# Appendix E

## LABORATORY REFERENCE VALUES

### HEMATOLOGY AND COAGULATION

| TEST | REFERENCE RANGE |
|---|---|
| **Hemoglobin:** | |
| Newborn | 16–23 g/dL |
| Children | 10–14 g/dL |
| Adult males | 13–17 g/dL |
| Adult females | 12–15 g/dL |
| **Microhematocrit:** | |
| Newborn | 51–60% |
| One year | 32–38% |
| Six years | 34–42% |
| Adult males | 42–52% |
| Adult females | 36–48% |
| **Reticulocyte Percentages:** | |
| Newborn | 2.5–6.5% |
| Adult | 0.5–1.5% |

**Erythrocyte Sedimentation Rate (ESR)**

*Wintrobe method (one-hour)*

| | |
|---|---|
| Children | 0–13 mm |
| Adult males | 0–9 mm |
| Adult females | 0–20 mm |

*One hour Sediplast® ESR*

| | | |
|---|---|---|
| Males | < 50 years | 0–15 mm |
| | > 50 years | 0–20 mm |
| Females | < 50 years | 0–20 mm |
| | > 50 years | 0–30 mm |

*ZSR (all ages)*

| | |
|---|---|
| Normal | 40–51% |
| Borderline | 51–54% |
| Elevated | ≥–55% |

| TEST | REFERENCE RANGE |
|---|---|
| **ACT (Hemochron Jr.)** | 89–153 sec |
| **Prothrombin Time** | 11–13 sec |
| **Partial Thromboplastin Time** | 31–39 sec |
| **Bleeding Time:** | |
| Ivy method | 2–9 min |
| Duke method | 1–3 min |
| **Leukocyte Counts:** | |
| Newborn | $9.0–30.0 \times 10^9/L$ |
| One year | $6.0–14.0 \times 10^9/L$ |
| Six years | $4.5–12.0 \times 10^9/L$ |
| Adult | $4.5–11.0 \times 10^9/L$ |
| **Erythrocyte Counts:** | |
| Adult males | $4.5–6.0 \times 10^{12}/L$ |
| Adult females | $4.0–5.5 \times 10^{12}/L$ |
| **Erythrocyte Indices:** | |
| Mean Corpuscular Volume (MCV) | 80–100 fL |
| Mean Corpuscular Hemoglobin (MCH) | 27–32 pg |
| Mean Corpuscular Hemoglobin Concentration (MCHC) | 32–37% |
| **Platelet Count** | $0.15–0.40 \times 10^{12}/L$ |

**Differential Leukocyte Count:**

| Leukocyte | one month | six-year-old | twelve-year-old | adult |
|---|---|---|---|---|
| Neutrophil (seg) | 15–35% | 45–50% | 45–50% | 50–65% |
| Neutrophil (band) | 7–13% | 0–7% | 6–8% | 0–7% |
| Eosinophil | 1–3% | 1–3% | 1–3% | 1–3% |
| Basophil | 0–1% | 0–1% | 0–1% | 0–1% |
| Monocyte | 5–8% | 4–8% | 3–8% | 3–9% |
| Lymphocyte | 40–70% | 40–45% | 35–40% | 25–40% |
| Platelets | An average of 7-20 platelets per oil immersion field is considered normal | | | |

# URINE REFERENCE VALUES

## URINE VOLUME:

| Age | Reference Range (mL/24 hours) |
|---|---|
| Newborn | 20–350 |
| One year | 300–600 |
| Ten years | 750–1500 |
| Adult | 750–2000 |

## COMPONENTS OF URINE SEDIMENT:

| | Reference Values |
|---|---|
| RBC/HPF | rare |
| WBC/HPF | 0–4 |
| Epith/HPF | occasional (may be higher in females) |
| Casts/LPF | occasional hyaline |
| Bacteria | negative |
| Mucus | negative to 2+ |
| Crystals | only crystals such as cystine, leucine, tyrosine, and cholesterol are considered clinically significant |

## PHYSICAL AND CHEMICAL CHARACTERISTICS OF URINE:

| | Reference Values |
|---|---|
| Color | straw to amber |
| Transparency | clear |
| Specific gravity | 1.005–1.030 |
| pH | 5.5–8.0 |
| Protein | negative–trace |
| Glucose | negative |
| Ketone | negative |
| Bilirubin | negative |
| Blood | negative |
| Urobilinogen | 0.1–1.0 EU/dL |
| Bacteria (nitrite) | negative |
| Leukocyte esterase | negative |

# CLINICAL CHEMISTRY REFERENCE VALUES

| Substance Measured | Reference Ranges | |
|---|---|---|
| | Conventional Units | SI Units |
| Alanine aminotransferase (ALT) | 3–30 U/L | |
| Albumin | 3.8–5.0 g/dL | 38–50 g/L |
| Alkaline phosphatase (ALP) | 20–130 U/L | |
| Aspartate aminotransferase (AST) | 6–25 U/L | |
| Bicarbonate ($HCO_3^-$) | 22–28 mEq/L | 22–28 mmol/L |
| Bilirubin (Total) | 0.1–1.2 mg/dL | 2–21 μmol/L |
| BUN | 8–18 mg/dL | 2.9–6.4 mmol/L |
| Calcium | 8.7–10.5 mg/dL | 2.18–2.63 mmol/L |
| Chloride | 98–108 mEq/L | 98–108 mmol/L |
| Cholesterol | 140–250 mg/dL (desirable level <200 mg/dl) | |
| Creatine kinase (CK) | 30–170 U/L | |
| Creatinine | 0.7–1.4 mg/dL | 62–125 μmol/L |
| Gamma glutamyl transferase (GGT) | 3–40 U/L | |
| Glucose | 70–110 mg/dL | 3.9–6.2 mmol/L |
| Iron | 65–165 μg/dL | 11.6–29.5 μmol/L |
| Lactate dehydrogenase (LD) | 125–290 U/L | |
| Phosphorus | 3.0–4.5 mg/dL | 0.96–1.44 mmol/L |
| Potassium | 3.5–5.4 mEq/L | 3.5–5.4 mmol/L |
| Sodium | 135–148 mEq/L | 135–148 mmol/L |
| $T_4$ | 5.5–12.5 μg/dL | 72–163 nmol/L |
| Total Protein | 6.0–8.0 g/dL | 60–80 g/L |
| Triglycerides | 10–190 mg/dL | 0.11–2.15 mmol/L |
| Uric Acid | 3.5–7.5 mg/dL | 0.21–0.44 mmol/L |

# Index